THE ECG IN ACUTE MI

AN EVIDENCE-BASED MANUAL
OF REPERFUSION THERAPY

THE ECG IN ACUTE MI

AN EVIDENCE-BASED MANUAL OF REPERFUSION THERAPY

Editor-in-Chief

STEPHEN W. SMITH, M.D.

Faculty Emergency Physician
Hennepin County Medical Center
Assistant Professor of Clinical Emergency Medicine
University of Minnesota School of Medicine
Minneapolis, Minnesota

Senior Editor

DEBORAH L. ZVOSEC, Ph.D.

Research Associate
Hennepin County Medical Center
Investigator
Minneapolis Medical Research Foundation
Minneapolis, Minnesota

Associate Editors

SCOTT W. SHARKEY, M.D.

Minneapolis Heart Institute
Minneapolis, Minnesota

TIMOTHY D. HENRY, M.D.

Director, Interventional Cardiology
Hennepin County Medical Center
Associate Professor of Medicine
University of Minneapolis School of Medicine
Minneapolis, Minnesota

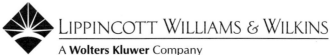

LIPPINCOTT WILLIAMS & WILKINS
A **Wolters Kluwer** Company
Philadelphia • Baltimore • New York • London
Buenos Aires • Hong Kong • Sydney • Tokyo

Acquisitions Editor: Anne M. Sydor
Developmental Editor: Joanne Bersin
Production Editor: Emily Lerman
Manufacturing Manager: Colin J. Warnock
Cover Designer: Patricia Gast
Compositor: Lippincott Williams & Wilkins Desktop Division
Printer: Maple-Vail

© 2002 by LIPPINCOTT WILLIAMS & WILKINS
530 Walnut Street
Philadelphia, PA 19106 USA
LWW.com

Printed in the USA

Library of Congress Cataloging-in-Publication Data

The ECG in acute MI: an evidence-based manual of reperfusion therapy / editor-in-chief, Stephen W. Smith ; senior editor, Deborah L. Zvosec ; associate editors, Scott W. Sharkey, Timothy D. Henry.
     p. ; cm.
   Includes bibliographical references and index.
   ISBN: 0-7817-2903-3 (alk. paper)
   1. Myocardial infarction—Handbooks, manuals, etc.   2. Electrocardiography—Handbooks, manuals, etc.   3. Myocardial reperfusion—Handbooks, manuals, etc.
I. Smith, Stephen W. (Stephen Wallner), 1958-
   [DNLM: 1. Myocardial Infarction—diagnosis.   2. Electrocardiography—methods.
3. Evidence-Based Medicine.   4. Myocardial Infarction—therapy.   5. Myocardial Reperfusion—methods.   WG 300 E17 2002]
RC685.I6 E295 2002
616.1′237—dc21   2002016160

Care has been taken to confirm the accuracy of the information presented and to describe generally accepted practices. However, the authors, editors, and publisher are not responsible for errors or omissions or for any consequences from application of the information in this book and make no warranty, expressed or implied, with respect to the currency, completeness, or accuracy of the contents of the publication. Application of this information in a particular situation remains the professional responsibility of the practitioner.

The authors, editors, and publisher have exerted every effort to ensure that drug selection and dosage set forth in this text are in accordance with current recommendations and practice at the time of publication. However, in view of ongoing research, changes in government regulations, and the constant flow of information relating to drug therapy and drug reactions, the reader is urged to check the package insert for each drug for any change in indications and dosage and for added warnings and precautions. This is particularly important when the recommended agent is a new or infrequently employed drug.

Some drugs and medical devices presented in this publication have Food and Drug Administration (FDA) clearance for limited use in restricted research settings. It is the responsibility of the health care provider to ascertain the FDA status of each drug or device planned for use in their clinical practice.

10 9 8 7 6 5 4 3 2 1

CONTENTS

CONTRIBUTING AUTHORS

Fred S. Apple, PhD Medical Director of Clinical Laboratories, Hennepin County Medical Center; Professor, Laboratory Medicine and Pathology, University of Minnesota School of Medicine, Minneapolis, Minnesota *(Chapter 29)*

William Brady, MD Associate Professor and Program Director, Department of Emergency Medicine and Associate Professor, Department of Internal Medicine, University of Virginia, Charlottesville, Virginia *(Chapter 1)*

Brian Erling, MD Chief Resident, Department of Emergency Medicine, University of Virginia, Charlottesville, Virginia *(Chapter 1)*

Timothy D. Henry, MD Director, Interventional Cardiology, Hennepin County Medical Center; Associate Professor of Medicine, University of Minnesota School of Medicine, Minneapolis, Minnesota *(Chapters 36 and 37)*

Farhana Kazzi, MD Instructor, Cardiology Division, University of Texas, Southwestern, Dallas, Texas *(Chapter 38)*

M. Bilal Murad, MD Division of Cardiovascular Medicine, Veteran's Administration Medical Center, Hennepin County Medical Center, Minneapolis, Minnesota *(Chapter 37)*

Rao Haris Naseem, MD Fellow, Cardiology, University of Texas, Southwestern, Dallas, Texas *(Chapter 36)*

Scott W. Sharkey, MD Minneapolis Heart Institute, Minneapolis, Minnesota

Stephen W. Smith, MD Faculty Emergency Physician, Hennepin County Medical Center; Assistant Professor of Clinical Emergency Medicine, University of Minnesota School of Medicine, Minneapolis, Minnesota *(Chapters 2–38)*

Kyuhyun Wang, MD Department of Medicine/Division of Cardiology, Hennepin County Medical Center, Minneapolis, Minnesota *(Many ECGs)*

Deborah L. Zvosec, PhD Research Associate, Hennepin County Medical Center; Investigator, Minneapolis Medical Research Foundation, Minneapolis, Minnesota *(Chapters 31 and 32)*

PREFACE

Reperfusion therapy, within which we include thrombolytic therapy and percutaneous coronary intervention (PCI), which includes angioplasty and stent placement, is the greatest advance in the treatment of acute myocardial infarction (AMI) since the advent of defibrillation and the establishment of Cardiac Care Units (CCUs). The decision to administer a thrombolytic agent or call an interventional cardiologist is a difficult decision that becomes more complex as new research increases our knowledge base and multiplies our options. Despite great technological advances in other diagnostic fields and in therapeutic procedures, the 12-lead electrocardiogram (ECG) remains the basis for the diagnosis and timely reperfusion of ST—elevation-AMI (STEMI). Consequently, advances in the recognition of candidates who may benefit from reperfusion therapy have been made primarily through increased sophistication in ECG interpretation.

Immediate reperfusion therapy is indicated primarily for ST elevation, with two well-defined and thoroughly discussed exceptions: (a) anterior ST depression indicative of posterior AMI and (b) hyperacute T waves. Because immediate PCI may be indicated for some cases of unstable angina and non—ST-Elevation AMI (UA/NSTEMI), we include a more limited discussion of these entities and their ECG findings. The diagnosis and management of UA/NSTEMI that presents with a nondiagnostic ECG is beyond the scope of this book.

Studies have shown that many patients with AMI who are eligible for reperfusion therapy do not receive it. Moreover, of those who do receive it, the time to administration of thrombolytic therapy, or "door-to-needle time" (DTNT), is often delayed, jeopardizing myocardium and leading to greater morbidity and mortality. Lack of physician confidence in ECG diagnosis and in analysis of risks versus benefits of thrombolytic therapy has been shown to be a significant contributing factor in these delays. The focus of this book is therefore on ECG interpretation and how this may be used to accurately diagnose AMI and to facilitate appropriate and timely therapy. Although we discuss fundamental concepts and developments in the field of reperfusion therapy, and we include brief chapters on choice of reperfusion therapy, adjunctive therapy, and therapy of UA/NSTEMI, we leave therapeutic details to other sources. In this way, we hope to offer you maximal coverage of sophisticated ECG interpretation and minimal obsolescence of therapeutic data.

Increased sophistication of ECG interpretation means that it is no longer adequate to simply recognize a massive anterior AMI and admit the patient to the CCU. It is no longer acceptable to recognize ST-segment elevation as the sole diagnostic criterion for AMI and for thrombolytic administration. Many patients have ST elevation without AMI, as a result of baseline electrocardiographic conditions such as early repolarization, left ventricular hypertrophy (LVH), left bundle branch block (LBBB), ventricular aneurysm, and pericarditis. How do we recognize the look-alikes, or pseudoinfarctions, so that we can, to the best of our abilities, avoid administering thrombolytics to a patient who is not having an AMI? In contrast, many patients **with** STEMI have subtle, nondiagnostic, or atypical ECGs, including borderline ST elevation, lateral AMI, posterior AMI, or AMI hidden in LVH or bundle branch block. How can we identify them? Furthermore, how can we recognize those patients who are having an AMI but for whom thrombolytic therapy is dangerous, as in cases of myocardial rupture? How do we use data from the ECG to evaluate the risk/benefit ratio of the administration of thrombolytics, particularly in patients for whom there are relative contraindications? The key to accurate and timely answers lies in our ability to interpret the ECG, and especially the subtle ECGs that are the primary focus of this manual.

Accurate ECG interpretation is dependent on factual knowledge and a familiarity with ECG morphology, or **pattern recognition**. The purpose of this book is to provide you with the tools to quickly and accurately recognize ECG morphologies and make appropriate therapeutic decisions. In Parts I through III, we provide guidelines for the **recognition of various ECG morphologies** of ischemia and infarction, and we illustrate diagnostic criteria with numerous ECGs, often several different examples of a given condition. Throughout the book, we focus on the difficult ECG, with many examples of both subtle infarction and pseudoinfarction. We give a **brief and pertinent case history** for each ECG so that it may be interpreted in clinical context and we highlight the important clinical considerations for each case as it relates to the reperfusion decision. In Part IV, we discuss pseudoinfarction patterns; in Part V we cover other important issues in the ECG diagnosis of AMI, and in Part VI we briefly cover therapeutics, including reperfusion treatment options, adjunctive therapy, and UA/NSTEMI.

HOW TO USE THIS BOOK

This manual is written as a **reference for quick use in a critical clinical situation**, as well as a reference for more detailed study. Most importantly, the book contains repetition of important points not only for reinforcement, but also so that any one section contains at least the essential information needed to manage your patient, avoiding the need to frequently flip pages back and forth. Chapters are easy to find. **Key points** are listed at the beginning of each chapter. Indexing and cross-referencing are used throughout so that you may locate information topically. **Common abbreviations are used and defined in Abbreviations,** with many less common terms defined in the **Glossary**. Citations in the text that are annotated in that chapter are cited in **boldface**. The second part of each chapter consists of cases and their corresponding ECGs. **Each ECG is coded with an "ECG Type"** (see Chapter 2) which corresponds to the indication for reperfusion therapy. An **annotated bibliography** is written in smaller type at the end of most sections.

This manual is **also designed for more leisurely and detailed study** in order to master fundamentals and fine-tune ECG interpretation. We begin with drawings made from MRI images of the heart to illustrate the anatomy and reciprocity of ECG leads so that you will be better able to understand and quickly interpret ECGs spatially and logically, rather than simply by rote memorization. We discuss **key points** in greater detail and with reference to relevant research in an annotated bibliography at the end of most sections, with the exception of some chapters that do not directly relate to the clinical interpretation of the ECG. Important **clinical trials of thrombolytics** are described in detail in the **Appendix**, so that the role of the ECG can be better understood in the context of the development of reperfusion therapy.

Our purpose is to provide a conceptual framework for interpreting ECGs in the context of the reperfusion decision.

We offer little theoretical discussion or electrophysiologic explication and we assume that the reader has a clinician's basic working understanding of electrocardiograms and terminology. We expect that expert electrocardiographers may find some points oversimplified, lacking discussion of exceptions and of electrophysiology, but our purpose is to keep discussion brief and focused on essentials of ECG interpretation in the context of the reperfusion decision. For more detailed and theoretical considerations, we refer you to an excellent text (1).

Lastly, it must be remembered that the ECG, albeit powerful, is only a test with **false positives and false negatives**, and must be interpreted in the **clinical context** (i.e., **the pretest probability**). ECGs are variable from patient to patient and concepts must be adapted to individuals. ST segments may rise early in one patient with occluded coronary arteries and later in another patient with apparently identical pathology. ST segments usually decrease quickly in TIMI grade 3 early reperfusion, but not always and sometimes not at all; T waves invert after AMI of all kinds, sometimes deeply and sometimes not. Any one patient may not conform to the concepts presented and must be approached individually by a prepared mind.

This manual is for all clinicians who treat patients with acute chest pain, and thus it is for all who may have to recognize and treat an AMI. Thus, this book is for **emergency physicians, cardiologists, intensivists, hospitalists, internists, family practitioners,** and **physician assistants** as well as **residents** and **medical students**. It is also meant for **nurses** in the Cardiac Care Unit or the Emergency Department. It will be useful for both study and on-the-job reference.

This book is really for all of our patients who may be suffering from AMI. We hope that it will improve their care.

ACKNOWLEDGMENTS

Special thanks to:

Kyuhyun Wang, M.D., for his years of teaching, his many ECG contributions, and his many suggestions.

Hennepin County Medical Center:
The institution and its commitment to excellent patient care, teaching, and research made everything possible.
The emergency physicians, whose devotion to excellent patient care and to teaching is unsurpassed.
The emergency department nurses, whose devotion to excellent patient care and support of research and education make our jobs both possible and rewarding.
The cardiology division, whose clinical excellence has always been an inspiration.

Our patients: You have taught us so much.

1

BASIC PRINCIPLES AND ELECTROPHYSIOLOGY

BRIAN ERLING
WILLIAM BRADY

KEY POINTS

- Knowledge of electrophysiology may aid in understanding the electrocardiogram (ECG).
- Pattern recognition remains the basis for most diagnosis and management.

GENERAL BACKGROUND

The most common method of electrocardiographic interpretation is pattern recognition, which requires limited knowledge of electrophysiology. However, changes of ischemia and infarction on the ECG can be variable and complicated. For those interested in a more complete utilization of the ECG, we discuss the basic electrophysiology that produces its waveforms.

There are two types of sensing electrodes used in clinical practice; these are the bipolar and unipolar leads. **Bipolar electrodes** have a positive and a negative electrode, as demonstrated in Figure 1-1; these reflect an electrical vector in relation to the vector of the leads. A **unipolar lead** consists of only one (positive) reading electrode. Unipolar leads came into use after it was discovered that removing the negative lead actually augments the normal deflection. The **12-lead ECG** is a combination of three bipolar leads (I, II, III) and nine unipolar leads (aVR, aVL, aVF, and V1–V6), all of which should be interpreted in concert using the vector concept of electrocardiography to provide the most complete electrical picture of the heart.

The **vector concept** assumes that the electrical activity of the heart is three-dimensional and originates in the center of the heart. All electrical activity will be reflected on each lead, depending on many factors, including the location and direction of the lead axis, the direction and amplitude of the electrical vector, and the distance of the leads from the electrical vector (Fig. 1-1). All vectors have direction, magnitude, and polarity such that a **positive vector toward a positive lead has a positive deflection on ECG.** The vector is the mean of electrical activity at any one point in time.

The modern scalar ECG (the familiar 12-lead ECG) is a composite of two-dimensional vectors that can be combined into a three-dimensional interpretation. Einthoven's bipolar limb leads (I, II, III) and the unipolar augmented leads (aVL, aVR, aVF) look at the heart in the frontal plane. The augmented limb leads increase Einthoven's triaxial system to a hexaxial system, without requiring additional lead placement. (It was discovered that removing the negative lead augments the deflection without changing vector direction.) Leads V1–V6, the unipolar precordial leads, add three-dimensionality to the ECG, all of which is shown in Figure 1-2. Additional precordial leads are occasionally performed to better record the right ventricle (RV) (V3R-V7R) or the posterior wall of the left ventricle (LV) (V8–V9).

NORMAL CARDIAC CELLULAR AND ELECTRICAL ACTIVITY

To best understand the ECG, one must understand the cellular activity of the heart. Cardiac cells have several remarkable properties known as **excitability, automaticity, conductivity, and contraction.** The **excitability** of the cells is due to the basic, and well-known, cellular action potential. This is a five-phase process as identified in Figure 1-3. All normal cardiac cells have a resting diastolic transmembrane potential of approximately −60 (sinoatrial node [SA]) to −90 millivolts (mV) (contractile cells) that is established by the sodium (Na^+)/potassium (K^+) adenosine triphosphate (ATP)-ase pump during phase 4 of the action potential. This pump generates an electrolyte gradient, with high K^+ concentration inside the cells and high Na^+ concentration outside of the cells. The charge on the cell membrane

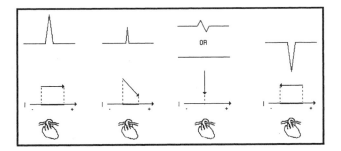

FIGURE 1-1. QRS in relation to depolarization vector and location of reading electrode. The waveform of the ECG depends upon the magnitude of the depolarization vector, and the direction with relation to the reading electrode, which in each case here is on the patient's right.

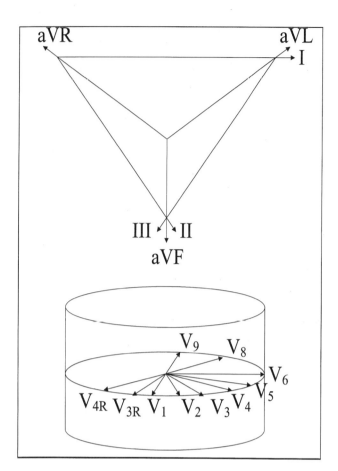

FIGURE 1-2. Two-dimensional planes of the 12-lead ECG. Above, the hexaxial system of the limb leads and the augmented leads. Below, the three-dimensionality of the ECG is established by the precordial leads. Also shown are the right-sided and posterior leads.

depends upon which of the two ions can freely cross the membrane. In diastole, the cell membrane is more permeable to K^+, which provides for the negative transmembrane potential.

Automaticity is generated in the noncontractile pacemaker cells of the heart because of a slowly depolarizing Na^+ leak into the cell during phase 4 (Fig. 1-3). The stable phase 4 diastolic

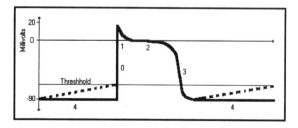

FIGURE 1-3. The four phases of cellular depolarization. Phase 0 is the rapid depolarization; phase 1 is the overshoot; phase 2 is the plateau; phase 3 is repolarization; phase 4 is the resting membrane potential. The dashed line represents phase 4 in cardiac cells with automaticity, slowly leaking toward the threshold for depolarization in a rhythmic, temporal manner.

transmembrane potential in contractile cells explains their lack of automaticity and is what allows for their stable diastolic polarization. This is what produces the cellular polarity that is the foundation for the electrical vectors that ultimately form the familiar QRS-T pattern on the ECG. When the membrane potential crosses a threshold, whether it is due to phase 4 leak or direct stimulus, fast Na^+ channels open and phase 0 depolarization occurs. The transmembrane potential overshoots initially in phase 1 depolarization, reaching around $^+20$ mV, and then plateaus at 0 mV during phase 2. This plateau is achieved by slow calcium channel influx balancing the slow K^+ efflux and allows for prolonged contraction in cardiac myocytes. During phase 3 repolarization, calcium channels close and K^+ efflux restores the negative resting membrane potential.

After the initial stimulus on the cell, the membrane does not completely and instantaneously depolarize throughout the length of the cell. Rather, it is a process that begins at the point of origin and continues three-dimensionally and temporally toward the other pole of the cell. **At rest,** the K^+ permeability gives the cell membrane a **negative potential,** which is analogous to having a **positive charge on the outside of the cell.** The cell membrane then **becomes negative after depolarization.** As depolarization progresses, a dipole is set up with the vector oriented from the negative (depolarized) direction toward the positive (resting) portion of the cell (Fig. 1-4). A single positive electrode on the resting side of the cell would show a positive electrical deflection, which would be greatest when the cell is halfway depolarized. In normal cells, **subsequent repolarization** starts at the same location where depolarization began and progresses from the newly repolarized positive side to the still depolarized portion that is negative (to reiterate, this negativity refers to the **outside** of the cell). On a cellular level, in contrast to the clinical ECG, the direction of the repolarization vector is oriented exactly opposite to the depolarization vector. Myocardial cells **contract** when depolarized, and their depolarization depolarizes succeeding cells, leading to **conductivity.**

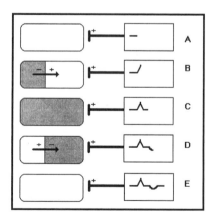

FIGURE 1-4. Cellular depolarization as interpreted by a single positive reading electrode. A is the rest state; **B** is cellular depolarization; **C** is depolarization completed; **D** is repolarization, originating from the same point as depolarization and progressing in the same direction, but with a negative vector; **E** is completed repolarization. (+) and (–) refer to the relative charge on the **outside** of the cell.

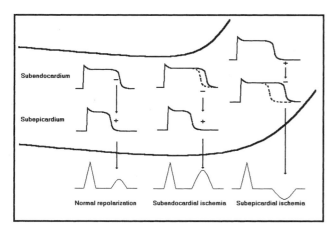

FIGURE 1-5. Electrical activity in normal and ischemic tissue. During normal repolarization, the intrinsic delay of the endocardium to repolarize generates a positive T wave, as shown on the left. During subendocardial ischemia, the further delay of the tissue to repolarize results in the hyperacute T wave, shown in the middle. During subepicardial ischemia, the delay to repolarization reverses the repolarization vector, resulting in an inverted T wave, as shown on the right.

On an organ level, the depolarization of the heart is represented electrocardiographically by the QRS and has a similar upright pattern as compared with cellular depolarization. Cardiac **repolarization,** however, is the **opposite of cellular depolarization,** with a vector (T wave) that is normally positive. This is due to a repolarization delay in the subendocardium resulting in a repolarization wave moving **away** from the positive electrode and progressing from the subepicardium to the subendocardium. This is demonstrated schematically on the left side of Figure 1-5. This delay is hypothesized to be due to a chronic hypometabolic state in the subendocardium secondary to poor blood supply, which behaves electrically like ischemic tissue. The result is the familiar upright QRS-T pattern of the ECG.

ISCHEMIC PROCESSES

A cascade of events occurs in **ischemic cells,** beginning with metabolic changes and subsequent electrical changes and alterations in contractility. Intracellular K^+ decreases because of the decreased activity of the Na^+/K^+ ATP-ase pump. This causes a decrease in diastolic transmembrane potential and results in delayed phase 3 repolarization. Additionally, in ischemic cells, repolarization originates at the **last** point in the cell membrane to depolarize, unlike a normal cell, in which repolarization begins at the same point that depolarization began. Therefore **in ischemia, the cellular repolarization vector will be opposite to that of a normal cell** and will be **delayed.**

Hyperacute T Waves and T-Wave Inversion

Subendocardial ischemia is the first pathologic process to have an ECG correlate during acute coronary syndrome (ACS). Endocardial ischemia results in delayed recovery of this area. Since repolarization normally proceeds from the epicardium to the endocardium, the direction of the repolarization vector does

not change, but the **amplitude** of the vector increases, resulting in a **"hyperacute" T wave. Subepicardial** ischemia results in a delay in subepicardial repolarization, and a reverse in direction of the repolarization vector; the result in this situation is **T-wave inversion** (Fig. 1-5). Subepicardial ischemia rarely occurs without involvement of the endocardium (transmural ischemia). However, the **ECG picture is dominated by the subepicardial ischemia.** This is due, most likely, to the closer proximity of the epicardium to the electrode, as well as to the relative mass of the subepicardium as compared with the endocardium. On the standard 12-lead ECG, this pattern holds true for inferior, lateral, and anterior ischemia, whereas the **reverse** is true for posterior wall ischemia. In the anterior leads (V1–V2), posterior subepicardial ischemia causes a positive T wave, whereas subendocardial ischemia results in a more negative T wave. The posterior leads (V8–V9) of the 15-lead ECG would show the usual pattern for posterior ischemia. Theoretically, T-wave inversions of transmural ischemia occur last during an infarction, after ST segment and Q-wave changes have been seen. In vivo, however, all can happen at once in different zones of tissue around an infarct.

ST Segment Changes: Two Theories

The **"current of injury" theory** has been proposed to explain the **ST segment changes** seen during myocardial injury. Damaged cells lose their membrane integrity resulting in a K^+ leak. The (outside of the) cells become more electrically negative, which **decreases the charge of the baseline, or isoelectric line.** If the damage is near the positive electrode, as in subepicardial/transmural injury, the baseline (TP segment) decreases in voltage and the ST segment is then elevated relative to this baseline (ST elevation). Since the cells still depolarize, the ST segment remains at the "normal" isoelectric line (Fig. 1-6). In subendocardial injury, the tissue becomes more negative at a dis-

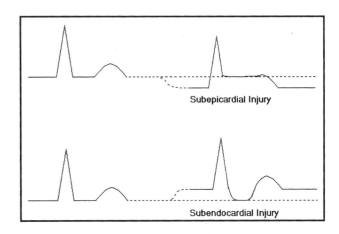

FIGURE 1-6. The "current of injury" theory of ST elevation and depression. The "current of injury" theory explains ST-segment changes as a result of changing isoelectric line charge, secondary to a decrease in charge of injured tissue. The ST segment remains at the "normal" isoelectric line, as the tissue is still able to depolarize. The result is ST-segment elevation or depression, depending on the proximity of the electrode to the site of injury.

tance from the electrode, resulting in a more positive vector for the isoelectric line. In this situation, the isoelectric line increases and the **ST segment appears depressed.**

The **"incomplete depolarization" theory** is based on the belief that damaged cells do not completely depolarize. If the electrode is in close proximity to these damaged cells, as in subepicardial/transmural injury, a more positive ST segment will be maintained during systole. The partial depolarization of subendocardial injury would result in **ST depression** in leads over the normally depolarizing epicardium. With this theory there is no change to the isoelectric line.

Reciprocal Changes

When transmural injury occurs, in addition to the ST elevations at proximate electrodes, distant electrodes may show ST depressions. These **"reciprocal changes"** of transmural injury can be explained by either of the preceding theories. **There must be ST elevation at some recording electrode for ST depressions** to be called reciprocal changes rather than simply subendocardial injury. The **exception** to this on the standard 12-lead ECG is with posterior wall subepicardial/transmural injury, as there are no directly posterior leads. The reciprocal changes of ST depression in V1–V2, and sometimes the inferior leads, may be misinterpreted unless the clinician suspects posterior wall injury and requests posterior leads (V8–V9).

Q Waves

QRS changes in the first 40 ms of depolarization can be due either to preexcitation or infarction. Usually, the degree of infarction necessary to result in pathologic Q waves is only seen in transmural infarctions. **Normal ventricular depolarization begins in the septum for the initial 20 ms; proceeds to the anterior, inferior, and lateral walls over the next 30 to 40 ms; and terminates in the posterior and high lateral walls.** In the case of infarction, the dead tissue becomes electrically silent. The vector for the initial 40 ms points away from this quiet tissue toward normal muscle, resulting in classic ECG changes. **In inferior and lateral infarcts,** the result is deep, pathologic (>1 mm wide and >3 mm deep) Q waves. **Anterior septal infarcts** will lose their R waves in V1–V3, with poor R-wave progression across the precordium (V1–V6), and loss of the initial "septal" Q waves in leads I, V5–V6. **Anterior wall infarcts** result in forces deviated to the right with an R wave in V1, while maintaining normal septal Q waves in leads I, aVL, V5, and V6. **High posterior wall infarcts** direct forces anteriorly with large R waves in leads V1–V3 and small or absent S waves. **Posterior basal wall infarct** is the exception to the rule, as the initial changes in the depolarization vector are deviated into the transverse and sagittal planes and are not detected by the standard 12-lead ECG.

For more detailed information on electrophysiology and electrical pathophysiology of ischemia and infarction, we refer you to several excellent texts (1–10).

TERMINOLOGY AND ECG TYPES IN ACUTE CORONARY SYNDROMES

KEY POINTS

- Acute coronary syndrome (ACS) is broadly differentiated by its ECG manifestations into ST-elevation myocardial infarction (STEMI) and unstable angina/non-ST-elevation myocardial infarction (UA/NSTEMI).
- Type 1a–1d ECG: The ECG meets commonly recommended "criteria" for reperfusion therapy. ST elevation (or hyperacute T waves or ST depression of posterior acute myocardial infarction (AMI) in V1–V4) is present but may or may not be due to AMI.
- Type 2 ECG: The ECG is diagnostic of UA/NSTEMI.
- Type 3 ECG: This is an abnormal ECG that is not diagnostic of any kind of ACS.
- Type 4 ECG: This is a normal ECG.

GENERAL BACKGROUND

ACS refers to any rupture of coronary atherosclerotic plaque or thrombotic event that results in symptomatic ischemia or infarction; there are also asymptomatic coronary events. Coronary thrombosis may be occlusive or nonocclusive. Total occlusion of the artery supplying the myocardium under the recording lead, without collateral circulation, usually results in ST elevation. It may result in ST depression if the lead is recording an opposite wall; an example is "anterior" ST depression (V1–V3) during posterior infarction. Nonocclusive thrombosis or occlusive thrombosis with good collateral circulation often results in ST depression because the ischemia involves primarily the more susceptible subendocardial region while sparing the subepicardium (nontransmural). If the area at risk is small, in an electrocardiographically silent area, or ischemic for a short time period, there may be no ECG changes. Absence of ECG changes may be due to failure to record at the right moment or due to actual absence of electrically detectable abnormalities.

Because of inconsistency in the relationship between ST elevation or depression and "subendocardial" or "transmural" infarction, these terms have been largely abandoned. Instead, **AMI is classified according to the presence or absence of ST elevation.** ST elevation helps to direct immediate therapy by identifying a population that clearly benefits from reperfusion therapy; this is because ST elevation discriminates well between those with and without complete **coronary thrombotic occlusion.** Thus the disease spectrum ranges, in increasing order of severity, from unstable angina (UA) to non-ST—elevation MI (INSTEMI) to ST-elevation MI (STEMI) (Fig. 2-1). Severity depends on the duration of coronary occlusion, complete versus partial occlusion, size of the area at risk, and presence of collateral circulation.

Q-wave MI and non–Q-wave MI are also commonly used terms that have little utility for the reperfusion decision because they describe the ECG **after** the infarct is complete. STEMI usually results in Q-wave MI, but also in non–Q-wave MI. Although unusual, ST elevation may result in no MI at all if the thrombotic occlusion is so brief that the infarction is aborted before irreversible damage and troponin release from tissue (transient ST elevation without MI, see Case 8-12). We outline

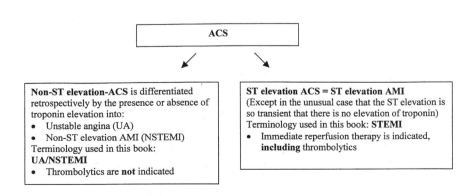

FIGURE 2-1. Disease spectrum of ACS.

the relationship between ECG manifestations (presence or absence of ST elevation or Q waves) and pathophysiologic correlates (total coronary occlusion, persistent occlusion vs. reperfusion, collateral circulation, area at risk, and presence of subendocardial or transmural AMI) at the end of this chapter.

The **distinction between UA and NSTEMI is made retrospectively** by the presence or absence of myocardial injury (cellular necrosis), which is determined by measurement of the biomarkers cardiac troponin I (cTnI) or cardiac troponin T (cTnT); **levels of these biomarkers sometimes are not elevated until 6 to 12 or more hours after symptom onset.** In ACS, an ischemic area is at risk for infarction. When coronary occlusion is complete, as in most STEMI, without collaterals and without reperfusion, the infarct area is a large proportion of the entire area at risk. With NSTEMI, the area of reversible ischemia is generally larger than the area of irreversible injury. By definition, in UA, serial troponin levels are ultimately normal. Thus all of the ischemia is ultimately proven to have been reversible.

Formerly, AMI was defined as elevation of the isoenzyme creatine kinase-MB (CK-MB) to greater than twice the normal levels in the context of 30 minutes of symptoms. CTnI and cTnT identify additional patients who have had myocardial injury (cellular necrosis) but who do not have diagnostic elevations of CK-MB. These patients with "minor myocardial damage" (11) are now classified as having sustained AMI (11,12). It is estimated that **30% of patients who were formerly classified as UA are now classified as NSTEMI** (11). Although both entities may represent a very large area of myocardium at risk, the **release of even a small amount of cardiac troponin is associated with a significantly greater incidence of future adverse cardiac events** (13,14).

Reperfusion therapy includes thrombolytic therapy and coronary angiography with or without percutaneous coronary intervention (PCI) (angiography ± PCI). Reperfusion therapy is distinguished from other anti-ischemic therapy by its cost, its significant risk (especially thrombolytics), and its invasive nature (PCI); these therapies must therefore be chosen with discrimination. With some exceptions, thrombolytics are not indicated unless there is ST elevation. The two terms, UA and NSTEMI, are linked because (a) the relevant distinction for the reperfusion decision is the presence versus absence of ST elevation; (b) neither NSTEMI nor UA has persistent ST elevation; and (c) UA cannot be clinically distinguished from NSTEMI until later confirmation by biomarkers. **Thus AMI is categorized as STEMI or UA/NSTEMI.**

Functions of the ECG in Patients with ACS

There are two essential functions of the ECG in patients with ACS, as follows:

1. **To identify patients with STEMI** (ST elevation and thrombotic occlusion) who are **candidates for acute reperfusion therapy** including thrombolytics (Types 1a, 1b, and, in many cases, Types 1c and 1d ECGs; see later).
2. **To identify patients with ACS** who, though they do not have STEMI and thus are not eligible for thrombolytics, are **candidates for aggressive medical therapy** (UA/NSTEMI, Type 2 ECG; see later); these patients may be eligible for angiography ± PCI.

(Note: The ECG does not exclude ACS.)

NEW ECG CLASSIFICATION

Much of the earlier literature divided ECGs into three confusing categories: diagnostic, nonspecific, and normal ECGs. These categories are poorly defined and too rarely based on therapeutic management. Therefore we promote the following classification (15).

- The ECG in AMI may manifest as Types 1 to 4.
  - Femsire **(16)** used a similar classification of Types 1 to 4, but did not break Type 1 into four subtypes.
- The ECG in UA/NSTEMI may manifest as Types 1c, 1d, and 2 through 4.
  - If Type 1a or 1b ST elevation is transient and biomarkers are negative, it is often called UA.

Type 1 ECG: Meets recommended "criteria" for reperfusion therapy (see Chapter 6).

ST elevation (or hyperacute T waves or ST depression of posterior AMI in V1–V4) is present but may or may not be due to AMI. If due to AMI, these are the **only indications for thrombolytics as well as angiography ± PCI.**

Type 1a ECG: Clearly diagnostic of AMI due to acute, thrombotic occlusion.

This is an indication for reperfusion therapy, **including thrombolytics and angiography ± PCI.** Nonexperts easily diagnose this type of AMI. It is the initial ECG type in approximately 45% of all AMIs (as measured by CK-MB, not troponin) (17, 18, **19**). Specificity of a Type 1a ECG for AMI is at least 94% (17).

ECG Characteristics

- ST elevation > 2 mm in two consecutive precordial leads or > 1 mm in two consecutive limb leads.
- No confounding factors, such as left ventricular hypertrophy (LVH), bundle branch block (BBB), early repolarization, pericarditis, and ventricular aneurysm.
- Typical morphology.

Important Aspects of Type 1a ECGs

Electrocardiographic acuity may be as important as history in determining time since onset (see Chapter 33). A large myocardial risk area increases mortality and increases the potential benefit of reperfusion therapy. ECG features help to roughly estimate infarct size and the benefit/risk ratio (see Chapter 6). This is particularly important when there are relative contraindications to thrombolytics.

Type 1b ECG: Diagnostic of AMI, but subtle and difficult.

Specificity for acute thrombotic occlusion may be approximately 90%. These ECGs are indications for reperfusion therapy, including **thrombolytics and angiography ± PCI.** Many ECGs that appear to be nondiagnostic of AMI are indeed diagnostic upon closer scrutiny if you know what to look for.

ECG Characteristics

- These ECGs may be due to lateral AMI, AMI with borderline ST elevation, ST elevation in one lead only, posterior AMI, hyperacute T waves, or AMI in the presence of confounding factors such as LVH, left bundle branch block (LBBB) or right bundle branch block (RBBB), early repolarization, pericarditis, or ventricular aneurysm.
- ST elevation is borderline because the ECG was recorded early in the course of AMI or AMI is in an electrocardiographically silent area, or there is good collateral circulation or intermittent occlusion. Borderline ST elevation, unless it is due to early or intermittent occlusion, is associated with lower risk.

Type 1c ECG: Equivocal

There is ST elevation that meets "criteria" for thrombolytics, but it is uncertain whether it is due to AMI or to another condition. **Additional information is necessary** to determine if reperfusion is indicated. **Angiography ± PCI is preferable,** if available.

- The ST elevation may be due to AMI or another abnormality, such as LVH, LBBB, early repolarization, ventricular aneurysm, or pericarditis.
- Additional information may include comparison with a previous ECG, serial ECGs, echocardiography, angiography, and/or biomarker levels. Some Type 1c ECGs will be reclassified as Type 3 if MI is eliminated as the source of the ST elevation.

Type 1d ECG: ST Elevation ± QS Waves

Type 1d ECG manifests ST elevation that is **diagnostic of AMI,** but there is also T-wave inversion indicative of **spontaneous reperfusion OR** QS waves and T-wave inversion indicative of **subacute MI.**

 Reperfusion therapy is indicated if

- An especially careful history clearly establishes symptom onset within less than 12 hours; be certain that this Type 1 ECG is due to **acute** infarction.
- Symptoms are unequivocally ongoing; be certain that this infarction has not already spontaneously reperfused.
- Angiography ± PCI may be the preferred reperfusion strategy.

 Note: Types 1b, 1c, and 1d, the subtle and difficult ECGs, are the focus of this book. They may be read as nondiagnostic by many clinicians or electrocardiographers or both. These ECGs could have been classified as diagnostic, nonspecific, or normal using previous literature classifications.

Type 2 ECG: Diagnostic of UA/NSTEMI.

The ECG has "primary" ST depression or T-wave inversion that is nondiagnostic of AMI but **is** diagnostic of myocardial ischemia. **Angiography ± PCI** may be indicated in these cases, but **thrombolytic therapy is not indicated.** "Primary" means that the ST-T changes cannot be completely explained as secondary to a depolarization, or QRS, disorder.

ECG Characteristics

- New or evolving ST depression, especially 1 mm or more, that is not posterior AMI.
- New or evolving T-wave inversion of 1 mm or more.
- These ECGs comprise approximately 25% to 35% of all AMIs (as measured by CK-MB, not troponin) most of which are non–Q-wave MI (18,20). Patients with Type 2 ECGs who do not develop elevated troponin receive a diagnosis of UA.

Management

Intensive monitoring and treatment for ACS (see Chapter 37) is indicated, which may include angiography ± PCI for ongoing symptoms that persist despite medical therapy, or for hemodynamic instability. **Consider serial ECGs, 12-lead monitoring, and posterior leads in order to detect STEMI.**

Type 3 ECG: Nonspecific ECG that is abnormal but nondiagnostic of any kind of ACS.

Angiography ± PCI, but not thrombolytic therapy, may be indicated for high clinical suspicion, especially with hemodynamic instability. Of all AMIs, 22.5% present with a "nonspecific" Type 3 ECG, and 8.6% of patients who present with ischemic symptoms and a Type 3 ECG rule in for AMI as measured by CK-MB (18,21). See Chapter 5 for more detail.

ECG Characteristics

- There may be one or more of the following: Q waves, LVH, or minor, nondynamic ST or T-wave abnormalities that are not suggestive of ischemia or infarction, such as ST depression of less than 1 mm or T-wave flattening or inversion of less than 1 mm that is unchanged from a previous ECG, especially if secondary to depolarization abnormalities (i.e., an abnormal QRS).
- Some of these with ST elevation may initially be Type 1c ECGs until diagnostic modalities rule out AMI as the source of the ST elevation.

Management

Intensive monitoring and possible angiography ± PCI for those with high clinical suspicion. See Case 26-2. Also consider serial ECGs, 12-lead monitoring, and posterior leads; see Chapter 5.

Type 4 ECG

The Type 4 ECG is a normal ECG. As measured by CK-MB, 6.4% of all AMIs manifest "normal" initial ECGs and 3.4% of patients with ischemic symptoms and a "normal" ECG "rule in" for AMI (as measured by CK-MB) (18,21,22). Many patients with UA are in this category.

Management

Consider **serial ECGs, 12-lead monitoring, and posterior leads** (see Chapter 5).

ECG Pathophysiologic Correlates and Development in ACS

ST elevation, ST depression, Q waves, and the correlation of each with subendocardial ischemia, subendocardial infarction, or transmural infarction depend on risk area, collateral circulation, and reperfusion. Some authors call the loss of R-wave voltage a "Q-wave" infarction.

Patients with thrombotic occlusion of a coronary artery:

- Usually develop ST elevation, but sometimes **do not,** especially with a small risk area.
- May have intermittent occlusion or spontaneously reperfuse. ST elevation may be transient. If reperfusion occurs before the first ECG, ST elevation may be missed.
- In the absence of reperfusion, usually develop Q waves and transmural infarction, but **may not,** depending on collateral circulation, risk area, size and ECG silence of risk area.

Patients with ST elevation usually have thrombotic occlusion. With very **early** reperfusion, they often do not develop Q waves and are unlikely to have transmural MI. With no reperfusion therapy, approximately 86% develop Q waves (23).

Patients without ST elevation on the initial ECG may have thrombotic coronary occlusion, but usually with good collateral circulation, small risk area, or a silent risk area. They may develop Q waves if there is no early reperfusion, but they are much less likely to do so than patients with ST elevation. **Of those with AMI** (as measured by CK-MB) without ST elevation, but **with ST depression,** 29% develop Q waves. And of those with AMI who present with no significant ST deviation, 24% develop Q waves (23).

Patients who develop Q waves may or may not have transmural infarction. Patients with transmural infarction may or may not develop Q waves. Patients with nontransmural (subendocardial) infarction may or may not develop Q waves. Q waves may resolve several months to years after a Q-wave infarction.

General Relationship of ST Elevation, Q Waves, and Transmural Infarction

- **AMI with ST elevation due to total occlusion** of an infarct-related artery (IRA) that does not reperfuse is very likely to result in transmural infarction and Q waves.

- Although there are many determinants of magnitude of ST elevation, in general, the higher the ST elevation, the more likely is the development of transmural infarction and Q waves (if there is no reperfusion).

Complexities and Shortcomings of ECG Research

Most ECG studies are of ECGs at one moment in time, as is the ECG you are interpreting. These studies often do not account for the changes that occur in the ECG over time and therefore miss transient abnormalities. They frequently do not account for reperfusion and reocclusion. Nor do they account for the presence of collateral circulation and individual anatomy, which affect the location of the AMI as well as ECG features of ST elevation, ST depression, and the development of Q waves. They infrequently correlate the ECG with angiography, and frequently correlate it with biochemical incidence of AMI. Given the critical importance of the ECG for the initial phases of ACS, much more and better research is needed.

ANNOTATED BIBLIOGRAPHY

See also annotated bibliography in Chapters 3, 5, and 6.

Fesmire FM, et al. Risk stratification according to the initial electrocardiogram in patients with suspected acute myocardial infarction, 1989.
   Methods: Fesmire et al. (24) studied 426 patients with suspected AMI who were admitted. They classified the initial ECG as "normal" (identical to Type 4), "abnormal" (identical to Type 3), or "positive" (corresponds to Type 1 or 2).
   Findings: Compared with normal (and abnormal) ECGs, respectively, patients with positive ECGs had a 2.9 (1.7) times greater risk of interventions, a 3.2 (2.6) times greater risk of life-threatening complications, and a 14.2 (4.9) times greater risk of AMI.

Fesmire FM. Which chest pain patients benefit from continuous ST-segment monitoring with automated serial ECG? 1999 (abstract).
   Methods and Findings: Fesmire (16) categorized patients by ECG in his study of automated serial ECGs (see annotation Chapter 10). Categories were as follows: 1 = ACS and eligible for reperfusion therapy; 2 = obvious ACS, but not a candidate for reperfusion therapy; 3 = possible ACS; and 4 = lower risk still, but warrants monitoring.

Fesmire FM, et al. Initial ECG in Q wave and non–Q wave myocardial infarction, 1989.
   Methods: Fesmire et al. (19) studied the initial and subsequent ECGs in 100 consecutive AMI patients. The number of patients undergoing reperfusion is not stated.
   Findings: Acute injury pattern (Type 1) was seen in 47%, with a positive predictive value (PPV) of 84%. "Ischemia" (Type 2) was seen in 15%, with a positive predictive value (PPV) of 39%. LVH with strain was seen in 11%, with a PPV of 19%. Q-wave AMI occurred in 43 patients, 72% of whose initial ECGs showed injury (Type 1). Fifty patients sustained non–Q-wave AMI, 38% of whose initial ECGs showed injury. Only 17% of patients with Q-wave infarct had an initial ECG with "ischemia or strain" (Types 2 or 3), compared to 36% of patients with a non–Q-wave AMI.

3

THE ROLE OF THE ECG IN REPERFUSION THERAPY

KEY POINTS

- Reperfusion therapy is underutilized and often delayed, largely due to difficulty in ECG interpretation.
- Suspect AMI and record an ECG for atypical symptoms.
- Learn to read the difficult ECGs.

GENERAL BACKGROUND

The ECG is critical in the reperfusion decision and must be interpreted in the context of a patient's history and physical exam (25,26,27,28). Efficacy of reperfusion therapy is greatest if administered less than 1 hour after symptom onset and decreases rapidly thereafter (29,30,31). **Many patients who should receive reperfusion therapy do not receive it,** and many others receive reperfusion therapy with **inappropriate delay (25,27,28,32,**33). These shortcomings are often due to physician uncertainty and error in ECG interpretation (19, 34,**35–40**). Furthermore, **computer algorithms are very insensitive for STEMI (**41–45,**46,**47). Thus the American College of Cardiology (ACC) states that, because ST segment criteria are insensitive and nonspecific for the reperfusion decision, skilled and confidant ECG interpretation are critical (48).

Physicians make more errors of omission (not administering reperfusion therapy when the patient has AMI) **than errors of commission** (administering reperfusion therapy when the patient does not have AMI) **and could save more lives by being more aggressive and treating more expeditiously (28,40,**49).

Priorities in the Care of AMI

1. Assess airway, breathing, circulation (ABCs).
2. Intravenous (IV), oxygen, cardiac rhythm monitor, vital signs.
3. Correct hemodynamically significant brady- or tachydysrhythmias.
4. Give aspirin and sublingual nitroglycerine (NTG) ± pain relief with morphine.
5. Record a 12-lead ECG.

6. Assess the patient's ECG and clinical presentation for indications and contraindications for reperfusion therapy. Interpreting the subtle ECG in the context of the clinical presentation (assessing the pre-test probability) is critical.
7. Assess the benefit/risk ratio.
8. **Give a thrombolytic bolus or call an interventional cardiologist.**

Assessment of Benefit/Risk Ratio in the Reperfusion Decision

See Chapter 35 for more detailed discussion.

Symptoms

Determine if symptoms are **typical or atypical** and the **time since symptom onset.**

History

Determine if there are **risk factors** for coronary artery disease (CAD) or bleeding or both. Assess for **contraindications** (absolute, major, significant, minor, or inconsequential) before administration of thrombolytics (see Table 34-4).

Physical Exam

Assess hemodynamic stability. What are the vital signs? Is there evidence of poor perfusion? Is there a new murmur or evidence of congestive heart failure (CHF) such as orthopnea, rales, or peripheral edema?

Determine the ECG Type: See Chapter 2 for detailed discussion.

- **Types 1a–1d ECG:** ECG meets "criteria" for reperfusion therapy. ST elevation (or hyperacute T waves, or ST depression of posterior AMI in V1—V4) is present but may or may not be due to AMI. **Reperfusion therapy including thrombolytics is indicated for Types 1a and 1b.** Types 1c and 1d depend upon further investigation.
- **Type 2 ECG:** Diagnostic of UA/NSTEMI.

- **Type 3 ECG:** An abnormal ECG that is not diagnostic of any kind of ACS.
- **Type 4 ECG:** A normal ECG.

COMMON REASONS FOR DELAYED OR MISSED REPERFUSION THERAPY

The following are situations in which patients may receive delayed reperfusion therapy or may not receive it at all. See also Table 3-1 for presentations of patients who commonly do not receive reperfusion therapy; many are due to ECG characteristics (**28**). **Systematic causes of delay** and suggestions for improvement are discussed in Chapter 32.

Missed Diagnosis of Unequivocal AMI

Atypical Symptoms

An ECG, which would be unequivocal, may not be obtained due to an **atypical presentation.** Such cases, if discovered, are only discovered later from a serial ECG or development of hemodynamic instability, dysrhythmias, CHF, elevated biomarker levels, or death.

Atypical symptoms include dyspnea, abdominal pain, and back, arm, hand, shoulder, and jaw pain. Additional symptoms include nausea, vomiting, or anxiety; dizziness or weakness; especially in the elderly; or uncontrolled hyperglycemia in diabetics. In AMI as diagnosed by CK-MB, 42% of patients more than 75 years of age and 63% to 75% of those of more than 85 years of age, **do not complain of chest pain (CP)** (50,51); 25% to 37% of those with STEMI beyond the age of 65 have no CP (**28,52**,53–55). See Table 3-2 for characteristics of AMI patients without CP (**52**).

- **Always obtain an ECG immediately for atypical symptoms, especially in elderly patients. If the ECG is unequivocally diagnostic, it is AMI until proven otherwise.**

There are also occasional pseudoinfarction patterns that manifest as a Type 1a ECG and are indistinguishable from STEMI, which we denote as Type 1a versus 1c. (See Cases 20-5, 20-6, 21-4, 22-2, 22-4, 24-5, 24-6, 24-8, and 24-9.) In general, atypical symptoms should not dissuade you from the diagnosis of AMI if the ECG is Type 1a. Because of occasional **false-positive** ECGs (both Types 1a and 1b), **it is acceptable that up to 10% of patients who receive thrombolytics will not, in retrospect, have STEMI** (15,17,**39**,41,46,49,56,57); we refer to this as **"inadvertent" thrombolytic therapy.** This percentage should be lower at institutions that have the option of angiography ± PCI.

Unstable physiologic states appear to occasionally result in **false-positives** (Type 1a ECGs without coronary occlusion). These include respiratory failure (see Cases 26-6 and 26-7), massive overdose (see Case 17-8), severe metabolic derangement (see Case 22-9), and severe hypertension (HTN) or LVH (see Cases 22-2 and 22-11). In such situations, **record a repeat ECG after stabilization.**

Unrecognized Unequivocal ECG

AMI may also be undiagnosed because **ST elevation is missed** or its significance is unappreciated, as in Type 1b, 1c, or 1d ECGs. See Case 3-1.

Delay in Diagnosis of Subtle AMIs

Delayed diagnosis of a subtle AMI may be due to (a) delayed recording of the ECG, especially in patients with atypical symptoms; (b) uncertainty in ECG interpretation when the recording is not delayed (Type 1b or 1c ECG); or (c) failure to record serial ECGs which would have become diagnostic. Table 3-3 shows the consequences of delayed therapy (**58**).

- Learn to recognize electrocardiographically subtle AMIs, obtain the patient's most recent previous ECG immediately, and obtain serial ECGs every 15 minutes or use continuous ST segment monitoring when suspicion of AMI is high. See Cases 3-2 and 3-3. See also Cases 5-2 and 5-4 and Chapters 9, 10, and 17 through 25.

Delay in Administration of Therapy

Delay may result from excessive time spent on diagnostic or therapeutic measures of lower priority (see Case 11-3) or inappropriate concern for **relatively** unimportant contraindications (see Case 16-5).

- **Aspirin and sublingual NTG** are the only two medications that should receive priority over the thrombolytic bolus. **NTG may abort STEMI before thrombolytics** (see Cases 5-4, 12-3, 31-1, 31-2, and 31-3).
  - Heparin, IV NTG, beta-blockers, and other medications are of lower priority and may be given after the thrombolytic bolus.
- IV NTG is not routinely indicated for patients undergoing thrombolysis and may be detrimental (59–63). Routine use of IV NTG with angioplasty, however, is acceptable. Use of IV NTG should never delay reperfusion therapy unless it is necessary to control HTN or CHF.
- If angiography ± PCI is planned, give heparin with or without glycoprotein (GP) IIb–IIIa inhibitor before the procedure.

Abortion of Treatment

Therapy may be inappropriately aborted due to symptom resolution, despite persistent ST elevation. **Resolution of ST elevation is the best predictor of reperfusion** (see Chapter 27). If symptoms are resolving, it is essential to record another ECG.

- **With increased, unchanged, or less than 25% ST elevation resolution, continue reperfusion therapy.**
- With 25% to 50% resolution, or terminal T-wave inversion, record serial ECGs and look for 50% ST resolution or more.
- With 50% to 100% resolution, it is appropriate to suspend reperfusion therapy pending further assessment, especially continuous ST monitoring.

TABLE 3.1. PRESENTATIONS OF PATIENTS LEAST LIKELY TO RECEIVE APPROPRIATE REPERFUSION THERAPY

Clinical variable	Adjusted OR (CI)	No. received thrombolytics/eligible	
LBBB	0.04; (0.01–0.17)	2/98	(2.0%)
CP > 6 hours	0.26; (0.17–0.38)	105/400	(26%)
History of coronary artery bypass graft	0.30; (0.14–0.65)	13/55	(24%)
No CP	0.31; (0.21–0.48)	56/279	(20%)
Q-waves	0.35; (0.17–0.69)	169/382	(44%)
≤6 mm total ST elevation	0.38; (0.24–0.60)	166/500	(33%)
ST elevation in 2 adjacent leads only	0.62; (0.41–0.98)	88/342	(26%)
Age 75 to 84 years	0.65; (0.54–0.77)	109/289	(38%)
Confusion	0.34; (0.14–0.80)	9/59	(15%)
Coma	0.07; (0.01–0.56)	1/22	(4.6%)
Age > 85 years	0.28; (0.18–0.43)	18/110	(16%)

OR, odds ratio; CI, confidence interval.
Adapted from Krumholz HM, Murillo JE, Chen J, et al. Thrombolytic therapy for eligible elderly patients with acute myocardial infarction. *JAMA* 1997;277:1683–1688, with permission. Copyrighted 1997, American Medical Association.

TABLE 3.2. CHARACTERISTICS OF AMI PATIENTS WITH AND WITHOUT CP

Characteristic	Without CP (33%)	With CP (67%)
Mean age	74 years	67 years
Received reperfusion therapy	25%	74%
Adjusted in-hospital mortality	23.3%	9.3%; OR: 2.17–2.26
Women	49.0%	38.0%
Prior stroke	14.1%	7.7%
Prior heart failure	26.4%	12.3%
Killip class I–II at presentation	82.4%	93.3%
Killip class III–IV	17.5%	6.6%
ST elevation on initial ECG	23.3%	47.3%
LBBB on initial ECG	9.7%	5.4%
Anterior AMI	24.0%	27.2%
Q-wave AMI	36.2%	51.7%
Non–Q-wave AMI	63.7%	48.3%

Adapted from Canto JG, Shlipak MG, Rogers WJ, et al. Prevalence, clinical characteristics, and mortality among patients with myocardial infarction presenting without chest pain. *JAMA* 2000;283:3223–3229, with permission. Copyrighted 2000, American Medical Association.

TABLE 3.3. ASSOCIATION OF DELAYS IN PRESENTATION AND TREATMENT WITH 30-DAY MORTALITY IN GUSTO

Presentation delay	30-day mortality	Treatment delay	Mortality
<1 hour	5.6%	<1 hour	5.4%
>4 hours	8.6%	>4 hours	8.1%

Reprinted with permission from the American College of Cardiology (ACC) from Newby LK, Rutsch WR, Califf RM, et al. Time from symptom onset to treatment and outcomes after thrombolytic therapy. GUSTO-1 Investigators. *J Am Coll Cardiol* 1996;27:1646–1655.

CASE 3-1

Atypical Symptoms Resulted in Delayed Diagnosis and Treatment of Electrocardiographically Unequivocal Anterior AMI

History

This 73-year-old man presented at 00:45 complaining of abdominal pain, nausea, vomiting, and bloating (**atypical symptoms**) that began at midnight, with no CP or dyspnea.

ECG 3-1 (Type 1a)

Not obtained until 02:07, shows an unequivocal **anterior AMI**.

Clinical Course

Due to atypical symptoms, physicians doubted the ECG diagnosis of AMI. Thrombolysis was delayed an additional 90 minutes, for a total treatment delay of 3 hours.

Conclusion

Do not doubt the diagnosis of AMI with a Type 1a ECG, even with atypical symptoms.

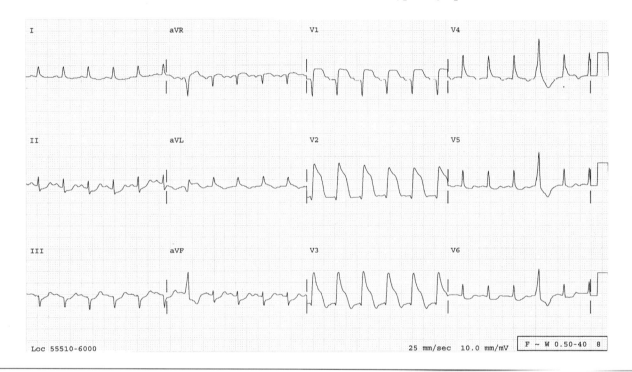

Loc 55510-6000   25 mm/sec   10.0 mm/mV   F ~ W 0.50-40 8

CASE 3-2

A Patient with "Reflux" Who Had Pain Relief After an Antacid and Then Sustained a Cardiac Arrest

History

This 62-year-old man complained of burning pain from epigastrium to throat, which he had never before experienced. He was otherwise healthy. His physical examination was normal.

ECG 3-2A (Type 3)

- No ST elevation.
- T waves: aVL, are larger than the entire QRS (hyperacute T wave), and, in V4–V6, are also large, which is abnormal but by no means diagnostic. It is also easily missed, as it was by 9 of 10 cardiologists at a later conference. However, you can find these abnormalities if you look for them. This difference in amplitude is not a result of differing QRS and T-waves axes, which are similar.

Clinical Course

The emergency physician misread the ECG as normal. The

patient experienced immediate and complete pain relief after receiving an antacid and viscous xylocaine. As he was being discharged, he suffered cardiac arrest from ventricular fibrillation.

ECG 3-2B (Type 1a)

Recorded after resuscitation, shows an obvious **anterolateral AMI**.

Clinical Course

Angioplasty opened an occluded proximal left anterior descending artery (LAD). The patient had a good outcome.

Conclusion

Look for subtle ECG signs of AMI. New substernal symptoms, no matter how atypical, may be due to ACS. Do not use a positive response to antacids or NTG as a diagnostic tool.

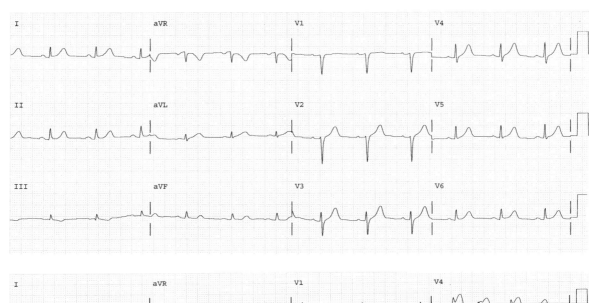

A

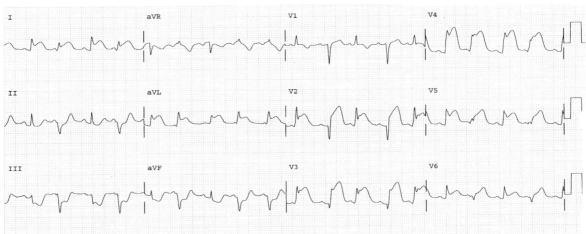

B

CASE 3-3

Inferoposterior STEMI Missed Because of ECG Changes of Previous MI and Subtle ST Deviation

History

This 48-year-old woman presented with CP one week after successful thrombolytic therapy for an inferior AMI. She had discontinued her medications and continued smoking.

ECG 3-3A (Type 1b)

At 20:19

- Q waves and T-wave inversions: II, III, aVL are indicative of a previous Q-wave MI.
- ST elevation: < 1 mm; II, III, and aVF, new since 1 week, is diagnostic of **inferior AMI** (previous ECG not shown).
- ST depression: V2–V3 is diagnostic of **posterior AMI.**
- The most recent previous ECG showed no residual ST elevation, but it was not sought for comparison. Thus this ECG was erroneously considered nondiagnostic of AMI.

ECG 3-3B (Type 1a)

At 21:59

- ST elevation: II, III, and aVF; and requisite reciprocal ST depression: aVL, make this diagnostic of **inferior AMI.**
- ST depression: V1–V3 is not anterior ischemia. In the presence of inferior AMI, it is **almost always** diagnostic of **posterior AMI.**
- Notice "pseudonormalized" (upright) T waves: III, aVF, diagnostic of **reocclusion.**

Clinical Course

Although clinicians administered thrombolytics appropriately, treatment was unnecessarily delayed 91 minutes.

Conclusion

Delay due to failure to recognize the AMI on the initial ECG could have been prevented with a prompt serial ECG. Record a repeat ECG every 15 minutes for 60 minutes or more, or perform continuous ST segment monitoring on any patient with a high clinical suspicion of AMI, even if the initial ECG is normal. Record a repeat ECG on any patient with a reasonable clinical suspicion of AMI whose initial ECG is normal.

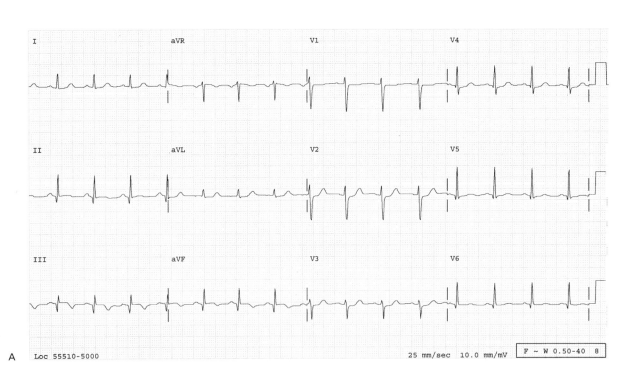

A   Loc 55510-5000   25 mm/sec   10.0 mm/mV   F ~ W 0.50-40 8

(continued on next page)

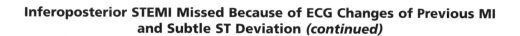

CASE 3-3

Inferoposterior STEMI Missed Because of ECG Changes of Previous MI and Subtle ST Deviation *(continued)*

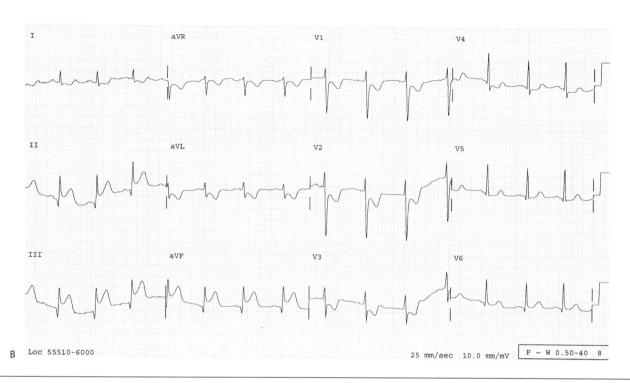

B   Loc 55510-6000   25 mm/sec   10.0 mm/mV   F ~ W 0.50-40   8

ANNOTATED BIBLIOGRAPHY

See also annotated bibliography in Chapter 6.

Atypical Symptoms

Canto JG, et al. Prevalence, clinical characteristics, and mortality among patients with myocardial infarction presenting without chest pain, 2000.

Methods: Canto et al. (52) analyzed data from 434,000 AMI patients in the National Registry of Myocardial Infarction-2 (NRMI-2) (see Appendix C).

Findings: Of all AMI patients, 33% presented without CP. Those without CP delayed their presentation to the ED longer and were less likely to receive a timely ECG. See Table 3-2 for additional characteristics.

Undertreatment

Thiemann DR, et al. Lack of benefit for intravenous thrombolysis in patients with myocardial infarction who are older than 75 years, 2000.

Methods: Thiemann et al. (32) analyzed data from the Cooperative Cardiovascular Project (CCP), from February 1994 until July 1995. All patients were more than 65 years of age. (See annotation in Chapter 34 for more detail.)

Findings: Only 74% of eligible patients 65 to 75 years of age and 60% of eligible patients 76 to 86 years of age received thrombolytics within 4 hours of presentation.

Berger AK, et al. Primary coronary angioplasty versus thrombolysis for the management of acute myocardial infarction in elderly patients, 1999.

Methods: Berger et al. (27) analyzed CCP data from 1994 to 1996. (See annotation in Chapter 34 for more detail.)

Findings: **Only 26% of eligible elderly patients more than 65 years of age** received reperfusion therapy.

Krumholz HM, et al. Thrombolytic therapy for eligible elderly patients with acute myocardial infarction, 1997.

Methods: Krumholz et al. (28) utilized CCP data (all patients more than 65 years of age) to identify 3,000 patients with AMI at nongovernmental acute-care hospitals in Connecticut between 1992 and 1993; they then reviewed the charts and ECGs.

Findings: Of 753 patients eligible for reperfusion and with no contraindications, **419 (56%) did not receive it**; 279 (37%) of the 753 patients had no CP. Multivariate analysis yielded the results listed in Table 3-1. Among all eligible patients, 30-day mortality in those who received thrombolysis was 14.7% versus 20.5% for those who did not receive it. **The only patients consistently treated appropriately were less than 75 years of age, with electrocardiographically large AMI and with CP for less than 6 hours. Even among this subset, however, 64 of 261 (25%) did not undergo thrombolysis.**

Barron HV, et al. Use of reperfusion therapy for acute myocardial infarction in the United States: Data from the NRMI 2, 1997.

Methods: Barron et al. (25) analyzed NRMI-2 data on 272,651 AMI patients of all ages (see Appendix C).

Findings: Of 272,651 AMI patients, the authors determined that 84,000 were unequivocally eligible for reperfusion therapy. Of these 84,000, approximately 24% did **not** receive it. These numbers **underestimate** the problem, however, because the group of "eligible" candidates did **not** include (a) patients who arrived more than 6 hours after onset of symptoms (41% of the total sample of 272,651), even though they **are** eligible for reperfusion up to 12 hours after onset; (b) patients with an initial nondiagnostic ECG, even if later ECGs were diagnostic; or (c) patients with any contraindication (3% of the total sample). Thus a very large proportion of excluded patients really were eligible.

Difficulties in Electrocardiographic Diagnosis

Sharkey SW, et al. Impact of the electrocardiogram on the delivery of thrombolytic therapy for acute myocardial infarction, 1994.

Methods: Sharkey et al. (39) prospectively studied the time from arrival to the ED to time of thrombolysis in 93 consecutive patients with suspected AMI.

Findings: In 83 patients with proven AMI, **time to thrombolysis correlated only with the sum of ST elevation; when that sum was not large, treatment was delayed.** In patients whose mean time to thrombolysis was more than 30 minutes versus less than 30 minutes, mean ST elevation sum was 11.5 mm versus 21.5 mm, respectively. Of patients who received thrombolytics, 11% did not have an AMI. These patients had ST elevation due to early repolarization, LVH, ventricular aneurysm, or conduction delay.

Hirvonen TP, et al. Delays in thrombolytic therapy for acute myocardial infarction in Finland, 1998.

Methods: Hirvonen et al. (38) studied 1,012 consecutive patients who received thrombolytics in Finland in 1995.

Findings: **Long diagnostic delays were often due to the ECG-related diagnostic difficulties** of emergency physicians and were especially associated with lower ST elevation. Patients with anterior AMI and a diagnostic delay had a mean sum of 0.7 millivolts (mV) (7 mm) of ST elevation versus 1.0 mV for those without delay. Patients with inferior AMI and delay had a mean of 0.3 mV of ST elevation versus 0.5 mV for those without delay.

Tandberg D, et al. Observer variation in measured ST-segment elevation, 1999.

Methods: Tandberg et al. (64) analyzed ST segment measurements by 52 physicians, residents, and medical students who unknowingly read identical pairs of ECG complexes.

Findings: **There was significant intraobserver variation;** interpretation by the same reader as to whether the same ST segment was < or ≥ 2 mm was inconsistent 14% of the time; 20% of the time a single reader differed by more than 0.5 mm for the same tracing.

Brady WJ, et al. Electrocardiographic ST segment elevation: correct identification of AMI and non-AMI syndromes by emergency physicians, 2000.

Methods: Brady et al. (37) showed a series of 11 ECGs to 458 emergency physicians. The ECG series manifested various AMI and pseudo-AMI morphologies in the context of a 45-year-old man with typical CP.

Findings: Appropriate thrombolysis was performed in 33% (atypical ST elevation) to 100% (RBBB and LBBB) of cases. Inappropriate thrombolysis ranged from none (LVH, RBBB, and ventricular paced rhythm) to 39% (ventricular aneurysm). **Physicians need more education on ECG discrimination of AMI and pseudoinfarction patterns.**

Brady WJ. ST segment elevation in ED adult chest pain patients: etiology and diagnostic accuracy for AMI, 1998.

Methods: Brady (65) analyzed ECGs from 902 CP patients for presence of ST elevation (≥1 mm in limb leads or ≥2 mm in precordial leads).

Findings: Of 902 patients, 202 (22.4%) had ST elevation, of which 171 (85%) had a non-AMI diagnosis; this included LVH, LBBB, early repolarization, and other pseudoinfarction patterns. The presence of reciprocal changes improved the specificity of ST elevation for AMI.

Brady WJ, et al. Errors in emergency physician interpretation of ST-segment elevation in emergency department chest pain patients, 2000.

Methods: Brady et al. (36) reviewed charts of 202 patients with ST elevation and CP. Initial interpretation by the emergency physician was compared with final interpretation by a cardiologist and supported by clinical findings.

Findings: There were two false-negative and 10 false-positive ECG readings; this is low relative to the total number of patients with CP and ST elevation (*n* = 202) but not low relative to the total with CP, ST elevation **and AMI** (*n* = 29).

Jayes RL, et al. Physician electrocardiogram reading in the emergency department—accuracy and effect on triage decisions: findings from a multicenter study, 1992.

Methods: Jayes et al. (35) performed a prospective observational study of patients with symptoms compatible with myocardial ischemia.

Findings: Emergency physicians, as compared with "expert" electrocardiographers, frequently misread the ST segment and T-wave abnormalities, with 41% and 36% false negatives, and 14% and 17% false positives, respectively. Follow-up showed that this error adversely affected the triage of these CP patients.

Chapman GD, et al. Minimizing the risk of inappropriately administering thrombolytic therapy, 1993.

Methods: Chapman et al. (66) studied all the patients from several thrombolytic trials who received thrombolytics but whose CK-MB levels subsequently ruled out AMI.

Findings: Only 20 (1.4%) of 1,387 patients who received thrombolytics ruled out for AMI.

Comment: No data were available regarding the number who should have received thrombolytics but did not. It is likely that predominantly patients with electrocardiographically obvious AMI (Type 1a) were entered into the study. The only certain conclusion from this study is that when limiting administration of thrombolytics to AMI patients manifesting unmistakable STEMI, the rate of inappropriate administration is low.

Computer Algorithms

See annotation of Massel et al. (41) in Chapter 6.

Kudenchuk PJ, et al. Accuracy of computer-interpreted electrocardiography in selecting patients for thrombolytic therapy, 1991.

Methods: Kudenchuk et al. (46) used ECGs and data from 1,189 patients entered into the Myocardial Infarction Triage and Intervention (MITI) trial (see Chapter 31) to compare diagnosis of STEMI by computer (Marquette 12 SL program, versions 4 to 6) with that of two electrocardiographers, whose differences were resolved in consensus with a third. In contrast to Massel et al. (41) (see annotation in Chapter 6), the final hospital diagnosis of AMI was used as the reference. In the presence of LVH, 4 mm of ST elevation was required for the ECG diagnosis of AMI.

Findings: Of 391 patients with a final diagnosis of AMI, 202 were identified by the computer (sensitivity, 52%), compared with 259 by the electrocardiographers (sensitivity, 66%). Of 798 patients without AMI, only 14 were identified by the computer as AMI (specificity, 98%; PPV, 94%), and 41 by the electrocardiographers (specificity, 95%; PPV, 86%). The sensitivity of the computer for STEMI, as compared with electrocardiographers, was 78%.

Factors and Outcomes Associated with Therapeutic Delay

Boersma E, et al. Early thrombolytic treatment in acute myocardial infarction: reappraisal of the golden hour, 1996.

Methods: Boersma et al. (31) analyzed outcomes of placebo-controlled thrombolytic trials from 1983 to 1993.

Findings: Number of lives saved per 1,000 patients treated was 65 if thrombolytics were given less than 1 hour after pain onset; 37 if given from 1 to 2 hours; 26, from 2 to 3 hours; and 29, from 3 to 6 hours.

Newby LK, et al. Time from symptom onset to treatment and outcomes after thrombolytic therapy, 1996.

Methods: Newby et al. (58) studied time intervals and corresponding outcomes in the GUSTO-I trial of 41,021 patients (see Appendix C).

Findings: Longer presentation and treatment delay were strongly associated with increased 30-day mortality, as shown in Table 3-3.

Berger AK, et al. Factors associated with delay in reperfusion therapy in elderly patients with acute myocardial infarction: analysis of the cooperative cardiovascular project, 2000.

Methods: Berger et al. (40) utilized CCP data from January 1994 until February 1996 to analyze factors associated with treatment times in 17,379 patients more than 65 years of age who were eligible for thrombolytic therapy and received it.

Findings: Only 22.2% of patients were treated within 30 minutes of hospital arrival. Some of the independent factors associated with delay included advancing age (OR = 1.15), female sex (OR = 1.30), LBBB (OR = 2.42), < 6 mm total ST elevation (OR = 1.5). Compared with those treated within 30 minutes, adjusted 1-year mortality was 1.09 for those treated between 30 and 90 minutes, and 1.27 for those treated between 91 and 360 minutes.

ANATOMIC CORRELATES OF THE ECG

KEY POINTS

- **Understanding ECG lead placement with respect to cardiac and coronary anatomy aids interpretation of ECG manifestations of coronary occlusion.**
- **Coronary anatomy is highly variable among patients.**

GENERAL BACKGROUND

Standard lead placement and patient positioning are essential when recording an ECG. Recording at one intercostal space (ICS) higher or lower, or with the patient upright instead of supine, can markedly alter the QRST complex. Lead placement is shown in Figure 4-1.

A firm understanding of ECG lead placement in relation to cardiac and coronary anatomy frees the clinician from dependence on rote memorization. Figures 4-2 to 4-4 illustrate the location of leads, relative to the heart, of the 12-lead ECG, plus leads V7–V9. Figure 4-5 and Table 4-1 demonstrate how ECG changes correlate with coronary artery occlusion and with the myocardial wall affected.

Lead III is the best lead for detecting the inferior wall and is therefore the most sensitive for detecting **inferior AMI** (Fig. 4-2). **Lead aVL** is most directly **opposite** to lead III.

- In **inferior AMI,** if there is ST elevation in lead III, there will be **ST depression in aVL unless** there is concurrent lateral injury causing lateral ST elevation. This contrasts with diffuse pericarditis (diffuse is the typical form), which exhibits inflammation and repolarization abnormalities around all walls of the heart, with no ST depression in aVL.

Lead aVL is the best for detecting the **high lateral wall** and is thus most sensitive for **lateral AMI.** Notice that the lateral wall is also detected by leads **I and V5–V6.**

Leads V1–V2 are placed in the third intercostal space, positioned over both the RV and the interventricular septum (Fig. 4-3).

- **Septal AMI** (usually in conjunction with anterior AMI) produces ST elevation in **V1.**
- **Anterior AMI** produces ST elevation in **V2–V4.**
- **RV AMI** often produces ST elevation in V1. In a **right-sided ECG,** V1 and V2 are reversed; therefore an RV AMI manifests ST elevation identical to V1 in **V2R.**

Leads V1–V2 (as well as **V3–V4**) are positioned **opposite** the posterior wall of LV.

- **Posterior AMI** manifests as **ST depression,** primarily in **V1–V3.** Remember that the ST elevation in V1 that may result from RV AMI may be **canceled out** by simultaneous posterior AMI.

Leads V3–V4 are positioned directly over the anterior wall. **Lead V3** is placed in the fourth intercostal space and V4–V6 in the fifth intercostal space (Fig. 4-4).

- Anterior AMI is best seen in leads **V2–V4.**

Leads V5–V6 are positioned directly over the lateral wall.

- **Lateral AMI** is very often seen in leads **V5–V6,** but is often **best seen in lead aVL** (see also Fig. 4-2).
- **Septal or RV AMI** may manifest **ST depression** here because V5–V6 are **opposite** the septum and the RV free wall.

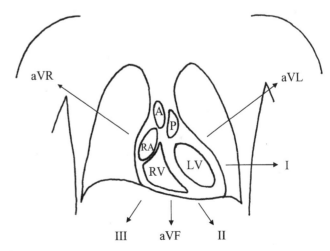

FIGURE 4-2. Placement and significance of the limb leads. (Abbreviations: A, aorta; P, pulmonary artery; RA, right atrium; RV, right ventricle; LV, left ventricle.)

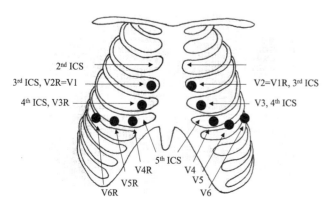

FIGURE 4-1. Lead placement.

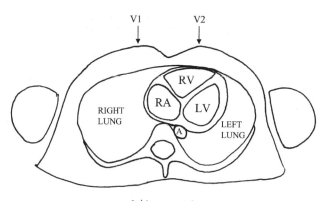

3rd intercostal space

FIGURE 4-3. Precordial leads V1 and V2.

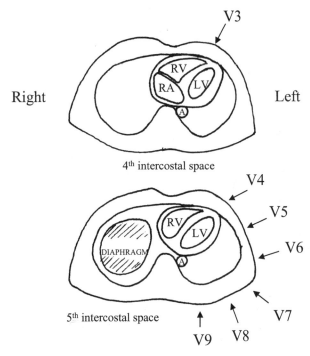

FIGURE 4-4. Precordial leads V3 (above) and V4–V9 (below).

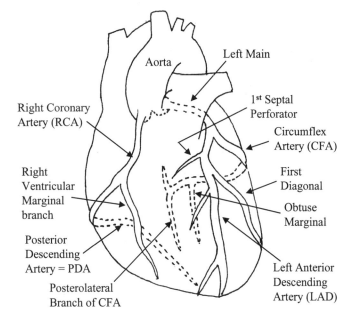

FIGURE 4-5. Coronary anatomy. Use this as a guide and remember that there is much variation among patients. Here the RCA is dominant, supplying the inferior wall, as in 85% of hearts.

TABLE 4.1. ST ELEVATION, LOCATION OF STEMI, AND CORRESPONDING CORONARY ARTERY^a

ST elevation	Coronary artery (See Fig. 4-5)	AMI location
II, III, aVF (reciprocal ST depression in aVL)	RCA or circumflex artery	Inferior AMI
II, III, aVF (reciprocal ST depression in aVL) plus V1 Right-sided ECG: V4R	RCA proximal to RV marginal branch	Inferior and RV AMI
II, III, aVF (reciprocal ST depression in aVL) plus ST depression in V1–V4	Dominant RCA (70%) Dominant circumflex (30%)	Inferoposterior AMI
II, III, aVF plus (I, aVL and/or V5, V6)	Dominant circumflex **or** dominant RCA with lateral branches	Inferolateral AMI
II, III, aVF plus (V5, V6) and/or (I, aVL) and ST depression any of V1–V6	Dominant RCA with lateral branches or dominant circumflex	Inferoposterolateral AMI
V2–V4	Mid-LAD	Anterior AMI
I, aVL, V5, and/or V6	First diagonal or circumflex or obtuse marginal artery	Lateral AMI
V1–V4	LAD distal to first septal perforator but proximal to first diagonal	Anteroseptal AMI
V1–V6, I, aVL	LAD proximal to first diagonal and first septal perforator	Anteroseptal-lateral AMI

^aThere is great variation among patients. Use this for guidelines only.

NORMAL AND NONSPECIFIC ECGS

KEY POINTS

- AMI and ACS may present with a nonspecific (Type 3) or normal (Type 4) ECG.
- Computer algorithms may misread ECGs as normal or nonspecific.
- Serial ECGs are necessary to identify high-risk patients who may ultimately need reperfusion therapy.
- If serial ECGs remain Type 3 or Type 4, further workup may be necessary to identify patients at risk for further coronary events.

GENERAL BACKGROUND

Clinical studies have shown that a normal initial ECG occurs in 6.4% of all AMIs and that a nonspecific initial ECG occurs in approximately 22% of all AMIs. These studies, however, were performed when the definition of AMI was based on CK-MB, not on troponin, as it is today (18,21,22). Further, these studies did not strictly define the term "normal" ECG. Thus in many studies "nonspecific/nondiagnostic ECGs" included (a) ECGs nondiagnostic of AMI but diagnostic of UA/NSTEMI; and (b) ECGs nondiagnostic of any kind of ACS. **Management of patients with these two types of "nonspecific" ECG types may be different.** Therefore, as described in Chapter 2, **we propose a new classification of ECG types based on therapeutic implications.** We distinguish between Type 2 ECGs, which are diagnostic of UA/NSTEMI, and Type 3 ECGs, which are nondiagnostic of any kind of ACS. Clinical experience and judgment are often necessary to distinguish between ST-T abnormalities of these two ECG types. Here we focus on **normal (Type 4) and nonspecific (Type 3) ECGs, both of which are nondiagnostic of any kind of ACS.** (See Chapter 8 for discussion of Type 2 ECGs.) Table 5-1 lists percentages of patients in two studies who were found to have normal or nonspecific ECGs and AMI as diagnosed by CK-MB (18,21). See Cases 5-1 through 5-5.

NORMAL ECG (TYPE 4 ECG)

Definition of a Normal ECG (Type 4 ECG)

- Sinus rhythm with normal p waves.
- ST elevation/depression < 0.5 mm relative to corresponding PR segments.
- No LVH, abnormal Q waves, or conduction abnormalities (QRS must be < 100 ms).
- Size of T waves is proportional to R waves and T wave axis is close to QRS axis.
- Normal R-wave progression.
- ST segment is neither up- nor downsloping.

Treatment Precautions in Patients with Type 4 ECGs

- A normal ECG is not unusual in **very early AMI.**
- A series of normal ECGs is common in ACS with minimal or no injury, especially if symptoms have resolved.
- Time since pain onset may not affect the negative predictive value (NPV) of the ECG (67).

TABLE 5.1. COMBINED FINDINGS OF TWO ECG STUDIES OF PATIENTS WHO PRESENTED WITH ISCHEMIC SYMPTOMS

Number of patients	11,805
Patients with AMI	1,962
Normal (nl) ECG	3,635
Normal ECG and AMI	125
	(6.4% of AMI)
	(3.4% of nl ECG)
	(1.06% of all patients)
Nonspecific ECG (NS)	5,191
NS ECG and AMI	442
	(22.5% of AMI)
	(8.6% of NS ECG)
	(3.7% of all pts.)
Nl or NS ECG	8,826
	(75% of all pts.)
Nl or NS ECG and AMI	567
	(4.8% of all patients)
	(29% of all AMI)
	(6.4% of all nl/NS ECG)

- A series of normal ECGs over 15 to 60 minutes is unusual in complete and persistent left anterior descending artery (LAD) or right coronary artery (RCA) occlusion, but it is **not** unusual in circumflex or branch vessel occlusion (68,69,**70**).
- **Posterior leads** may detect a posterior AMI that would otherwise show no ST deviation (71,72).
- **A Type 4 ECG may develop into a diagnostic (Type 1 or 2) ECG with serial ECGs.**
- **Record a repeat ECG every 15 minutes** for 60 minutes or more, or perform continuous ST segment monitoring on any patient with a **high clinical suspicion** of AMI, even if the initial ECG is totally normal. Record a **repeat ECG** on any patient with a **reasonable clinical suspicion** of AMI if the initial ECG is totally normal.

NONSPECIFIC ECG (TYPE 3 ECG)

We define a nonspecific (Type 3) ECG as **abnormal but nondiagnostic of any ACS,** neither AMI nor UA/NSTEMI. Although angiography ± PCI may be clinically indicated, **thrombolytics are NOT indicated.** A Type 3 ECG may be nonspecific because of the presence of Q waves, LVH, or minor, nondynamic ST or T-wave abnormalities that are not suggestive of ischemia. These include ST depression and T-wave inversion of < 1 mm and unchanging. These abnormalities are still defined as nonspecific even if changed from a previous ECG (18), although the probability of AMI is double if there is such a change (**73**). **A Type 3 ECG is not unusual** (a) **early** after thrombotic coronary occlusion; (b) in thrombotic occlusion with excellent collateral circulation; (c) with nonocclusive or intermittently occlusive thrombus; (d) after thrombotic occlusion with spontaneous reperfusion; (e) after thrombotic occlusion with injury of an electrocardiographically silent area of myocardium; or (f) with injury of a small area of myocardium.

Treatment Precautions in Patients with Type 3 ECGs

- All Type 3 ECGs are **abnormal.**
- A Type 3 ECG is much more likely to occur in AMI than a normal ECG (22% versus 6.4%) (**18,21**).
- In the reperfusion era, **a Type 3 ECG in the presence of AMI does not necessarily reflect lower mortality than a Type 1 ECG.** AMI patients with Type 3 ECGs are not eligible for thrombolysis and may have a higher mortality than AMI patients whose ECGs meet eligibility requirements for thrombolytics and receive them (**74**). In the **prethrombolytic era,** AMI patients with a "negative" ECG (approximately Type 3 or 4) had a much better prognosis than those with a positive ECG (Type 1 or 2) (75). **Consider immediate**

angiography ± PCI in cases of high clinical suspicion, especially if there is hemodynamic instability or pulmonary edema (see Case 26-2).
- A series of Type 3 ECG is common in ACS with minimal or no injury.
- **An initial Type 3 ECG may be followed by a diagnostic ECG** (Type 1 or Type 2) on serial ECGs.
- **Record serial ECGs** every 15 minutes for 60 minutes or more, or perform continuous ST segment monitoring on any patient with an initial Type 3 ECG but **high clinical suspicion** of AMI.
- **Record a serial ECG** on any patient with an initial Type 3 ECG with **continued symptoms and reasonable clinical suspicion** of AMI.

ECG COMPUTER ALGORITHMS

ECG computer algorithms have inadequate sensitivity for STEMI (41–47). These "normal ECG" misreads may occur with ST elevation that is less than standard "thrombolytic criteria" (less than 1 to 2 mm in two consecutive anterior leads and less than 1 mm in two consecutive inferior leads). The computer may also misinterpret ST elevation of AMI as another condition, especially early repolarization. **You must learn to read the ECG yourself. Look for ST deviation and dynamic and/or resolved ST and T-wave changes.**

MANAGEMENT

Specific details of managing patients with persistent Type 3 and Type 4 ECGs are beyond the scope of this book. Fundamentally, however, with Type 3 and Type 4 ECGs and some clinical suspicion:

- **Examine prehospital rhythm strips** (see Cases 12-3 and 31-1 to 31-3).
- **Compare with a previous ECG.** Obtain earlier ECGs from other institutions by fax.
- **Record serial ECGs.** Record a repeat ECG every 15 minutes for 60 minutes or more, or perform continuous ST segment monitoring on any patient with a **high clinical suspicion** of AMI, even if the initial ECG is totally normal or nondiagnostic.
- Consider **posterior leads** and **echocardiography.**
- Patients at moderate risk for ACS should undergo a standard CP unit evaluation. Consider treatment for ACS. Obtain serial biochemical markers, preferably cTnI or cTnT. Observe. Further work-up may include stress electrocardiography, stress echocardiography, sestamibi scanning, or stress nuclear testing, as dictated by institutional protocols. Electron beam computed tomography (CT) may prove valuable.

CASE 5-1

Typical Symptoms and a Nonspecific (Type 3) ECG Misread as Normal

History
This 39-year-old construction worker presented with typical CP in less than 1 hour.

ECG 5-1 (Type 3)
Read as "normal" by the computer.
- ST elevation: 1 mm, V2, not due to early repolarization because the other precordial leads are not consistent.
- Tall T wave: V2, suggestive of posterior reperfusion. (See Chapters 16 and 27.)
- ST downsloping: V5–V6, not completely normal.
- II, III, aVF are normal.

Clinical Course
The patient was sent home, his CK-MB levels returned elevated, and he was called back. He did not develop Q waves and remained stable through angioplasty, which opened a 99% RCA stenosis.

Conclusion
Failure to observe this patient and record serial ECGs could have had dire results.

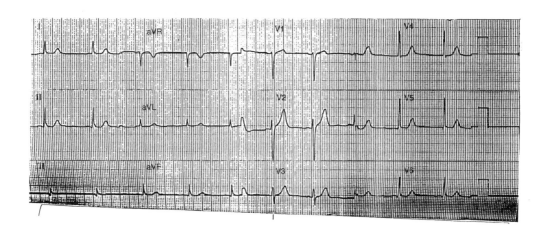

CASE 5-2

Atypical Symptoms and a Nonspecific (Type 3) ECG Misread As Normal

History

This 44-year-old man with no risk factors complained of epigastric burning, "just like my ulcer." He received antacids and viscous xylocaine and his symptoms resolved immediately.

ECG 5-2 (Type 3), was misread as "normal" by the computer.

- ST elevation: almost 1 mm, I and aVL. This is an **abnormal ECG** (although it could be baseline for this patient).

Clinical Course

This patient was released and returned later with recurrent symptoms. An ECG (not shown) revealed a very large **anterolateral AMI** that was treated with tPA.

Conclusion

AMI could have been suspected earlier with close inspection of this "normal" ECG. However, it remains uncertain whether the findings in I and aVL were related to ischemia or not. Only comparison with a previous ECG could confirm it.

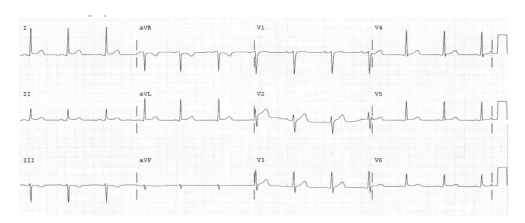

CASE 5-3

Young Woman with CP and a Normal (Type 4) ECG Followed by a Nonspecific (Type 3) ECG that Renormalized 7 Days Later

This young woman returned with Wellens' syndrome 3 weeks later.

History

This 32-year-old woman smoker and cocaine user complained of 30 minutes of severe substernal pain radiating to her left arm. This was the fourth such episode in 3 days, all associated with dyspnea and exertion, resolving after 15 minutes. This episode persisted, so she called 911. Paramedics administered aspirin and sublingual NTG, with improvement of pain. Pain then resolved in the emergency department (ED) after three additional NTG. She arrived at 12:09.

ECG 5-3A (Type 4)

At 12:36

- This is a normal ECG.

Clinical Course

A repeat ECG at 13:58 was unchanged. No prehospital strips were available for analysis. She was admitted to telemetry. A cTnI drawn at 13:52 was 0.1 ng/mL.

ECG 5-3B (Type 3)

At 19:57, V1–V6 only

- Inversion of the latter part of T-waves: subtle, V1–V3. Such a change may be the only clue to significant coronary disease.

(continued on next page)

CASE 5-3

Young Woman with CP and a Normal (Type 4) ECG Followed by a Nonspecific (Type 3) ECG that Normalized 7 Days Later *(continued)*

Clinical Course

This change was not noticed. A cTnI from 23:35 returned at 0.2 ng/mL (elevated). Urine was positive for cocaine. A cTnI from 04:21 the next morning was 0.1 ng/mL. The patient was discharged home with CP of uncertain etiology and a stress echocardiogram was scheduled for the following day, which she missed. She returned to the ED 7 days later with identical CP. Clinicians recorded a third ECG, which was **significantly changed back to normal** from the most recent previous ECG (ECG 5-3b), and was essentially the same as ECG 5-3a. She was admitted again, had negative cTnI (less than 0.1 ng/mL), and urine positive for cocaine. She was discharged. She returned 3 weeks later with identical CP of 10 minutes duration that resolved as she was running to the phone to call 911.

ECG 5-3C (Type 2)

At 20:43, V1–V6 only

■ Terminal T-wave inversion (Wellens' syndrome, see Chapter 8). This indicates severe LAD stenosis.

Clinical Course

Treated for UA/NSTEMI (see Chapter 37), admitted. Had recurrent 7/10 pain 7 hours later.

ECG 5-3D (Type 4)

V1–V3 only

■ T waves upright: **"pseudonormalization,"** indicates probable reocclusion of severe LAD stenosis.

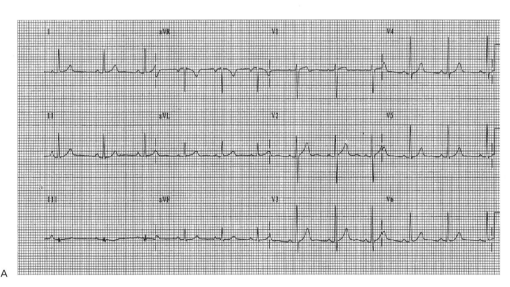

A

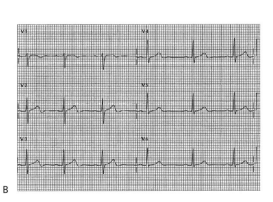

B

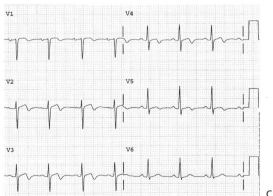

C

(continued on next page)

CASE 5-3

Young Woman with CP and a Normal (Type 4) ECG Followed by a Nonspecific (Type 3) ECG that Normalized 7 Days Later *(continued)*

Clinical Course

Sublingual NTG was given, pain resolved, and a repeat ECG was recorded.

ECG 5-3E (Type 2)

V1–V3 only

■ T waves with terminal inversion suggests **reperfusion** again. (See Chapters 8 and 27).

Clinical Course

CTnI returned at 2.2 ng/mL. Angiography several hours later showed a severe ostial LAD lesion, for which coronary artery bypass graft (CABG) was undertaken uneventfully.

Conclusion

Normal and nonspecific (Type 3 and 4) ECGs can offer much information if they are interpreted in the context of sequences of ECGs. Out of context, ECG 5-3b is simply nonspecific; in the context of the clinical data and ECG 5-3a, it is suspicious for ischemia. Similarly, ECG 5-3d is nearly normal out of context, but **in the context of serial recordings, it helps to reveal the pathology.**

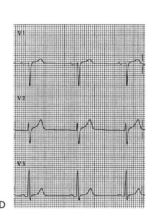
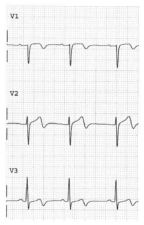

CASE 5-4

Subtle Lateral AMI, Not Yet a Thrombolytic Candidate, Reperfuses with Sublingual NTG

History

This 56-year-old man with several risk factors for coronary disease presented with 1 hour of typical CP with radiation to left arm and diaphoresis. Blood pressure (BP) = 210/108 and P = 48.

ECG 5-4A (Type 3)

- ST elevation, < 1 mm: aVL, V5–V6.
- Slightly downsloping reciprocal ST segments: II, III, aVF; unusual ST segment in V2, V3.

Clinical Course

ECG findings not commented upon, but sublingual NTG × 3 completely relieved the symptoms, with resolution of the nonspecific abnormalities.

ECG 5-4B (Type 4)

- T-wave inversions: aVL and V2
- Normal when viewed alone, but abnormal in its change.

Clinical Course

Aspirin, heparin, NTG drip, and metoprolol were administered. Echocardiography revealed lateral wall motion abnormality (WMA). Troponin I (cTnI) peaked at 10.4 ng/mL. Angiography revealed a 95% first diagonal culprit lesion, as well as 80% LAD stenosis. Revascularization was planned.

Conclusion

Though thrombolytics may not be indicated, the ECG and symptoms suggest coronary occlusion. If treatment for NSTEMI does not relieve symptoms, immediate angiography may be indicated.

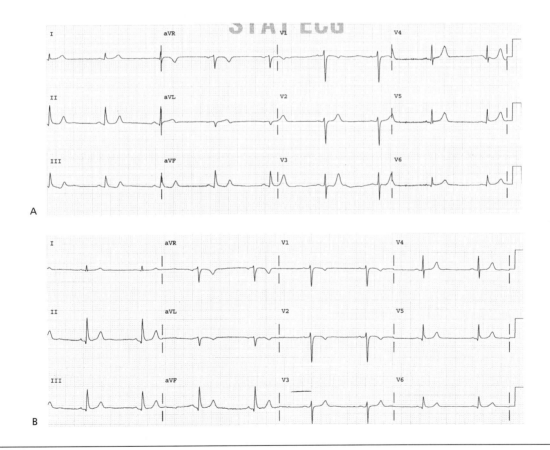

CASE 5-5

Type 1b ECG Missed, Patient Sent Home and Died

History
This 39-year-old man presented with CP.

ECG 5-5 (Type 1b)
- ST elevation: II, III, aVF, although very **suspicious,** was missed. Inferior ST depression: aVL, minimal, increases **suspicion** of inferior AMI.
- ST depression: V2–V5, subtle, is **suspicious** for posterior AMI.
- Although all these suspicious findings add up to a subtly diagnostic ECG (Type 1b), it was read as normal by the computer and the emergency physician.

Clinical Course
The patient was discharged, arrested, and died. Autopsy revealed inferior AMI.

Conclusion
This ECG is clearly abnormal and is an indication for reperfusion therapy. Even if not recognized immediately as a Type 1 ECG, it should be clear that it is not a Type 4 ECG and that, at a minimum, additional ECGs and diagnostic steps are necessary.

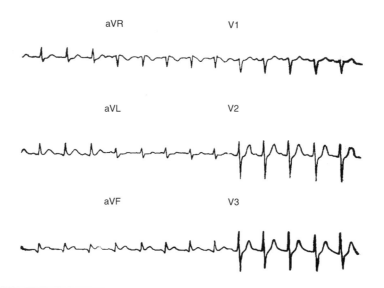

ANNOTATED BIBLIOGRAPHY

Unless otherwise noted, the following studies used the presence of elevated blood levels of CK-MB for the definitive diagnosis of AMI.

Christian TF, et al. Exercise tomographic thallium-201 imaging in patients with severe coronary artery disease and normal electrocardiograms, 1994.
   Methods: Christian et al. (76) studied 411 patients with thallium exercise tests and subsequent angiography; all had normal resting ECGs.
   Findings: Of 298 patients with significant CAD, 77 (26%) had left main or three-vessel disease. Concurrent thallium scintigraphy demonstrated that 25% of these 77 patients had normal ECGs while they were having ischemia. This indicates that **ECGs are relatively insensitive, at least for nonocclusive ischemia.**

Studies of Normal and Nonspecific ECGs and AMI
Rouan GW, et al. Clinical characteristics and outcome of acute myocardial infarction in patients with initially normal or nonspecific electrocardiograms, 1989 and Karlson BW et al. Early prediction of acute myocardial infarction from clinical history, examination and electrocardiogram in the emergency room, 1991.
   Methods: Rouan et al. (18) analyzed data from 7,115 consecutive CP patients (admitted or discharged) in the Multicenter Chest Pain Study. Patients were included if they had CP unexplained by chest wall or chest radiographic findings. Investigators defined nonspecific ST or T-wave changes to be minor ST or T-wave abnormalities not suggestive of ischemia or strain, even if changed from a previous tracing. Karlson et al. (21) studied 4,690 CP patients admitted to the hospital. Pain was **NOT** subcategorized into ongoing or resolved in either study. Although the ECGs in both studies were presumably initial ECGs, this is not explicitly stated, nor is it specified whether serial ECGs were recorded. **Incidence of unstable angina and occurrence of long-term cardiac endpoints were not measured.**
   Findings: See Table 5-1. Karlson et al. (21) also found that of the 466 patients (10%) for whom the physician had "no suspicion of MI," six patients (1.5%) had an AMI. Rouan et al. (18) found that 461 (45%) of 1,024 AMI patients had classic ECG findings (Type 1a). Of the 17% with nonspecific (Type 3) ECGs, 7% had nonspecific ST-T abnormalities, 5% had old infarction, and 5% had "other" abnormali-

ties, including LVH and atrial abnormalities. "Normal" ECGs (Type 4) were found in 3.5%. In comparison with AMI patients with a diagnostic ECG (Type 1), if the ECG was Type 3 or Type 4 and the patient was admitted, the total CK was lower (643 IU/L versus 1,032 IU/L), mortality was lower (6% versus 12%), there was less cardiogenic shock, dysrhythmia, atrioventricular (AV) block, CHF, and most often, involvement of the circumflex artery. Confidence intervals (CIs) of the relative risk (RR) for AMI for patient characteristics were as follows: age more than 60 years (1.5 to 2.3); male (1.2 to 1.6); "pressure" (1.4 to 1.9), radiation (1.2 to 1.8); diaphoresis (1.1 to 1.9); and history of prior MI or angina and normal ECG (1.0 to 1.8). Of 42 patients with normal ECGs and all characteristics, 8 (17%) ruled in for AMI. Of 551 patients with normal ECGs and none of the characteristics, none ruled in for AMI. Of 285 patients with nonspecific ECGs and none of the characteristics, one ruled in for AMI. Use of reperfusion therapy is not mentioned; data were apparently gathered in the prereperfusion era.

Slater DK, et al. Outcome in suspected acute myocardial infarction with normal or minimally abnormal admission electrocardiographic findings, 1987.

Methods: Slater et al. (22) studied 775 patients **admitted** to the hospital with symptoms "suggestive of acute MI." Pain was not subcategorized into ongoing or resolved. The ECG was presumably the first and only ECG obtained, although this is not explicitly stated.

Findings: Of 775 patients, 262 (34%) ruled in for AMI. Of 107 patients (14%) with normal ECGs, 11 (10%) ruled in for AMI (4.2% of total AMI), one with complications. Of 73 patients (9%) with nonspecific ECGs, six (8%) ruled in for AMI (2.3% of all AMI), four with complications. Thus 6.5% of AMI patients had either Type 3 or Type 4 ECGs, which is far less than the 28.9% in Table 5-1. This, together with the high rate of rule-ins, suggests hidden methodologic differences from studies by Rouan et al. (18) and Karlson et al. (21) described earlier.

Patients with Cardiac Ischemia Mistakenly Sent Home from the ED

Pope JH, et al. Missed diagnosis of acute cardiac ischemia in the emergency department, 2000.

Methods: From May to November 1993, Pope et al. (77) conducted a multicenter prospective study of all patients presenting with CP or other symptoms suggesting acute cardiac ischemia. Patients who were discharged returned at 24 to 72 hours for repeat evaluation, ECG, and CK-MB measurement.

Findings: There was 30-day follow-up in 99% of patients. Of 10,689 patients, 8% ruled in for AMI by CK-MB levels, 7% met criteria for UA, 21% had other cardiac problems, and 55% had noncardiac problems. Of 889 AMI patients, **19 (2.1%) were discharged home; when retrospectively examined, 17 of these ECGs showed "no evidence of ischemia" and two were "normal."** Of 966 patients with UA, 22 (2.3%) were mistakenly discharged; retrospective examination of these ECGs revealed that none showed evidence of ischemia and two were normal ECGs. **Nonwhite ethnicity, female sex, chief complaint of dyspnea, and a normal ECG all correlated with mistaken discharge.**

Lee TH, et al. Clinical characteristics and natural history of patients with acute myocardial infarction sent home from the emergency room, 1987.

Methods: Lee et al. (78) conducted a prospective study of 3,077 patients with precordial or left-sided CP (including pleuritic and nontraumatic chest wall pain) unexplained by obvious local trauma or radiographic abnormalities. Pain was not subcategorized into ongoing or resolved.

Findings: Of 1,794 admitted patients, 459 (26%) had AMI, 55 (12%) of whom died. Of 1,283 patients sent home, 35 (2.5%) had

AMI (7% of total AMIs). Of the 35 AMI patients sent home, 13 (37%) had ECG evidence of acute ischemia, five (14%) were less than 42 years of age, and nine (26%) died (0.7% of all CP patients). Of the nine sent home who died, six (67%) had ECGs that were misread.

McCarthy BD, et al. Missed diagnosis of acute myocardial infarction in the emergency department: results from a multicenter study, 1993.

Methods: McCarthy et al. (79) studied 5,773 CP patients, 1,000 of whom had AMI as determined by CK-MB. Pain was not subcategorized into ongoing or resolved.

Findings: Of 1,000 AMI patients, 20 (2%) were discharged from EDs. Five (25%) of those sent home (0.5% of total AMI patients) suffered cardiac arrest; some were resuscitated. Five (25%) of the 20 patients sent home had ST elevation ≥ 1 mm that was missed, and an additional five (25%) had a diagnosis of UA.

Singer AJ, et al. Effect of duration from symptom onset on the negative predictive value of a normal ECG for exclusion of acute myocardial infarction, 1997.

Methods: Singer et al. (67) studied 526 patients with CP or associated symptoms.

Findings: Time from onset of CP to the first ECG did not affect the predictive value of a "negative" ECG for AMI.

Smith SW. ECG abnormality in acute myocardial infarction, 1998.

Findings: Smith (80) notes that Singer's study (67) did not classify time of onset as time of onset of **constant** pain. It also did not address how many had a completely normal ECG or whether those patients who presented earlier had larger AMIs.

Fesmire FM, et al. Diagnostic and prognostic importance of comparing the initial to the previous electrocardiogram in patients admitted for suspected acute myocardial infarction, 1991.

Methods: Fesmire et al. (73) studied 258 patients admitted for suspected AMI.

Findings: A patient with a "negative" ECG, if changed from a previous "negative" ECG, had double the likelihood of receiving an intervention.

Cragg DR, et al. Outcome of patients with acute myocardial infarction who are ineligible for thrombolytic therapy, 1991.

Methods: Cragg et al. (74) studied 1,471 AMI patients, as diagnosed by CK-MB.

Findings: **Nearly 50% had ECGs nonspecific for AMI and thus were not eligible for thrombolysis.** Mortality for this group was 14% compared with 4% for patients with an ECG that met eligibility requirements **AND** who thus received thrombolytics.

Comment: Although Rouan et al. (18), described earlier, found **lower** mortality for patients with "nonspecific" ECGs, that study appears to have been done in the prethrombolytic era.

Christian TF, et al. Noninvasive identification of myocardium at risk in patients with acute myocardial infarction and nondiagnostic electrocardiograms with technetium-99m-sestamibi, 1991.

Methods: Christian et al. (70) did sestamibi scans on 113 consecutive AMI patients.

Findings: Of 113 patients, 14 (12%) had AMI without ST elevation. Of these 14, all but three initial ECGs appear to have been, by description, **either** Type 1b ECGs (all with ST depression in V1–V4), Type 1c (LBBB), or Type 2 (ST depression or T-wave inversions). The mean size of perfusion defects (indicating myocardium at risk) was 20% of the LV, and, in one case, 50%. Eleven of 14 patients had total coronary occlusion with no reperfusion. Of 13 patients in whom the infarct related artery (IRA) could be identified, it was the **circumflex artery** in six.

6

AMI AND ST-SEGMENT ELEVATION

KEY POINTS

- ST elevation measurement is not standardized; measurement relative to the PR segment is most accurate.
- ST elevation ≥ 1 mm in two consecutive leads is the standard "criterion" for reperfusion therapy in AMI. Unfortunately, measurement alone without interpretation is insensitive and nonspecific.
- Computer algorithms are insensitive for STEMI.
- Height and extent of ST elevation correlate with prognosis and potential benefit of thrombolysis.

GENERAL BACKGROUND

Measuring ST Elevation and Depression

The best and easiest method for determining ST deviation is to **measure the ST segment relative to the PR segment** (Fig. 6-1). Atrial repolarization occurs in the opposite direction from the p wave, lasts until 40 to 80 ms after the end of the QRS, and frequently depresses the PR segment at baseline. Thus relative to the isoelectric TP segment, the PR segment may be depressed as a normal condition (81,82). If it is thus depressed, the ST segment at the J point (junction of the QRS and ST segments) should be equally depressed. Because atrial repolarization lasts a maximum of 80 ms after the J point, an alternative method is **to measure the ST segment relative to the TP segment at 60 ms (83,84) or 80 ms (85) after the J point.** Case 6-1 illustrates the false-positive ST elevation that results from an inverted p wave with an upright atrial repolarization wave.

Thrombolytic trials rarely specify the method or location of ST measurement (29,86). Electrocardiographers, when diagnosing STEMI, might use any combination of baselines and locations for measurement (41). This is problematic, because measurement of ST elevation may be very different depending on location of measurement, especially if the ST segment slurs into the T wave without first flattening. Thus the ST segment at 60 to 80 ms after the J point may be significantly higher than at the J point (see ECGs 9-1b and 9-2b) (84). In any case, **subjective interpretation** of the appearance of the ST segment leads to **more accurate, especially more sensitive, diagnosis of STEMI than measured ST elevation (41).**

ST-Segment Morphology

A **straight ST segment** is the most common finding in anterior AMI. **Upward concavity** is the next most common finding, but this is also the most common finding in the nonpathologic state. **Upward convexity is likely to be STEMI.** Although upward convexity is less common than upward concavity or straight morphologies in AMI, it is often present and it is associated with larger infarct and lower ejection fraction (EF) at discharge (87). See Figure 6-2 for examples of ST deviation.

In inferior or lateral AMI, ST elevation with a straight or upwardly convex morphology ("non-concave") is highly specific for STEMI (87.5).

Evolution of an STEMI

Nonreperfused Complete Coronary Occlusion

A nonreperfused complete coronary occlusion, without good collateral circulation, demonstrates a typical sequence of ECG changes (if they are recorded) as follows (Fig. 6-3; also Fig. 8-3, 1A to 9A):

- **T-wave enlargement,** in both width and height, sometimes with depressed ST takeoff (88,89).
- **ST elevation,** which may fluctuate (90,91).
- **Q-wave formation or loss of R-wave amplitude.** A Q wave may begin to form in less than 1 hour, be reversible for up to 6 hours, and be completely formed by 12 hours (92,93).
- **ST stabilization,** often with persistent elevation, usually within the first 12 hours (93).
- **T-wave inversion before ST resolution** (in contrast with pericarditis, in which the ST segment normalizes first, before T-wave inversion); the T wave inverts within 72 hours and is usually < 3 mm (94).
- **ST resolution,** which may occur over 12 to 72 hours, or may never completely resolve, especially in anterior AMI (95).
  - ST reelevation may occur due to infarct extension, reocclusion in a partially reperfused AMI, or postinfarction pericarditis.
- Established Q waves disappear in days, weeks, or months in 15% to 30% of AMI (2).
- T waves may normalize over days, weeks, or months (2).

Reperfused Coronary Occlusion

See Chapters 8 and 27.

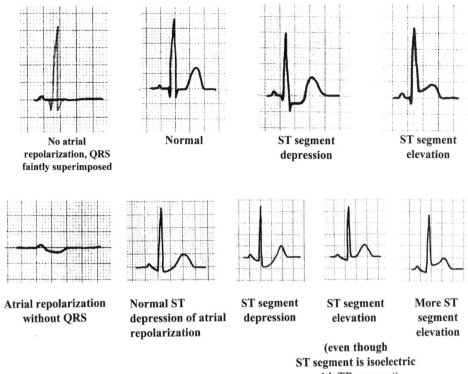

No atrial repolarization, QRS faintly superimposed

Normal

ST segment depression

ST segment elevation

Atrial repolarization without QRS

Normal ST depression of atrial repolarization

ST segment depression

ST segment elevation

More ST segment elevation

(even though ST segment is isoelectric with TP segment)

FIGURE 6-1. ST elevation and depression (above) with no atrial repolarization wave, and (below) with a (negative) atrial repolarization wave.

- Earlier ST normalization and stabilization.
- T-wave inversion may accelerate.
  - Because it begins while the ST segment remains elevated, the early morphology is of **terminal** T-wave inversion (see Chapter 8).
- T waves usually deepen symmetrically over time.
- Compared to no reperfusion, Q-wave development that is less pronounced or even absent. This depends in part on the timeliness of reperfusion therapy.

ST Elevation of Early Repolarization

Some ST elevation in precordial leads is seen in up to 90% of normal subjects (2,96). Many subjects have a higher degree of ST elevation known as **early repolarization** (see Chapter 20), which demonstrates the following:

- ST segments are highest in V2–V3, up to 3 mm.
- Upwardly concave ST segments, not convex (Figs. 6-2b, 6-2c, and 6-2f).
- ST elevation is seldom > 0.5 mm in leads V5–V6.
- ST elevation is seldom > 2 mm in people beyond 45 years of age.
- ST elevation is more pronounced in younger people, possibly also in African-American men (97).
- T waves are tall, but not wide and not much taller than the R wave (versus hyperacute T waves).
- Early repolarization is much less common in people beyond the age of 55 years.

Anterior AMI may mimic early repolarization. Small degrees of ST elevation, even < 1 mm, may represent anterior AMI. Look for hyperacute T waves, consult a previous ECG, and rule out other pathologic causes of ST elevation (Table 6-1). (See Cases 12-4, 12-5, 20-9, and 20-10.)

ST ELEVATION AND REPERFUSION THERAPY

Criteria for Thrombolytic Therapy

Clinical trials of thrombolytic therapy used different criteria for amount of ST elevation (1 or 2 mm) and for number of leads required (one or two leads). See Table 6-2 for "criteria" from GISSI-1 (29), GISSI-2 (98), GUSTO (86), TIMI (99,100), TAMI (101), ISIS-2 (102), ISIS-3 (103), and the Minnesota Code (104). **The ACC/American Heart Association (AHA) Guidelines use as "criteria" only 1 mm of ST elevation in precordial leads** (105). However, it is important to remember, that, as measured by either the clinician or the ECG computer algorithm, **ST-segment criteria are relatively crude instruments for the identification of AMI.** ST elevation on the initial ECG has been found to be only 45% sensitive for all AMI diagnosed by CK-MB (18,20,24). Thus, many AMIs are not eligible for thrombolysis using these criteria. Sensitivity may be improved to as high as 69%, with some loss of specificity, by using less strict criteria (**17**). Sensitivity is especially poor for circumflex occlusions with resultant lateral or posterior AMI or both (68). Computer algorithms are consistently insensitive for

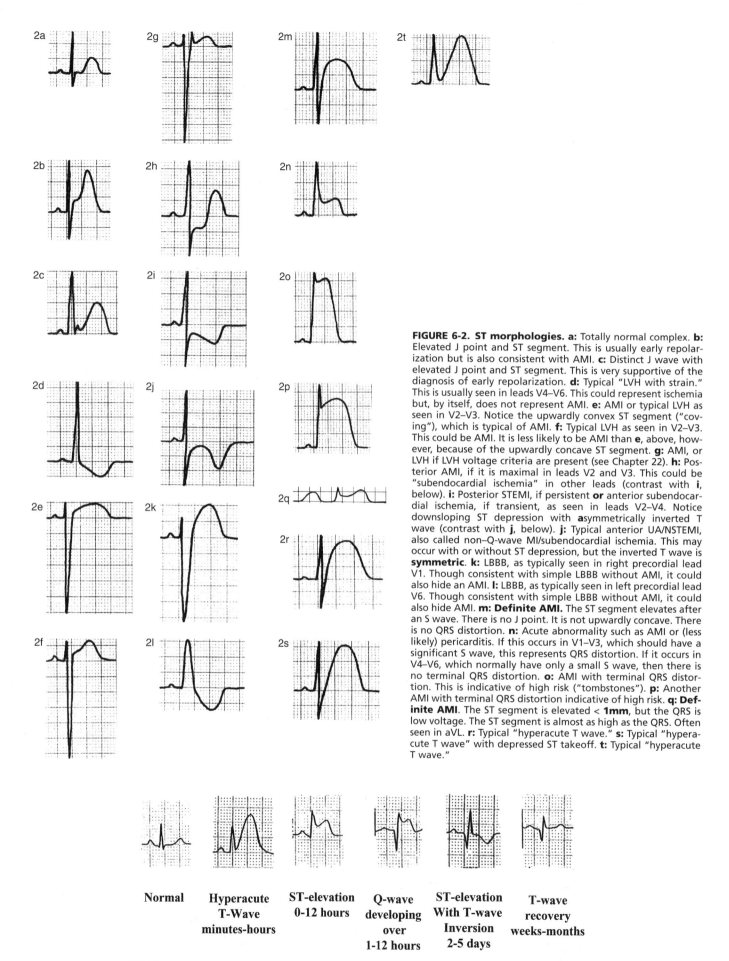

FIGURE 6-2. ST morphologies. a: Totally normal complex. **b:** Elevated J point and ST segment. This is usually early repolarization but is also consistent with AMI. **c:** Distinct J wave with elevated J point and ST segment. This is very supportive of the diagnosis of early repolarization. **d:** Typical "LVH with strain." This is usually seen in leads V4–V6. This could represent ischemia but, by itself, does not represent AMI. **e:** AMI or typical LVH as seen in V2–V3. Notice the upwardly convex ST segment ("coving"), which is typical of AMI. **f:** Typical LVH as seen in V2–V3. This could be AMI. It is less likely to be AMI than **e**, above, however, because of the upwardly concave ST segment. **g:** AMI, or LVH if LVH voltage criteria are present (see Chapter 22). **h:** Posterior AMI, if it is maximal in leads V2 and V3. This could be "subendocardial ischemia" in other leads (contrast with **i**, below). **i:** Posterior STEMI, if persistent **or** anterior subendocardial ischemia, if transient, as seen in leads V2–V4. Notice downsloping ST depression with **a**symmetrically inverted T wave (contrast with **j**, below). **j:** Typical anterior UA/NSTEMI, also called non–Q-wave MI/subendocardial ischemia. This may occur with or without ST depression, but the inverted T wave is **symmetric**. **k:** LBBB, as typically seen in right precordial lead V1. Though consistent with simple LBBB without AMI, it could also hide an AMI. **l:** LBBB, as typically seen in left precordial lead V6. Though consistent with simple LBBB without AMI, it could also hide AMI. **m: Definite AMI.** The ST segment elevates after an S wave. There is no J point. It is not upwardly concave. There is no QRS distortion. **n:** Acute abnormality such as AMI or (less likely) pericarditis. If this occurs in V1–V3, which should have a significant S wave, this represents QRS distortion. If it occurs in V4–V6, which normally have only a small S wave, then there is no terminal QRS distortion. **o:** AMI with terminal QRS distortion. This is indicative of high risk ("tombstones"). **p:** Another AMI with terminal QRS distortion indicative of high risk. **q: Definite AMI.** The ST segment is elevated < **1mm**, but the QRS is low voltage. The ST segment is almost as high as the QRS. Often seen in aVL. **r:** Typical "hyperacute T wave." **s:** Typical "hyperacute T wave" with depressed ST takeoff. **t:** Typical "hyperacute T wave."

| Normal | Hyperacute T-Wave minutes-hours | ST-elevation 0-12 hours | Q-wave developing over 1-12 hours | ST-elevation With T-wave Inversion 2-5 days | T-wave recovery weeks-months |

FIGURE 6-3. Progression of a nonreperfused Q-wave ("transmural") AMI. (ECG reproduced from unpublished data with permission from K. Wang, M.D).

TABLE 6.1. PATHOLOGIC CAUSES OF ST SEGMENT ELEVATION

AMI
LVH
Left ventricular aneurysm
Pericarditis
LBBB
Hyperkalemia
Critical illness, including neurologic conditions such as subarachnoid hemorrhage, may result in ST elevation and T-wave inversion, with echocardiographic wall motion abnormalities (WMAs) that mimic AMI.

STEMI (41–47). Massel et al. compared computer algorithm interpretation with the consensus opinion of three cardiologists on 75 ECGs and found that dependence on the computer algorithm would have lead to significant **underuse** of thrombolytics; the computer program had 100% specificity but **only 62% sensitivity for STEMI.** They also found that the use of strict measurement criteria at 1 mm by the cardiologists would have lead to significant **overuse** of thrombolytics (**41**). Thus we recommend that you **always consider ST deviation within the larger context of overall ECG morphology and clinical presentation.**

Inaccurate Diagnosis with Use of ST-Segment "Criteria" Alone

There may even be significant **intra**-observer variation in measurement of ST elevation. In one study of unwitting, repeat, blinded readings, 14% of ECGs were inconsistently classified by the same interpreters as meeting, or not meeting, criteria (64).

In AMI, the ST segment may have only minimal elevation in a lead with low QRS voltage; you must therefore **assess ST elevation relative to QRS voltage** (Fig. 6-2q).

Underdiagnosis may occur because early STEMI or STEMI in an electrocardiographically silent area of the heart may result in < 1 mm of ST elevation. Criteria of 2 mm in precordial leads are insensitive for many early anterior STEMIs (**41**) and are especially insensitive for AMI manifesting in V5 and V6, where ST elevation > 1 mm is unusual as a normal condition (96,104). Posterior AMI, for which thrombolysis is indicated (105), may manifest ST depression only.

Overdiagnosis may occur due to alternative causes of ST elevation, such as normal variant or non-AMI pathologic conditions, as listed in Table 6-1. In one prehospital study, 25% of CP patients had ≥ 1 mm of ST elevation on two contiguous leads, but only 49% had AMI by CK-MB (106). In another study, only 15% of those with ST elevation ≥ 1 mm in two contiguous limb leads or ≥ 2 mm in two contiguous precordial leads had AMI (65). The majority of these patients had pseudoinfarction patterns. **The presence of reciprocal changes improves the specificity** of ST elevation for AMI (42,44,45,47,65,106), although such changes may also manifest in LVH and LV aneurysm. Dependence on reciprocity lessens the sensitivity for STEMI (17).

Predictors of Outcome and Thrombolytic Benefit

ECG predictors of poor outcome and, therefore, of greater potential benefit from reperfusion therapy, include:

- **Location** of ST changes. **Anterior location** correlates with large myocardial area at risk and great potential benefit from reperfusion (101–106,**107–110**). GISSI-1 data showed no mortality benefit of streptokinase (SK) in small inferior AMI (with ST elevation in only two or three leads, no reciprocal changes, and no RV AMI) (109). Fibrinolytic Therapy Trialists (FTT) data demonstrated statistically significant thrombolytic benefit for "other" AMIs, presumably lateral (30), even though these AMIs were frequently described as small.
- **High ST score** (sum of ST elevation, in mm, from all leads with ST elevation); > 12 mm for anterior AMI and > 6 mm for inferior AMI (**111**).
- **Greater number of leads** with reciprocal ST depression. Mortality increases by 35% for each 0.5 mV (5 mm) of summed ST depression (**112**).
- **Total sum** of absolute ST deviation, whether positive or negative. Although ST deviation does correlate with worse outcome and greater potential benefit to reperfusion therapy,

TABLE 6.2. ST ELEVATION REQUIREMENTS FOR SOME MAJOR THROMBOLYTIC TRIALS

Study	Number of consecutive leads required	Number of mm required in limb leads	Number of mm required in precordial leads
GISSI-1	1	1	2
GISSI-2	1	1	2
GUSTO	2	1	2
TIMI	2	1	1
AHA/ACC recommendations	2	1	1
TAMI	2	1	1
ISIS-2, ISIS-3	None, "suspected MI" only		
Minnesota Code	1	1 mm in I, II, III, aVL, aVF, V5, V6 2 mm in V1–V4	

there is **wide variation** (111,113,114,115). Thus some patients with a low ST score or ST deviation in only a few leads may nevertheless have a very large amount of myocardium at risk.

■ **Terminal QRS distortion** by the ST segment (see Figs. 6-2, o and p). In leads that normally have little or no ST elevation, look for a J point of 50% or more of the R-wave height. In leads with RS configuration, look for disappearance of the S wave. See Cases 6-2 and 6-3.

■ **Presence of new Q waves.** (They do not necessarily reflect late presentation. See Chapter 11).

It is also important to consider **clinical predictors** of poor outcome and greater potential benefit from reperfusion therapy.

These include **systolic BP < 90, P > 100 bpm,** presence of **rales** on physical exam, and **increased age (116)**.

Transient STEMI

ST elevation may resolve spontaneously, or after administration of aspirin or heparin or both. This ST elevation may or may not be recorded on the initial ECG. Echocardiography may reveal a WMA even after ST resolution. Although there may be subsequent development of T-wave inversion (see Chapter 8), there also may be no T-wave inversion, particularly in the unusual case of occlusion so brief that there is no injury, as demonstrated by a normal troponin level. See Case 6-4.

CASE 6-1

Inferior ST Elevation Due to an Upright Atrial Repolarization Wave

History
This 24-year-old man presented with atypical CP.

ECG 6-1 (Type 3)
■ Inverted P wave: II, with short PR interval. There is a pacemaker high in the AV node.
■ ST elevation: V2–V6 (due to early repolarization), and also in II, III, aVF, maximal in II, but **without** reciprocal ST depression in aVL. In the context of an inverted P wave, ST elevation may be due to upright atrial repolarization wave, which here persists well beyond the end of the QRS due to the very short PR interval. An ECG

recorded 19 minutes earlier had normal upright P waves and isoelectric ST segments.

Clinical Course
Clinicians did not administer reperfusion therapy. CTnI levels were normal.

Conclusion
Junctional rhythm may lead to false-positive ST elevation: a short PR interval and retrograde depolarization of the atrium with a resulting inverted P wave combine to result in a late and positive atrial repolarization wave that elevates the ST segment.

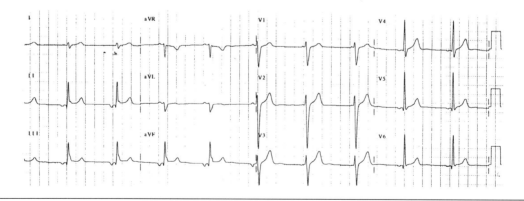

CASE 6-2

Extensive Anterolateral AMI

History
This 45-year-old smoker presented with typical CP.

ECG 6-2 (Type 1a)
- ST elevation: V1–V6, I, II, aVL, maximal in V4 (20 mm); ST depression: III; **ST score:** approximately 60; distorted terminal QRS: V1–V6, I, aVL; minimal Q waves: V2–V5. This ECG is diagnostic of an extensive **anterolateral AMI.**

- Note also "giant R waves" in V3–V5, in which the ST segment is as high as the R wave.

Conclusion
An ECG with a high ST score has high mortality and great potential benefit from reperfusion therapy. This may be mistaken for ventricular tachycardia on a single lead monitor.

ECG reproduced from unpublished data with permission of K. Wang, M.D.

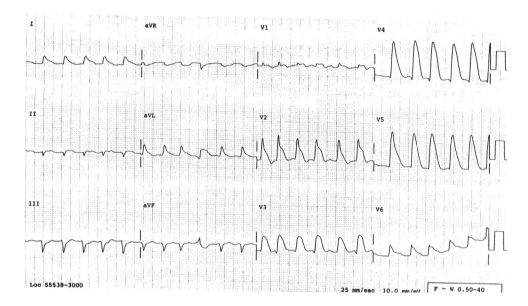

CASE 6-3

Left Main Coronary Occlusion

History
This 42-year-old man experienced onset of CP at 07:00, followed by syncope. Vital signs were BP = 100/60, P = 100, and oxygen (O_2) saturation = 89% on room air.

ECG 6-3 (Type 1a)
- Profound ST abnormalities: nine leads; ST elevation: V1–V5, I, aVL, maximal V3–V4 (approximately 10 mm); moderately large ST score; ST depression: deep, II, III, aVF; and distorted terminal QRS: V2–V5, I, aVL are diagnostic of **anterolateral AMI.** An ECG such as this is common in patients with left main coronary occlusion who survive to the hospital.
- Q waves: V1–V4, I, and aVL are common in **early** anterior AMI.

- **Total ST deviation is very high.**

Clinical Course
The patient developed hypotension but improved quickly with hydration administered after a chest film indicated no pulmonary edema. He received thrombolytics, aspirin, and hirudin and was taken to the catheterization (cath) lab. Angiography revealed an 80% left main coronary occlusion, with TIMI-2 flow. An intra-aortic balloon pump was placed and the patient survived subsequent emergency CABG.

Conclusion
This ECG is indicative of high acuity, a very large amount of myocardium at risk, high mortality, and great potential benefit from reperfusion therapy.

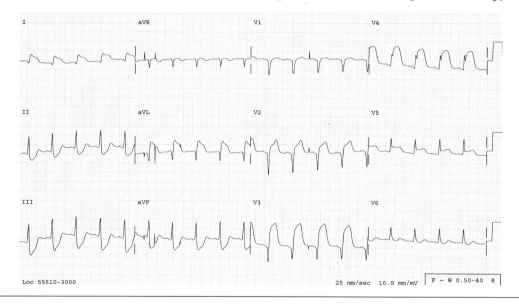

Loc 55510-3000   25 mm/sec   10.0 mm/mV   F ~ W 0.50-40   8

CASE 6-4

Transient STEMI

History
This 49-year-old man presented with atypical CP. The initial ECG at 10:54 was a Type 3 ECG, with nonspecific ST elevation in V1–V4. The patient received aspirin.

ECG 6-4A (Type 1a)
V1–V6 only, at 12:20, was the second ECG
- ST elevation: V1–V4 is diagnostic of **anterior AMI**.

Clinical Course
Clinicians began preparation for reperfusion, but the pain resolved spontaneously. A third ECG at 12:42 showed ST resolution. Clinicians administered heparin and admitted the patient to the CCU.

ECG 6-4B (Type 2)
V2 only, at 15:29, was the fourth ECG
- ST resolution
- Minimal terminal T-wave inversion: V2 only (Wellens' syndrome, Pattern A)

Clinical Course
CTnI rose from less than 0.1 ng/mL to 0.4 ng/mL and then fell back to 0.1 ng/mL, indicating AMI with "minor myocardial injury." Nonemergent angiography revealed a 99% mid-LAD stenosis (with thrombus), which was opened and stented.

ECG 6-4C (Type 2)
V1–V6 only, was the fifth ECG, the next morning
- Deepening terminal T-wave inversion: V2–V4 (Wellens' syndrome, Pattern A)

Conclusion
Transient STEMI may occur and often results in terminal T-wave inversion, especially if myocardium is injured. In this case, if ECG 6-4b had been the first ECG recorded, it would be identical to "Wellens' syndrome," which is associated with a very tight LAD stenosis (see Chapter 8). In the absence of ECG 6-4a, the label NSTEMI would have been applied.

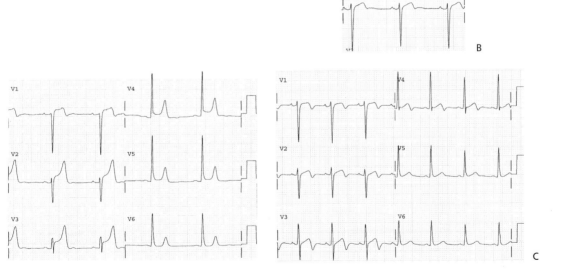

ANNOTATED BIBLIOGRAPHY

See also the annotated bibliography of Chapter 3.

Measurement of the ST Segment
Menown IB, et al. Optimizing the initial 12-lead electrocardiographic diagnosis of acute myocardial infarction, 2000.

> *Methods:* Menown et al. (17) studied the sensitivity and specificity of various criteria from the initial ECGs of 1,041 patients presenting with CP and an additional 149 from a cohort of healthy subjects without CP. AMI was diagnosed by CP of more than 20 minutes' duration and by CK-MB or new Q waves or new persistent T-wave inversions. Subjects were randomly divided into a training set (n = 587) and a validation set (n = 603). ST elevation was measured relative to the PR segment, but location of measurement is not specified.

> *Findings:* The best model used optimum ST elevation of ≥ 1 mm in one or more of leads II, III, aVL, aVF, V5, V6, and I, or ≥ 2 mm in one or more of leads V1–V4 (Minnesota Code criteria, 104), with 55.8% sensitivity and 94.0% specificity. The criteria selected resulted in wide variation in sensitivity and specificity: 45.4% and 98.1% to 68.6% and 81.2%, respectively. The incidence of "significant" ST elevation without AMI was 13%.

Rude RE, et al. Electrocardiographic and clinical criteria for recognition of acute myocardial infarction based on analysis of 3,697 patients, 1983.

> **Methods:** Rude et al. (20) correlated ECG findings with diagnosis of AMI by total CK in 3,697 patients with CP for more than 30 minutes.
>
> **Findings:** Presence of either ST elevation of 1 mm (**NOT** 2 mm) in any two consecutive leads, ST depression, new Q waves, or new LBBB, was 81% sensitive and 69% specific for AMI. Prevalence of AMI was 49% in this entire group and the PPV was 72% for any single criterion. ST elevation alone was only 46% sensitive but 91% specific for AMI. ST elevation **OR** depression was 75% sensitive and 77% specific for AMI.

Massel D, et al. Strict reliance on a computer algorithm or measurable ST-segment criteria may lead to errors in thrombolytic therapy eligibility, 2000.

> **Methods:** Massel et al. (41) had three cardiologists interpret 75 ECGs on two separate occasions by two methods: (a) formal measurement of ST elevation of ≥ 1 mm in two contiguous leads; and (b) criterion (a) plus subjective interpretation. By intention, they made no mention of where or how the ST elevation was to be formally measured. The final interpretation by each method was arrived at by consensus. The two methods were compared, and compared with the computerized interpretation by a Marquette 12 SL system. Because there is no "gold standard" for STEMI, Massel et al. chose to use the cardiologists' interpretation rather than biomarker diagnosis as the reference, reasoning that a positive CK-MB may simply be diagnostic of NSTEMI.
>
> **Findings:** Interrater agreement was good for both methods, but **better for subjective interpretation** (94.7% agreement between any pair of raters) than for formal measurement (87% to 93% agreement). By measured criteria, 49% were eligible for thrombolytics; by interpretive criteria, 35% were eligible. Use of the cardiologists' **measured** criteria would, therefore, have led to **overuse**, with 11 of 49 patients without AMI (as determined by interpretive criteria) receiving thrombolytics. Compared with 26 diagnoses of STEMI by interpretive criteria, the computer had sensitivity of only 62%, with specificity of 100%, and would have led to inappropriate withholding of thrombolytics in 10 of 26 STEMI patients. **The computer was insensitive, and measured criteria were nonspecific, for the diagnosis of STEMI.**

Q Waves, R Waves, and Terminal QRS Distortion

Raitt MH, et al. Appearance of abnormal Q waves early in the course of acute myocardial infarction: implications for efficacy of thrombolytic therapy, 1995.

> **Methods:** Raitt et al. (92) pooled data from 695 patients in four prospective thrombolytic trials. Patients had no previous history of MI and their admission ECGs allowed prediction of infarct size based on myocardium at risk.
>
> **Findings:** Of patients with an initial ECG recorded within 1 hour of symptom onset, 53% **already had abnormal Q waves** on the initial ECG. Thrombolysis saved as much myocardium in these patients as in patients without such Q waves. Vermeer et al. (117) support these findings (see later).

Bar FW, et al. Development of ST-segment elevation and Q- and R wave changes in acute myocardial infarction and the influence of thrombolytic therapy, 1996.

> **Methods:** Bar et al. (93) analyzed serial ECGs of 358 patients with reperfused and nonreperfused AMI.
>
> **Findings:** Mean magnitude of fully developed Q waves or loss of R wave did not change after 9 hours in nonreperfused cases. **ST elevation was stabilized by 5 hours and normalized slowly, over days.**

Birnbaum Y, et al. Prognostic significance of the admission electrocardiogram in acute myocardial infarction, 1996.

> **Methods:** Birnbaum et al. (118) analyzed data from 2,603 patients who received thrombolytics and whose ECGs showed ST elevation and positive T waves in ≥ 2 adjacent leads.
>
> **Findings:** In-hospital mortality and mean peak total CK were 6.8% and 1,617 IU/L for 1,371 patients with terminal QRS distortion, and 3.8% and 1,080 IU/L for 1,232 patients without QRS distortion. Although QRS distortion was an independent predictor of mortality, Birnbaum et al. did not investigate whether it was independent of ST-segment height. A very small study by Hasdai et al. (119), supported by data from Garcia-Rubira et al. (120), suggests that **QRS distortion** is

more important than total ST elevation; the greater the ST-segment height, the more distorted the QRS.

Madias JE. The "giant R waves" ECG pattern of hyperacute phase of myocardial infarction, 1993.

> **Findings:** Madias (121) describes **"giant R waves"** (identical to those in Case 6-2) and suggests that they may represent abnormal propagation of ventricular activation and that they are a marker of the hyperacute phase, at which time thrombolysis is most beneficial.
>
> **Comment:** Alternatively, they may simply represent very high ST elevation, which causes such QRS distortion that the end of the QRS is not definable.

Infarct Location and ST Deviation: Relation to Risk Area, Outcomes, and Reperfusion Benefit

> **Comment:** ST score is consistently defined as sum, in mm, of the ST elevations from all leads. The ST score is measured on the initial diagnostic ECG, which may not be the optimum moment. Bear in mind that the method and location of ST-segment measurement, although not consistently stated in the studies described below, have been found to affect the results. In one study, the mean sum of ST displacement was 16 mm when measured **at** the J point, and 23 mm when measured 60 msec **after** the J point (84).

Hands ME, et al. Prognostic significance of electrocardiographic site of infarction after correction for enzymatic size of infarction, 1986 and Stone PH, et al. Prognostic significance of location and type of MI: independent adverse outcome associated with anterior location, 1988.

> **Methods:** These studies (107,108) compared outcomes from 651 anterior AMI patients and 617 inferior AMI patients; none received reperfusion therapy.
>
> **Findings:** For any given infarct size, anterior AMI resulted in a lower EF (approximately 40% versus 56%) and a greater incidence of CHF; short and long term mortality of anterior AMI were more than twice that for inferior AMI.

Mauri F, et al. Prognostic significance of the extent of myocardial injury in acute myocardial infarction treated by streptokinase (GISSI Trial), 1989.

> **Methods:** Mauri et al. (109) classified ECGs from 8,731 GISSI-1 patients (randomized to SK or placebo, see Appendix C) with ST elevation and no previous infarct into four groups: (a) small (ST elevation in two or three leads, 41% of patients); (b) modest (four or five leads, 25%); (c) large (six or seven leads, 19%); and (d) extensive infarct (eight or nine leads, 15%). ST depression and height of ST segments were not addressed.
>
> **Findings:** Of large or extensive infarcts, 100% were anterior or multiple site and of small infarcts, 93% were inferior. Although infarct size, mortality, ultimate development of Q wave or loss of R wave, and benefit from SK correlated with location (anterior infarction was the worst), they **correlated more strongly with number of leads involved.** Small AMI (three leads or less) did not correlate with significant mortality benefit from SK.

Bar FW, et al. Value of admission electrocardiogram in predicting outcome of thrombolytic therapy in acute myocardial infarction, 1987.

> **Methods:** Bar et al. (111) analyzed data from 488 patients randomized to intracoronary SK or control.
>
> **Findings:** Patients with anterior location, high ST score (**> 12 mm for anterior, > 6 mm for inferior**), marked ST depression, or presence of Q waves had the greatest limitation of infarct size as measured by radionuclide left ventriculography and CK. For both anterior and inferior locations, in the absence of concomitant Q waves, **no significant limitation was seen in patients with low ST score, BUT confidence intervals were wide.**

Lee KL, et al. Predictors of 30-day mortality in the era of reperfusion for acute myocardial infarction: results from an international trial of 41,021 patients, 1995.

> **Methods:** Lee et al. (122) analyzed GUSTO-1 data (see Appendix C).
>
> **Findings:** Mortality was 9.9% for all anterior AMIs versus 5.0% for all inferior AMIs (all patients received thrombolytics).
>
> **Comments:** This study does NOT reflect the heterogeneity of inferior MI; although low for simple inferior MI, **mortality is high for inferoposterior, infero-RV, and inferolateral MI.**

Vermeer F, et al. Which patients benefit most from early thrombolytic therapy with intracoronary streptokinase? 1999.

Methods: Vermeer et al. (117) analyzed ECGs, radionuclide left ventriculography and enzyme-release data from 533 patients randomized to intracoronary SK versus control (no SK).

Findings: Thrombolysis with SK resulted in the greatest limitation of infarct size in patients with electrocardiographically larger AMIs (large new Q waves, high ST elevation, reciprocal depression, and anterior AMI) or in those admitted within two hours of symptom onset. Among all patients with an **ST score < 12 mm**, those who received SK more than 2 hours after symptom onset demonstrated no beneficial effects on mortality, LV function as measured by radionuclide left ventriculography, or enzymatic infarct size, over those who did not receive thrombolytics.

Gwechenberger M, et al. Prediction of early complications in patients with acute myocardial infarction by calculation of the ST score, 1997.

Methods: Gwechenberger et al. (123) conducted an observational study of 243 patients who presented with anterior or inferior AMI and received thrombolytics.

Findings: Increased ST score was associated with an increased rate of complications. A cutoff of **9 mm for inferior AMI and 13 mm for anterior AMI** predicted worse outcome.

Peterson ED, et al. Prognostic significance of precordial ST-segment depression during inferior myocardial infarction in the thrombolytic era: results in 16,521 patients, 1996.

Methods: Peterson et al. (112) analyzed clinical and angiographic outcomes of 16,521 patients with inferior AMI who received thrombolytics in the GUSTO-1 trial (see Appendix C).

Findings: **Greater reciprocal ST depression correlated strongly with poor outcome.**

Willems JL, et al. Significance of initial ST-segment elevation and depression for the management of thrombolytic therapy in acute myocardial infarction, 1990.

Methods: Willems et al. (84) analyzed data on enzyme release, ventriculographic EF, and wall motion from 665 patients in the ECSG trial of tPA for treatment of AMI (see Appendix C).

Findings: In-hospital mortality was greater, but benefit from thrombolytics as measured by mortality and by limitation of infarct size was also greater, with a total sum of ST elevation (as measured 60 ms after the J point) of > 20 mm. The sum was significantly different when measured at the J point or 60 msec after the J point (mean, 16 ± 9 mm versus 23 ± 11 mm).

Hathaway WR, et al. Prognostic significance of the initial electrocardiogram in patients with acute myocardial infarction, 1998.

Methods: Hathaway et al. (116) analyzed clinical and ECG findings from GUSTO-1 (see Appendix C). All patients received thrombolytics.

Findings: The strongest independent **overall predictors** of 30-day mortality were **age, systolic BP, and Killip class.** The strongest independent **ECG predictors** were **absolute ST deviation** (in precordial and limb leads), **HR, QRS duration, AND ECG evidence of previous infarct.** The study does not comment on thrombolytic benefit in these instances. Data from Nixdorff et al. (124) and Sugiura et al. (125) support these findings.

ST Score May Have Wide Variability in Prediction

Hick JL, et al. Clinical utility of the electrocardiogram for prediction of myocardium at risk in acute myocardial infarction, unpublished.

Methods: Hick et al. (114) injected sestamibi within 60 minutes of the diagnostic ECG (BUT before reperfusion therapy) in 105 AMI patients, and again before hospital discharge. From this they identified ECG correlates of myocardium at risk (MAR) and myocardial salvage (MS), and evaluated these findings as predictors of final infarct size.

Findings: In anterior versus other infarcts, MAR (45 ± 2% versus 16 ± 1.5%) and MS (30 ± 2% versus 8.5 ± 1.3%) was greater. However, although the correlation coefficients (r) between MAR and ST values were significant, they were weak ($r = 0.18$ for ST score, $r = 0.23$ for total ST displacement, $r = 0.24$ for number of leads with ST elevation, $r = 0.37$ for number with ST displacement). Calculation of Aldrich score

(see later, 126), did not add to predictive value. **Patients with ST elevation ≥ 20 mm had perfusion defects from 5% to 75% of the LV. Defects ranged from 5% to 62% in patients with ST elevation in six leads, and from 0 to 47% for patients with ST elevation in two leads.**

Christian TF, et al. Estimates of myocardium at risk and collateral flow in acute myocardial infarction using electrocardiographic indexes with comparison to radionuclide and angiographic measures, 1995.

Methods: Christian et al. (113) injected sestamibi in 67 AMI patients before angioplasty, and again before hospital discharge, to determine ECG correlates of myocardium at risk, collateral flow, and time to reperfusion, and to evaluate these findings as predictors of final infarct size.

Findings: Anterior infarct location correlated most strongly, and ST score correlated weakly, with a large amount of myocardium at risk. ST score showed a moderate inverse correlation with collateral flow. These two variables, as well as time from onset of CP to ECG evidence of reperfusion, correlated independently with infarct size, but the confidence intervals were wide. This suggests that **ST score is a weaker predictor of myocardium at risk than is anterior infarct location, and there is large individual variation.**

Wilkins ML, et al. Variability of acute ST segment predicted myocardial infarct size in the absence of thrombolytic therapy, 1994.

Methods: Wilkins et al. (90) analyzed prehospital and ED ECGs of 185 AMI patients.

Findings: Due to the instability of ST segments, calculation of infarct size depended on the precise moment of the ECG.

ST Morphology

Kosuge M, et al. Value of ST-segment elevation pattern in predicting infarct size and left ventricular function at discharge in patients with reperfused acute anterior myocardial infarction, 1999.

Methods: Kosuge et al. (87) assessed the predictive value of ST morphology in lead V3. They studied 77 patients with first anterior AMI due to total LAD occlusion; angioplasty opened all occlusions by 6 hours.

Findings: ST segments were upwardly concave in 24 cases, straight in 41, and upwardly convex in 12. At discharge, the mean EF was 58%, 48%, and 41%, respectively. Peak CK was 2,287 U/L, 4,371 U/L, and 5,322 U/L, respectively. Time to reperfusion was 3.6, 3.8, and 4.3 hours, respectively. Convex morphology was associated with larger infarct and worse EF in patients with LAD occlusion. It is uncertain whether this is due to differing collateral circulation, differing time to reperfusion, or larger risk area.

Prediction of Infarct Size

Selvester RH. The 12-lead ECG and the initiation of thrombolytic therapy for acute myocardial infarction, 1993.

Methods: Selvester (110) analyzed GISSI, ISIS-2, and ECSG data to determine ECG risk subsets (see Appendix C).

Findings: Although combining all inferior and lateral AMIs indicated no benefit from thrombolysis, certain subsets did show benefit, including **inferoposterior AMI and infero-RV AMI.**

Aldrich HR, et al. Use of initial ST-segment deviation for prediction of final electrocardiographic size of acute myocardial infarcts, 1988.

Methods: Aldrich et al. (126) correlated initial ECGs in nonreperfused STEMI (68 anterior AMI and 80 inferior AMI) with final infarct size as estimated by Selvester QRS score (110). They then developed formulas using the initial ECG to predict final infarct size as a percentage of myocardium that will necrose without reperfusion, as follows:

Findings: Anterior: 3 × (1.5 × (number of leads with ST elevation) − 0.4) = % of myocardium necrosing

Inferior: 3 × (0.6 × (sum of ST elevation in II, III, aVF) + 2) = % of myocardium necrosing

Comment: Unfortunately, due to ST-segment instability, this number depends on the precise moment of the ECG (90). Furthermore, because this method does not account for the presence of reciprocal changes, posterior AMI or RV AMI, its accuracy and utility especially for inferior AMI are very suspect.

RECIPROCAL ST DEPRESSION

GENERAL BACKGROUND

The general term "reciprocal depression" includes the following three contexts in which ST depression occurs in leads distant from ST elevation of AMI: (a) most commonly, **true reciprocal changes,** which refers to ST depression in leads registering the opposite ECG view of the ST elevation (the amount of reciprocal depression correlates with the amount of ST elevation); (b) **simultaneous posterior AMI,** if it occurs maximally in V2–V3, representing a second area of STEMI; and (c) less commonly, simultaneous subendocardial ischemia in a different coronary artery distribution.

Reciprocal depression is significant because **ST elevation is much more likely to indicate AMI if it is accompanied by reciprocal ST depression** (17,65,106). Additionally, reciprocal depression generally indicates a **larger infarct area at risk,** with a higher risk of mortality and complications, and greater potential benefit from thrombolytics.

RECIPROCAL DEPRESSION IN INFERIOR AMI

Inferior AMI nearly always manifests **ST elevation in leads II, III, and/or aVF, and reciprocal ST depression manifests in aVL.** Notice in Figure 4-2 that leads III and aVL are 150° opposite each other. In inferior AMI, ST elevation is usually greatest in lead III, ST depression is usually greatest in aVL, and ST depression in lead I is common because leads I and III are oriented 120° apart. ST depression in aVL may be a more powerful predictor of inferior AMI than inferior ST elevation (127) (see Case 7-1). See Case 20-3 for ST elevation in II, III, and aVF, without reciprocal depression in aVL, due to early repolarization.

Inferoposterior AMI manifests ST elevation in II, III, aVF, and reciprocal ST depression in aVL due to inferior AMI, **PLUS** reciprocal ST depression in any of leads V1–V4, and often out to V6. The prognosis in these cases, which generally worsens in proportion to the total sum of ST depression, is worse than that in inferior AMI without ST depression (84,112,128,129). Thus there is greater benefit from reperfusion therapy (see Case 7-2).

Inferolateral AMI manifests **ST elevation in II, III, aVF, V5 and V6, and ST elevation** (see Case 7-3) **OR ST depression in aVL** (see Case 13-5). The expected ST elevation in aVL due to lateral AMI and the expected reciprocal depression in aVL due to inferior AMI may **cancel each other out,** leaving aVL isoelectric, depressed, or elevated. Inferior AMI with ST elevation in V5 and/or V6, or with less reciprocal depression in leads I and/or aVL, correlates with concurrent lateral AMI and the circumflex as the culprit artery (130,131).

Inferior AMI Versus Pericarditis

Pericarditis may be mistaken for inferior AMI. However, **there is no reciprocal ST depression in pericarditis.** Concurrent inferior and lateral inflammation cause inferior ST elevation and lateral ST elevation, **NOT** ST depression. Additionally, the ST elevation of pericarditis is almost always **DIFFUSE,** greatest in lead II, and typically manifested in at least some precordial leads (see Case 7-4).

Localized pericarditis (less common) may also mimic inferior AMI when local inflammation of the inferior wall manifests as **inferior ST elevation with reciprocal ST depression in aVL** (see Cases 24-4 to 24-6). Since the ECG of localized pericarditis may be identical to that of inferior AMI, the diagnosis must be based also on clinical suspicion and ancillary studies such as echocardiography.

Reciprocal Changes in Limb Leads

Other conditions may cause **reciprocal changes in limb leads,** similar to those of inferior AMI. **Ventricular aneurysm** (see Chapter 23) and **LVH** (see Chapter 22), for example, occasionally cause ST elevation in III with reciprocal ST depression in aVL (see Case 7-5).

RECIPROCAL DEPRESSION IN LATERAL AMI AND ANTERIOR AMI

Lateral AMI manifests **ST elevation in aVL,** and possibly in I, V5–V6, with **reciprocal ST depression in leads II, III, and/or aVF.**

These reciprocal changes are due to the electrically opposite view of lateral wall infarct. Such ST depression in the context of lateral ST elevation must be assumed to be reciprocal to lateral STEMI and **NOT** due to inferior subendocardial ischemia with reciprocal elevation in aVL. See Case 7-6. (See also Case 14-1, of inferior ST depression in lateral AMI.)

Anterior AMI manifests **ST elevation in V1–V4 (especially in V2–V3)**, which may be accompanied by **reciprocal depression in II, III, and aVF.** This inferior ST depression is most commonly due to an electrically opposite view of proximal LAD occlusion in the high anterior wall (132,133). **ST depression ≥ 1 mm** in inferior leads correlates with (**a**) proximal LAD occlusion (often with ST elevation in I and aVL due to occlusion proximal to the first diagonal branch and concurrent lateral AMI); (**b**) larger anterior AMI; (**c**) higher precordial ST elevation; and (**d**) worse prognosis (Case 7-7). (See also Case 6-3, which demonstrates anterior ST elevation with deep reciprocal ST depression in II, III, and aVF due to left main coronary occlusion.)

CASE 7-1

Inferior AMI with Reciprocal Changes

History
This 72-year-old man presented with typical CP.

ECG 7-1 (Type 1a)
- ST elevation: II, III, and aVF; with reciprocal ST depression: aVL. The ST elevation is more marked in III than in II, which is consistent with inferior AMI rather than pericarditis or early repolarization. This ECG is diagnostic of **inferior AMI.**

Clinical Course
The patient received tPA immediately and reperfused successfully.

ECG reproduced from unpublished data with permission of K. Wang, M.D.

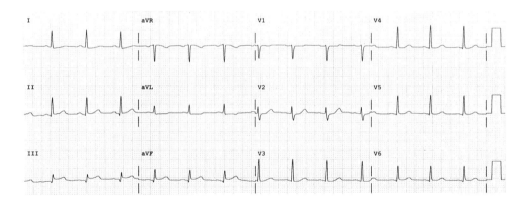

CASE 7-2

Inferior AMI with Concurrent Posterior AMI and RV AMI

History

This 52-year-old man with history of coronary artery disease (CAD) presented with intermittent CP.

ECG 7-2 (Type 1a)

- ST elevation: II, III, aVF; with reciprocal depression in aVL, is diagnostic of **inferior AMI.**
- ST depression: V2–V6, is diagnostic of **posterior AMI.**
- ST elevation: V1, is **suspicious** for RV AMI.

Clinical Course

A right-sided ECG showed **ST elevation in all right-sided leads, confirming RV AMI. Without RV AMI, posterior AMI probably would have manifested ST DEPRESSION in V1.** ST depression in V5–V6 may be reciprocal to right-sided ST elevation.

Conclusion

This AMI has a moderately high risk of complications and death, with corresponding potential benefit from timely reperfusion therapy.

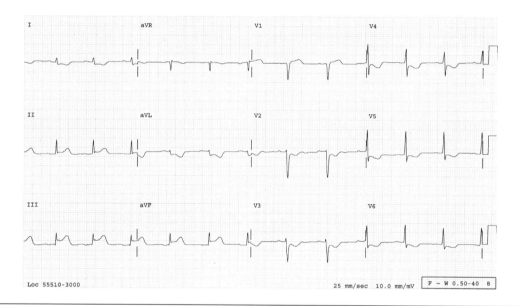

Loc 55510-3000   25 mm/sec 10.0 mm/mV   F ~ W 0.50-40 8

CASE 7-3

Inferolateral AMI with Minimal Reciprocal Depression in aVL, Initially Misdiagnosed as Pericarditis

History

This 39-year-old man presented with CP.

ECG 7-3 (Type 1b)

■ ST elevation: II, III, aVF, V5–V6 may be due to pericarditis or inferolateral AMI. Findings that favor inferolateral AMI include: (a) ST elevation in III ≥ II; (b) **reciprocal ST depression in aVL,** (which is **present, though minimal** due to cancellation by lateral ST elevation); and (c) absence of ST elevation in V2–V4 (which would raise the likelihood of pericarditis). This is a difficult ECG, but **diagnostic of STEMI.**

Clinical Course

The computer missed this inferolateral AMI and read it as "pericarditis." Physicians were uncertain and ordered echocardiography, which revealed inferolateral hypokinesis. Thrombolytics were given, with reperfusion. A stress test was negative and the patient was discharged. He returned 6 months later with recurrent inferolateral AMI; angiography revealed occlusions of the first diagonal and of the posterolateral branch of the RCA, as well as 80% stenosis of both obtuse marginal arteries. The culprit artery was difficult to ascertain.

Conclusion

This case shows the difficulty of differentiating inferolateral AMI from pericarditis.

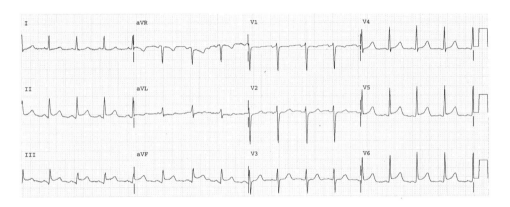

CASE 7-4

Inferior ST Elevation with No Reciprocal Changes, Due to Pericarditis

ECG 7-4 (Type 3)

Ignore artifactual V5 and V6.

- ST elevation: diffuse, greater in II than in III; absence of reciprocal changes between III and aVL; and PR segment depression make this ECG highly suggestive of pericarditis.
- Though large infero-antero-lateral AMI is possible, it is unlikely because R waves are much taller than T waves,

there is PR depression, and ST elevation in II is greater than that in III.

ECG reproduced from unpublished data with permission of K. Wang, M.D.

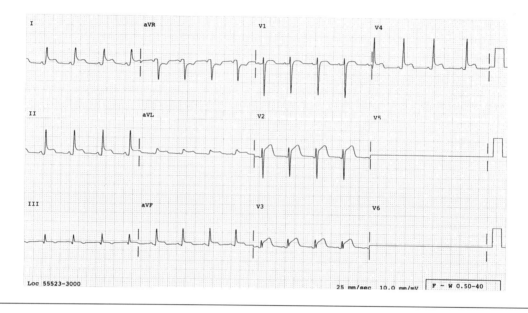

CASE 7-5

Inferior ST Elevation with Reciprocal Depression in aVL: Patient with Ventricular Aneurysm Who Received Thrombolytics

History

This 67-year-old man with a history of MI presented with CP.

ECG 7-5 (Type 1c)

- ST elevation: II, III, aVF; with reciprocal depression: I, aVL
- QS waves: V1–V5
- Qr waves (very small R waves): II, III, aVF, without large T waves

Clinical Course

The patient received thrombolytics for inferior AMI but biochemical markers were negative. Comparison with a previous ECG revealed that this was the patient's post-MI baseline. The diagnosis was **inferior ventricular aneurysm**.

Conclusion

Although the ST elevation could be new and due to AMI, the deep Q waves, with flat or inverted T waves, especially in the context of previous MI, should alert the clinician to the likelihood of ventricular aneurysm (see Chapter 23).

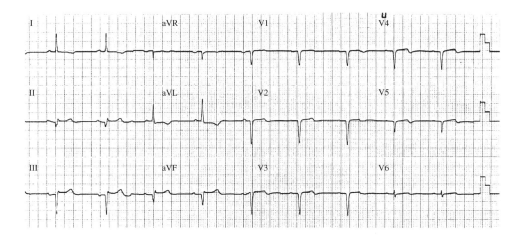

CASE 7-6

Lateral AMI with Reciprocal Changes More Prominent than ST Elevation

History
This 31-year-old man presented with CP.

ECG 7-6 (Type 1b)
■ **Hyperacute T wave:** aVL; ST elevation: aVL, < 1 mm, but the QRS is low voltage and ST segment voltage is almost as high, which is as high as it can be; and **reciprocal ST depression:** II, III, aVF, make this ECG diagnostic of **lateral AMI.**

Clinical Course
The computer missed this AMI. Physicians diagnosed it as "inferior ischemia." A repeat ECG 30 minutes later showed very obvious ST elevation of AMI.

Conclusion
Minimal lateral ST elevation combines with inferior reciprocal depression to make this ECG diagnostic of AMI; failure to recognize this delayed thrombolysis by 70 minutes.

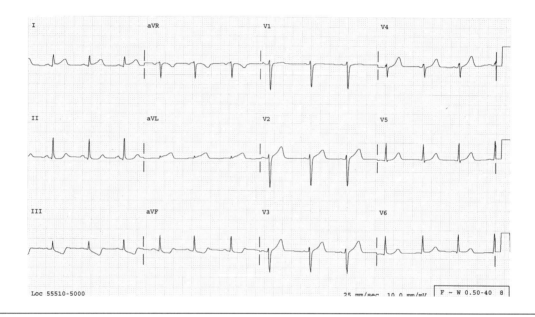

Loc 55510-5000   25 mm/sec   10.0 mm/mV   F ~ W 0.50-40   8

CASE 7-7

Anterolateral AMI from Proximal LAD Occlusion with Inferior Reciprocal Depression

History
This 51-year-old man presented with 1 hour of CP.

ECG 7-7 (Type 1a)
- ST elevation: V2–V5, I, aVL; with reciprocal ST depression: II, III, aVF, is diagnostic of **anterolateral AMI.**

Clinical Course
Angioplasty opened an LAD occlusion proximal to the first diagonal artery.

Conclusion
The ST depression in II, III, and aVF is due to an electrically opposite view of ST elevation in the lateral leads due to infarction, **NOT** to inferior subendocardial ischemia. A high ST score (based on the ST elevation in six leads and the degree of elevation) and terminal QRS distortion indicate that this is a high-risk AMI.

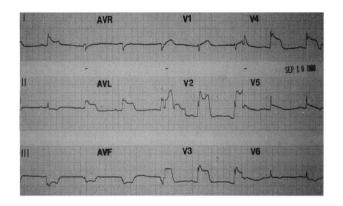

ANNOTATED BIBLIOGRAPHY

Reciprocal Depression in Anterior and Inferior AMI
See annotations in Chapter 12 (132–137) and Chapter 13 (138–141).

Higher Mortality in AMI with Reciprocal Changes
Savonitto S, et al. Prognostic value of the admission electrocardiogram in acute coronary syndromes, 1999.
   Methods: Savonitto et al. (142) studied 12,142 CP patients.
   Findings: Thirty-day mortality was 5.5% for patients with T-wave inversion, 9.4% for patients with ST elevation, 10.5% for patients with ST depression, and **12.4% for patients with ST elevation AND ST depression.**

Willems JL, et al., Significance of initial ST segment elevation and depression for the management of thrombolytic therapy in acute myocardial infarction, 1990.
   Methods: Willems et al. (84) analyzed data from the 655 patients in the ECSG trial whose QRS duration was < 120 ms. This trial (see Appendix C) randomized patients with AMI in any location to placebo or tissue plasminogen activator (tPA).
   Findings: In-hospital mortality was greater, but benefit from thrombolytics as measured by mortality and by limitation of infarct size was also greater, when the sum of ST deviations (ST depression plus ST elevation) was greater.

Hasdai D, et al. Prognostic significance of maximal precordial ST segment depression in right (V1–V3) versus left (V4–V6) leads in patients with inferior wall acute myocardial infarction, 1994.
   Methods: Hasdai et al. (128) studied the ECGs and clinical outcomes of 213 patients with early inferior AMI (before T-wave inversion).
   Findings: Forty-three patients had no precordial ST depression, 46 patients had precordial ST depression maximal in leads V1–V3, and 124 patients had precordial ST depression maximal in V4–V6. In-hospital mortality was 12%, 10%, and 41%, respectively. **ST depression in V4–V6 independently predicted in-hospital mortality,** with an OR of 4.9 (1.93 to 12.26).
   Comment: ST depression in leads V4–V6 may represent RV AMI (reciprocal to right side), which is known to have high mortality.

Birnbaum Y, et al. Prognostic significance of precordial ST segment depression on admission electrocardiogram in patients with inferior wall myocardial infarction, 1996.
   Methods: Birnbaum et al. (129) studied 1,321 GUSTO-1 patients in Israel (see Appendix C).
   Findings: As with Hasdai et al. (128) earlier, **ST depression in V4–V6 was an independent predictor of mortality,** with an **OR** of 2.78 (1.26 to 6.13), which was, again, significantly higher than for leads V1–V3.

Peterson ED, et al. Prognostic significance of precordial ST segment depression during inferior myocardial infarction in the thrombolytic era: results in 16,521 patients, 1996.
   Methods: Peterson et al. (112) analyzed GUSTO-1 data from 16,521 inferior AMI patients who received thrombolytics (see Appendix C).
   Findings: For each 0.5 mV of summed ST depression in V1–V6, 30-day mortality increased by 36%. Unlike findings by Hasdai et al. (128) and Birnbaum et al. (129) described earlier, Peterson et al. found no difference in 30-day mortality between patients with summed ST

depression in V1–V3 versus V4–V6. Thirty-day mortality among patients with and without any ST depression in V1–V6 was 4.7% versus 3.2%. **One-year mortality in patients with and without any ST depression was 7.0% versus 4.6%, respectively. ST depression in V1–V3 correlated with much higher CK levels, greater infarct size, and circumflex occlusion.**

Krone RJ, et al. Long-term prognostic significance of ST segment depression during acute myocardial infarction, 1993.

    Methods: Krone et al. (23) studied 1,234 AMI patients in the Multicenter Diltiazem Postinfarction Trial, which enrolled patients between 1983 and 1986.

    Findings: Of 951 patients (77%) with ST elevation, location was anterior in 437 and inferior in 514. Ten percent had only ST depression, and 13% had neither ST elevation nor depression. Q-wave MI occurred in 896 patients and non–Q-wave MI, in 338. The **number of leads with reciprocal ST depression correlated highly with mortality and complications.** In STEMI, 1-year mortality was 10.3% for those with reciprocal ST depression versus 5.6% for those without it. For anterior AMI with reciprocal ST depression (36% of anterior AMI), mortality was 13.6% versus 6.9% without; for inferior AMI (64% of inferior AMI), the difference was **11.0% versus 1.8%.**

Shah A, et al. Comparative prognostic significance of simultaneous versus independent resolution of ST segment depression relative to ST segment elevation during acute myocardial infarction, 1997.

    Methods: Shah et al. (143) used continuous ST segment monitoring to study 261 patients who underwent thrombolysis and whose arteries reperfused.

    Findings: Following reperfusion, in-hospital mortality was 13% among patients in whom ST depression failed to resolve simultaneously with resolving ST elevation; this compared with 1% mortality for patients **with** simultaneous resolution. In-hospital mortality for patients without any reciprocal ST depression was 0.

ST DEPRESSION AND T-WAVE INVERSION

GENERAL BACKGROUND

ST depression and T-wave inversion may result from a variety of conditions. First, they may be secondary to depolarization abnormalities (which manifest as an abnormal QRS) such as LVH, LBBB, RBBB, right ventricular hypertrophy (RVH), or Wolff-Parkinson-White (WPW), in which case they are called **"secondary ST-T-wave abnormalities."** If they are in the context of normal depolarization, ST depression and T-wave inversion are **"primary."** In the context of symptoms or signs of acute ischemia, primary ST depression or T-wave inversion MUST be assumed to be manifestations of ischemia and/or infarction. Primary and secondary ST-T-wave abnormalities may coexist, resulting in difficult ECG interpretation. It is important to know the morphology of secondary ST-T abnormalities associated with abnormal depolarization in order to recognize simultaneous primary abnormalities.

ECG characteristics that are most strongly suggestive of ischemia and infarction are the following:

- **Marked ST depression** (> 1 mm, or 0.1 mV). The greater the depth of ST depression, the more likely is ischemia and/or infarction.
- **Deep T-wave inversion** (> 1 mm). The deeper the inversion, the more likely is ischemia and/or infarction.
- **Dynamic ST depression or T-wave inversion**: change from a previous ECG or change during serial ECGs.

- In the presence of QRS abnormalities, **disproportionate** ST depression or T-wave inversion (e.g., ST depression in V4–V6 disproportionate to the voltage of LVH).

ST depression or T-wave inversion are NOT indications for thrombolysis, even as a manifestation of ischemia due to ACS. **Posterior AMI is the ONLY exception to this rule** (Figs. 8-1a and 8-1c; see also Chapter 16). In early placebo-controlled, randomized thrombolytic trials, patients with ST depression or T-wave inversion (in contrast to patients with ST elevation) who underwent thrombolysis did **not** show decreased overall mortality (**30**,99). However, in these studies all ST depression was grouped together regardless of location, depth, or persistence. Thus ST depression should not be ruled out as an indication for

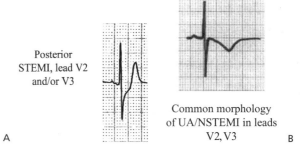

In leads V2-V3, the morphologies below could represent either posterior STEMI or anterior UA/NSTEMI

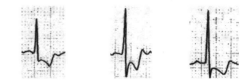

FIGURE 8-1. Interpretation of ST depression in V1–V4. In any other leads (e.g., lateral or inferior), ischemic ST depression must be assumed to be UA/NSTEMI unless it is reciprocal to ST elevation elsewhere. **A:** ECG complex diagnostic of posterior STEMI. Notice that the J point is depressed (i.e., the QRS has not returned to the baseline before the takeoff of the depressed ST segment) and the T wave is upright. **Even when isolated** (no ST elevation elsewhere on the ECG), this is usually due to occlusion of the circumflex artery and is an indication for reperfusion therapy, including thrombolytics. **B:** Likely to represent UA/NSTEMI in any lead, even in V2 and V3. Notice that the QRS returns to baseline before downsloping ST depression and that the T wave is symmetrically inverted. **C:** Again, ST depression in which the QRS does not return to baseline but the T wave is not entirely upright. This is likely to represent posterior wall STEMI, but also possibly anterior UA/NSTEMI. If **persistent** in V1–V4, it is an indication for reperfusion therapy, including thrombolytics.

thrombolysis in all cases. In fact, despite a lack of randomized trials, **precordial ST depression due to posterior injury (STEMI) is considered an indication for thrombolytic therapy** (see later) (105).

T-wave inversion is a sign of ischemia and often of AMI. It is also a common manifestation of "minimal myocardial injury," or AMI as diagnosed by troponin but with a negative CK-MB. If T-wave inversion occurs at the end of upsloping ST elevation, it is "terminal" because it comprises the latter part of the T wave, giving it a biphasic appearance. Terminal T-wave inversion generally develops into deeper, symmetric T-wave inversion as the ST segment normalizes. **T-wave inversion by itself is not an indication for reperfusion therapy (30).** Because terminal T-wave inversion may signify either reperfused myocardium or AMI that is relatively late in its course, it may complicate reperfusion therapy for STEMI; this is a Type 1d ECG (see later).

ST DEPRESSION

Measuring ST Depression

Measure the ST segment relative to the PR segment. (For detailed discussion, see Chapter 6.) Alternatively, compare the ST segment at 60 to 80 ms after the J point with the TP segment (see Figs. 6-1a and 6-1 b). Figure 8-2 illustrates atrial repolarization and why ST depression is frequently a baseline condition of the first 40 to 80 ms of the ST segment.

Etiologies of ST Depression

Noncardiac causes of ST depression include **atrial repolarization** (which is corrected if the ST segment is measured relative to the PR segment), therapeutic **digitalis** use, **tachycardia,** electrolyte or metabolic abnormalities, especially **hypokalemia.** Some individuals also have normal baseline ST depression of < 1 mm. However, in the context of ischemic symptoms, such abnormalities usually represent ischemia.

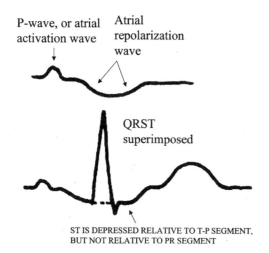

FIGURE 8-2. Atrial repolarization. This schematic illustrates atrial repolarization that depresses the PR and ST segments relative to the TP segment, which is frequently a baseline condition. For this reason it is more accurate to measure the ST segment relative to the PR segment.

Cardiac causes of ST depression may be "primary" (due to ischemia) or secondary to other disorders such as **postcardioversion** (Case 8-1), **LVH, RVH** (Case 8-2), and **WPW** (Case 8-3). WPW and RVH may mimic posterior AMI.

ST DEPRESSION DUE TO ISCHEMIA

ST depression due to ischemia may indicate (a) posterior STEMI, (b) reciprocal depression of STEMI, or (c) subendocardial ischemia, which may be a result of ACS or of secondary ischemia or sympathetic overload.

ST Depression of Posterior AMI (Posterior STEMI)

In the context of typical AMI symptoms, **isolated ST depression in V1–V4** that is maximal in V2–V3, especially if **persistent** for 30 minutes on serial ECGs or continuous monitoring, is diagnostic of **isolated posterior AMI** (Case 8-4). Posterior STEMI usually manifests the morphology shown in Figure 8-1a, but may also manifest the morphologies shown in Figure 8-1c.

- Do not assume that persistent ST depression limited to V1–V4 is anterior subendocardial ischemia/infarction (UA/NSTEMI) (83,144,145).
- Anterior subendocardial ischemia/infarction (UA/NSTEMI) manifests more commonly across all precordial leads (V1–V6) and is more transient (dynamic). It may manifest the morphologies shown in Figure 8-1c, although these are at least as likely to be due to posterior STEMI. **If the QRS returns to the baseline** and then has downsloping ST depression, especially if ending in a deep, symmetrically inverted T wave (Fig. 8-1b), ST depression in V1–V4 is likely due to anterior UA/NSTEMI.

Management

Although posterior AMI does not meet the ST elevation "criteria" of thrombolytic trials, the **ACC/AHA recommends thrombolysis "when marked ST segment depression is confined to leads V1 through V4"** (105). Thus isolated ST depression ≥ 2 mm in two or more leads, confined to V1–V4 and maximal in V2–V3, **IS an indication for reperfusion therapy, including thrombolytics** (48,105). If you suspect posterior AMI, see Chapter 16 for details on diagnosis and management.

Beware: Posterior STEMI Look-Alikes

Conduction disturbances such as RVH and WPW may manifest secondary ST depression and/or T-wave inversion that **mimics** ACS, including posterior AMI.

- **RVH** is differentiated by the presence of a **very** large and wide R wave in V1, right axis deviation, and/or S waves in I, V5, V6 (see Case 8-2).
- **WPW** is differentiated by the presence of delta waves (slurred QRS upstroke), a short PR interval (usually), and other ST and T-wave changes (see Case 8-3).

Reciprocal ST Depression of STEMI

ST depression may occur in leads reciprocal to leads manifesting ST elevation of STEMI (Type 1 ECG), as discussed in Chapter 7. This ST depression is morphologically identical to the ST depression of subendocardial ischemia.

ST depression in inferior leads II, III, and aVF may be reciprocal to **anterior** or **lateral AMI.** If this is present, scrutinize V2–V4 and aVL for ST elevation, however minimal. In the case of lateral AMI, inferior ST depression may be more impressive than lateral ST elevation (see Cases 7-6 and 14-1).

ST depression in lateral leads I and aVL may be reciprocal to **inferior AMI.** If this is present, scrutinize II, III, and aVF for ST elevation.

ST depression in V5–V6 may be reciprocal to **RV AMI** because leads V5–V6 are electrically opposite the RV (138). Record right-sided leads to detect RV AMI. Look for **inferior ST elevation or Q waves** as well, because RV AMI usually occurs in the presence of inferior MI, either acute or old.

Management

AMI with reciprocal depression carries **a worse prognosis and improves the benefit/risk ratio** of reperfusion therapy. Thrombolysis or angiography ± PCI are indicated.

ST Depression Due to Subendocardial Ischemia

ST depression of subendocardial ischemia may be due to: (a) **ACS,** in which there is a nonocclusive thrombus or an occlusive thrombus that has collateral circulation or (b) **secondary causes,** including sympathetic overload (see later). You cannot distinguish these two etiologies from the ECG alone. ST depression of subendocardial ischemia (UA/NSTEMI):

- Is transient and dynamic.
- May or may not also have T-wave inversion.
- Is not reciprocal to ST elevation elsewhere.
- Usually has flat or downsloping ST segments.

ACS

Although ST depression of UA/NSTEMI does not represent complete coronary occlusion, as does STEMI, it is **associated with high mortality and morbidity (146,147).** It typically represents severe stenosis without occlusion or complete occlusion with some (inadequate) collateral blood supply. **ST depression > 2 mm and presence in three or more leads** is associated with a **high probability of CK-confirmed infarction and a 30-day mortality of approximately 10%,** whether or not it is due to complete coronary occlusion (**142**). ST depression, along with a positive troponin, remains a strong predictor of adverse outcome and is one of the strongest markers for benefit from an early invasive management strategy (148). See Cases 8-5 and 8-6. (See also Case 37-1, of dyspnea, pulmonary edema, and transient ST depression in V3–V6 and see Case 22-7.)

Management
See Chapter 37.

Secondary Ischemia

Secondary causes of infarction/ischemia are **NOT** due to unstable coronary plaque with fissuring and thrombosis. **Inadequate myocardial oxygenation** may be due to **excess myocardial oxygen demand.** This excess oxygen demand, similar to an exercise stress test, may be caused by conditions including valvular disease, or high cardiac output states (e.g., sepsis), Addison's disease, hyperthyroidism, or high catecholamine states with tachycardia and hypertension (HTN). **Inadequate myocardial oxygen supply** may result from inadequate coronary perfusion pressure due to hypotension from any cause, usually associated with **fixed** coronary stenosis, or it may result from anemia, hypoxemia, or toxins such as carbon monoxide. Secondary causes of ischemia may also, as with ACS, lead to myocardial necrosis and resultant troponin elevation; this typically results in a subendocardial and non–Q-wave AMI (see Case 8-7).

Secondary ischemia also includes **ST depression due to sympathetic overload,** which occurs in such conditions as **subarachnoid hemorrhage, sepsis, respiratory failure, and overdose** and may be confused with ACS (including posterior STEMI) (see Case 8-8). However, these conditions **more commonly manifest T-wave inversion** (see Case 8-9). In the case of subarachnoid hemorrhage, epicardial coronary arteries are neither stenotic nor in spasm (149), although there may be global small-vessel ischemia due to sympathetic overload. As with ACS, echocardiography often reveals global or regional dysfunction (150). Clinical presentation is the best way to differentiate subarachnoid hemorrhage from myocardial ischemia.

Management
Correct the underlying condition.

T-WAVE INVERSION

Characteristics of a Normal T Wave

- The normal T vector is leftward, inferior, and anterior.
- The T wave should be positive in lead II. **Inversion in lead I in the presence of a positive QRS is always abnormal. In a normal ECG, T waves in V5–V6 should ALWAYS be upright.**
- Inversion in either lead III or aVL may be normal.
- Lead aVF may be slightly negative.
- Lead V1 is commonly negative.
- Of leads V2–V4, normal inversion is rare in V2, more rare in V3, and most rare in V4.

NONISCHEMIC T-WAVE INVERSION

Causes of Nonischemic T-Wave Inversion

Nonischemic T-wave inversion may be due to pathologic causes, as are listed in Table 8-1, or may be nonpathologic. **Nonpathologic causes include** hyperventilation (151), orthostatic changes, "postprandial" T waves, electrolyte abnormalities, and normal variant (see Chapter 20).

Normal variants include the following:

TABLE 8.1. PATHOLOGIC NON-ACS CAUSES OF T-WAVE INVERSION

Metabolic disturbances
Conditions of posttachycardia and postpacemaker
Intracranial disease such as subarachnoid hemorrhage
Myocardial disease such as pericarditis
Pulmonary embolus or pneumothorax
LVH, RVH, WPW
Conduction defects such as LBBB, RBBB, intraventricular conduction delay (IVCD), left anterior fascicular block (LAFB), left posterior fascicular block (LPFB)
Many critical illnesses may manifest T-wave inversion and other ECG changes mimicking ACS, as well as regional WMAs. The exact etiology in all cases is unclear but probably involves small-vessel ischemia.

1. **Persistent juvenile pattern** (151). This pattern is more common in young African-Americans, especially women. Look for:
   - T-wave inversion, without ST elevation, in right precordial leads (V1–V3) with normal R-wave progression and normal presence of S waves.
2. **"Benign T-wave inversion:"** This is more common in young African-American men and in trained athletes. Look for:
   - Terminal T-wave inversions in precordial leads V3–V5, often in association with the ST elevation of early repolarization (see Case 20-11), and short QT$_c$ interval (almost always < 430 ms).
   - This may be mistaken for the very malignant Wellens' syndrome, which manifests more commonly in V2–V4 and without short QT$_c$ interval.
   - Benign T-wave inversion can only be established with certainty if there are identical ECGs both before and days to weeks after the ECG in question.

T-WAVE INVERSION DUE TO ISCHEMIA

T-wave inversion is a result of delayed repolarization of the ischemic zone. Because of delayed repolarization, the **QT$_c$ is usually increased** or is at the upper end of normal range. T-wave inversion due to ACS in the absence of preceding ST elevation (witnessed or not) **may represent reversible ischemia** (see Case 21-1). Alternatively, it may **evolve during STEMI.** T-wave inversions due to ACS are generally narrow and symmetric, in contrast to those associated with stroke or Stokes-Adams attacks. In **STEMI** (whether the IRA is reperfused early, late, or not at all), if there is at least minimal injury (infarction) as measured by troponin, T-wave inversion will almost always evolve over a variable time course such that it may only be evident on serial ECGs (Fig. 8-3). The earliest T-wave inversions begin before ST normalization, and thus the T wave appears to be turned down ("terminal" T-wave inversion, Pattern A). T-wave inversion associated with AMI is believed to be a result of ischemia surrounding the infarct zone.

T-wave inversion may be induced by **non-ACS causes,** such as subarachnoid hemorrhage (see Case 8-9), pulmonary embolism (see Case 8-10), Stokes-Adams attack (see Case 8-11), or other conditions. For many non-ACS etiologies, T-wave

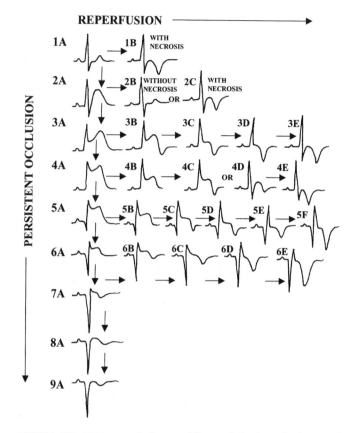

FIGURE 8-3. ECG morphology with persistent occlusion and with reperfusion occurring at progressively later stages of anterior AMI in leads V2 or V3. Similar patterns occur in other locations. Complexes 1A to 9A represent the progression of persistently occluded LAD. Tracings across the page from left to right (**A–F**) represent morphology development after reperfusion occurs at the stage of development at the far left: **1A,** before LAD occlusion; **1B,** after some minimal necrosis from partial or brief occlusion (non–Q-wave MI, intervening complex may have had some ST depression or elevation, some terminal T-wave inversion, or none at all). **2A,** hyperacute T wave; **2B,** after reperfusion and without or, **2C,** with necrosis. **3A,** ST elevation; **3B,** shortly after reperfusion, with terminal T-wave inversion (T-wave inversion Pattern A); **3C,** still more time since reperfusion, continuing on through stage **3D** to **3E,** in which T-wave inversion becomes progressively more deep and symmetric. **4A,** persistent occlusion with higher ST elevation; **4B,** reperfusion, with some recovery of ST segment; **4C,** terminal T-wave inversion without or, **4D,** with reestablishment of S wave; **4E,** deep, symmetric T-wave inversion. **5A,** development of small Q wave (schematically indicating necrosis, but in the case of the precordial leads it may only represent a reversible conduction disturbance); **5B–5F,** representing progression from 5A after reperfusion: from decreased ST elevation to terminal T-wave inversion to deep T-wave inversion; **6A,** persistent occlusion with falling ST segment and deeper Q wave; **6B–6E,** similar to 5B–5F but with lower ST segment and deeper Q wave. **7A,** persistent occlusion, with slowly recovering ST segment, shallow T-wave inversion, and deeper Q wave. **8A,** persistent occlusion, now with QS wave (probable transmural necrosis), some residual ST elevation and shallow T-wave inversion. **9A,** complete necrosis, ST elevation resolved (complete resolution occurs in about 50%), QS wave, shallow T-wave inversion.

inversion is presumed to be a result of sympathetically mediated ischemia. Although T-wave inversions due to stroke are described as widely splayed, blunted, and bizarre (1), they are often indistinguishable from those due to ACS.

On an initial ECG, T-wave inversion, especially ST elevation with terminal T-wave inversion, often represents spontaneous

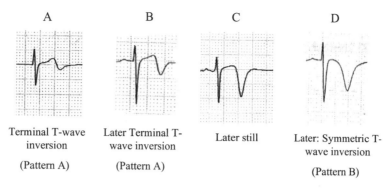

A   B   C   D

Terminal T-wave   Later Terminal T-   Later still   Later: Symmetric T-
inversion   wave inversion   wave inversion

(Pattern A)   (Pattern A)   (Pattern B)

FIGURE 8-4. Progression from Wellens' pattern A (terminal) to pattern B (deep, symmetric) T-wave inversion over hours.

reperfusion of STEMI (Fig. 8-3, images 3B–D, 4C–E, 5C–F, 6B–E and Fig. 8-4). In the context of ischemic symptoms, **look for pseudonormalization and reelevation of ST segments** (Fig. 8-5), which indicate **reocclusion** (see Case 8-12).

Shallow T-wave inversion, in the presence of **deep QS waves** usually represents late presentation with completed injury (Fig. 8-3, images 7A, 8A, 9A); in this situation, even with remaining ST elevation, it may be too late for reperfusion therapy (Type 1d ECG).

Evolution of T-Wave Inversion in a Nonreperfused STEMI

A nonreperfused STEMI due to total occlusion of a coronary artery with poor collateral supply typically produces **QS waves and GRADUAL T-wave inversion over 72 hours** (Fig. 8-3, images 1A–9A). T-wave inversion occurs before full normalization of the ST segment. (This contrasts with **pericarditis,** in which the T wave typically inverts after ST normalization.) Depth of T-wave inversion is typically ≤ 3 mm, in contrast to T-wave inversion in the context of **ischemia with less extensive infarction** (due to reperfusion or good collateral circula-

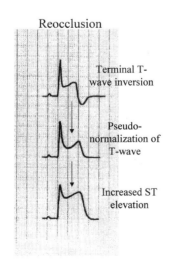

Reocclusion

Terminal T-wave inversion

Pseudo-normalization of T-wave

Increased ST elevation

FIGURE 8-5. Pseudonormalization of inverted (pattern B) T wave.

tion), which manifests as deep (> 3 mm) symmetrical inversions (94) (Fig. 8-3, images 1B, 2C, 3D, 3E, 4E, 5E, 5F, 6D, 6F).

Normalization of inverted T waves within a few hours may indicate **reocclusion** of the IRA. Gradual normalization starting at least 48 hours from onset of AMI, especially in the context of pleuritic CP, indicates **postinfarction regional pericarditis (PIRP)** (see Chapter 28). Normalization over weeks to months is common.

ST Elevation with T-Wave Inversion in the Presence of a QS Wave

The presence of a QS wave with T-wave inversion is suggestive of **sub**acute MI, the evolution of which may be too far progressed for reperfusion therapy to be beneficial; this is a Type 1d ECG (Fig. 8-3, images 7A to 9A, and Case 8-13).

ST Elevation with T-Wave Inversion in the Presence of Persistent R Waves

In contrast to a completed QS-wave AMI, as described earlier, ST elevation may occur with T-wave inversion in the presence of persistent R waves, in which case the T-wave inversion appears as "terminal" T-wave inversion. This is **Wellens' syndrome** Pattern A and is representative of reperfused STEMI (transient ST elevation due to spontaneous reperfusion [152,153]). The same morphology is often found after therapeutic reperfusion (see Chapter 27).

Wellens' Syndrome: T-Wave Inversion Patterns A and B

"Wellens' syndrome" refers to angina and T-wave inversion in **V2–V4 (152,**153–155). It appears to represent LAD occlusion (transient STEMI) that spontaneously reperfused before the tracing. It is associated with a high incidence of critical narrowing of the proximal LAD and indicates an **LAD lesion at risk for reocclusion and recurrent STEMI.** Identical T-wave morphology occurs after approximately 60% of cases of successful reperfusion therapy for anterior STEMI (156,157). These patterns of T-wave inversion may occur in any coronary distribution (e.g., inferior or lateral) but Wellens' syndrome was originally described in the LAD distribution. (See Cases 5-3 [ECG 5-3c] and 12-3 of spontaneous reperfusion of anterior AMI.)

Pattern A: Terminal T-Wave Inversion or Biphasic T Waves (Fig. 8-3, images 3B, 4C, 4D, 5C, 6B; Fig. 8-4 A and B; and Fig. 8-6).

As stated earlier, biphasic or **terminal** T-wave inversion implies some ST elevation preceding the downturn of the T wave. This pattern is associated with **recent reperfusion** of total coronary occlusion (94,156,158). It may also occur due to improved collateral flow. Both spontaneous and therapeutic reperfusion often cause **rapid terminal T-wave inversion or ST normalization or both** (156,159). Terminal T-wave inversion is usually present without full ST normalization, and develops into deep T-wave inversion over hours to days, as the ST segment resolves (94) (Fig. 8-3, images 3B to 3E, 4C to 4E, 5C to 5F, 6B to 6E and Fig. 8-4D).

Pattern B: Deeply Inverted Symmetric T Waves (Fig. 8-3, images 1B, 2C, 3E, 4E, 5F, 6E, and Fig. 8-4D).

The pattern of deep symmetric T-wave inversion has been called **non–Q-wave MI,** or "subendocardial MI", although it may occasionally be a result of completely reversible ischemia. It is

possible that there was unwitnessed ST elevation before the recording and that the ECG indicates reperfusion of complete coronary occlusion. Deep, symmetric T-wave inversion is usually preceded by, and is usually less recent than, terminal T-wave inversion (94,156). It is usually seen after the ST segment has nearly normalized. Mortality is lower than that in patients whose initial ECG manifests ST depression (160). T-wave inversions diagnostic of UA/NSTEMI (Type 2 ECG) are almost always associated with troponin elevation, and, if so, will ultimately be labeled a "non–Q-wave MI" if no Q waves develop. See Cases 8-12 and 8-14.

Management of Wellens' Syndrome

Management requires aggressive therapy for UA/NSTEMI (see Chapter 37). Consider immediate angiography ± PCI for refractory symptoms.

- **Monitor for reocclusion** (Fig. 8-5), ideally with continuous ST-segment monitoring. Terminal T-wave inversion may be dynamic, with repeated reocclusion and reperfusion. Reocclusion manifests as ST segment reelevation and normalization of terminal T-wave inversion, called **"pseudonormalization"**, because the T wave flips upright (see Cases 5-3d, 8–12).
- **Thrombolysis or angiography ± PCI are indicated** in cases of reocclusion.

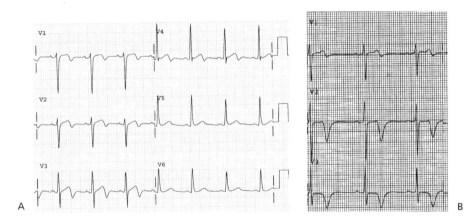

FIGURE 8-6. Wellens' syndrome. A: Pattern A as seen in leads V1–V6 in a patient with resolved CP. Twelve hours previously, the patient had CP and transient 4 mm ST elevation recorded in leads V2–V4, which then immediately and spontaneously resolved before reperfusion therapy. Nonemergent angiography revealed a 99% LAD stenosis. **B: Pattern B** as seen in leads V1–V6 exactly 22 hours after thrombolytics led to immediate reperfusion of anterior STEMI. A 90% proximal LAD stenosis was demonstrated.

CASE 8-1

Transient Precordial ST Depression Following Cardioversion of Ventricular Tachycardia

History

This 41-year-old man presented with 2 hours of weakness and palpitations with no CP. A rhythm strip showed ventricular tachycardia at a rate of 213 bpm. He was electrically cardioverted.

ECG 8-1 (Type 3 or Type 2)

Immediately after cardioversion

- Normal sinus rhythm, rate 100 bpm.
- ST depression: V2–V6, II, III, aVF.

Clinical Course

A repeat ECG recorded 7 minutes later was **normal**, which confirmed transient ST depression of cardioversion. The final diagnosis was idiopathic cardiomyopathy without CAD. Coronary arteries were large and normal.

Conclusion

Though this ECG may appear to represent posterior AMI, the findings are **transient**; reperfusion is **not** indicated.

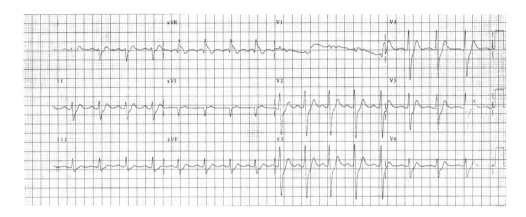

CASE 8-2

RVH That Is Almost Indistinguishable from Posterolateral STEMI

History
This 45-year-old woman presented with atypical CP.

ECG 8-2 (Type 1c)
- ST depression: V2–V5, maximal V2–V3; asymmetric T-wave inversion; and tall R waves: V1–V3, make this ECG **suspicious** for posterior AMI.
- ST elevation: aVL; and ST depression: II, III, aVF, are **suspicious** for lateral AMI.
- Very large, wide R wave: V1; right axis deviation; and S wave: I, V5–V6 are diagnostic of RVH.

Clinical Course
Previous ECGs confirmed no change. Serial CK-MB levels were normal and serial ECGs over 3 days were identical.

Conclusion
ST deviation and T-wave inversion may be a result of RVH. In the right clinical context, further evaluation with serial ECGs, ultrasound, or angiography would be indicated with this ECG.

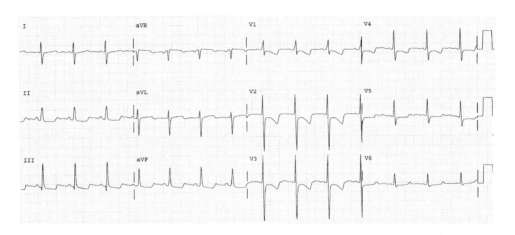

CASE 8-3

ST Abnormalities of WPW Following Conversion of PSVT Mimic Posterolateral AMI

History

This 21-year-old woman had just converted from paroxysmal supraventricular tachycardia (PSVT) at a rate of 217 bpm moments before ECG 8-3 was recorded.

ECG 8-3 (Type 3)

- ST elevation: aVL, with reciprocal depression in II, III, aVF is **suspicious** for lateral AMI.
- ST depression: V2–V6, deep; and tall R waves: V1–V3 are **suspicious** for posterior AMI.
- Very short PR interval (80 ms); and "delta waves" (slurred upstroke of R wave): II, III, aVF, make this ECG diagnostic of **WPW**.

Clinical Course

On a repeat ECG 15 minutes later, ST depression was largely resolved and serial cTnI were normal.

Conclusion

WPW may manifest ST depression. Transient ST depression is common after conversion from tachydysrhythmias. The two phenomena overlap on this ECG to produce profound ST abnormalities that mimic posterolateral STEMI.

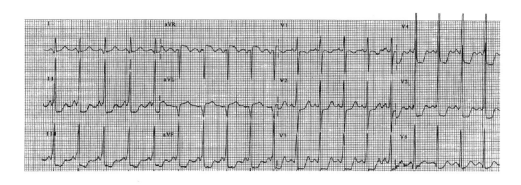

CASE 8-4

ST Depression and Tall R Waves Representing Posterior STEMI:
Brief, Limited Bedside Echocardiography Indicates Myocardial Rupture.

History

This 83-year-old man presented with CP.

ECG 8-4 (Type 1b)

- Tall R waves: V1–V3; ST depression: V1–V3; and borderline ST elevation: V5–V6 and aVL make this ECG diagnostic of **posterior AMI.**

Clinical Course

A brief, routine bedside echocardiogram detected a large amount of unsuspected pericardial fluid. Clinicians sus-pected myocardial rupture, withheld thrombolytics, and sent the patient for emergency surgical repair. Angiography revealed circumflex occlusion with posterior AMI. The patient survived and was discharged with good cardiac and cerebral function.

Conclusion

ST depression in V1–V3, especially with an upright T wave, is diagnostic of posterior AMI. Such "reciprocal" ST elevation indicates transmural ischemia due to coronary occlusion and can lead to myocardial rupture.

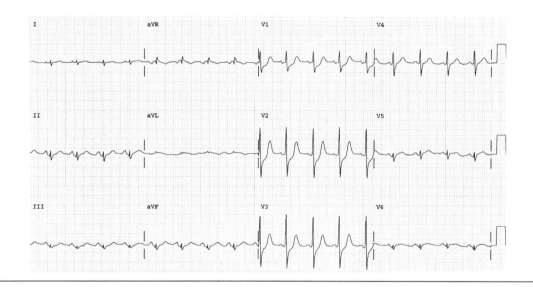

CASE 8-5

Primary ST Depression of Reversible Ischemia
Misread as ST Depression Purely Secondary to LVH

History

This 69-year-old woman presented with nausea, dyspnea, hypoxia, and worsening CHF. She had a history of diabetes, severe CAD, and was status post-rotary ablation of three LAD lesions. She had experienced no CP with previous ischemic episodes.

ECG 8-5 (Type 2)

Day 1, meets criteria for LVH.

■ ST depression: V3–V6, downsloping; the computer and the cardiologist read this as LVH.

■ **Concordant ST depression** V3 (in the same direction as the majority of the QRS). This is a strong indication that the ST depression is due to **ischemia**, not LVH. The ST depression in V4–V6 is also **disproportionate** to the QRS

voltage and thus **should not be assumed to be due to LVH only.**

Clinical Course

Echocardiography revealed acute lateral and apical WMA but no LVH. CTnI peaked at 1.1 ng/mL, indicative of a non–Q-wave MI. Angiography revealed new 90% stenosis of the first diagonal artery and of the obtuse marginal artery. The patient underwent three-vessel CABG. An ECG on Day 4 (not shown) showed complete resolution of both ST depression and the WMA.

Conclusion

Although this ST depression, at first glance, appears to be secondary to LVH, there are characteristics indicative of primary ST depression due to ischemia.

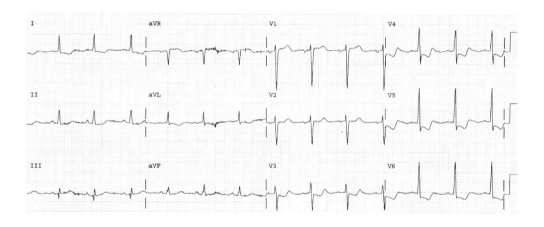

CASE 8-6

Dynamic ST Depression in V2–V6, Maximal in V4–V6, Due to Anterior UA/NSTEMI

History

This 50-year-old man presented with 24 hours of CP that was never completely relieved by 24 NTG tablets. Prior angiography had revealed a 60% LAD lesion proximal to the first diagonal artery with diffuse distal disease as well, a 60% RCA lesion, and diffuse disease of the circumflex artery.

ECG 8-6 (Type 2)

- Diffuse ST depression: **not** maximal in V1–V4; therefore moderately likely to represent posterior AMI. Thrombolytics are **not** indicated.

Clinical Course

Clinicians treated the patient for UA/NSTEMI. Symptoms resolved but then recurred. The patient underwent immediate angioplasty of a 95% LAD lesion and ruled out for MI by CK-MB. Echocardiography revealed an anteroapical WMA.

Conclusion

Precordial ST depression maximal in lateral precordial leads is often due to anterior wall UA/NSTEMI. Thrombolytics are not indicated; emergent angiography ± PCI is indicated for ischemia refractory to medical therapy.

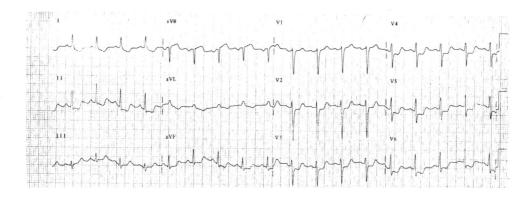

CASE 8-7

ST Depression of Anterolateral Ischemia Due to Secondary Causes

History

This 67-year-old woman was found comatose, severely dehydrated. P = 130 to 140 bpm, BP = 220 mm Hg systolic.

ECG 8-7 (Type 2)

■ ST depression: 2 mm, V2–V6, maximal V3–V5.

■ ST depression: 1 mm, II, III, aVF.

Clinical Course

Following rehydration and lowering of P and BP, a repeat ECG showed ST resolution. Subsequent echocardiography showed no WMA and cTnI peaked at 2.0 ng/mL.

Conclusion

Ischemic ST depression of primary causes (ACS) and secondary causes are indistinguishable. The response to fluids indicates a secondary etiology, rather than ACS; that is, it was not due to unstable coronary plaque.

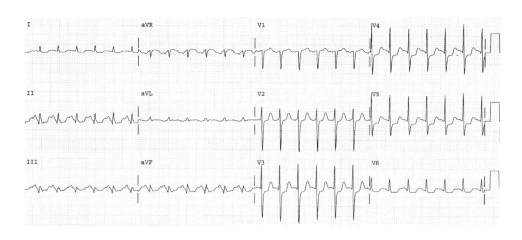

ST Depression Due to Subarachnoid Hemorrhage

History
This 40-year-old woman presented with severe headache and CP.

ECG 8-8 (Type 3)
- Very prolonged QT_c interval (approximately 600 ms).
- ST depression: V2–V6, maximal V2–V3, is **suspicious** for posterior AMI. LVH is also present.

Clinical Course
A repeat ECG showed resolution of ST depression and new T-wave inversions in inferior leads, consistent with **reperfusion of inferoposterior non—Q-wave AMI**. CT scan of the patient's head was diagnostic of subarachnoid hemorrhage, cTnI peaked at 3.0 ng/mL, and echocardiography performed after the resolution of ST depression showed no WMA.

Conclusion
Subarachnoid hemorrhage may manifest ST depression that mimics posterior AMI. It may also result in cardiac ischemia and injury in the absence of ACS or coronary spasm. The QT interval is frequently very prolonged.

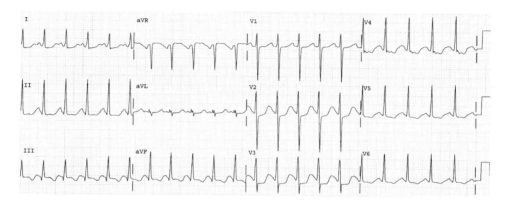

T-Wave Inversion as a Result of Subarachnoid Hemorrhage

History
This 60-year-old woman presented with sudden severe headache and dizziness. Her previous ECG was normal.

ECG 8-9 (Type 2)
Prolonged QT_c (483 ms)
- T-wave inversion: I, aVL, V2–V6; no ST elevation or depression.

Clinical Course
A head CT scan revealed subarachnoid hemorrhage, and cerebral angiography revealed anterior communicating artery aneurysm. CTnI was 9.8 ng/mL. Coronary angiography was normal.

Conclusion
Subarachnoid hemorrhage can result in T-wave inversion and elevated cTnI in the absence of coronary disease.

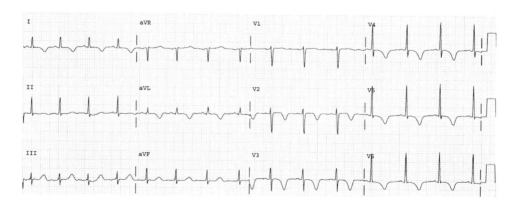

CASE 8-10

T-Wave Inversion Due to Pulmonary Embolus

History
This 44-year-old man, status post circumflex artery and LAD stent for UA, presented with 12 hours of severe left-sided CP similar to his previous angina. His previous ECG was normal.

ECG 8-10 (Type 2)
Prolonged QT$_c$ (480 ms)
- Sinus tachycardia
- T-wave inversion: **V1–V3**, without ST elevation or depression, is suggestive of anterior wall ischemia.

Clinical Course
Echocardiography revealed normal LV function, inferior WMA, and RV dysfunction. Right heart catheterization and angiography revealed a large pulmonary embolus. CTnI was 1.6 ng/mL.

Conclusion
Pulmonary embolus may result in T-wave inversion.

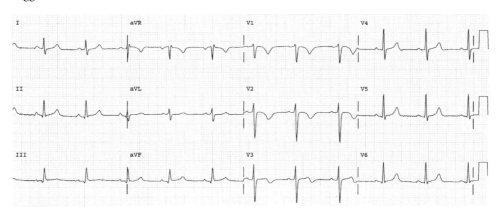

CASE 8-11

Large Flipped T Waves of Stokes-Adams Attack

History
This 75-year-old man presented with syncope. A previous ECG showed LBBB.

ECG 8-11 (Type 2)
Prolonged QT$_c$ (482 ms), bradycardia with third-degree AV block, RBBB.

■ T-wave inversion: V1–V4, wide and bizarre; T waves typical of Stokes-Adams attacks.

Conclusion
Alternating LBBB and RBBB suggest intermittent complete AV block associated with Stokes-Adams attacks, with which such T-wave inversions may be associated. The etiology is uncertain.

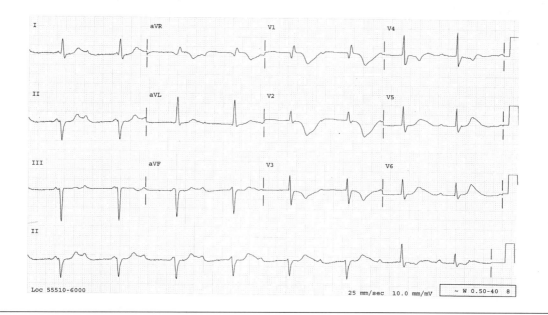

Loc 55510-6000   25 mm/sec   10.0 mm/mV   ~ W 0.50-40   8

CASE 8-12

Pseudonormalization of Deeply Inverted T Waves

History
This 49-year-old man presented with CP.

ECG 8-12a (Type 2)
- T-wave inversion: II, III, aVF, V4–V6; probable previous inferolateral (non–Q-wave) MI.
- Tall R wave and large T wave: V2, possible posterior (non–Q-wave) MI.
- This ECG shows non–Q-wave MI, probably due to subacute or remote reperfusion. Reperfusion is probably not acute (less than 2 hours), because T waves are symmetrically inverted, not terminally inverted. The patient's CP continued.

ECG 8-12b (Type 1a)
20 minutes later shows **reocclusion**
- Upright T waves: II, III, aVF, and V4–V6 is **pseudonormalization.**

- ST elevation: II, III, aVF, also V5, V6, diagnostic of **inferolateral AMI.**
- Inverted T waves and ST depression: V2, V3 diagnostic of **posterior AMI.**

Clinical Course
Angiography demonstrated a spontaneously reperfusing thrombotic occlusion of a dominant RCA, which was opened and stented. Serial troponins were ultimately normal.

Conclusion
These ECGs indicate dynamic occlusion and spontaneous reperfusion occurring before acute necrosis but overlaying a baseline of previous MI.

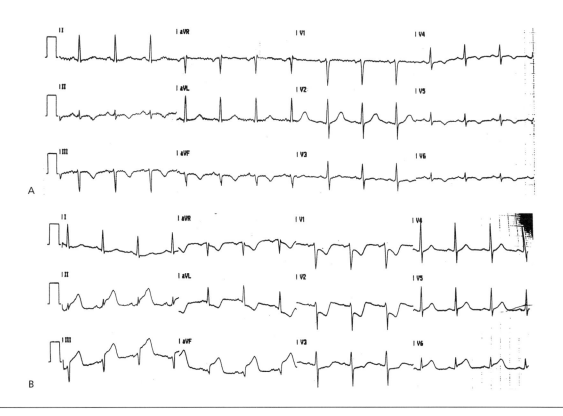

CASE 8-13

Prolonged CP and ST Elevation: QS waves with T-wave inversions are consistent with prolonged duration of AMI (similar to Case 33-7)

History

This 37-year-old man presented with 30 hours of CP following cocaine use. He had presented to another ED 24 hours earlier and was discharged without an ECG.

ECG 8-13 (Type 1d)

- ST elevation: V1–V3, is diagnostic of **anterior MI**.
- QS waves: V1–V3; inverted T waves: V2–V5. These findings are consistent with prolonged symptoms and indicate either a **completed, subacute MI, or late reperfusion**.
- Notice that ST elevation is not resolved.

Clinical Course

Total CK was 4,819 IU/L at the time of ECG 8-13 and peaked at 5,615 IU/L. CTnI 5.5 hours later was 256 ng/mL. Angioplasty opened an occluded LAD.

Conclusion

Despite ST elevation, **thrombolytics are NOT indicated**. The duration of coronary occlusion is too prolonged, as indicated by symptom duration and confirmed by the lack of ECG acuteness, as indicated by the presence of QS waves and T-wave inversions.

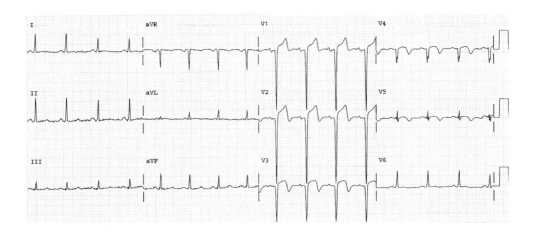

CASE 8-14

Wide and Deeply Inverted T Waves of Non–Q-Wave MI

History
This 67-year-old woman presented with dyspnea, CHF, and femoral artery occlusion. An angiogram 2 weeks earlier for CP had revealed diffuse moderate coronary disease and an echocardiogram was without WMA.

ECG 8-14 (Type 2)
■ New, deep, wide symmetric T-wave inversions: V1–V6, II, III, aVF; no ST elevation, no posterior AMI (no anterior ST depression); QT_c prolonged at 510 ms.

Clinical Course
Echocardiography showed a **new** WMA affecting anterolateral, distal, septal, and apical areas, with moderately decreased systolic function. Symptoms improved with medical therapy. CTnI peaked at 1.7 ng/mL (normal < 0.3 ng/mL). Repeat echocardiography showed WMA resolution. In later ECGs, T-wave inversion continued but was shallower. No angiography was done. Thus it is uncertain whether the electrocardiographic and echocardiographic evidence of ischemia is due to ACS or to perhaps sympathetic overload from respiratory distress.

Conclusion
This T-wave inversion resulted from mostly reversible ischemia, with a small non–Q-wave MI. Angiography ± PCI would be indicated for symptoms refractory to medical therapy (see Chapter 37).

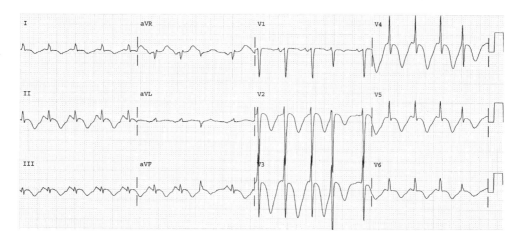

ANNOTATED BIBLIOGRAPHY

More literature on reciprocal ST depression, and ST depression of posterior AMI, can be found in Chapter 7 (23,84,112,128,**142**,143), Chapter 12 (132–137), Chapter 13 (138–141), and Chapter 16. Literature on management of patients with ST depression and T-wave inversion who are not thrombolytic candidates (UA/NSTEMI) can be found in Chapter 37.

High Mortality of ST Depression
Schechtman KB, et al. Risk stratification of patients with non–Q-wave myocardial infarction: the critical role of ST segment depression, 1989.

Methods: Schechtman et al. (147) studied the ECGs of 515 patients who survived hospitalization for non–Q-wave AMI. The ST segment was measured at 80 msec after the J point and ST depression was defined as ≥ 1 mm. If an old ECG was available (50% of patients), a 1-mm change was required. If LVH criteria were present, 2 mm of ST depression was required.

Findings: One-year adjusted mortality was 5.5% in patients with **no** ST depression of ≥ 1 mm, 10.1% in those with either admission or discharge ST depression, and 22.2% (26 of 117) in those with both admission and discharge ST depression.

The FTT Collaborative Group, Indications for fibrinolytic therapy in suspected acute myocardial infarction: collaborative overview of early mortality and major morbidity results from all randomized trials of more than 1,000 patients, 1994.

Methods: The FTT Collaborative Group (30) analyzed data from nine trials of thrombolytic versus control in patients with suspected AMI (see Appendix C). Each trial had more than 1,000 patients, and the vast majority of patients were confirmed for AMI.

Findings: **Thirty-five-day mortality of patients with ST depression was very high** (14.5%); this was higher than mortality in patients with inferior or "other" infarction, and nearly as high as in patients with anterior infarction. Mortality was not decreased by thrombolytic therapy.

Lee HS, et al. Patients with suspected myocardial infarction who present with ST depression, 1993.

Methods: Lee et al. (146) studied 136 consecutive patients with suspected AMI and ST depression ≥ 1 mm **at the J point, AND** a horizontal or downsloping ST segment, and no ST elevation. They then measured the ST segment at 80 msec after the J point.

Findings: Of 136 patients, 74 (54%) were ruled in for AMI by CK-MB. One-year mortality was 35% for patients who did not receive thrombolytics (*n* = 49) versus 24% for those who did (*n* = 25). **Mortality and incidence of MI were much higher if the ST depression**

> 2 mm or manifested in three leads or more. These patients were older and more likely to have previous MI. One-year mortality for patients with ST depression ≥ 2 mm was 39%, and for patients with ST depression in **three leads or more** it was 30%; mortality for those with 1 mm ST depression or ST depression in two leads or less was 14% and 11%, respectively.

Savonitto S, et al. Prognostic value of the admission electrocardiogram in acute coronary syndromes, 1999.

Methods: Savonitto et al. (142) retrospectively studied the presenting ECGs and the clinical course of 12,142 patients in the GUSTO-IIb trial (comparing heparin to desirudin), who had symptoms of cardiac ischemia at rest. ECG signs of ischemia (ST elevation or depression ≥ 0.5 mm, or T-wave inversion of > 1 mm) were required for entry.

Findings: T-wave inversion (without ST elevation) was present on 22%; ST elevation, on 28%; ST depression only on 35%; and both ST elevation and depression in 15% of presenting ECGs. Thus 43% had any ST elevation (62% of whom received thrombolytics) and 50% had any ST depression. Incidence of AMI, as measured by elevated total CK at 16 hours, and 30-day mortality (with independent risk of death relative to T-wave inversion only) was:

■ **32% and 5.5%** (1.00 independent risk, IR, of death) **for patients with T-wave inversion**
■ 81% and 9.4% (1.68 IR, CI: 1.36–2.08) for those with ST elevation
■ **48% and 10.5% (1.62, IR, CI: 1.32–1.98) for those with ST depression only**
■ 89% and 12.4% (2.27, CI: 1.80–2.86) for those with ST elevation **and** ST depression.

Thrombolytics for ST Depression

(See also Chapters 7 and 16.) Most patients with ST depression are older, have a history of MI, and have severe coronary disease and a poor prognosis (161). Autopsy studies in the prereperfusion era (162) show that most patients with subendocardial infarction had ST depression on the presenting ECG and many had previous MI. In clinical trials, thrombolytics have not been proven beneficial for patients with ischemic syndromes and ST depression (UA/NSTEMI) (30,**163, 164**). Therefore thrombolytics are generally not indicated for ST depression alone. However, these trials included unselected patients: any age, with or without previous MI or known severe CAD, with ST depression in only one lead, in any location, and of any depth (161). **Thus their findings do not necessarily apply to the previously healthy patient with persistent isolated ST depression in V1–V4 (indicative of posterior STEMI), a group for whom no randomized trial of thrombolytics has been done.** The basis for thrombolytics in these patients is rationale, not proof, and is based on surrogate endpoints (other than mortality endpoints in randomized trials) and on data demonstrating that the etiology of their syndrome is usually occlusion of the coronary artery supplying the posterior wall. See Chapter 16.

White HD, et al. Effects of streptokinase in patients presenting within 6 hours of prolonged chest pain with ST segment depression, 1995.

Methods: White et al. (165) randomized 112 patients with ischemic CP and ST depression ≥ 1 mm in any one lead, without ST elevation, to SK or placebo. Only 63% of patients received aspirin (equal in both groups).

Findings: Thirty-day and 1-year endpoints (death, AMI, early angiography, or positive exercise test) were the same in both groups, 82% and 75%, respectively. ST depression ≥ 3 mm was 90% specific for AMI.

FTT Collaborative Group

The FTT Collaborative Group (30) is described earlier. (Also see Appendix C.)

Findings: ECG analysis revealed no significant difference between treatment with thrombolytics (mostly SK) and that with placebo for patients with ST depression. However, patients were not differentiated according to location, depth, or **persistence** of ST depression.

Roberts MJD, et al. Double-blind randomized trial of alteplase versus placebo in patients with chest pain at rest, 1993.

Methods: Roberts et al. (164) randomized 80 patients with CP at rest and ST depression ≥ 1 mm in any lead to immediate treatment with tPA versus placebo. Angiography was performed in 73 patients.

Findings: There was no significant difference in outcome or angiographic parameters.

Anderson HV, et al. One-year results of the Thrombolysis in Myocardial Infarction (TIMI) IIIB clinical trial: a randomised comparison of tissue-type plasminogen activator versus placebo and early invasive versus early conservative strategies in unstable angina and non-Q wave myocardial infarction, 1995.

Methods: The TIMI investigators, in the TIMI-IIIA (99) and TIMI-IIIB (see Anderson et al. [163] and TIMI IIIB Investigators [166]) randomized 306 and 1,473 patients, respectively, with ischemic-type CP at rest and **either** ECG changes diagnostic of ischemia but not diagnostic of STEMI **or** known CAD (these are typical entry criteria into UA trials) to tPA or placebo along with standard therapy for ACS. In TIMI-IIIB, they further randomized patients to early invasive management (coronary angiography at 18 to 48 hours followed by revascularization if appropriate) versus early conservative management (without routine angiography or revascularization). **Patients with ongoing or recurrent ischemia were excluded because they all underwent angiography.**

Findings: ST depression was present in 32%. In TIMI-IIIA there was modest improvement in the culprit lesion with the use of tPA. However, there was no difference between tPA and placebo in the combined clinical endpoint of death, AMI, or provokable ischemia at 6 weeks (166). Nor did TIMI-IIIB demonstrate a 1-year mortality difference between early conservative or early invasive treatment (163). However, time to angioplasty was not immediate, and patients with early invasive treatment had shorter hospital stays, fewer readmissions, less ischemia, and fewer subsequent symptoms. By the end of the year, the numbers in each group who had undergone invasive management was approximately equal. **Thus in this study, thrombolytics were not beneficial for UA/NSTEMI, but early invasive management may be the preferred strategy. For patients with ongoing or recurrent ischemia, invasive management is clearly preferred.**

Langer A, et al. Late Assessment of Thrombolytic Efficacy (LATE) Study: Prognosis in patients with non-Q wave myocardial infarction, 1996; and Braunwald E, et al. Non-Q-wave and ST segment depression myocardial infarction: Is there a role for thrombolytic therapy? 1996.

Methods: Langer et al. (167), with Braunwald et al. (168), performed a post hoc analysis of data from the LATE trial (169) (see Appendix C).

Findings: Of 5,711 patients, 1,480 patients presented with ST depression without elevation; 4,759 of 5,711 patients (83%) ruled in for AMI by a CK enzyme level twice normal. Of these 4,759, 1,309 (28%) had non–Q-wave AMI, of whom 528 (40%) had **isolated ST depression ≥ 2 mm.** Thirty-five-day mortality in this group was 8.6% (tPA) versus 16.6% (placebo). One-year mortality was 20.1% (tPA) versus 31.9% (placebo). In fact, this analysis indicated that **ALL the benefit of tPA demonstrated in the LATE study was in this subgroup of isolated ST depression ≥ 2 mm.** Patients with ST elevation who were treated more than 6 hours following the onset of symptoms appeared not to benefit.

Anatomic Significance of ST Depression

See references in Chapter 16 .

T-Wave Inversion

See Chapter 27 for discussion of T-wave inversion and its relation to persistently occluded or reperfused coronary arteries after AMI.

De Zwaan C, et al. Angiographic and clinical characteristics of patients with unstable angina showing an ECG pattern indicating critical narrowing of the proximal LAD coronary artery, 1989.

Methods: In follow-up to their previous study (153), de Zwaan et al. (152) studied the 180 patients, out of 1,260 consecutive admissions for UA, who had abnormal ST segments and negative T waves in

V2–V3 in the absence of pathologic Q waves. Most also had the same findings in V1 and V4, and sometimes V5–V6. In 108, the findings were present at admission; in 72, they developed while in the hospital. Because 75% of such patients went on to anterior AMI in the authors' previous series (153), all patients underwent aggressive therapy, including early revascularization.

Findings: Forty-four patients manifested "pattern A" (terminal) T-wave inversion (isoelectric or minimally elevated takeoff of the ST segment and a symmetrically inverted T wave) and 136 patients manifested "pattern B" (takeoff of the ST segment below the isoelectric line followed by a convex ST segment passing into a deep, symmetrically inverted T wave). **All patients had abnormalities of the LAD, with mean stenosis of 85%. Collateral circulation was present in all 33 totally obstructed arteries.** A small increase in total CK (mean, 294 IU/L) was found in 21 patients.

Comment: If this study was repeated in the troponin era, it is likely that nearly all would have a positive troponin. Because Wellens was the senior author of both papers, the term *Wellens' syndrome* was coined (154).

Thrombolytics for T-Wave Inversion
Langer et al. (167) (see earlier).

Findings: There was no benefit of thrombolytics for patients with T-wave inversions alone (i.e., without concurrent ST elevation or depression) in two leads or more.

The FTT Collaborative Group
The FTT Collaborative Group (30) is described earlier. (Also see Appendix C.)

Findings: Thrombolytic therapy provided no significant benefit to 10,000 patients with "other abnormalities," which included inverted T waves or some other nonspecific pattern suggestive of acute ischemia.

9

SUBTLE ECG ABNORMALITIES AND HYPERACUTE T WAVES

KEY POINTS

Look for borderline ST elevation and hyperacute T waves.
- When AMI is possible but the ECG is subtle:
  - Compare with a previous ECG.
  - Obtain serial ECGs at 15-minute intervals OR use continuous ST-segment monitoring OR monitor with rhythm leads III and MCL$_{2-3}$.
  - Use additional diagnostic tools (echocardiography, angiography, biomarkers).

GENERAL BACKGROUND

Subtle ECG abnormalities include **borderline ST elevation and hyperacute T waves.** These findings may represent STEMI but do not necessarily fit the "criteria" for thrombolytics developed from major placebo-controlled thrombolytic trials. Although, on average, patients with lower ST segments have lower overall mortality than those with a high ST score (see Chapter 6), there is great individual variability. These patients may have significant mortality and morbidity and should receive reperfusion therapy if the diagnosis is certain. Moreover, the ECG in a very large AMI may be subtle simply because the ECG is recorded **early** after coronary occlusion. Computer algorithms vary, but all have inadequate sensitivity for STEMI. The sensitivity of one was only 62%; its use would lead to significant undertreatment with thrombolytics (41).

BORDERLINE ST ELEVATION

ST elevation ≥ 1 mm in two consecutive leads is considered a criterion for thrombolysis (105), although some studies required 2 mm or greater in precordial leads (86). In leads **V1–V4,** ANY ST elevation < 2 mm is borderline. However, **ST elevation < 1 to 2 mm may indicate AMI** (see Chapter 6 for details).

Key Considerations in Borderline ST Elevation

- **Upward convexity** strongly suggests AMI; upward concavity **may** be AMI.
- With **low QRS voltage,** ST elevation < 1 mm may be diagnostic. This frequently occurs in lead aVL. (See Chapter 14 and Fig. 6-2q.)
- **Early** in the course of AMI, ST elevation may be minimal; serial ECGs are critical.
- The presence of **reciprocal ST depression** makes minimal ST elevation much more significant and much more likely to represent AMI.
- **Any ST elevation may be an AMI** if a patient's baseline ECG has an isoelectric (or nearly isoelectric) ST segment, even if the ST elevation appears to be early repolarization. Obtain previous ECGs, serial ECGs, or both.
- When the ST segment is **depressed** on a baseline ECG, minimal elevation may be ≥ 1 mm of **change,** and this may be diagnostic.
- **Lateral ST elevation** is commonly missed; therefore lateral AMI is commonly missed.

Confounding Conditions

LVH, ventricular aneurysm, and pericarditis may cause ST elevation that mimics AMI (see Chapters 22 to 24). **Early repolarization** is the most common confounding condition; it may also have ≥ 2 mm of ST elevation at baseline. In contrast with subtle ST elevation of AMI, the **ST elevation of early repolarization:**

- Is highest in V3–V4, up to 3 mm (rarely ever higher).
- Is upwardly concave, not convex.
- Shows J-point elevation.
- Rarely occurs with a low-voltage QRS.
- Is rarely > 1 mm in lateral precordial leads.
- Is more pronounced in younger individuals; seldom > 2 mm in people more than 45 years of age.
- Is not seen in aVL.

See Cases 9-1 to 9-5 for examples of subtle STEMI. (See also Case 7-6 of a subtle lateral AMI with reciprocal changes; Case 3-3 of subtle inferior ST elevation superimposed on inferior Q-wave MI; Case 14-3 of subtle lateral AMI; and Case 11-2 of tiny Q waves that help to make the diagnosis of **acute anterior MI**.)

HYPERACUTE T WAVES

Alteration in T-wave morphology and/or amplitude may be the first ECG sign of coronary occlusion. "Hyperacute T waves" may form as soon as 2 minutes after experimental or clinical coronary occlusion, as follows (**170,171**,172–175,**176**).

- The first change may be merely an **oblique straightening** of the ST segment (see leads V2 and V3 of ECG 9-5a) (1).
- There may be **subtle enlargement** of the T wave, disproportionate to the QRS; that is, with low QRS voltage, a small T wave may be hyperacute (see Case 3-2) (1).
- Hyperacute T waves are often **bulky and wide,** without much upward concavity (**176**,177,178) and are **localized** to the area of infarct.

- The QT interval is usually prolonged.
- **The J point may become depressed** and the ST segment upsloping, with the T wave appearing to have its take-off below the isoelectric line (see Cases 9-6 and 9-7) (1,88).

Hyperacute T waves are distinct from T waves due to **early repolarization,** which show more upward concavity than hyperacute T waves and are asymmetric (steeper downward than upward). Hyperacute T waves typically are NOT narrow based, peaked, and tented, as are the T waves of **hyperkalemia,** which also have a short QT interval in the absence of QRS prolongation; check the potassium level.

We classify an **ECG with hyperacute T waves as a Type 1b ECG, for which reperfusion therapy may be indicated** (105). See Cases 9-1 and 9-5 through 9-9 for examples of hyperacute T waves. (See also Case 3-2 of a very subtle hyperacute T wave in lead aVL; Case 7-6 of a hyperacute T wave in aVL; Case 12-5 of hyperacute T waves mimicking early repolarization; Case 24-7 of a large AMI with hyperacute T waves that was misdiagnosed as pericarditis; Case 18-12 of LBBB with developing hyperacute T waves and ST elevation; and Case 10-1 of subtle hyperacute T waves [ECG Type 1c] developing into ST elevation on a repeat ECG.)

CASE 9-1

A Type 3 ECG Followed by a Type 1b ECG: the Change Is Especially Diagnostic

History

This 48-year-old obese woman with diabetes mellitus (DM) and hyperlipidemia presented with atypical CP.

ECG 9-1A (Type 3)

At 03:21.

- Nonspecific, poor R-wave progression. The patient's CP continued. She was admitted to the CCU before serial ECGs were recorded.

ECG 9-1B (Type 1b)

At 05:52.

- ST elevation: V1–V3 (1 mm at the J point but 2 mm at 80 ms after the J point); and hyperacute T waves: V2 V5,

definitely new. **This ECG alone is diagnostic of AMI but is especially remarkable when compared with ECG 9-1a.**

Clinical Course

Although the computer printout read "consider anterior infarct," clinicians interpreted ECG 9-1b as normal. Anterior AMI was obvious on a follow-up ECG, and a distal 100% LAD occlusion was opened with angioplasty at 12:00 hours. Total CK peaked 20 hours after presentation at 700 IU/L with cTnI of 16.8 ng/mL.

Conclusion

Immediate angiography ± PCI is indicated.

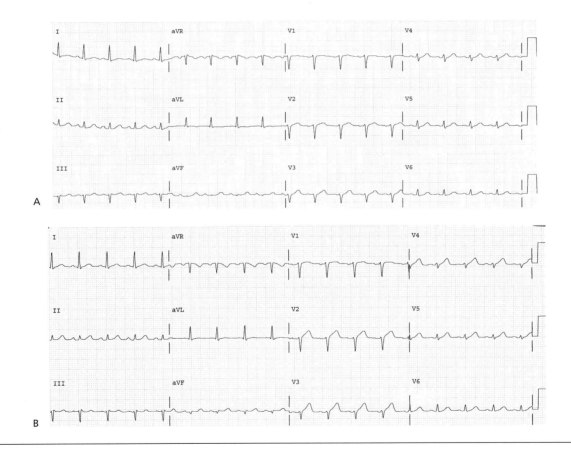

CASE 9-2

Anterior AMI Misdiagnosed as Early Repolarization

History
This 62-year-old non–English-speaking woman presented with CP.

ECG 9-2A (Type 4)
This is a previous ECG of leads V1–V3 only; this was available but not sought for comparison.

■ There is NO ST elevation.

ECG 9-2B (Type 1b, but Type 1a when compared with previous ECG)

■ ST elevation: V1–V3 (2 mm at the J point but 4 mm at 80 ms after the J point), is **diagnostic of anterior AMI by itself,** but especially when compared with ECG 9-2A.

Due to the elevated J point and upward concavity, clinicians misdiagnosed this as early repolarization.

Clinical Course
The patient was admitted to the CCU. A repeat ECG showed increased ST elevation. After thrombolysis, ST segments completely normalized to baseline. Subsequent reocclusion was treated with LAD angioplasty. Convalescent EF was 50%.

Conclusion
Reperfusion therapy was delayed 90 minutes because of misdiagnosis as early repolarization. Comparison with ECG 9-3A would have made the diagnosis obvious.

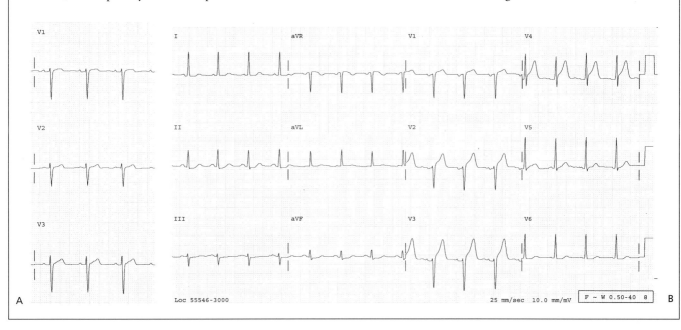

A   Loc 55546-3000   25 mm/sec   10.0 mm/mV   F ~ W 0.50-40 8   B

CASE 9-3

Subtle Inferoposterior AMI

History

This 41-year-old man with risk factors for AMI presented with typical CP.

ECG 9-3 (Type 1b)

- ST elevation: almost 1 mm, II, III; very large T waves; slight ST elevation with low QRS voltage: aVF; reciprocal depression: aVL. This ECG is diagnostic of **inferior AMI.**
- ST depression: minimal, V2–V4, is **suspicious** for posterior AMI.

Clinical Course

The computer algorithm and clinicians missed this AMI. A repeat ECG 80 minutes later showed more pronounced changes and tPA was given. Echocardiography revealed an inferoposterior WMA but good LV function. An ECG the next day revealed inferior QS waves. Total CK peaked at 1,363 IU/L. Angioplasty opened a tight mid-circumflex stenosis.

Conclusion

Reperfusion therapy was delayed due to failure to diagnose a subtle inferior posterior AMI.

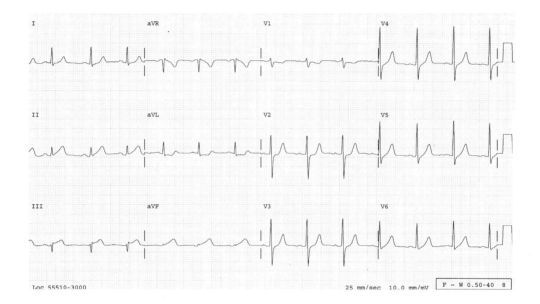

Loc 55510-3000   25 mm/sec   10.0 mm/mV   F ~ W 0.50-40 8

CASE 9-4

Subtle Infero-Lateral Posterior AMI

History

This 65-year-old woman presented with 2 hours of typical CP.

ECG 9-4A (Type 1c)

■ Left anterior fascicular block (LAFB) (see Chapter 17).
■ ST elevation: subtle, II, III, aVF, I, V5–V6; reciprocal depression: subtle, aVL, V1–V3. This ECG is **suspicious** for a subtle infero-lateral-posterior AMI.

ECG 9-4B (Type 3)

A previous ECG was obtained.
■ LAFB; and ST segments are isoelectric at baseline. Comparison with this ECG confirms that ECG 9-4a is diagnostic of **infero-lateral posterior AMI.**

Clinical Course

Clinicians did not recognize this AMI. An ECG recorded 20 minutes later showed 1-mm ST elevation in II, III, aVF with increased reciprocal depression, but it was overlooked again. At 14 hours after pain onset, cTnI peaked at 63 ng/mL and total CK at 1,150 IU/L. Although indicated, reperfusion therapy was not administered. Angiography 36 hours after presentation showed that the circumflex consisted predominantly of a large second obtuse marginal, which was occluded with thrombus. It could not be opened with angioplasty and thus was treated with a GP IIb–IIIa inhibitor.

Conclusion

Clinicians missed this infero-lateral posterior AMI despite typical symptoms, comparison with an old ECG, and a follow-up ECG.

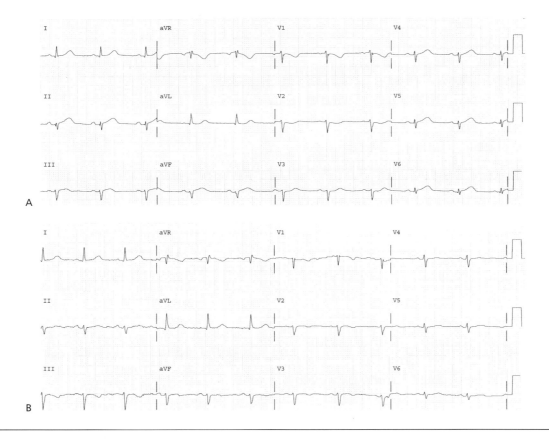

CASE 9-5

Subtle Anterior AMI

History
This 81-year-old man presented with less than 1 hour of typical CP.

ECG 9-5A (Type 1c)
- LAFB: right axis deviation and large S waves: II, III, aVF (see Chapter 17).

- Notice the minimally elevated J point: V1–V3; this could be normal.
- Large T wave: V2, **suspicious** for possibly being hyperacute; T wave: V1 is larger than in V6, favoring AMI over early repolarization; and septal Q wave: V2, is also suspicious.

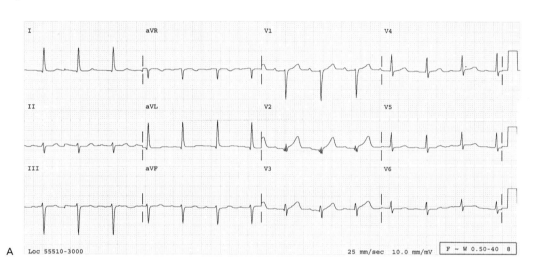

A   Loc 55510-3000   25 mm/sec 10.0 mm/mV   F ~ W 0.50-40 8

(continued on next page)

CASE 9-5

Subtle Anterior AMI *(continued)*

ECG 9-5B (Type 3)

A previous ECG was obtained; V1–V6 only shown.

■ **ST segments are isoelectric** at baseline. Comparison with this previous ECG enabled clinicians to determine that ECG 9-5A was diagnostic of **anterior AMI.**

Clinical Course

Thrombolytics were administered. An ECG recorded after reperfusion therapy was identical to ECG 9-5B (the baseline ECG), with no Q waves, and a normalized T wave in V2.

Troponin (cTnI) and total CK were confirmatory but minimally elevated. Convalescent echocardiography revealed no WMA and normal LV function.

Conclusion

So little myocardium was lost in this rapidly treated AMI that there were no lingering repolarization abnormalities, such as T-wave inversion. **Timely diagnosis and treatment in this case were facilitated by recognition of subtle signs of AMI and prompt comparison with a previous ECG.**

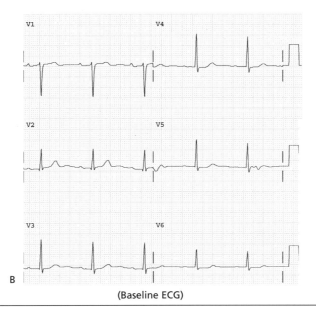

(Baseline ECG)

CASE 9-6

Hyperacute T Waves and Depressed ST Takeoff Not Recognized

History

This 42-year-old man presented with 45 minutes of CP.

ECG 9-6A (Type 2)

At 10:40, 40 minutes after arrival

- Disproportionately large T waves: V2–V4; and ST depression: V2–V6 are **suspicious** for anterior AMI. Frequent serial ECGs are indicated.

Clinical Course

Clinicians did not suspect AMI and did not record frequent serial ECGs. The patient was admitted to the CCU. Although tPA was ultimately administered 5.25 hours after pain onset, the ECG that prompted thrombolytic therapy was not found.

ECG 9-6B

The patient ruled in for a large anterior MI with deep Q waves, V1–V5. Echocardiography revealed a new anteroseptal and apical WMA.

Conclusion

Hyperacute T waves may be preceded by a depressed takeoff of the ST segment (see also ECG 9-7A). Diagnosis and thrombolysis of this extensive anterior AMI were delayed by hours because the significance of the ST segments and T waves was not appreciated. Earlier repeat ECGs are indicated.

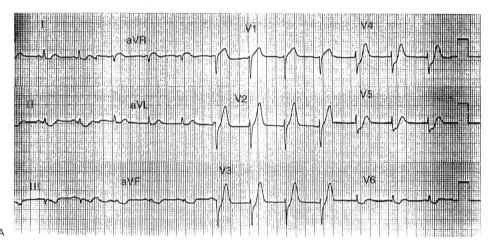

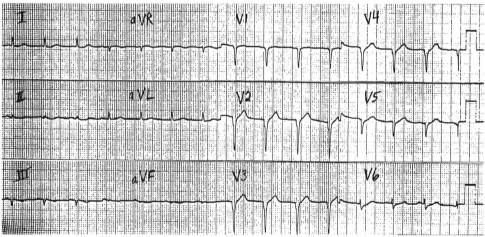

CASE 9-7

Classic Hyperacute T Waves, Also with Depressed ST Takeoff

History
This 56-year-old man presented with CP of short duration.

ECG 9-7A (Type 1b)
- ST elevation: minimal, V1 only; and profound hyperacute T waves: V2–V3 are diagnostic of **anterior AMI.**

ECG 9-7B (Type 1a)
Twelve minutes later
- ST elevation: V2–V4; subtle but diagnostic of **anterior AMI.**

Clinical Course
An ECG 27 minutes later had 4 mm of anterior ST elevation. Thrombolysis resulted in successful reperfusion, with a small elevation of CK-MB and no complications.

Conclusion
Clinicians' suspicion of AMI and confirmation with a serial ECG enabled timely thrombolysis and minimization of myocardial damage.

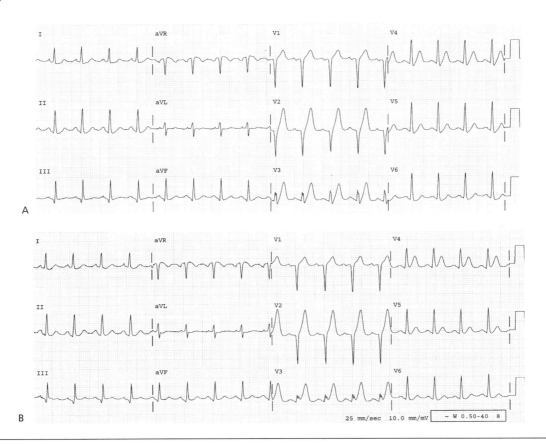

CASE 9-8

Hyperacute T Waves with LVH, Obscured by Half Standard Calibration

History

This 36-year-old diabetic man presented with 45 minutes of CP.

ECG 9-8A (Type 1b)

At 14:46, is half standard calibration in the precordial leads (0.1 mV = 0.5 mm amplitude, versus full standard calibration of 0.1 mV = 1.0 mm). See step-down box at far right.

- Q waves and high voltage: V1–V3, probably due to LVH, since there is no evidence of previous MI.
- ST (J point) elevation: 1 to 2 mm, V2–V3, and minimal in aVL; hyperacute T waves: I, aVL, V2–V4. Although this ECG might be misinterpreted as LVH with or without old anterior MI, it is diagnostic of **anterior AMI.** A serial ECG at 15:27, at half standard calibration, was identical to ECG 9-8A.

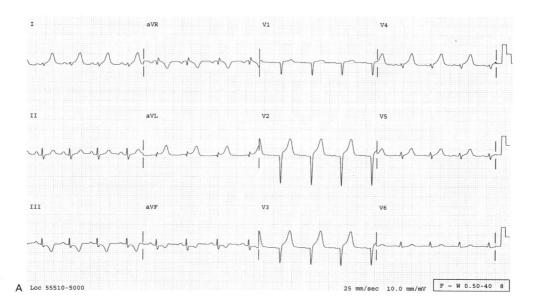

A Loc 55510-5000   25 mm/sec 10.0 mm/mV   F ~ W 0.50-40 8

(continued on next page)

CASE 9-8

Hyperacute T Waves with LVH, Obscured by Half Standard Calibration
(continued)

ECG 9-8B (Type 1a)

Also at 15:27, is full standard calibration.

- Massively hyperacute T waves: V2–V5. These were present all along, but obscured by the half standard calibration.

Clinical Course

The patient received thrombolytics; total CK peaked 7 hours later at 4,000 IU/L.

Conclusion

Failure to recognize hyperacute T waves resulted in delayed thrombolysis.

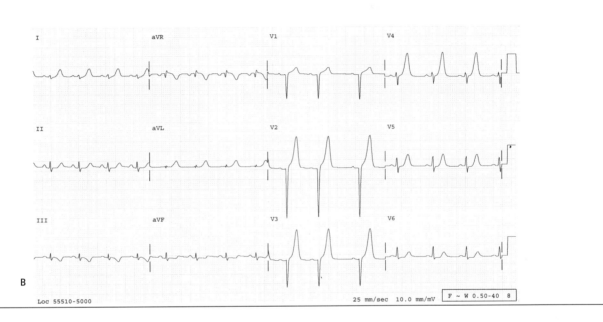

B

Loc 55510-5000

25 mm/sec   10.0 mm/mV   F ~ W 0.50-40   8

CASE 9-9

Very Peaked Hyperacute T Waves Missed by Clinicians

History

This 65-year-old man complained of 1 hour of typical CP.

ECG 9-9A (Type 4)

This is a baseline normal ECG from 4 days earlier.

ECG 9-9B (Type 1a)

- **T waves:** large, V2–V4. A potassium level of 4.5 mEq/L (normal) indicates that these are not due to hyperkalemia. Therefore this ECG is diagnostic of **anterior** AMI and reperfusion therapy is indicated.

Clinical Course

Clinicians missed this AMI, but fortunately the artery spontaneously reperfused. An ECG 6 hours after ECG 9-9B was normal. A second serial ECG recorded 9 hours after ECG 9-9B showed anterior terminal T wave inversion, nearly identical to Fig. 8-6 (Wellen's syndrome). Angioplasty opened a 99% LAD stenosis the next day.

Conclusion

Failure to recognize hyperacute T waves could have resulted in complete anterior wall necrosis had there not been spontaneous reperfusion.

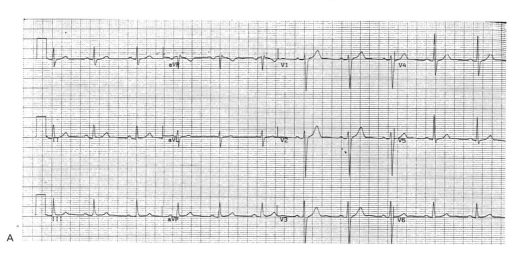

A

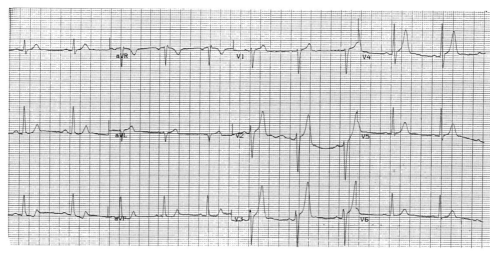

B

ANNOTATED BIBLIOGRAPHY

Collins MS, et al. Hyperacute T-wave criteria using computer ECG analysis, 1990.

Methods: Collins et al. (179) utilized computer analysis of ECGs to develop criteria for differentiating hyperacute T waves from the tall, peaked T waves of early repolarization.

Findings: The following features correlated with hyperacute T waves: (a) J-point amplitude/T-wave amplitude > 25%; (b) T-wave amplitude/QRS amplitude of more than 75%; (c) J-point elevation > 0.3 mV; and (d) age of more than 45 years.

Hochrein J, et al. Higher T-wave amplitude associated with better prognosis in patients receiving thrombolytic therapy for acute myocardial infarction (a GUSTO-1 substudy), 1998.

Methods: Hochrein et al. (180) studied the relationship between T-wave amplitude and thrombolytic outcome, independent of historical time since pain onset.

Findings: High T-wave amplitude correlated independently with clinically and statistically significant better outcome. **Patients with high T-wave amplitude, as a marker of very early AMI, are very likely to benefit from reperfusion therapy.**

Smith FM. The ligation of coronary arteries with electrocardiographic study, 1918.

Methods: Smith (170) studied ECG effects of coronary ligation in dogs.

Findings: T-wave height increased immediately after ligation.

Bayley RH, et al. Electrocardiographic changes (local ventricular ischemia and injury) produced in the dog by temporary occlusion of a coronary artery, showing a new stage in the evolution of myocardial infarction, 1944.

Methods: Bayley et al. (171) studied T waves after experimental coronary occlusion.

Findings: **T waves peaked within minutes and preceded ST elevation.**

Pinto IJ, et al. Tall upright T waves in the precordial leads, 1967.

Methods: Pinto et al. (176) studied 110 cases of precordial T waves > 10 mm.

Findings: Thirty-five cases involved ischemic heart disease. Ischemia was associated with wide, tall T waves, in contrast to narrow tented T waves in patients with hyperkalemia.

10

SERIAL ECG COMPARISON AND CONTINUOUS ST-SEGMENT MONITORING

KEY POINTS

- The ECG in AMI may be dynamic, with rising and falling ST segments that may be missed by a single ECG. Comparison with serial ECGs can document or confirm the changes of STEMI.
- Absence of evolution on serial ECGs may aid confirmation of pseudoinfarction.
- Continuous ST monitoring (preferably automated 12-lead or two-lead ST-segment monitoring, but including rhythm monitoring with attention to the ST segment as well as the rhythm) may detect ST elevation or depression that would otherwise go unnoticed.

GENERAL BACKGROUND

Comparison with serial static ECGs or continuous ST monitoring can document or confirm new ST elevation that is not reflected on a single initial ECG. Any patient with **continued suspicious symptoms, especially ongoing typical CP, and a Type 2, 3, 4, 1c, or 1d ECG requires continued attention to ST segments.** Use either serial static ECGs or continuous ST monitoring. In cases of Type 1b ECGs in which a subtle AMI is unrecognized, these modalities may also hasten diagnosis and facilitate timely treatment. **Comparison with a previous ECG, if available, is equally important.**

T-wave evolution of STEMI may aid in the diagnosis but is seldom rapid enough to aid in reperfusion therapy. However, pseudonormalization of inverted T waves may be diagnostic of reocclusion in STEMI. Rapid terminal inversion of upright T waves is indicative of reperfusion (see Chapters 8 and 27).

Type 2, 3, and 4 ECGs: No ST Elevation

Approximately 25% of patients with AMI have an initially "negative" ECG (normal or nondiagnostic [i.e., roughly, Type 3 or 4 ECGs]) (18,19). This may be because

- The ECG was recorded **too early** in the coronary event to show **any** ST elevation.
- The ECG was recorded **too early** in the coronary event to show **diagnostic** ST elevation.
- The ECG **never develops Type 1 changes** (ST elevation) because the infarct is too small or in a silent area. This is frequently the case with occlusion of the circumflex artery or one of its branches.
- The IRA reperfused spontaneously, and ST segments are back to baseline.
- **Unstable** ST segments are rising and falling due to intermittent occlusion (**181**).

See Cases 10-1 to 10-4. (See also Case 8-12 of T-wave pseudonormalization.)

Type 1b ECGs: Subtle but Diagnostic

Ideally, subtle Type 1b ECGs are recognized as diagnostic by the astute clinician. However, they are often overlooked. Timely serial ECGs can prevent treatment delays. See Cases 10-5 and 10-6.

Type 1c ECGs: Nondiagnostic ST Elevation

Additional information is necessary for Type 1c ECGs to be diagnostic of AMI. You may suspect that ST elevation is baseline (normal variant, LVH, or other) **or** you may suspect very early AMI; comparison with a previous or serial ECGs may confirm either suspicion (see Case 10-7).

Monitor for increasingly elevated ST segments; ST depression or inverting T waves may detect UA/NSTEMI. Diagnostic changes may also be seen with LBBB (**182**) (Figs. 18-3, 18-4, and Case 18-12) or intraventricular conduction delay (IVCD) (see Case 18-13).

Although the **absence of diagnostic changes** helps to rule out STEMI (see Case 10-8), it is **not infallible** (**183**). (See Case 11-2 of a very large anterior AMI with subsequent cardiogenic shock and subtle ST elevation that did **not** increase over time). **If high clinical suspicion persists, use other diagnostic modalities.**

Type 1d ECGs: ST Elevation and T-Wave Inversion

Type 1d ECGs may indicate spontaneously reperfused AMI in cases of intermittent coronary occlusion, subtotal occlusion, or occlusion with collaterals. These patients are **at risk for reocclusion,** for which timely intervention may be critical. Reocclusion manifests as pseudonormalization of inverted T waves with or without reelevation of the ST segment. The **absence of deepening T-wave inversion over many hours** is evidence, though not definitive, that the findings are not acute (see Case 20-11).

MANAGEMENT

First, **compare the ECG with a previous ECG.** If none is available, **record serial ECGs every 15 minutes to 1 hour,** depending on clinical suspicion, or perform **continuous ST monitoring.** Monitor for diagnostic changes, including ST elevation or pseudonormalization of inverted T waves, with or without recurrent or increased ST elevation. For low-risk ED patients, with atypical or resolved CP and no recurrence, continuous monitoring is low yield (**184,185**).

CONTINUOUS ST MONITORING

Continuous monitoring of the ST segments, as opposed to frequent static ECGs, is ideal because (a) the clinician is aware of dynamic ST elevation or depression as it occurs; (b) there is no dependence on the availability of ECG technicians; and (c) there is no need to remember to reorder ECGs. Monitoring for reperfusion or reocclusion may be accomplished with frequent static ECGs, but they are not as accurate as continuous monitoring (**185,186**). Continuous ST monitoring may also alert the clinician to ischemia or infarction even in patients whose symptoms have resolved, because ST segments may elevate before or without pain.

Automated Continuous 12-Lead or Two-Lead ST-Segment Monitoring

Continuous ST-segment monitoring may be two-lead or 12-lead. **Two-lead monitoring** is useful if there are **particularly suspicious leads** on the 12-lead ECG that can be **targeted** for monitoring. Unlike rhythm monitoring, an alarm sounds for ST elevation, and it can plot time versus ST elevation. Disadvantages include greater cost and complexity than rhythm monitors. (See Case 27-3.)

If the initial 12-lead is normal **or** there are no particularly suspicious leads, and high suspicion of AMI persists, multiple leads are useful to screen for changes. Unlike rhythm monitoring, 12-lead monitoring can detect reciprocal depression,

which improves the specificity for STEMI (65,106). These units may be simple and portable, can store ECGs at predetermined intervals, perform frequent computer analysis, detect ST changes from baseline, and have ST-segment alarms (186).

Continuous monitoring may be used to monitor for reperfusion or reocclusion (186,**187**) (see Chapter 27). Detection of reperfusion, and especially **failure** of reperfusion, is essential. Patients who fail to reperfuse should be taken for rescue PCI. Continuous monitoring for **reocclusion after reperfusion therapy** is useful **because symptoms may be absent** (69).

Rhythm Monitoring for Detection of ST Shifts

Rhythm monitoring may be performed using three or four limb leads or with a fifth "modified chest lead" (MCL). Rhythm monitoring, using routinely applied leads in all CP patients, has never been formally studied for efficacy in identifying patients with STEMI.

- Placement: right arm, left arm, right leg, and left leg. MCL is on the precordium.
- Strips produced: I, II, III, aVR, aVL, aVF, and any single precordial lead, which is the MCL, depending on where you place that lead.

Monitors that can display three leads simultaneously should display leads III, MCL-2 (V2), and MCL-3 (V3) (**83**). In these leads:

- ST elevation in MCL_{2-3} (V2/V3) suggests anterior AMI.
- ST elevation in lead III suggests inferior AMI.
- ST depression in MCL_{2-3} suggests posterior AMI.
- ST depression in III suggests lateral AMI.
- Substituting MCL-5 (V5) for MCL-3 (V3) may be more sensitive (**188**).

If ST elevation or depression develops, with or without recurrent CP, record a 12-lead ECG. See Cases 10-9 through 10-12 for examples of rhythm monitoring. (See also Case 12-3, in which prehospital ST elevation in MCL-3 resolved after NTG; and Cases 31-1 to 31-3.)

Disadvantages of Rhythm Monitoring

If there are no ST alarms, you must actively observe the ST segments. There are also technical problems with rhythm monitoring. ST elevation may be so pronounced that it completely obscures the QRS, mimicking a wide-complex rhythm. When accompanied by tachycardia, this may appear on the monitor to be ventricular tachycardia (Case 10-12). Gain settings are nonuniform, so the measurement of ST segments is nonuniform. The diagnostic utility of the reciprocal changes seen in 12-lead ECGs is lost and pseudoinfarction patterns such as LVH and LBBB readily result in false positives.

CASE 10-1

A Type 3 ECG with Suggestive Hyperacute T Waves
Followed by a Type 1a ECG

History
Unknown.

ECG 10-1A (Type 3)
At 07:33.
- This is a nondiagnostic ECG. The P waves are artifactual.
- Hyperacute T waves: subtle, V4–V5; and reverse R-wave progression: V2–V3 are **suspicious** for anterolateral AMI.

ECG 10-1B (Type 1a)
At 08:14, 41 minutes later.
- ST elevation: V1–V6, aVL; and reciprocal ST depression: II, III, aVF are diagnostic of **anterolateral AMI.**

Clinical Course
Clinicians administered thrombolytics.

Conclusion
Serial ECGs enabled timely diagnosis.

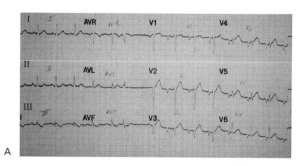
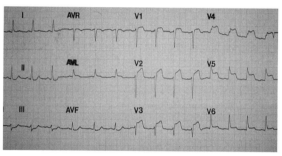

CASE 10-2

Very Atypical Symptoms, Very Subtle ECGs, with a Diagnostic Change

History
This 56-year-old man with one risk factor complained of burning from the epigastrium to the throat, which he reported experiencing every time he lay down to sleep at night.

ECG 10-2A (Type 3)
- No significant ST elevation.
- T-wave inversions: I, II, III, aVL, aVF, V4–V6; ST depression: minimal, II, aVF, V5–V6, suggestive of ischemia, possibly in the distant past.
- The patient's burning pain resolved with antacid given in the ED but recurred later.

ECG 10-2B (Type 1b)
80 minutes later
- Pseudonormalization of T waves in all leads in which they were abnormally inverted.

- ST elevation: II, III, aVF, of less than 1 mm but **at least** a 1-mm change from ECG 10-3a; and reciprocal ST depression: aVL, V2–V4, are diagnostic of AMI.

Clinical Course
The emergency physician missed this ST elevation, but it was recognized in the CCU. Angioplasty opened a fully occluded second obtuse marginal branch of the circumflex artery. Total CK peaked at 2,403 IU/L with an MB fraction of 157 ng/mL. Convalescent echocardiography demonstrated a 55% EF and a posterolateral WMA.

Conclusion
A serial ECG identified the need for reperfusion despite atypical symptoms.

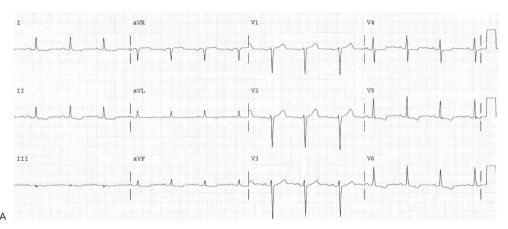

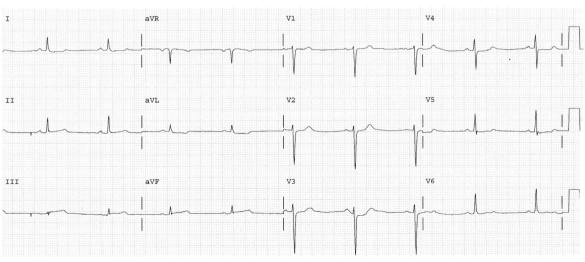

CASE 10-3

Initial Nondiagnostic ECG Followed by a Second ECG Diagnostic of Inferior AMI

History

This 55-year-old woman presented with 1 hour of CP, which persisted in spite of sublingual NTG and aspirin.

ECG 10-3A (Type 3)

At 12:32.

- Minimal ST elevation: II, III.

ECG 10-3B (Type 1a)

Not obtained until 2 hours later.

- ST elevation: II, III, aVF with reciprocal depression in aVL is diagnostic of **inferior AMI.**

- ST depression: V2–V3 is diagnostic of **posterior AMI.**

Clinical Course

The patient underwent immediate angioplasty of an occluded RCA. The infarct resulted in inferior hypokinesis but normal LV function.

Conclusion

Although a serial ECG facilitated diagnosis and treatment, it was unnecessarily delayed by 2 hours.

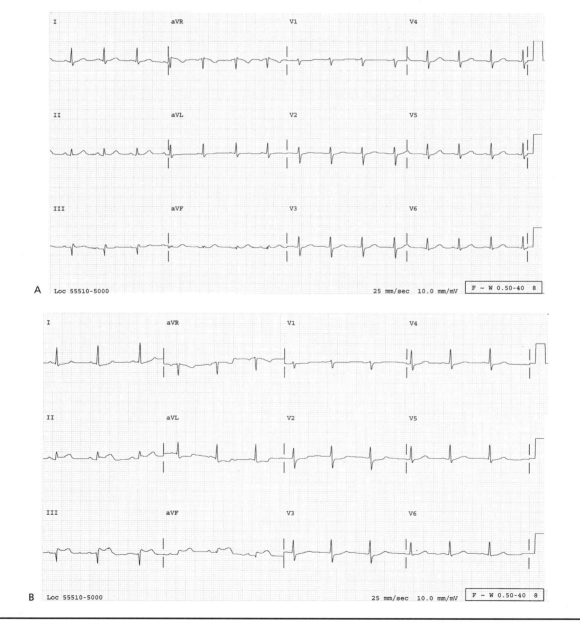

CASE 10-4

Subtle Inferior ST Elevation with No Reciprocal Depression in aVL; the Absence of Change on Serial ECGs Helps to Rule Out AMI

History

This 41-year-old man presented with atypical CP. He was 3 years status post CABG as a result of left main stenosis, but he had no history of MI. Four days earlier he had presented with crushing CP. With an ECG identical to the one below, and despite concurrent echocardiography that found no WMA, he had received thrombolytics. All ECGs since 1994 were identical and the patient ruled out for MI by enzymes in all five admissions.

ECG 10-4 (Type 3)

■ ST elevation: II, III, aVF, but no reciprocal depression in aVL. This ECG is identical to all the previous ECGs.

Clinical Course

Two ECGs over the next 2 hours remained identical to ECG 10-4. Clinicians did not administer thrombolytics.

Conclusion

The absence of change on serial ECGs helped to confirm the absence of AMI.

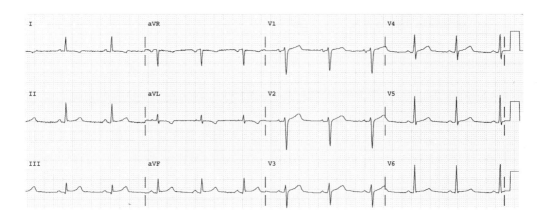

CASE 10-5

"Early Repolarization," Subtly Diagnostic Made Obviously Diagnostic 18 Minutes Later with a Serial ECG

History
This 51-year-old man presented with 1 hour of CP that radiated to both arms.

ECG 10-5A (Type 1b)
At 16:37, V1–V6 only.
- ST elevation: V1–V4; and J-point elevation.
- The computer read this as early repolarization. However, in spite of upwardly concave ST segments, this ECG is diagnostic of **anterior AMI** because the **ST elevation is disproportionate to the QRS** and a diagnosis of early repolarization in a **patient more than 40 years of age** must be suspect.

ECG 10-5B (Type 1a)
16:55, 18 minutes later, V1–V6 only.
- ST segment "**coving**" (upward convexity): V2, is obviously diagnostic of **anterior AMI.** Never attribute this to early repolarization.

Clinical Course
Clinicians performed rapid thrombolysis, which resulted in complete reperfusion and a maximum total CK = 357 IU/L.

Conclusion
A serial ECG of an unrecognized subtle AMI (Type 1b ECG) enabled rapid diagnosis and treatment.

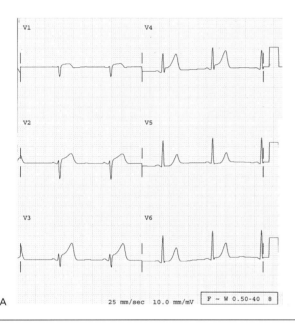

A   25 mm/sec   10.0 mm/mV   F ~ W 0.50-40 8

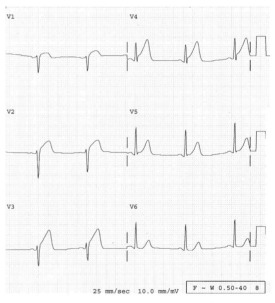

25 mm/sec   10.0 mm/mV   F ~ W 0.50-40 8   B

CASE 10-6

Serial ECGs Read Independently Are Subtly Diagnostic of AMI: Together, the Change Makes the Diagnosis More Obvious

History

This 62-year-old man presented with "grippy" substernal chest tightness that increased to severe pain over 2 hours, radiating to the interscapular area, with no associated symptoms.

ECG 10-6A (Type 1b)

At 05:06.

■ J-point elevation: V1–V5, with an upwardly concave ST segment, is suggestive of early repolarization. However, the patient's age (>60 years) makes this unlikely.

■ ST elevation: minimal, aVL, is very **suspicious** for lateral AMI.

■ The preceding features, in addition to reciprocal ST depression: II, III, aVF, and hyperacute T waves: V2–V4, make this ECG diagnostic of **anterior AMI.**

ECG 10-6B (Type 1b)

16 minutes later, V1–V3 only.

■ On comparison with ECG 10-6A, it is evident that the ST elevation has **increased** in V2 (still < 2 mm) and is **new** in V3, making the diagnosis of anterolateral AMI much more obvious.

Clinical Course

Clinicians administered thrombolytics immediately. Subsequent echocardiography showed an anterior WMA and the patient ruled in for AMI by biochemical markers.

Conclusion

An ECG from 1 year earlier showed isoelectric ST segments. In cases such as this, recognition of a subtle AMI in the first ECG is optimal. However, when missed, comparison with a timely serial ECG, also subtly diagnostic, may hasten diagnosis and treatment.

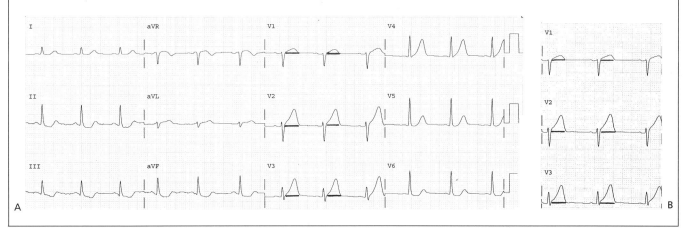

CASE 10-7

Type 1c ECG with Subtle ST Elevation Became Diagnostic of Anterior AMI with a Serial ECG

History

This 60-year-old man presented with 2.5 hours of CP.

ECG 10-7 (Type 1c)

At 02:26.

- ST elevation: V1–V3, looks like early repolarization, but be suspicious of AMI in patients more than 40 years of age.
- ST depression: minimal, II, III, aVF, is **suspicious** for reciprocal changes of anterior AMI.

Clinical Course

The patient was admitted to the CCU. A repeat ECG 2.5 hours later was obviously diagnostic of **anterior AMI,** with increased ST elevation and development of Q waves; tPA was given. **Later comparison with a previous ECG confirmed that ST elevation on ECG 10-7 was new.**

Conclusion

A serial ECG made the diagnosis, although this Type 1c ECG was diagnostic **when compared with a previous ECG.** Severe symptoms should prompt repeat ECGs every 15 minutes.

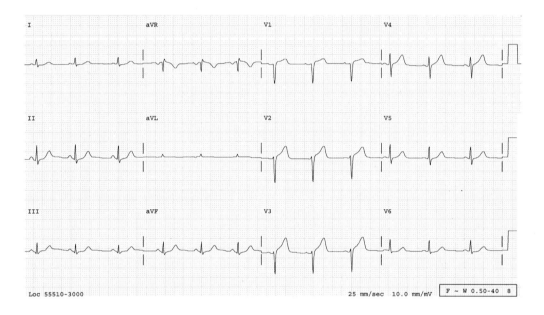

CASE 10-8

Type 1c ECG Very Suspicious for AMI, but Slightly Atypical; Serial ECGs Helped to Prevent Unnecessary Thrombolysis

History
This 35-year-old man presented with 40 minutes of pleuritic CP and chest tightness that radiated to the throat, accompanied by dyspnea. A chest x-ray showed pulmonary edema. The patient vehemently denied cocaine use.

ECG 10-8 (Type 1b Versus 1c)
At 00:51.
■ ST elevation: V2–V3, consistent with anterior AMI but T-wave amplitude is atypically low.

Clinical Course
Unconvinced of STEMI, the physician did not give throm-

bolytics immediately. Serial ECGs were recorded every 15 minutes for 1 hour, and all were identical. Immediate echocardiography revealed concentric LVH but no WMA. Pulmonary edema was apparently due to diastolic dysfunction. A urine drug screen revealed cocaine metabolites. CTnI remained less than 0.3 ng/mL over 24 hours and the ECG normalized 6 hours later.

Conclusion
The diagnosis is uncertain but was possibly cocaine-related reversible ischemia. Although coronary disease was not definitely ruled out, serial ECGs helped to prevent thrombolysis that, at least in retrospect, was unnecessary.

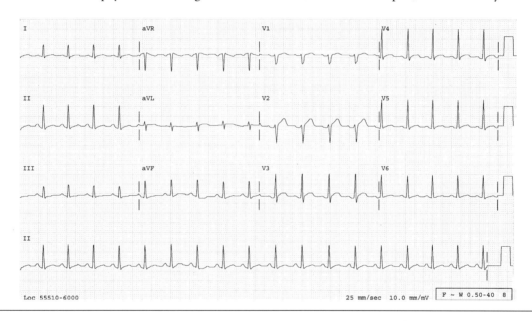

Loc 55510-6000   25 mm/sec 10.0 mm/mV   F ~ W 0.50-40 8

CASE 10-9

Prehospital ST Elevation in MCL-3 (in the Area of V3)

Prehospital ST elevation in MCL-3 (in the area of V3) alerted paramedics to anterior AMI and decreased door-to-needle time (DTNT).

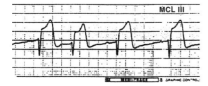

CASE 10-10

ED Rhythm Strip: Lead II Makes Obvious Diagnosis of Inferior AMI

A 12-lead ECG obtained immediately after this strip revealed less inferior ST elevation, but additional ST elevation in V4. Angioplasty opened an occluded "wraparound" LAD.

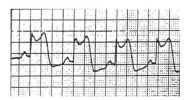

CASE 10-11

MCL-1 in the ED Alerted Clinicians to Developing RV (and Inferior) AMI

History
This 65-year-old man presented with CP.

ECG 10-11A
This is an ED rhythm strip.

■ ST elevation: MCL-1, is suspicious for AMI and alerted clinicians.

ECG 10-11B (Type 1a)
■ ST elevation: II, III, and aVF, diagnostic of **inferior AMI.**
■ ST elevation: V1, diagnostic of **RV AMI.**

Clinical Course
A right-sided ECG confirmed RV AMI, tPA was immediately administered, with reperfusion. Angiography revealed a patent RCA with a moderately stenotic proximal culprit lesion and EF of 56%.

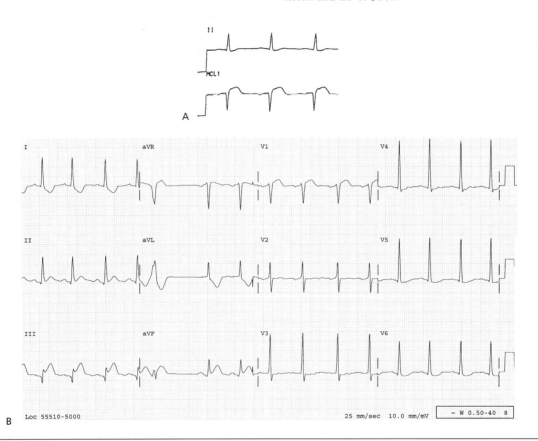

CASE 10-12

On the Monitor, ST Elevation Mimics Ventricular Tachycardia

History
This 60-year-old critically ill woman with sepsis and an initially nondiagnostic ECG was in a monitored bed when the alarm sounded. A Lead II rhythm strip showed heart rate (HR) = 149, with apparent wide complex.

ECG 10-12 (Type 1a)
Lead II rhythm strip is shown at bottom. Could be mistaken for ventricular tachycardia, but P waves are visible and the complex is narrow in V5.

■ ST elevation: II, III, aVF, 10 mm, also V6; and ST depression: V1–V5 are diagnostic of **inferoposterior** AMI.

Clinical Course
Immediate echocardiography confirmed inferoposterior WMA. Catheterization revealed severe three-vessel disease and a thrombus in the mid-RCA, which was stented.

Conclusion
High ST elevation on a rhythm strip may mimic a wide QRS. Look carefully at all leads.

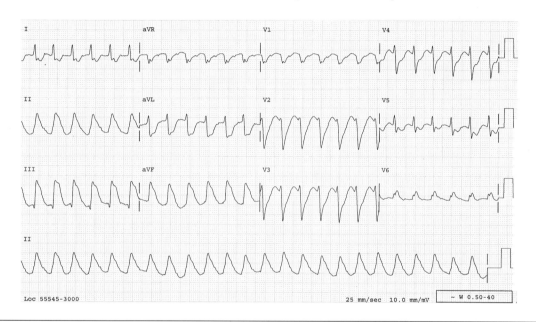

Loc 55545-3000   25 mm/sec   10.0 mm/mV   ~ W 0.50-40

ANNOTATED BIBLIOGRAPHY

Continuous ST-Segment Monitoring
ST segments may elevate before pain onset and often without any pain at all.

Wilkins ML, et al. Variability of acute ST-segment predicted myocardial infarct size in the absence of thrombolytic therapy, 1994.
   Methods: Wilkins et al. (90) compared prehospital and ED ECGs of 155 STEMI patients.
   Findings: ST segments in 33% of the patients were unstable, rising and falling, before thrombolysis.

Krucoff MW, et al. Quantitative and qualitative ST-segment monitoring during and after percutaneous and transluminal coronary angioplasty, 1990; Krucoff MW, et al. The portable programmable microprocessor-driven real-time 12-lead electrocardiographic monitor: a preliminary report of a new device for the noninvasive detection of successful reperfusion or silent coronary reocclusion, 1990; Krucoff MW, et al. Stability of multilead ST-segment "fingerprints" over time after percutaneous transluminal coronary angioplasty and its usefulness in detecting reocclusion, 1988; and Krucoff MW, et al. Noninvasive detection of coronary artery patency using continuous ST-segment monitoring, 1986.

   Methods: Krucoff et al. (187,189–191) used continuous 12-lead ST-segment monitoring on inpatients and on patients undergoing angioplasty in order to detect STEMI, reperfusion, and reocclusion.
   Findings: ST-segment changes on continuous monitoring were strongly correlated with both thrombotic occlusion and angioplasty balloon inflation. Repeat occlusion of the same artery in the same location produced consistent ECG changes, called an "ischemic fingerprint."

Fesmire FM, et al. Instability of ST segments in the early stages of acute myocardial infarction in patients undergoing continuous 12-lead ECG monitoring, 1995.
   Methods: Fesmire et al. (181) studied the use of automated continuous 12-lead ECGs in the ED.
   Findings: ST segments in early AMI were unstable, alternately rising and falling. Therefore, any single ECG may miss the ST elevation of AMI. Fesmire also reported the case of a monitored ED patient who suffered silent cardiac arrest preceded by unstable ST segments (192).

Monitoring High-Risk Patients
Record serial ECGs or perform continuous ST-segment monitoring on high-risk patients during at least the first hour of presentation.

Fesmire FM. Which chest pain patients benefit from continuous ST-segment monitoring with automated serial ECG? 1999.

Methods: Fesmire (16) performed continuous ST-segment monitoring with automated serial ECGs on 706 ED CP patients classified into four risk categories, as follows: 1 = ACS and eligible for reperfusion therapy; 2 = obvious ACS but not a candidate for reperfusion therapy; 3 = possible ACS; and 4 = lower risk still but warrants monitoring. The automated serial ECGs were initiated at 21 ± 20 minutes after ED presentation and continued for a mean of 116 ± 44 minutes.

Findings: Of 28 patients in Category 1, treatment was changed as a result of serial ECGs in four patients, all of whom were sent for rescue angioplasty after continuous monitoring failed to reveal ECG signs of reperfusion (see Chapter 27). Of 136 patients in Category 2, new ST elevation was detected by serial ECGs in 20 patients at a mean of 24 ± 32 minutes (i.e., these 20 patients' ECGs became Category 1 during continuous monitoring). All 20 patients received reperfusion therapy.

Fesmire FM, et al. Usefulness of automated serial 12-lead ECG monitoring during the initial emergency department evaluation of patients with chest pain, 1998.

Methods: Fesmire et al. (183) studied 60-minute automated serial 12-lead monitoring during the initial ED evaluation of 1,000 CP patients.

Findings: CK-MB confirmed AMI in 204 patients, of whom 107 (52.5%) had ED reperfusion therapy. ST elevation on the **initial ECG was only 46% sensitive for AMI** (93 of 204) and was "positive" in another 13 cases that ultimately did not have MI (only four were not ACS). ST elevation on **automated serial 12-lead monitoring improved sensitivity for CK-MB confirmed AMI to 62%** (126 of 204) and also showed ST "injury" (Type 1) pattern in 19 patients who did not have positive CK-MB (17 of these 19 were later diagnosed with UA). Automated serial monitoring was also much more sensitive for (Type 2) changes diagnostic of UA/NSTEMI. This 60-minute monitoring was also **very useful for identifying patients with false-positive ECGs.** Only two of 19 patients with initially diagnostic ECGs but no evolutionary changes ruled in for AMI.

Silber SH, et al. Serial electrocardiograms for chest pain patients with initial nondiagnostic electrocardiograms: implications for thrombolytic therapy, 1996.

Methods: Silber et al. (193) reviewed charts of 114 patients with a discharge diagnosis of AMI.

Findings: Only 20 of 114 patients had initial ECGs that met thrombolytic criteria. Of the 94 remaining patients, 19 subsequently developed ECG changes that met thrombolytic criteria, seven within the first 8 hours. **Serial ECGs facilitated appropriate reperfusion in these cases.**

Zalenski RJ, et al. The emergency department electrocardiogram and hospital complications in myocardial infarction patients, 1996.

Methods: Zalenski et al. (194) retrospectively studied 65 patients with CK-MB diagnosis of MI.

Findings: Twenty-seven patients had initially negative ECGs (Type 3 or 4 by our classification), and 38 were initially positive (Type 1 or 2). There was no significant difference in complication rate between the groups. More important, of the patients with initially negative ECGs who did suffer complications, almost all (83%) evolved ECG changes beforehand. **Without serial ECGs these patients might not be identified in a timely manner.**

Leads to Monitor

Bush HS, et al. Twelve-lead electrocardiographic evaluation of ischemia during percutaneous transluminal coronary angioplasty and its correlation with acute reocclusion, 1991.

Methods: Bush et al. (83) performed continuous ST-segment monitoring during angioplasty balloon occlusion in 43 patients.

Findings: Of all 12 leads, **V2 and V3** were the best monitor leads for **LAD occlusion** (ST elevation), **V2 and V3 (NOT aVL)** were best for detecting **circumflex occlusion** (ST depression), and **lead III** was best for **RCA occlusion.** Of 43 circumflex artery balloon inflations, 32 (74%) resulted in ST depression in V2, and 35 (81%) resulted in ST depression in V2 and/or V3. Fifty-five of 62 balloon inflations of the LAD (88%) resulted in ST elevation in V2, and 59 of 62 (95%) in V2 and/or V3.

Mizutani M, et al. ST monitoring for myocardial ischemia during and after coronary angioplasty, 1990.

Methods: Similar to Bush et al. mentioned earlier, Mizutani et al. (188) performed continuous ST-segment monitoring during angioplasty balloon occlusions in 70 patients.

Findings: Selecting only leads III, V2, V3, or V5, they found either ST elevation or depression during 100% of balloon occlusions. The LAD was involved in 33 cases, the RCA in 19 cases, and the circumflex artery in 18 cases. **The best three-lead combination to detect any or all AMI was III, V2, and V5.** Observing for ST depression or elevation in these three leads detected more than 90% of LAD occlusions and 100% of RCA or circumflex occlusions.

Jernberg T, et al. ST-segment monitoring with continuous 12-lead ECG improves early risk stratification in patients with chest pain and ECG nondiagnostic of acute myocardial infarction, 1999.

Methods: Jernberg et al. (195) analyzed 9-hour continuous 12-lead monitoring of 630 **inpatients** with CP.

Findings: Of 630 patients, 100 (15.9%) manifested an "ST episode," defined as ST depression or elevation ≥ 1 mm lasting at least 1 minute. An ST episode was associated with a relative risk of 6.7 for AMI or death at 30 days. An episode of ST **elevation** occurred in 13 (2.1%) patients.

Comment: The incidence of ST episodes may diminish after the first hour in the ED has passed, and is low in patients without continued CP.

Holmvang L, et al. Relative contributions of a single-admission 12-lead electrocardiogram and early 24-hour continuous electrocardiographic monitoring for early risk stratification in patients with unstable coronary artery disease, 1999.

Methods: Holmvang et al. (196) performed 24-hour continuous vectorcardiographic monitoring on 308 patients with unstable coronary disease.

Findings: Change in ST vector magnitude was a very good independent predictor of 30-day outcomes. Further study for use in reperfusion therapy is warranted.

Continuous Monitoring of Low-Risk Patients

Gibler WB, et al. A rapid diagnostic and treatment center for patients with chest pain in the emergency department, 1995.

Methods: Gibler et al. (184) retrospectively studied 1,010 patients observed in a CP unit over 32 months. All had serial CK-MB testing and continuous 12-lead ST-segment trend monitoring.

Findings: Only 11 patients developed evidence of ischemia or evolving AMI, but only 43 patients overall were discharged with a diagnosis of ACS. Thus 26% of the patients with ischemia were identified.

Comment: In this very-low-risk group, continuous monitoring was infrequently positive.

Hedges JR, et al. Serial ECGs are less accurate than serial CK-MB results for emergency department diagnosis of myocardial infarction, 1992.

Methods: Hedges et al. (185) recorded ECGs at presentation and 3 to 4 hours later on 261 patients monitored in a CP unit. Initial ECGs were apparently Types 4, 3, 2, and 1c. The authors did not specify whether symptoms were ongoing.

Findings: At 3 to 4 hours, serial ECG changes only detected two STEMIs. Over this time period, CK-MB sampling was both more sensitive and more specific for identifying any MI than serial ECG changes.

Comment: Serial monitoring of an unselected population (low pretest probability) has a low yield.

Q WAVES

GENERAL BACKGROUND

The electrophysiology of Q waves is discussed in Chapter 1. There are normal Q waves that occur due to the normal sequence of depolarization, starting with the septum (Fig. 11-1). An abnormal Q wave results from a lack of electrical activity under the recording lead, usually representing infarction. See Table 11-1 for conditions other than AMI that manifest with Q waves (usually QS waves) (197). See Table 11-2 for correlation of Q waves on the ECG with anatomic location of old MI. The analysis of Q waves in this book is not meant to be exhaustive. **Our focus is the impact of Q waves on the reperfusion decision.**

Definitions

Abnormal Q waves include the following (2,111):
- **V2:** any Q wave.
- **V3:** almost any Q wave.
- **V4:** abnormal if more than 1 mm deep **or** larger than the Q wave in V5 **or** at least 0.02 sec (0.5 mm wide) (111).
- **Any Q wave ≥ 0.03 sec** (30 ms, 0.75 mm), **except** in leads III, aVR, or V1, which may have wide and deep Q waves in normal subjects.
- **aVL:** Q wave of more than 0.04 sec **or** > 50% of the amplitude of the QRS in the presence of an upright P wave (2).
- **Lead III:** Q wave ≥ 0.04 sec. A Q wave with a depth > 25% of R-wave height is often quoted as diagnostic, but width is more important than depth (2) (Fig. 11-2).
- Q waves are more likely in inferior leads **II, III, and aVF** when the QRS axis is vertical.

(NOTE: All succeeding mention of Q waves refers to abnormal Q waves unless otherwise stated.)

Abnormal R-wave progression may be an ECG sign of infarction. R waves should increase in amplitude from V1–V4; absence of this increase indicates a loss of R-wave progression. Reverse R-wave progression is demonstrated when R waves decrease in amplitude from V1–V4.

A QR wave is a Q wave followed by an R wave (**qR**- implies that the R wave is significantly larger than the Q wave and **Qr**- implies the opposite). A QR wave generally indicates smaller infarct area than a QS wave but it may indicate myocardium at

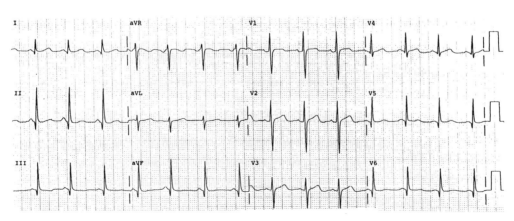

FIGURE 11-1. Normal septal Q waves. Q waves in leads II, III, aVF, and V4–V6 are not wide enough or deep enough to be abnormal. (ECG reproduced from unpublished data with permission of K. Wang, M.D.)

TABLE 11.1. CONDITIONS OTHER THAN INFARCTION THAT MAY MANIFEST Q WAVES

LVH (V1–V4, usually QS waves), also hypertrophic cardiomyopathy
RVH (qRS in right precordial leads V1–V3)
Cor pulmonale (QS in right precordial leads V1–V3)
Cardiomyopathy (QS waves)
LBBB (small or no R waves in right precordial leads V1–V3)
LAFB (leads I, aVL, and occasionally middle to right precordial leads)
WPW (negative delta wave)
Pulmonary embolism (lead III)

risk. If a QR—or qR—wave is present in anterior leads during early anterior AMI, it is commonly due to ischemia of the conduction system and is usually reversible (92). If a QR or qR with a tall R wave manifests in leads V1–V3, consider RBBB.

A **QS wave** is a Q wave that is **NOT** followed by an R wave. It generally indicates completed infarction and larger infarct area. If it is old, then less viable myocardium is at risk in this coronary artery distribution. A patient with a QS wave (even more than a patient with a QR wave) is at **greater risk** of morbidity and mortality from AMI in a new myocardial risk area; in general, **there is less myocardium to spare than in a patient whose ECG has R waves.**

Q WAVES AND REPERFUSION THERAPY IN AMI

Q-Wave MI and Non–Q-Wave MI

In AMI, the distinction of Q wave versus non–Q wave is based on the appearance of the ECG **after** the AMI is complete and has little utility in the reperfusion decision (see Chapter 2). In STEMI, reperfusion of the IRA (especially when it occurs early) makes evolution of subsequent Q waves less likely (**93**). Among patients who do undergo thrombolysis, those who do not develop Q waves have a better prognosis, quality of life, and overall health status, and use fewer resources, than those who do develop Q waves (198).

Q Waves and AMI

Q waves in leads with ST elevation of uncertain etiology (Type 1c ECG) support the diagnosis of AMI. Q waves in leads without ST elevation (due to old MI) indicate the presence of CAD, which increases the likelihood of new AMI. Absence of Q waves does **NOT,** of course, rule out CAD or even previous MI.

TABLE 11.2. LOCATION OF Q WAVES OR R WAVES DUE TO AMI

Q wave in II, III, aVF: **inferior MI**
Q wave in V2–V4: **anterior MI**
Q wave in V5–V6, I, aVL: **lateral MI**
Q wave in V1–V4: **anteroseptal MI**
Large R waves in V1–V3 (R in V1 > S in V1, or R in V2 > S in V2):
　　posterior AMI

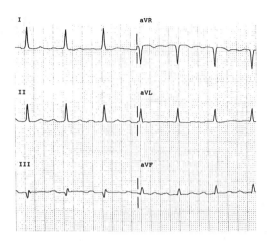

FIGURE 11-2. Old inferior MI with small Q waves diagnostic of old MI. The Q wave in III is small but diagnostic of old MI because the width is more than 0.04 sec. (ECG reproduced from unpublished data with permission of K. Wang, M.D).

Never let Q waves alone dissuade you from initiating reperfusion strategies. The presence of Q waves in leads with ST elevation is often cited incorrectly as evidence that the onset of infarction is too remote for reperfusion to be indicated. **Q waves are present or R waves are absent after only 1 hour of coronary artery occlusion in approximately 50% of anterior AMI,** possibly as a result of ischemia of the conduction system. Without reperfusion, Q waves are completely formed by 12 hours (**92**).

Q waves **by themselves** are a **poor predictor of AMI duration.** In leads **with** ST elevation, a **QS pattern** (as opposed to a QR pattern) is likely due to **old** MI, or AMI that is very late in its course (see Case 33-3), but a **QR pattern** is as likely due to **acute** MI as to old MI. In leads **without** ST elevation, a QR pattern is due to **old** MI. QS may be due to other causes (Table 11-1).

Of all AMI patients, those with NEW Q waves (almost always QR) in leads with ST elevation are older, present later, have larger AMIs with more myocardium at risk, involve greater mortality, and have equal, or possibly greater, mortality benefit from reperfusion therapy than those without Q waves (**92,199**).

Q waves may disappear with reperfusion (**92**).

See Cases 11-1 through 11-4 for examples of Q waves. (See also Case 3-3 of an **acute** inferior MI superimposed on an inferior Q-wave MI; Case 15-3 of old inferior Q waves and new anterior ST elevation representing new proximal RCA occlusion and RV AMI; and Case 33-8 of well-developed Q waves of **subacute** MI in a patient who presented after 12 hours of CP.)

Significance of New ST Elevation and Q-Wave Infarction

New ST elevation in a lead with a previous Q-wave infarction, especially a QS-wave infarction, indicates AMI in the same location as previous MI and limited potential benefit of thrombolytic therapy because there is less remaining myocardium.

Beware also that such ST elevation may be due to **ventricular aneurysm,** which can **mimic** AMI (see Chapter 23).

New ST elevation in a lead DISTANT from previous Q-wave infarction indicates new infarction that is more likely to lead to LV dysfunction. Therefore, **reperfusion is more urgent.**

Q Waves in Management

- A **new QR wave** in leads with **new** ST elevation indicates **potential benefit** from thrombolysis at least equal to the benefit in situations without this new Q wave.
- A **new QS wave** in leads with **new** ST elevation indicates **limited benefit** from thrombolysis; many are due to well-developed AMIs. Be sure the ECG findings are definitely new, and not due to ventricular aneurysm. Reassess symptom duration because duration of occlusion may be > 12 hours. **Do not withhold thrombolytics simply because Q waves are present.**

- **Old QR waves** in leads with **new** ST elevation may indicate **some** limitation of benefit from thrombolysis because some myocardium is already infarcted.
- **Old QS waves** in leads with **new** ST elevation indicate that benefit from thrombolysis may be **very limited.** Suspect that ST elevation may also be old (ventricular aneurysm).
- **Old QR or QS waves** in leads **distant** from new ST elevation may be associated with **extra mortality benefit** from reperfusion, due to greater dependence on remaining myocardium.

Inferior Q Waves

In the setting of suspected AMI, **inferior Q waves** (old inferior MI), as well as **inferior ST elevation** (**acute** inferior MI), should alert the clinician to the possibility of **RV AMI. Record a right-sided ECG** (see Case 15-3).

CASE 11-1

Well-Developed Acutely Formed Q Waves Early in Large Anterolateral AMI

History
This 55-year-old man presented with 2 hours of CP.

ECG 11-1 (Type 1a)
- Well-developed, acutely formed Q waves: aVL, V2–V3; terminal QRS distortion: V2–V4; and reciprocal ST depression: II, III, aVF are clearly diagnostic of a large **anterolateral AMI.**

Conclusion
Thrombolytics offer much benefit in this case. The presence of Q waves does **not** imply less benefit to thrombolytics. In fact, this ECG manifests very high acuteness, and reperfusion is indicated regardless of symptom duration (see Chapter 33).

ECG reproduced from unpublished data with permission of K. Wang, M.D.

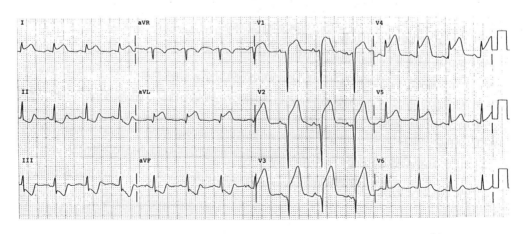

CASE 11-2

Tiny Q Waves and Reverse R-Wave Progression with Very Subtle ST Elevation Help to Make the Diagnosis of ACUTE MI

History

This 47-year-old man complained of 7 hours of constant typical CP, partly relieved with NTG. He reported a history of "two strokes" that he said were only treated in the ED and had not caused headache, and he stated that he had no remaining weakness or numbness. No previous records or ECG were available. BP = 120/80 mm Hg and P = 110 beats per minute (bpm).

ECG 11-2 (Type 1b)

■ ST elevation: < 2 mm, V1–V5, possibly due to early repolarization, although V5 morphology is more typical of AMI; and Q waves: tiny, V2–V4, larger in V5 and V6. These Q waves are not part of early repolarization but, rather, **support** the diagnosis of **anterolateral AMI**, although they could be due to previous MI.

Clinical Course

Subsequent ECGs never developed high ST elevation. Clinicians administered **thrombolytics** immediately, solely on the basis of the initial ECG. The patient continued to have pain and the ECG did not show significant ST recovery. Within 1 hour, the patient became hypotensive. Immediate angiography revealed an EF of 25%, anterior and api-cal akinesis, and severe multivessel disease with high-grade LAD stenosis necessitating an intra-aortic balloon pump and CABG. The patient's CK and cTnI at the specified time intervals were, respectively, 335 IU/L and 4.1 ng/mL at 17:41 on Day 0 (time of presentation), 3,070 IU/L and 402 ng/mL at 21:45 on Day 0, 4,229 IU/L and 526 ng/mL at 01:30 on Day 1, 4,374 IU/L and 369 ng/mL at 05:46 on Day 1, 829 IU/L and 84 ng/mL at 15:46 on Day 2.

Conclusion

Q waves, including reverse R-wave progression, may appear very early in AMI and may help distinguish early AMI from look-alikes. The increased cTnI concentration (4.1 ng/mL) at admission confirmed the diagnosis of AMI; this should bolster the confidence of a physician who is uncertain of the ECG interpretation (especially if the result can be obtained within 5 minutes), although **this ECG is diagnostic** (Type 1b) to the trained interpreter. This also demonstrates that the patient's onset of myocardial ischemia was at least 4 hours before the time of presentation. Furthermore, the rapid increase of cTnI to 402 ng/mL over the initial period following thrombolytic therapy suggests that there was successful reperfusion. For discussion of biomarkers, see Chapter 29.

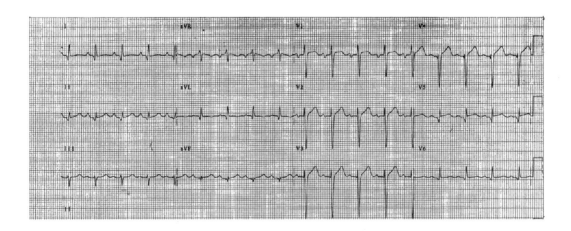

CASE 11-3

Acute Anterolateral AMI with Deep Q Waves in V2–V3

History

This 60-year-old man presented with 2 hours of constant CP.

ECG 11-3 (Type 1a)

At 16:16.

- ST elevation: aVL, V2–V5; reciprocal depression: II, III, aVF; and hyperacute T waves: V2–V5 are diagnostic of **anterolateral AMI.**
- Q waves (QS pattern): V2–V3.
- The differential diagnosis when viewing precordial leads includes old anterior MI with acute reinfarction, and anterior AMI with acutely formed Q waves. Ventricular aneurysm (old anterior MI with persistent ST elevation) would not have such hyperacute T waves (see Chapter 23).

Clinical Course

Because of hypotension resulting from use of IV NTG, clinicians spent 80 minutes managing the hypotension before giving thrombolytics. Angiography immediately following thrombolytics showed severe LAD stenosis with reperfusion and an EF of 54%. ST segments normalized with ensuing T-wave inversion and persistent Q waves 48 hours later. **One year later, R waves had replaced all Q waves and the ECG was normal.**

Conclusion

ST elevation in aVL, absence of Q wave in V4, and hyperacute T waves all help to make this ECG diagnostic of **acute MI.** Treatment was unnecessarily delayed by inappropriate administration of IV NTG before thrombolytics.

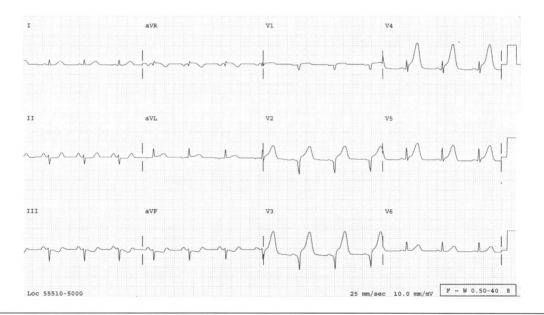

Loc 55510-5000   25 mm/sec   10.0 mm/mV   F ~ W 0.50-40 8

CASE 11-4

Inferior ST Elevation, even with Pathologic Q Waves, Is AMI until Proven Otherwise

History

This 66-year-old man with no history of MI but with history of aortic aneurysm repair and HTN, presented with dyspnea and diaphoresis. His initial BP = 220/152 and a chest x-ray revealed pulmonary congestion.

ECG 11-4 (Type 1c)

- IVCD
- ST elevation: II, III, aVF; and ST depression: V2–V5, are highly **suspicious** of inferoposterior AMI.
- qR waves with well-formed Q waves, but also well-formed R waves: II, III, aVF.
- Possible ventricular aneurysm, but probable AMI.

Clinical Course

Records showed that the Q waves were old but the ST elevation was **new.** Serial ECGs revealed increasing ST elevation and depression. Angioplasty opened a 100% acute RCA occlusion.

Conclusion

Inferior QR waves with ST elevation can be difficult to interpret, but unless there is good historical information to the contrary or an immediate ultrasound that confirms ventricular aneurysm, they should be assumed to be a manifestation of AMI. This is especially true in the presence of simultaneous precordial ST depression.

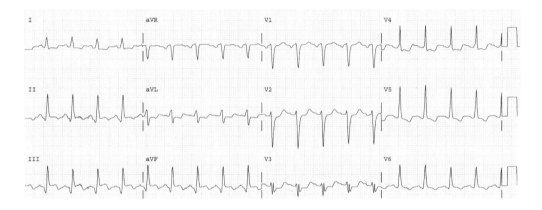

ANNOTATED BIBLIOGRAPHY

Raitt MH, et al. Appearance of abnormal Q waves early in the course of acute myocardial infarction: implications for efficacy of thrombolytic therapy, 1995.

Methods: Raitt et al. (92) studied 695 patients with first AMI who were admitted to thrombolytic trials and whose admission ECG allowed prediction of myocardial risk area using the Aldrich score (126). Thallium scintigraphy measured final LV infarct size in 436 patients.

Findings: Of these 436 patients with AMI whose ECG was recorded within 1 hour of pain onset, 53% already had abnormal Q waves. **Infarct size was larger in patients with Q waves on the initial ECG;** these patients showed **benefit** from thrombolytics equal to that of patients lacking such Q waves. Q waves were more common in early **anterior** AMI and may be due to a potentially reversible electrical phenomenon arising from ischemia of the conduction system. Vermeer et al. (117) and Bar et al. (111) support these findings (see Chapter 6).

Bar FW, et al. Development of ST-segment elevation and Q- and R-wave changes in acute myocardial infarction and the influence of thrombolytic therapy, 1996.

Methods: Bar et al. (93) analyzed serial ECGs of 358 patients with reperfused and nonreperfused AMI.

Findings: Mean magnitude of developed Q waves or loss of R wave remained constant after 9 hours in nonreperfused cases.

Birnbaum Y, et al. Abnormal Q waves on the admission electrocardiogram of patients with first acute myocardial infarction: prognostic implications, 1997.

Methods: Birnbaum et al. (199) studied ECGs of 2,370 patients with first AMI who received thrombolytics.

Findings: **Abnormal Q waves** on the admission ECG were associated with **higher peak CK, higher prevalence of heart failure, and higher mortality in patients with anterior, but not inferior, AMI.**

12

ANTERIOR AMI

KEY POINTS

- Anterior AMI is associated with the highest mortality and complication rate of AMIs and carries the greatest urgency for timely reperfusion.
- Even ST elevation of < 1 mm may represent early anterior AMI.
- Anterior AMI may mimic early repolarization and be missed.
- When clinical suspicion is high and there is any ST elevation, OBTAIN PREVIOUS AND SERIAL ECGs; anterior AMI may only become apparent upon comparison.

ANATOMY

The **left main coronary artery** supplies the **left anterior descending artery (LAD)** and the **circumflex artery.** Occlusion of the left main coronary artery (Fig. 12-1) usually leads to

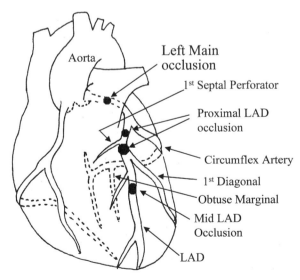

FIGURE 12-1. Occlusions of the left main coronary artery, and proximal and mid left anterior descending artery (LAD).

cardiogenic shock and death unless there is reperfusion. The **LAD** supplies the anterior wall, the anterolateral wall, and most of the septum. It may also extend around to the inferior wall, in which case it is called a "**wraparound LAD.**" Myocardium at risk in anterior AMI depends on proximal versus distal site of occlusion and the supply of collateral coronary arteries.

- **Proximal LAD occlusion** (Fig. 12-1) affects the first diagonal artery and/or the first septal perforator, causing **anterolateral AMI, anteroseptal AMI, or antero-septal lateral AMI.**
- **Mid-LAD occlusion** (Fig. 12-1) causes **anterior AMI.**

GENERAL BACKGROUND

Anterior AMI carries the highest mortality and complication rate of AMIs (122). The amount of myocardium at risk is greater in anterior AMI than for other locations (110,126). Postinfarction ejection fraction (EF) is also worse in anterior AMI than with AMI in other locations, even when controlled for size as calculated by creatine kinase (CK) release. Thus anterior AMI shows the **greatest urgency for timely reperfusion therapy.**

ECG DIAGNOSIS OF ANTERIOR AMI
Locations of ST Elevation in Anterior AMI

- **Anterior AMI** manifests ST elevation in **V2–V4,** maximal in V2–V3.
- **Anterolateral AMI** is generally due to proximal LAD occlusion and accounts for approximately 50% of anterior infarctions (132). It manifests as ST elevation in **V1 (or V2) – V4,** and ST elevation in **V5, V6, and/or I, aVL.** ST elevation in aVL > 0.5 mm is very sensitive for, and > 1.0 mm is very specific for, occlusion proximal to the first diagonal artery.
- **Anteroseptal AMI** manifests ST elevation in **V1–V4,** maximal in V2–V3. **Any** ST elevation in **aVR** is 43% sensitive and 95% specific for LAD occlusion proximal to the first septal perforator artery (133).
- **Anteroinferior AMI** is caused by occlusion of a wrap-around LAD when this is the primary artery supplying the inferior wall. It manifests ST elevation in **V2–V4** (with or without ST

elevation in V1, V5, I, aVL) **AND** in **II, III, aVF.** Anteroinferior AMI may be **mimicked** by "pseudoanteroseptal AMI," and it may mimic pericarditis. (See Case 24-7.)

See Cases 12-1 to 12-3 for examples of anterior AMI. (See also Cases 3-1 and 3-2, which show the ECG manifestations of proximal LAD occlusion.)

Pseudoanteroseptal AMI

Pseudoanteroseptal AMI looks like an anterior AMI but is actually a **large, high-risk right ventricular (RV) AMI** due to proximal right coronary artery (RCA) occlusion (200,201). Pseudoanteroseptal AMI:

- Manifests ST elevation in **V1–V3 (± V4–V5).**
- Causes up to 7% of cases with ST elevation in V1 to V5 (201).
- Usually occurs with **concomitant inferior AMI,** which manifests ST elevation in II, III, aVF (200,201). ST elevation is greatest in V1 and decreases from V1–V5 (see Case 13-3).
- May also show development of Q waves in V1–V3 (200).
- In the presence of right ventricular hypertrophy (RVH), may be nearly indistinguishable from anterior AMI (see Case 15-6).

Reciprocal Inferior ST Depression in Anterior AMI

Inferior ST depression in anterior AMI, **especially > 1 mm in lead II,** is highly **predictive of LAD occlusion proximal to the first diagonal (132,133).** This may indicate a true reciprocal view of high anterior infarction (**136**) **or** concurrent high lateral infarction, and is especially likely if there is also ST depression in lead III. Look for **ST elevation in aVL and I, in addition to inferior reciprocal depression.**

ST depression in **lead III** ≥ ST elevation in aVL is very accurate for occlusion proximal to **both** the first septal perforator and the first diagonal (**202**).

The presence of reciprocal changes is associated with **higher precordial ST elevation and with worse prognosis** than anterior AMI without reciprocal changes. See Lew et al. (**203**), Mittal et al. (**134**), and Haraphongse et al. (**135**) for alternative etiologies of reciprocal ST depression in II, III, and aVF in the context of anterior ST elevation.

Anterior AMI Look-Alikes

Anterior AMI can mimic early repolarization and be overlooked (see Case 12-4). Conversely, early repolarization, LVH, ventricular aneurysm, and, occasionally, pericarditis are common pseudoinfarction patterns that mimic anterior AMI

(see Chapters 20, 22–24). Consult a previous ECG, record serial ECGs and look for diagnostic changes (see Case 12-5).

ST Elevation of < 1 to 2 mm May Represent Anterior AMI

ST elevation "criteria" for thrombolysis in AMI are **GUIDELINES ONLY.** Many studies use 2 mm ST elevation in two leads or more. The American College of Cardiology (ACC) and American Heart Association (AHA) (105) and TAMI and TIMI study groups use 1 mm ST elevation (see Chapter 6). **If the patient's baseline ST segments show no elevation, early anterior ST-elevation MI (STEMI) may present with < 1 mm ST elevation on the initial ECG.** See Case 12-6. (See also Case 9-5 of a very subtle anterior AMI; and Case 11-2 in which tiny Q waves in a very subtle ECG aid diagnosis of anterior AMI.)

AREA AT RISK IN ANTERIOR AMI

Selvester's study (110) (prereperfusion era) of AMI size in 312 patients with LAD occlusion indicated the following:

13% massive	>30% of left ventricle (LV)	EF < 30%
18% large	21% to 30% of LV	EF 30% to 39%
40% moderate	11% to 20% of LV	EF 40% to 49%
29% small	<10% of LV	EF >50%

Predictors of Larger AMI and Greater Mortality

Overall mortality of anterior AMI in patients treated with thrombolytics is 9.9%, versus 5.5% for all inferior AMI (122). Predictors of larger AMI and greater mortality include the following:

- Greater **number** of leads with ST elevation
- Greater **height** of ST segments
- Presence of **reciprocal ST depression**
- **Sum** of absolute ST segment deviation (positive or negative) greater than 1.2 mV (**12 mm**)
- **Terminal QRS distortion** by the ST segment (see Figs. 6-2n–p)

These factors also indicate **increased benefit of reperfusion therapy.**

MANAGEMENT

Compare equivocal ECGs with previous tracings and serial tracings. Know the pseudoinfarction patterns. Treat aggressively with reperfusion therapy.

CASE 12-1

ECG Diagnostic of Antero-Septal Lateral AMI Despite ST Elevation < 2 mm

History
This 60-year-old man with no medical history presented with 5 hours of typical CP. Physical exam detected rales. A chest x-ray indicated congestive heart failure (CHF).

ECG 12-1A (Type 1c)
- ST elevation: **< 2 mm,** V1–V3 (whether measured at or 80 ms after the J point); there is no distinct J point or tall T wave of benign early repolarization and more than 45 years of age makes this diagnosis unlikely.
- Q wave: V2; poor R-wave progression; ST depression: minimal, II, III, aVF, probably reciprocal to minimal ST elevation in aVL. The computer (1998 program) read this ECG as a "possible old anteroseptal MI."

ECG 12-1B (Type 4)
ECG from 2 years prior
- This normal ECG faxed from another hospital demonstrates that ECG 12-1A shows clear changes and is diagnostic of **antero-septal lateral AMI.**

Clinical Course
Clinicians administered tissue plasminogen activator (tPA). The ECG showed no improvement at 90 minutes post treatment, so the patient was taken for angiography and possible percutaneous coronary infarction (PCI). A 95% LAD stenosis proximal to the first diagonal and first septal perforator arteries was dilated and stented. Cardiac troponin I (cTnI) and total CK were 3.5 ng/mL and 700 IU/L on arrival, respectively, and peaked at 560 ng/mL and 7,600 IU/L. Convalescent echocardiography revealed moderately decreased LV function and a moderate to severe wall motion abnormality (WMA) in anterior and lateral walls and the distal septum and apex.

Conclusion
ST elevation ≥ 2 mm is not a necessary condition for reperfusion therapy in anterior AMI. Despite small total ST deviation in this case, the infarct was very large.

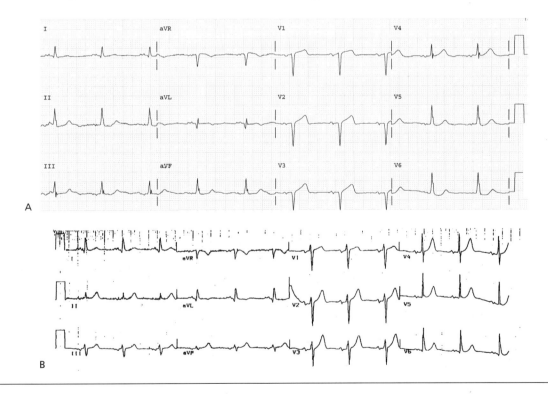

CASE 12-2

Antero-Lateral-Septal AMI

History

This 78-year-old man presented with 1 hour of CP and vomiting. He had a history of proximal LAD and circumflex artery disease and recent atherectomy of the mid-LAD.

ECG 12-2 (Type 1b)

- ST elevation: **< 2 mm at the J point, V1–V5 but 5 mm at 80 msec past the J point,** is diagnostic of **anterior AMI.**
- ST elevation: aVL; with reciprocal ST depression: II, III, aVF, V6. This confirms the diagnosis of **anterolateral**

AMI and is indicative of LAD occlusion proximal to the first diagonal artery. ST elevation: **aVR and V1**, indicates **septal** involvement.

Clinical Course

Immediate thrombolysis was followed by resolution of ST elevation and symptoms.

Conclusion

A proximal LAD lesion was presumed but angiography was not performed.

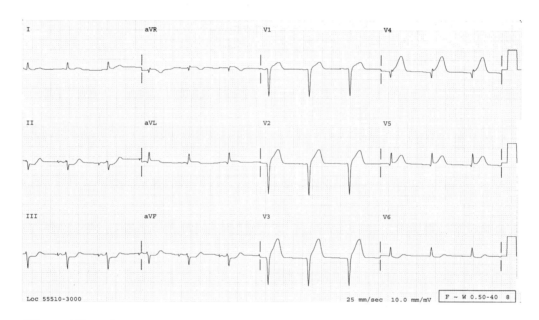

Loc 55510-3000   25 mm/sec   10.0 mm/mV   F ~ W 0.50-40   8

CASE 12-3

Spontaneously Reperfused Anterior AMI with Terminal T-Wave Inversion (Wellens' Syndrome)

History

This 51-year-old woman with history of RCA angioplasty and stent arrived by ambulance after 48 hours of stuttering CP and 1 hour of constant CP.

ECG 12-3A (Prehospital Rhythm Strip)
- ST elevation: MCL III (equivalent to V3), is **suspicious** for anterior AMI.

ECG 12-3B (Prehospital Rhythm Strip)
- Reciprocal depression: III, is **suspicious** for concurrent anterior or lateral AMI or for inferior ischemia. The patient received four sublingual nitroglycerine (NTG) and her pain resolved.

ECG 12-3C (Prehospital Rhythm Strip)

Fifteen minutes later, while pain-free
- Resolution of ST elevation in modified chest leads (MCL) III; reperfusion is probable.

ECG 12-3D (Type 2)

In the emergency department (ED):
- Terminal T-wave inversion: V2–V4, due to spontaneously reperfused anterior AMI; this is **Wellens' syndrome.** This morphology is also seen after therapeutic reperfusion.
- ST depression: minimal, II, III, aVF, remains.

Clinical Course

A previous ECG showed no T-wave morphology such as is seen in ECG 12-3D. The patient received aspirin, unfractionated heparin, metoprolol, intravenous (IV) NTG, and a glycoprotein (GP) IIb-IIIa inhibitor. Peak cTnI was 1.5 ng/mL, indicative of a very small amount of myocardial necrosis. Interventionalists successfully angioplastied and stented a 95% occluded mid-LAD, 85% occluded distal LAD and 95% occluded distal RCA.

Conclusion

Acute coronary syndrome (ACS) and ST elevation with terminal T-wave inversion (Wellens' syndrome) signifies spontaneous reperfusion of an occluded (usually critically narrowed) coronary artery.

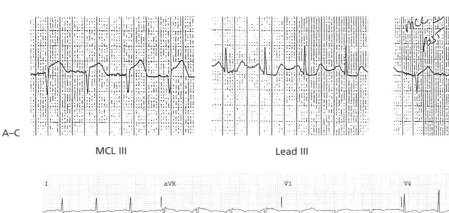

A–C   MCL III   Lead III   MCL III

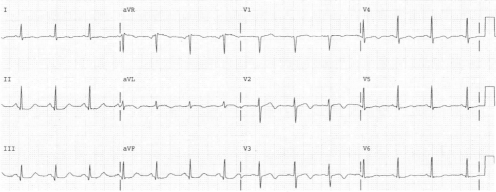

D

CASE 12-4

STEMI Mimics Early Repolarization but Is Due Entirely to Anterior AMI

History
This 56-year-old man presented with severe crushing CP with radiation to both arms, diaphoresis, and shortness of breath (SOB).

ECG 12-4A (Type 1c)
Recorded at 10:12
- ST elevation: V2–V3, consistent with early repolarization or STEMI.

ECG 12-4B (Type 1c by itself, but Type 1b after comparison with 12-4A)
Recorded at 10:28, V1–V6 only
- ST elevation: increased.

Clinical Course
Immediate bedside echocardiography confirmed severe anterior WMA. Clinicians administered tPA, with rapid and complete relief of symptoms.

ECG 12-4C (Type 4)
Recorded 32 minutes later, V1–V3 only
- All ST segments are at baseline.

Clinical Course
Maintained on heparin and aspirin. Peak cTnI was 13.3 ng/mL. Subsequent ECGs developed T-wave inversion. Angiography confirmed a 90% proximal LAD culprit lesion. Repeat echocardiography was normal.

Conclusion
For a patient with zero ST elevation at baseline, any ST elevation may be AMI. Do not assume early repolarization, and use serial ECGs and echocardiography if necessary.

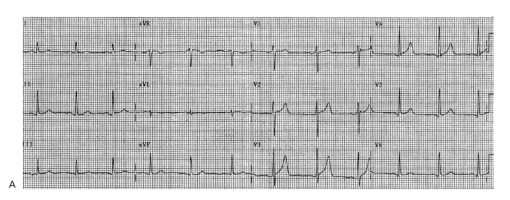

A

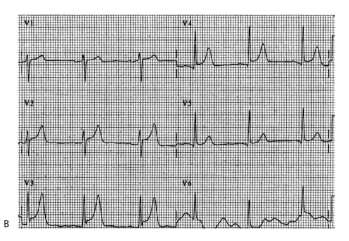

B

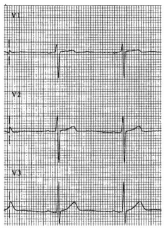

C

CASE 12-5

Hyperacute T Waves Mimic Early Repolarization in This Anterior AMI
Due to a Mid-LAD Occlusion

History
This 76-year-old Russian-speaking man with a history of CAD presented with 1 hour of CP.

ECG 12-5A (Type 1c)
■ ST elevation: V2–V4, 1 to 2 mm (although > 2 mm at 80 msec after the J point). Although this ECG looks like early repolarization, this is unlikely because the patient is 76 years old, there is no early transition, and the T wave is greater than the R wave in V2–V4.

ECG 12-5B (Type 3)
ECG from 3 days prior, V1–V6 only

■ This previous ECG confirms clear changes, making ECG 12-4a diagnostic of **anterior AMI.**

Clinical Course
Clinicians performed immediate successful PCI on an occluded mid-LAD. Peak cTnI was only 0.6 ng/mL and convalescent echocardiography was normal.

Conclusion
Do not attribute ST elevation to early repolarization if it occurs in the context of a typical AMI history. Prompt comparison with a previous ECG facilitates rapid diagnosis and treatment. Perform immediate angiography ± PCI and/or serial ECGs if there is no previous ECG available.

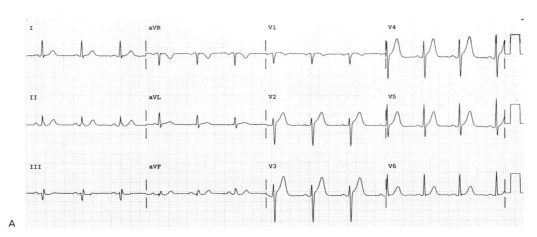

A

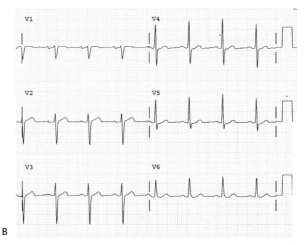

B

CASE 12-6

Subtle Anterior AMI with ST Elevation in V3–V4 Obscured, and Thus Missed, by Half-Standard Voltage

History

This 49-year-old man with risk factors for CAD (smoking, hyperlipidemia, concentric LVH) presented with 8 hours of severe intermittent typical CP.

ECG 12-6A (Type 1b)

At 01:13:

- ST elevation: 1 mm, V2–V4.
- Q waves: small, V3–V4, and also II, III, aVF, diagnostic of **old** inferior MI.
- Precordial leads are recorded at **half standard**, with 1 mm = 0.2 mV (see step-down boxes at right). The **ST elevation is 0.2 mV and is significant in comparison with the QRS magnitude.** This is **not** early repolarization, which would have large R waves in V2–V4. This ECG is diagnostic of **anterior AMI.**

ECG 12-6B (Type 1d)

Eighty minutes later, is **not** half standard.

- ST elevation: 2 to 3 mm (2 mm at the J point and 3 mm at 80 msec after the J point), V3–V4 (0.2 to 0.3 mV); and terminal T-wave inversions: V2–V5, confirm the diagnosis of **anterior AMI,** and suggest spontaneous reperfusion.

Clinical Course

The patient confirmed ongoing pain. Acute reperfusion therapy was not undertaken. He ruled in for AMI with cTnI of 51 ng/mL, a total CK of 990 IU/L, and development of diagnostic T-wave inversions. Angiography the next day revealed a 100% mid-LAD occlusion and a 95% stenosis of the first diagonal; PCI opened and stented both lesions. The patient's convalescent EF was 50% to 55% with concentric LVH and no WMA.

Conclusion

Subsequent deep T-wave inversions and relatively low enzymes, in spite of a persistently occluded vessel, suggest good collateral circulation. Fortunately, this infarct was small, with no significant WMA despite failure to perform acute reperfusion therapy. However, ventricular function was significantly impaired. **Remember to account for ECG calibration and assess ST elevation relative to QRS magnitude.**

For more examples of anterior AMI, see Chapters 6, 9, and 10.

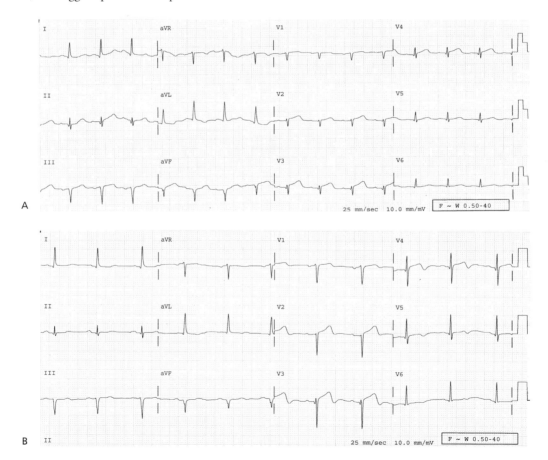

ANNOTATED BIBLIOGRAPHY

Reciprocal Changes and AMI Localization
See also Chapter 7.

Engelen DJ, et al. Value of the electrocardiogram in localizing the occlusion site in the left anterior descending coronary artery in acute myocardial infarction, 1999.
Methods: Engelen et al. (133) studied 100 patients who underwent angiography for first anterior AMI. ST segments were measured at the J point and relative to the TP segment.
Findings: Occlusion was proximal to the first diagonal artery in 41 patients and distal in 59. Occlusion was proximal to the first septal perforator in 42 patients and distal in 58. ST elevation of any amount (especially < 1 mm) in aVR was 43% sensitive and 95% specific for occlusion proximal to the first septal perforator, with a positive predictive value (PPV) of 86%. ST depression > 1 mm in lead II was only 34% sensitive but 98% specific for occlusion proximal to the first diagonal artery.

Tamura A, et al. Inferior ST segment depression as a useful marker for identifying proximal left anterior descending artery occlusion during acute anterior myocardial infarction, 1995.
Methods: Tamura et al. (137) studied 47 patients with proximal LAD occlusion and 59 patients with distal LAD occlusion.
Findings: One millimeter of ST depression in all three inferior leads at once (II, III, and aVF) was 77% sensitive and 78% specific for proximal LAD occlusion.

Birnbaum Y, et al. Prediction of the level of left anterior descending coronary artery obstruction during anterior wall acute myocardial infarction by the admission electrocardiogram, 1993.
Methods: Birnbaum et al. (132) studied 107 patients with anterior AMI who underwent angiography.
Findings: Occlusion was proximal to the first diagonal artery in 48 patients and distal in 59 patients. ST elevation > 1 mm in aVL was 46% sensitive for LAD occlusion proximal to the first diagonal and had a PPV of 81%. ST depression > 1 mm in inferior leads, especially aVF, was a useful indicator of LAD occlusion proximal to the first diagonal; it was 82% sensitive and had a PPV of 87%.

Tamura A, et al. Emergent coronary angiographic findings of patients with ST depression in the inferior or lateral leads, or both, during anterior wall acute myocardial infarction, 1995.
Methods: Tamura et al. (85) studied ECGs and angiograms of 106 anterior AMI patients.
Findings: Presence of **ST depression in inferior and/or lateral leads** occurred in 81 patients and was associated with **proximal LAD occlusion, greater infarct size, and a poorer prognosis.**

Kosuge M, et al. Electrocardiographic criteria for predicting total occlusion of the proximal left anterior descending coronary artery in anterior wall acute myocardial infarction, 2001.
Methods: Kosuge et al. (202) evaluated ECGs and angiograms of 128 anterior AMI patients with first AMI and complete LAD occlusion. LAD occlusion was proximal to the first diagonal and the first septal perforator artery in 33 patients, proximal to either in 51, and distal to both in 44 patients. ST elevation was measured at the J point and relative to the TP segment.
Findings: ST elevation ≥ 0.5 mm in aVL was 100% sensitive and 44% specific for proximal LAD occlusion. ST depression in lead III was 97% sensitive and 45% specific. **The most accurate predictor** of occlusion proximal to **both the first diagonal and the first septal perforator** was **ST depression in lead III >** ST elevation in aVL, with 85% sensitivity and 95% specificity.

Norell MS, et al. Significance of "reciprocal" ST segment depression: left ventriculographic observations during left anterior descending coronary angioplasty, 1989.
Methods: Norell et al. (136) evaluated ECGs and ventriculography of 27 patients with single vessel coronary artery disease (CAD) during balloon inflation of the LAD.
Findings: Patients with reciprocal inferior ST depression did **not** have inferior wall ventriculographic hypokinesis. They **did** have worse overall LV function, "anterobasal" (high anterior wall) hypokinesis and anterior and apical hypokinesis. The mean amount of anterior ST elevation in patients with reciprocal inferior ST depression was 5.0 mm versus 1.5 mm in patients without reciprocal depression. The authors conclude that **inferior reciprocal depression during anterior AMI is a reciprocal view of anterobasal ST elevation,** not a manifestation of inferior wall ischemia.

Lew AS, et al. Inferior ST segment changes during acute anterior myocardial infarction: a marker of the presence or absence of concomitant inferior wall ischemia, 1987.
Methods: Lew et al. (203) performed angiography on 60 anterior AMI patients.
Findings: The ABSENCE of inferior ST depression indicated concomitant inferior infarction, with the inferior wall collaterally dependent on the LAD. By their analysis, the ST elevation of inferior AMI canceled out reciprocal depression of the anterior AMI. This data suggests that inferior reciprocal depression in anterior AMI indicates a smaller AMI. Although this data is interesting, it is contrary to the vast majority of data that indicates that reciprocal ST depression signifies a larger AMI.

Haraphongse M, et al. Inferior ST segment depression during acute anterior myocardial infarction: clinical and angiographic correlations, 1984.
Methods: Haraphongse et al. (135) studied 33 anterior AMI patients.
Findings: Reciprocal ST depression in II, III, and aVF was associated with RCA or circumflex artery disease and greater mortality and complications. Patients lacking reciprocal depression were less likely to have other CAD.

Simultaneous RV AMI
Mittal SR, et al. Electrocardiographic diagnosis of infarction of the right ventricular anterior wall, 1996.
Methods: Mittal et al. (134) performed echocardiography and angiography on 50 patients with AMI manifesting in anterior leads.
Findings: Of 50 patients, 12 suffered **RV** AMI as well as LV anterior AMI. The presence of "reciprocal" ST depression in the inferior leads was highly sensitive and specific for infarction of the RV **and** LV anterior walls. This inferior "reciprocal" ST depression was present in 10 of 12 patients with both RV-anterior wall and LV-anterior wall AMI (sensitivity = 83%). Of 32 patients with **only LV**-anterior AMI, only two had inferior ST depression (specificity = 94%). Right-sided chest leads were insensitive for AMI in this area of the RV. Andersen et al. (204) also found significant association of RV AMI with anterior (LV) AMI and found that the right-sided leads were not as sensitive for this type of RV AMI as for RV AMI associated with inferior AMI (see Chapter 15).

Pseudoanteroseptal AMI
See annotations of Khan et al. (200) and Geft et al. (201) in Chapter 15.

Prognosis of Anterior AMI, Benefit of Reperfusion Therapy, and ST Score
See annotations in Chapter 6 (111,114,117,122,123,126).

13

INFERIOR AMI

KEY POINTS

- The hallmark of inferior AMI is ST elevation in II, III, and aVF, with concurrent ST depression in aVL.
- ALWAYS look for CONCURRENT RV AMI: look for ST elevation in V1; also ST depression in V5–V6.
  - Record a RIGHT-SIDED ECG: look for ST elevation in V2R–V7R, especially V4R. Use IV NTG with caution before ruling out concurrent RV AMI.
- A small inferior AMI in a patient with a previously normal EF has low mortality and may receive limited benefit from thrombolytics. Consider this in patients at high risk for bleeding.

ANATOMY

The **RCA** supplies the inferior wall in 80% to 85% of people; this is called a "right dominant system" (130,131) (Fig. 13-1) Alternatively, the **circumflex artery** supplies the inferior wall through the posterior descending artery in 15% to 20% of people; this is called a "left dominant system" (Fig. 13-2). The **RV marginal branch** of the RCA supplies the RV. The lateral and posterior walls are associated myocardial areas at risk with either right or left dominant systems.

- **RCA occlusion** is the most common cause of **inferior AMI** (**205**,206). **Proximal RCA occlusion** (Fig. 13-1a) results in **inferior AMI and concurrent RV AMI.** RCA occlusion distal to the RV marginal branch spares the RV (Fig. 13-1b). Occlusion of an RCA with a large posterolateral branch leads to **inferolateral, inferoposterior, or infero-postero lateral AMI.**
- **Circumflex artery occlusion** in a left dominant system is a less common cause of inferior AMI than RCA occlusion in a right dominant system; however, it may be a more common cause of **inferolateral AMI** than RCA occlusion (130,131). In inferior AMI, an isoelectric or elevated lead I (131), less reciprocal ST depression in lead aVL (130,131), and at least 0.5 mm ST elevation in leads V5 and V6 (130) is most commonly due to circumflex occlusion. ST elevation in II ≥ III predicts the circumflex as the culprit artery with 97% sensitivity and 90% specificity (131).

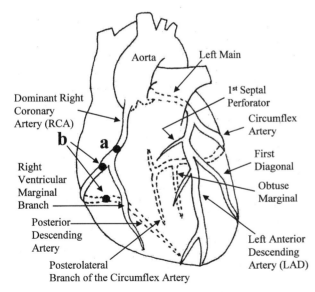

FIGURE 13-1. Coronary anatomy and sites of occlusion of dominant RCA ("right dominant system"). Occlusion at site **a** leads to inferior and RV AMI. Occlusion at sites labeled **b** spares the RV.

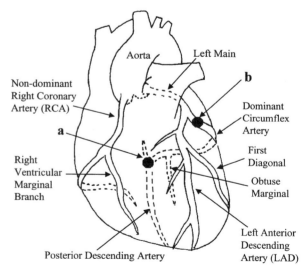

FIGURE 13-2. Coronary anatomy and sites of occlusion of a dominant circumflex ("left dominant system"). Occlusion at site **a** leads to inferior AMI. More proximal occlusion, as at **b** may affect the lateral and posterior walls.

ECG DIAGNOSIS OF INFERIOR AMI
ST Elevation in II, III, aVF

ST elevation < 1 mm in inferior leads may be a baseline finding, but ST elevation ≥ 0.5 mm should be considered **abnormal** until proven otherwise by any or all of the following:

■ **No change** from an old ECG.
■ **No change** in serial ECGs or ST segment monitoring.
■ **No ST depression in aVL;** baseline reciprocal ST depression is rare.

See Cases 13-1 and 13-2.

Other ST Elevation in Inferior AMI

ST elevation in V1 indicates RV AMI. Left-sided ST elevation may extend from **V1–V5,** with decreasing height of ST segments (200,201). This may mimic anterior AMI ("pseudoanteroseptal AMI," see Cases 13-3 and 15-6). Record right-sided chest leads to confirm RV AMI (207). Look for **ST elevation in V2R –V7R,** especially **V4R** (V2R is the same position as V1) (see Chapter 15). **ST elevation in lateral leads I, aVL, and/or V5–V6** indicates **inferolateral AMI** and is a result of occlusion of a **very large RCA** or of a **very large circumflex artery** (205) (see Case 7-3).

ST elevation in posterior chest leads V7–V9 indicates a larger infarct with greater incidence of adverse events and greater benefit from reperfusion therapy (**208**).

ST Depression in Inferior AMI

ST depression in aVL (and often in lead I) that is reciprocal to ST elevation in lead III is a very important diagnostic feature. Lead aVL is 150° opposite lead III and has an electrically opposite view. Lead I is 120° opposite lead III (see Fig. 4-2). Almost all inferior AMIs have reciprocal ST depression in aVL. This is not "lateral wall ischemia." **Exception:** Concurrent lateral AMI may elevate aVL to isoelectric or to actual elevation and obscure reciprocal depression in aVL (see Case 7-3).

ST depression in aVL helps to distinguish inferior AMI from diffuse pericarditis and early repolarization, which do not have ST depression in aVL. Diffuse pericarditis may lead to ST elevation in aVL. Pericarditis also typically shows maximal ST elevation in lead II, not lead III. Thus pericarditis and inferior AMI due to circumflex occlusion are very difficult to differentiate (see Chapter 24).

ST depression in precordial leads V1–V6 concurrent with inferior ST elevation reflects a larger amount of myocardium at risk, higher mortality, and greater potential benefit of reperfusion (**112,128,129,209**). This ST depression is generally due to concurrent posterior wall injury **(inferoposterior AMI), not** due to anterior subendocardial ischemia (**138–141,209**). See Case 13-4. (See also Cases 16-9 and 16-10.) ST depression in V5–V6 **may** reflect **RV AMI.** (See Cases 15-2 and 15-4.)

ST depression in V1–V3 concurrent with lateral ST elevation, in conjunction with inferior ST elevation, indicates **infero-posterior lateral AMI** (see Case 13-5).

Even minimal ST depression in **V1–V5** helps to confirm that subtle inferior ST elevation is due to inferior AMI. (See Case 5-5, which describes a patient who was discharged and died due to a subtle inferoposterior AMI that was missed.)

Inferior Pseudoinfarction

ST elevation of early repolarization is infrequent in inferior leads II, III, and aVF. ST elevation in inferior leads is **not** early repolarization unless it is also present in anterior precordial leads. ST elevation of early repolarization does **not** manifest with reciprocal ST depression. **Pericarditis** frequently mimics inferolateral AMI, especially the less common **localized** pericarditis (see Chapter 24). WPW may also mimic inferior AMI.

AREA AT RISK IN INFERIOR AMI
Infarct Size

Selvester's pre-reperfusion era study (**110**) of inferior AMI size in 301 patients indicated:

1% massive	>30% of LV	EF < 30%
6% large	21% to 30% of LV	EF 30% to 39%
35% moderate	11% to 20% of LV	EF 40% to 49%
58% small	<10% of LV	EF >50%

Predictors of Larger AMI and Greater Mortality

Large inferior AMIs have high mortality. Mortality in patients given thrombolytics is 5% for all inferior AMI versus 9.9% in anterior AMI (122; see annotation in Chapter 6). Predictors of larger size, greater mortality, and therefore greater potential benefit from reperfusion therapy include (**128,129,207,210**):

■ **Concurrent RV AMI,** especially as indicated by V4R.
■ **Greater number** of leads with **reciprocal ST depression.**
■ **Greater number** of leads with **ST elevation.**
■ **Greater height** of ST segments.
■ **Greater total sum** of absolute ST-segment deviation, positive and negative. A total sum of more than 1.2 mV (12 mm) is high risk (117).

MANAGEMENT

■ **Small inferior AMIs,** in patients with normal EFs, have low overall mortality. Therefore there is **less potential benefit** from thrombolytics if the AMI shows ST elevation **only** in II, III, aVF, and ST depression **only** in aVL (29,**30**). With **major relative contraindications to thrombolytics** and an AMI more than 6 hours old, thrombolytics may not be indicated. Angiography ± PCI is recommended, if available, to avoid risk of intracranial hemorrhage.
■ Record a right-sided ECG to look for concurrent RV AMI (see Chapter 15).
■ Use IV NTG with caution in the presence of suspected RV AMI (see Chapter 15).

CASE 13-1

Thrombolytics Delayed in a Patient with a Small Inferior AMI

History

This 68-year-old woman presented after 3 hours of CP. She had no relative contraindications to thrombolysis.

ECG 13-1 (Type 1b)

■ ST elevation: subtle, II, III, aVF; ST depression: subtle, aVL; hyperacute T waves: II, III, aVF. Despite a low ST score and ST elevation in only three leads (plus the obligatory reciprocal depression in aVL), this ECG is diagnostic of **inferior AMI**.

Clinical Course

A subsequent right-sided ECG was negative. The patient had no contraindications to thrombolysis. However, physicians did not recognize this AMI. A second ECG revealed increased ST deviations. Clinicians administered thrombolytics 108 minutes after presentation. Total CK peaked at 380 IU/L despite the delay.

Conclusion

This ECG, with a small ST score, represents a small AMI; nevertheless, prompt thrombolytic therapy is indicated.

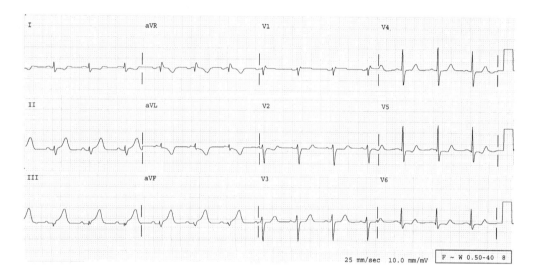

25 mm/sec 10.0 mm/mV   F ~ W 0.50-40 8

Inferior AMI and Delayed Reperfusion Therapy

History
This 56-year-old woman presented with 45 minutes of CP.

ECG 13-2 (Type 1b)
- ST elevation: subtle, II, III, aVF; and ST depression: subtle, aVL, are diagnostic of **inferior AMI.**

Clinical Course
Physicians did not recognize this AMI and sent the patient to a telemetry unit without reperfusion therapy. A repeat ECG 2 hours later was clearly diagnostic of AMI. Thrombolytics were administered and the artery reperfused. Angioplasty subsequent to reocclusion opened a mid-RCA occlusion. Convalescent echocardiography revealed an inferior WMA, but the EF was within normal limits.

Conclusion
Reperfusion therapy was unnecessarily delayed by 2 hours.

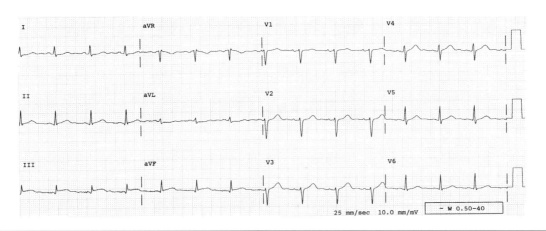

Pseudoanteroseptal AMI

History
This 52-year-old man presented with 2 to 3 days of intermittent epigastric burning, followed this day by dyspnea and syncope. Systolic BP = 70 to 80.

ECG 13-3 (Type 1a)
- ST elevation: II, III, aVF; and reciprocal ST depression: aVL, are diagnostic of **inferior AMI.**
- ST elevation: V1–V3, maximal in V2. This is **NOT** anterior AMI.

Clinical Course
IV fluids improved the BP. Angiography revealed RCA occlusion proximal to the RV branch. PCI with stenting resulted in TIMI-3 flow and immediate ST resolution.

Conclusion
This is an **inferior AMI** with a **large RV AMI** that, if untreated, could result in Q waves that mimic anterior MI.

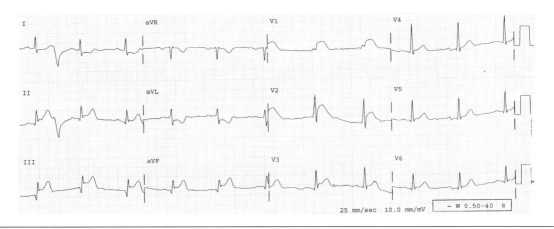

CASE 13-4

Inferoposterior AMI with Reperfusion and Reocclusion

History

This 52-year-old man presented with syncope and 80 minutes of CP.

ECG 13-4A (Type 1a)

At 03:00 on Day 1.

- ST elevation: II, III, aVF; and reciprocal ST depression: aVL, are diagnostic of **inferior AMI.**
- ST depression: deep, V2–V6, is diagnostic of **posterior AMI.**

Clinical Course

Clinicians administered thrombolytics.

ECG 13-4B (Type 2)

At 04:31 on Day 1.

- All ST deviations in ECG 13-3A are more than 50% resolved, indicating **reperfusion.**

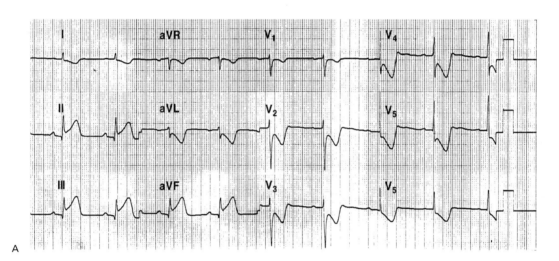

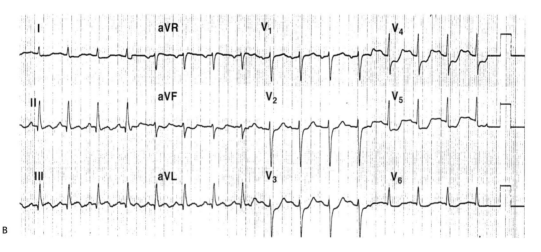

(continued on next page)

CASE 13-4

Inferoposterior AMI with Reperfusion and Reocclusion *(continued)*

ECG 13-4C (Type 1a)
At 07:56 on Day 2
- Third-degree atrioventricular (AV) block, with wide escape.
- Recurrent ST elevation: II, III, aVF, indicates **reocclusion.**
- V1–V3: Premature ventricular contractions (PVCs) and escape both have ST depression of **posterior AMI.**

Clinical Course
Angioplasty opened a high-grade lesion of a dominant RCA.

ECG 13-4D (Type 2)
At 08:20 on Day 2
- ST resolution: II, III, aVF, and V1–V6.
- Symmetric T-wave inversion > 3 mm: II, III, aVF, typical of reperfused MI.
- Tall precordial T waves, typical of **reperfusion** of posterior AMI.

Conclusion
Close monitoring of this large inferior AMI detected reperfusion and reocclusion.

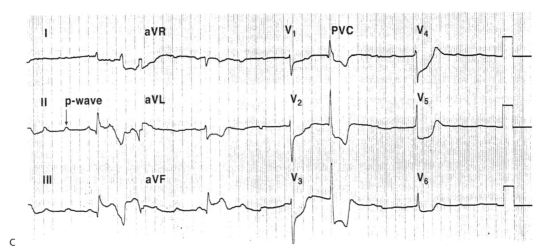

C

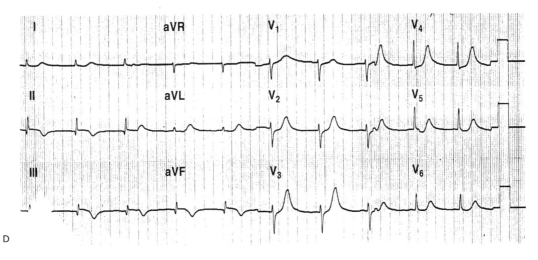

D

CASE 13-5

Large Infero-Posterolateral and RV AMI

History

This 68-year-old woman presented hypotensive and brady-cardic after 30 minutes of prehospital CP. She received atropine, and rhythm strips showed 8 mm of ST elevation in lead II.

ECG 13-5 (Type 1a)

- ST elevation: 6 mm, II, III, aVF; and reciprocal depression: I, aVL, are diagnostic of **inferior AMI.**
- ST depression: V1–V4, maximal in V3, is diagnostic of **posterior AMI.**
- ST elevation: V5–V6, is diagnostic of **lateral AMI.**
- ST score: 18 mm (1.8 mV) or 33 mm if the anterior ST depression is counted as ST elevation of posterior AMI. This is a **large AMI.**

Clinical Course

A subsequent right-sided ECG showed ST elevation in V4R. The patient was intubated, externally paced, and given thrombolytics within 18 minutes of arrival. Her dominant RCA reperfused and she recovered well. Subsequent angiography revealed "CAD of RCA and LAD," inferior akinesis, and mildly decreased LV function, but convalescent echocardiography revealed **no WMA and a normal EF.**

Conclusion

Rapid diagnosis and treatment enabled a good outcome despite a large AMI. Reciprocal changes are evident in aVL because the tendency to elevate the ST segment in aVL (due to lateral AMI) is "overpowered" by aVL's reciprocity to the electrically opposite lead III (due to inferior AMI).

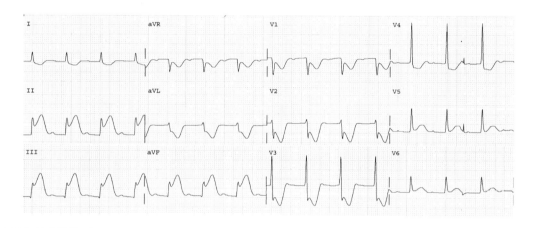

ANNOTATED BIBLIOGRAPHY

Benefit of Thrombolytic Therapy in Inferior AMI
See also annotation of Mauri et al. (109) in Chapter 6.

GISSI. Effectiveness of intravenous thrombolytic treatment in acute myocardial infarction, 1986 and ISIS-2. Randomised trial of intravenous streptokinase, oral aspirin, both, or neither among 17,187 cases of suspected acute myocardial infarction, 1988.
   Methods: GISSI-1 (29) and ISIS-2 (102) randomized patients with AMI to streptokinase (SK) versus control (see Appendix C).
   Findings: GISSI-I: Thirty-five-day mortality for all inferior AMI was 7.2% for controls and 6.8% for the SK group, which is not a statistically significant difference. ISIS-2: Thirty-five-day mortality for all inferior AMI in ISIS-2 was 8.8% for controls and 7.2% for the SK group. This represents 16 lives saved per 1,000 patients treated. The confidence interval (CI) was approximately 0 to 28.

FTT Collaborative Group. Indications for fibrinolytic therapy in suspected acute myocardial infarction: collaborative overview of early mortality and major morbidity results from all randomised trials of more than 1,000 patients, 1994.
   Methods: The FTT study (30) analyzed data on 58,600 patients in nine trials of thrombolytic therapy versus placebo (see Appendix C). Most patients received SK.
   Findings: All 13,000 inferior AMI patients were grouped together, with and without reciprocal depression, RV MI, or posterior AMI, and regardless of time from symptom onset to treatment. There was only a trend toward decreased mortality for inferior AMI at 35 days (8.4% versus 7.5%).
   Comment: Findings suggest that patients with small AMIs, usually inferior infarctions with no RV or posterior involvement, who present late and have one or more relative complications, may not benefit from streptokinase.

LATE Study Group. Late assessment of thrombolytic efficacy (LATE) study with alteplase 6 to 24 hours after onset of acute myocardial infarction, 1993.
   Methods: LATE (169) was a randomized, double-blind, placebo-controlled trial of tPA in 5,711 patients presenting late with symptoms and ECG findings consistent with AMI (see Appendix C).
   Findings: Thrombolytic therapy of inferior AMI patients from 6 to 12 hours after symptom onset showed no significant benefit.

Selvester RH. The 12-lead ECG and the initiation of thrombolytic therapy for acute myocardial infarction, 1993.
   Methods: Selvester (110) analyzed GISSI-1, ISIS-2, and ECSG data (see Appendix C) for risk subsets.

Findings: Although data from all inferior AMIs combined and all lateral AMIs combined showed no mortality benefit from thrombolytics, some subsets showed benefit; with inferior AMI **concurrent** with posterior or RV AMI, thrombolysis decreased mortality.

ST Score

See annotations in Chapter 6 (111,117,122,123,126).

Inferior AMI With Lateral Precordial ST Deviation

See annotations of Hasdai et al. (128), Birnbaum et al. (129), and Peterson et al. (112) in Chapter 7.

Assali AR, et al. Comparison of patients with inferior wall acute myocardial infarction with versus without ST-segment elevation in leads V5 and V6, 1998.

> **Methods:** Assali et al. (205) studied 141 patients with first AMI, located **inferiorly,** who underwent angiography during the acute hospitalization. A "**mega-artery**" was defined as a circumflex or RCA with large posterolateral branches **with** a small or medium sized LAD.
>
> **Findings:** ST elevation in V5–V6 occurred in 34 patients and was associated with **worse prognosis, larger infarct related artery (IRA), and greater benefit to reperfusion.** Among these patients, 65% demonstrated RCA occlusion and 30% circumflex occlusion. A mega-artery was found in 32 of the patients with lateral ST elevation, but in only two of 107 patients without this ECG finding, for a PPV of 94% and negative predictive value (NPV) of 98%.

Pseudoanteroseptal AMI

See annotations of Khan et al. (200) and Geft et al. (201) in Chapter 15.

Inferior AMI with Reciprocal Anterior Precordial ST Depression (Concomitant Posterior AMI)

See also Chapter 7.

Shah PK. New insights into the electrocardiogram of acute myocardial infarction, 1991.

> **Methods:** Shah (138) reviewed literature prior to 1990, with focus on the significance of precordial ST depression in inferior AMI.
>
> **Findings:** Most studies indicated that inferior AMI patients with reciprocal ST depression in V1–V4 had **larger infarcts, more extensive WMAs, lower EFs, and worse hemodynamics** than inferior AMI patients without precordial reciprocal ST depression. Findings do not support the notion that precordial reciprocal ST depression is caused by anterior subendocardial ischemia of the LAD distribution. The **magnitude** of ST depression or elevation in V1–V4 was found to depend primarily on the **presence of concurrent posterolateral AMI,** which depresses the precordial ST segment, and on RV AMI, which elevates it.

Bates ER, et al. Precordial ST segment depression predicts a worse prognosis in inferior infarction despite reperfusion therapy, 1990.

> **Methods:** Bates et al. (210) studied complication rates after thrombolysis in 583 AMI patients.
>
> **Findings:** Mortality was 8% for anterior AMI, 6% for inferior AMI with anterior reciprocal ST depression, and 5% for inferior AMI without anterior reciprocal ST depression.

Ruddy TD, et al. Anterior ST segment depression in acute myocardial infarction as a marker of greater inferior, apical, and posterolateral damage, 1986.

> **Methods:** Ruddy et al. (139) studied 67 inferior AMI patients with radionuclide imaging.
>
> **Findings:** At the time of imaging, 33 patients (49%) had concurrent ST depression in leads V1–V4 versus 34 (51%) who did not. Mean global EF was 5% lower (p = 0.02) in those with ST depression. There was no difference between groups in presence or absence of anterior WMAs, but the group with ST depression had significantly more posterolateral WMAs. Data necessary to calculate sensitivity and specificity of ST depression for posterior AMI are not provided. The literature discussed in the study further supports the idea that **ST depression in V1–V4 indicates posterolateral AMI, not remote (anterior) subendocardial ischemia.**

Edmunds JJ, et al. Significance of anterior ST depression in inferior wall acute myocardial infarction, 1994.

> **Methods:** Edmunds et al. (140) studied ECGs and angiographic findings of 41 inferior AMI patients.
>
> **Findings:** ST depression > 2 mm in V1–V4 occurred in 22 (54%) patients, none of whom had anterior perfusion defects. **Angiography detected no difference in prevalence of LAD or three-vessel disease** between patients with or without this ST depression. Four of five patients with circumflex involvement were in the ST depression group. The percentage of myocardium at risk was significantly greater (23% versus 15%) in patients with ST depression.

Wong CK, et al. Usefulness of continuous ST monitoring in inferior wall acute myocardial infarction for describing the relation between precordial ST depression and inferior ST elevation, 1993.

> **Methods:** Wong et al. (141) performed continuous ST-segment monitoring on 19 inferior AMI patients.
>
> **Findings:** The magnitude of precordial ST depression did not strictly correlate with the magnitude of inferior ST elevation. This indicates that **precordial ST depression during inferior AMI is NOT a simple electrical phenomenon.** Rather, it is an indication of infarction of another (i.e., posterior) wall.

Shah PK, et al. Noninvasive identification of a high-risk subset of patients with acute myocardial infarction, 1980.

> **Methods:** Shah et al. (209) utilized radionuclide ventriculography to study 44 inferior AMI patients with no prior infarction. Patients were divided into those with (Group A, n = 24) or without (Group B, n = 20) > 1 mm ST depression in at least two of six precordial leads. The study was conducted in the pre-reperfusion era.
>
> **Findings:** Incidence of the following findings in Group A versus Group B, respectively, was as follows: depressed EF (76% versus 10%), severe anteroseptal WMAs (50% versus 15%,), LV failure (50% versus 0), peak serum CK-MB (167 versus 84 ng/mL), and mortality (19% versus 0).
>
> **Comment:** In this small study, concurrent precordial ST depression was associated with anterior wall involvement.

Matetzky S, et al. Significance of ST segment elevation in posterior chest leads (V7–V9) in patients with acute inferior myocardial infarction: application for thrombolytic therapy, 1998.

> **Methods:** Matetzky et al. (208) recorded posterior chest leads in 87 patients with first inferior AMI.
>
> **Findings:** Posterior elevation in 46 inferior AMI patients was associated with larger AMIs and more adverse events. See Chapter 16 for a more detailed description.

14

LATERAL AMI

KEY POINTS

- Isolated lateral AMI is frequently MISSED.
- Myocardium at risk is sometimes large and may be preserved with reperfusion therapy.
- Lateral AMI frequently shows ST elevation < 1 mm OR it may ONLY show ST elevation in aVL, which is often overlooked.
- New ST elevation in aVL ONLY (one lead) IS an indication for reperfusion therapy if the diagnosis is certain, especially with reciprocal ST depression in lead III.
    - Angiography ± PCI is preferable, if available. Perform thrombolysis if there are no significant contraindications.

ANATOMY

The **lateral wall** of the LV is supplied by the **circumflex artery** and its obtuse marginal branches and by the **first diagonal**

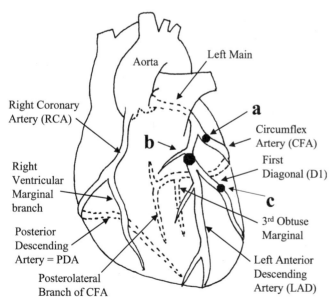

FIGURE 14-1. Coronary anatomy with circumflex occlusion (a), proximal LAD occlusion (b), and first diagonal (c) occlusion.

artery of the LAD (**Fig. 14-1**). Branches of a large dominant RCA may also supply the lateral wall (205).

- Occlusion of the **circumflex artery** and its **obtuse marginal branches** (**Fig. 14-1**) cause **lateral AMI**, often with involvement of inferior and posterior walls (inferolateral or posterolateral AMI).
- LAD occlusion proximal to the first diagonal artery (**Fig. 14-1**) causes **anterolateral AMI**.
    - Occlusion of the **first diagonal artery** (**Fig. 14-1**) causes **lateral AMI**.
- Occlusion of a **dominant RCA** with posterolateral branches (not shown) commonly causes **inferolateral AMI** (205).
- Occlusion of any of the **obtuse marginal branches** of the circumflex artery may also cause **(postero)lateral AMI.**

GENERAL BACKGROUND

The overall sensitivity of the initial 12-lead ECG for detecting STEMI **and** non-ST-elevation MI (NSTEMI) (as confirmed by CK-MB in all locations) using: (a) diagnostic ST elevation; (b) ST depression; and (c) T-wave inversion **combined,** is **70% to 75%** (18,20,21). The sensitivity of **ST elevation alone** for detection of AMI (as diagnosed by CK-MB) in any location is approximately **45%.** The sensitivity of ST elevation for detection of complete coronary occlusion, however, appears to be significantly higher (**68,69**). The sensitivity of ST elevation for **detection of lateral AMI is significantly lower** because the **circumflex artery supplies an electrocardiographically silent area of the myocardium.** Complete circumflex occlusion manifests (a) any ST elevation at all in only 36% of cases; (b) ST elevation > 2 mm in only 5% of cases; (c) ST depression alone in 30% of cases; (d) ST elevation or ST depression or both in approximately 67% of cases; and (e) neither ST elevation nor ST depression in 33% of cases (**68,69**,72,144,211). This contrasts markedly with complete LAD occlusion (anterior AMI) or RCA occlusion (inferior AMI), which manifest ST elevation in at least 70% to 92% of cases (**68,69**).

ECG DIAGNOSIS OF LATERAL AMI

Lateral AMI

Lateral AMI manifests ST elevation in **aVL, I, and/or V5–V6.** It frequently shows **ST elevation < 1 mm** (0.1 mV) **or NO ST**

elevation at all. It may also manifest ST elevation in **aVL only** (high lateral infarction), which is often overlooked. See Cases 14-1 and 14-2. (See also Case 7-3 of a lateral AMI that was mistaken for pericarditis; Case 7-6 of a lateral AMI with reciprocal ST depression more prominent than the ST elevation; and Case 21-3 of a patient with extremely subtle ST elevation that resolved twice without thrombolysis.)

Posterolateral AMI

In addition to the ST elevation in lateral leads, **posterolateral AMI manifests ST depression in V1–V3 and ST elevation in V7–V9.** It is usually due to circumflex occlusion but may be the result of occlusion of an RCA with posterolateral branches (see Cases 14-3–14-6).

Inferolateral AMI

Inferolateral AMI manifests **ST elevation in II, III, aVF AND in at least one of leads I, aVL, or V5–V6.** Remember that ST elevation in aVL **may be canceled out** by reciprocal depression due to inferior AMI (see Case 14-7).

Anterolateral AMI

Anterolateral AMI manifests ST elevation in **V2–V4 AND in at least one of leads I, aVL, or V5–V6.**

Pseudoinfarction

There may also be **rare** cases in which a patient's **baseline ECG findings** are consistent with lateral AMI (see Case 14-8).

MANAGEMENT

Reperfusion Therapy for Lateral AMI

The size of the area at risk in lateral AMI varies widely. The mean size appears to be larger than that of inferior AMI (**68**), and a large amount of myocardium may be preserved with reperfusion therapy of the circumflex artery (**206**). Mortality benefit from reperfusion therapy is greater for lateral AMI than for all inferior AMIs grouped together (**30**).

Reperfusion therapy is indicated for **ANY new ST elevation in lateral leads.** Because many lateral AMIs have < 1 mm ST elevation in lateral leads, which is often due to a low-voltage QRS, **< 1 mm ST elevation may be an adequate** indication for **reperfusion therapy IF** the diagnosis is certain (**212**). Either thrombolysis or angiography ± PCI is appropriate. Similarly, because lateral AMI may manifest only in aVL, **NEW ST elevation in aVL (one lead only)** is an indication for **reperfusion therapy IF** the diagnosis is certain, especially if there is **reciprocal ST depression in lead III** (**30**). In cases with ST elevation in one lead only, angiography ± PCI is preferable, if available. Thrombolytics are indicated if there are no significant contraindications.

CASE 14-1

Lateral Transient STEMI Easy to Misread as Early Repolarization, Resolved with Sublingual NTG

History

This 41-year-old man with a history of inferior MI presented with 5 hours of severe stuttering anginal pain.

ECG 14-1A (Type 1a)

The computer did not detect inferior or lateral ST abnormalities.

- Q waves: II, III, aVF, also present on a previous ECG indicate old inferior MI.
- ST elevation: nonspecific, V2–V4, probably early repolarization, also present on past ECGs.
- ST elevation: aVL; and reciprocal depression: I, II, III, aVF, are **new** and diagnostic of **lateral AMI.**

Clinical Course

Symptoms were relieved with sublingual NTG, but the ECG did not change. The patient was taken for immediate angiography, which revealed an **old** occlusion of the RCA. A **new**

99% stenosis of the second obtuse marginal was opened. Severe circumflex disease and moderately severe (50% to 70%) LAD lesions were also revealed.

ECG 14-1B

After angioplasty.
- ST elevation: decreased.

Clinical Course

Echocardiography 2 days later revealed inferior, posterior, and lateral akinesis and mild to moderately decreased LV function. Peak cTnI was only 0.4 ng/mL.

Conclusion

The anterior ST elevation is probably due to early repolarization, but the inferior ST depression is reciprocal to lateral STEMI. It is **NOT** due to inferior ischemia.

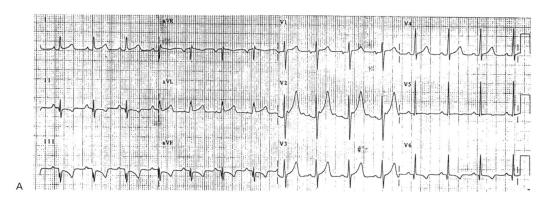

A

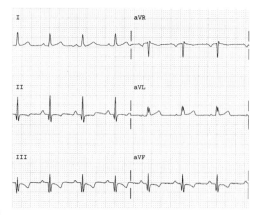

B

CASE 14-2

Subtle Lateral AMI in a Patient's Thirty-fifth CP Presentation

History
This 61-year-old woman presented with 45 minutes of CP. The patient had a known long-standing history of three-vessel CAD, but she had "ruled out" for AMI on 34 prior admissions. Angiography 3 months prior revealed severe circumflex and second obtuse marginal disease. Previous ECGs were available for comparison.

ECG 14-2 (Type 1b)
- New Q wave: aVL.
- New ST elevation: aVL; and new reciprocal depression: II, III, aVF are diagnostic of **lateral AMI.** Anterior leads are unchanged from old ECGs.

Clinical Course
The patient successfully reperfused after rapid administration of tPA. Total CK peaked at 746 IU/L. Angiography was not performed.

Conclusion
Obtuse marginal, or even circumflex, occlusion may present with ST elevation in aVL only; thrombolytics are indicated. First diagonal occlusion cannot be ruled out.

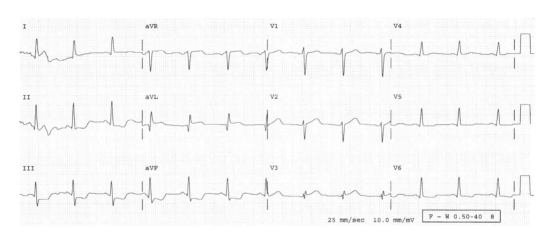

25 mm/sec   10.0 mm/mV   F ~ W 0.50-40 8

CASE 14-3

Subtle but Large Posterolateral AMI

History
This 56-year-old man with multiple risk factors and history of LAD angioplasty presented after sudden severe CP while walking. An old ECG showed no baseline ST elevation.

ECG 14-3A (Type 1c)
At 15:33
- ST elevation: diffuse, I, II, V4–V6, and 0.5 mm in aVL; and no reciprocal depression, are highly suspicious for **lateral AMI.**
- ST depression: slight, V1–V2, is **suspicious** for posterior involvement.

ECG 14-3B (Type 1a)
At 15:50
- ST elevation: increased, I, II, V4–V6; ST elevation: minimal, aVL; and **ST depression: V1, V2** are diagnostic of **posterolateral AMI.**

Clinical Course
Both ECGs show 0.5 mm of ST elevation in aVL and a total QRS < 2 mm. Although the **computer read this as "pericarditis,"** clinicians recognized that the ST depression in V1 was diagnostic of posterolateral AMI and gave thrombolytics. A repeat ECG 2.5 hours later showed complete ST resolution. Total CK peaked at 1,912 IU/L and CK-MB peaked at 127 ng/mL 25 hours after treatment; this delayed peak suggests that reperfusion was partial or absent (see Chapter 29). Echocardiography revealed a posterolateral WMA. Angiography performed 3 years later confirmed moderately severe circumflex disease.

Conclusion
A large lateral AMI may show only 0.5 mm of ST elevation in aVL when the QRS is small.

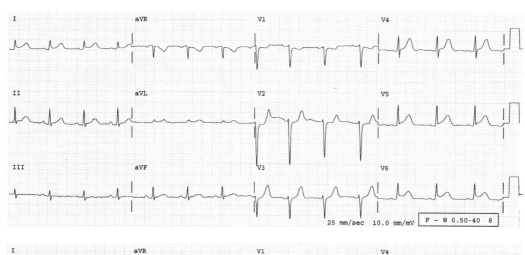

A   25 mm/sec   10.0 mm/mV   F ~ W 0.50-40   8

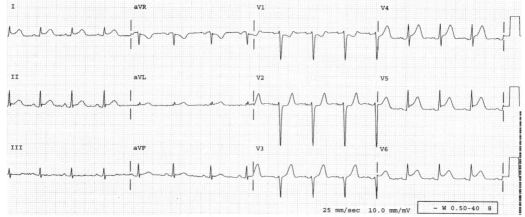

B   25 mm/sec   10.0 mm/mV   ~ W 0.50-40   8

Large Posterolateral AMI with Reciprocal Depression in Inferior Leads

History
This 50-year-old patient presented with CP and hypotension.

ECG 14-4 (Type 1a)
- Tachydysrhythmia, probably sinus tachycardia.

- Severe QRS distortion: I, aVL.
- ST depression: V1–V3, is diagnostic of **posterior AMI.**
- ST elevation: I, aVL, V5–V6; and reciprocal ST depression: III, aVF (electrically opposite aVL) are diagnostic of **lateral AMI.**

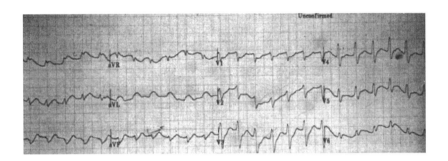

Large Posterolateral AMI with a Subtle but Diagnostic ECG

History
This 63-year-old man presented with exactly 2 hours of substernal chest pressure.

ECG 14-5 (Type 1b)
- ST elevation: I, aVL; and ST depression: III, aVF, V1–V3, are subtle but diagnostic of **posterolateral AMI.** The computer and clinicians missed this AMI.

Clinical Course
A repeat ECG 18 minutes later showed no change. Although reperfusion therapy was indicated, the patient received aspirin and was admitted to the CCU on a NTG drip. Serial ECGs revealed increased ST elevation in I and aVL, and clinicians gave thrombolytics. CK peaked at 3,200 IU/L and CK-MB peaked at 264 ng/mL, with a relative index of 8% (large AMI). Subsequent angiography revealed a persistently occluded obtuse marginal.

Conclusion
Thrombolytics were delayed 5.5 hours from pain onset because this **large** lateral AMI was **electrocardiographically subtle.**

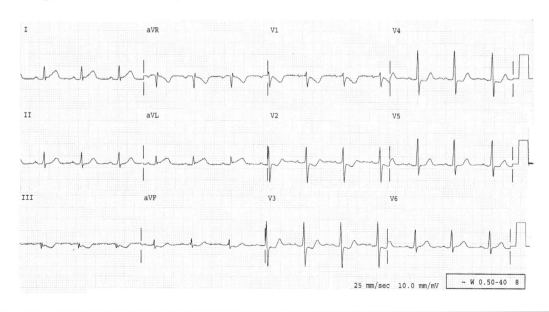

25 mm/sec 10.0 mm/mV ~ W 0.50-40 8

CASE 14-6

Subtle but Diagnostic ECG of Large Posterolateral AMI, Missed in Spite of Serial Tracings

History
This 53-year-old woman presented with 2 hours of CP unrelieved by aspirin and sublingual NTG.

ECG 14-6 (Type 1b)
At 07:38
- ST elevation: I, aVL; and reciprocal ST depression: III, aVF, are diagnostic of **lateral AMI.**
- ST depression: V1–V3, is diagnostic of **posterior AMI.**

Clinical Course
Immediate reperfusion therapy, including thrombolytics, was indicated, but the computer and clinicians missed the

AMI on this and serial ECGs. Clinicians diagnosed it after admission and gave SK. Total CK peaked at 1,030 IU/L, with CK-MB of 82 ng/mL (relative index = 8.0%). Later angioplasty dilated a severely stenotic culprit lesion of the first diagonal artery. Convalescent EF was 60%.

Conclusion
Thrombolytics were delayed 3 hours after the first diagnostic ECG (recorded 5.5 hours after pain onset), despite diagnostic serial ECGs. In this case (as compared with Case 14-5), the **subtle** findings corresponded to a **moderately sized risk area.**

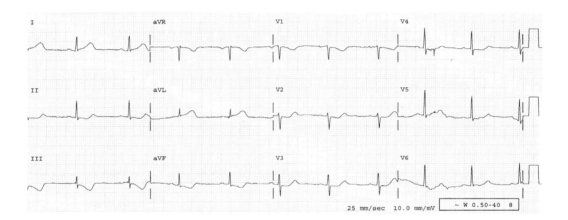

25 mm/sec   10.0 mm/mV   ~ W 0.50-40 8

CASE 14-7

Large Infero-Posterolateral AMI with ST Depression in aVL Reciprocal to the Inferior ST Elevation

History

This 54-year-old man presented with 1 hour of typical CP.

ECG 14-7 (Type 1a)

- ST depression: V1–V3, is diagnostic of **posterior AMI.**
- ST elevation: V5–V6, is diagnostic of **lateral AMI.** There is **no ST elevation in aVL.**
- ST elevation: II, III, aVF; and reciprocal ST depression: aVL are diagnostic of **inferior AMI.**

Clinical Course

Clinicians administered tPA. An ECG and angiography confirmed reperfusion and a culprit lesion in a left dominant circumflex.

Conclusion

Reciprocal depression of a large concurrent inferior AMI may cancel out the typical manifestation of lateral AMI (ST elevation in I and aVL). This is a very large, high-risk infarct, requiring immediate reperfusion therapy.

ECG reproduced from unpublished data with permission of K. Wang, M.D.

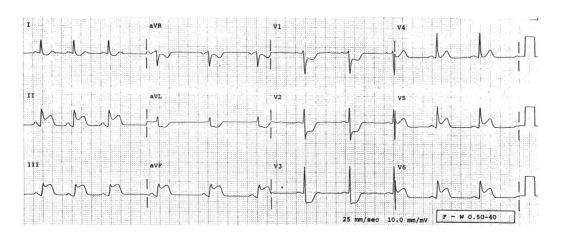

CASE 14-8

Baseline ECG Consistent with Lateral AMI (Rare)

History

This 40-year-old man presented with atypical CP. He had received thrombolytics for CP with identical ECGs twice before and both times had ruled out for AMI.

ECG 14-8 (Type 1b)

- ST elevation: I, aVL; and reciprocal depression: III and aVF, are identical to old ECGs.

Clinical Course

Due to atypical symptoms and the past history of two false-positive presentations for AMI, clinicians ordered

immediate echocardiography. No WMA was identified and clinicians withheld reperfusion therapy. Because angiography was not performed, there is no way to confirm the presence of normal coronary arteries. Comparison with old ECGs, however, showed no change and the patient ruled out for AMI.

Conclusion

It may be critical to obtain old tracings to avoid unnecessary thrombolysis.

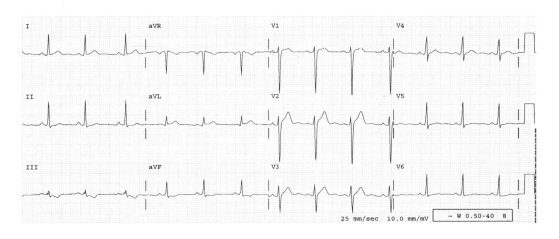

ANNOTATED BIBLIOGRAPHY

Huey BL, et al. A comprehensive analysis of myocardial infarction due to left circumflex artery occlusion: comparison with infarction due to right coronary artery and left anterior descending artery occlusion, 1988.

Methods: Huey et al. (68) studied ECGs of 241 consecutive AMI patients with no severe complications who were admitted to their CCU and agreed to undergo angiography. It is not stated whether any or all patients received reperfusion therapy. However, because the manuscript was submitted late in 1987 and makes no reference to thrombolysis, it is likely that no patients received it. All patients underwent radionuclide ventriculography to identify WMA and angiography to identify the IRA.

Findings: Of 40 patients with the **circumflex as the IRA, only 48% manifested ST elevation and 38% had neither ST elevation nor ST depression** on the initial ECG. This contrasted with the RCA and LAD, which manifested ST elevation in 71% (RCA, *n* = 107) and 72% (LAD, *n* = 94), and neither ST elevation nor depression in 21% and 20%, respectively. Despite its comparative invisibility on the ECG, **consequences of circumflex occlusion** (as assessed by Killip class and frequency of in-hospital complications) **did not differ significantly** from those of either **RCA or LAD occlusion.** During long-term follow-up, the probability of recurrent cardiac events was also similar. Huey et al. utilized 1 mm as the criterion for ST elevation; it is unknown how many patients demonstrated smaller amounts of ST elevation.

Comment: Angiography revealed that many of these IRAs were not totally occluded. The number of IRAs totally occluded at the time of the initial ECG is unknown; there is a significant rate of spontaneous

reperfusion before angiography. Nevertheless, the relative difference in sensitivity of the ECG between the circumflex and the LAD and RCA is significant.

Berry C, et al. Surface electrocardiogram in the detection of transmural myocardial ischemia during coronary artery occlusion, 1989.

Methods: Berry et al. (69) recorded ECGs of 56 patients during angioplasty balloon occlusion, including 25 LAD, 19 circumflex artery, and 12 RCA occlusions.

Findings: **Only six (32%) of patients with circumflex occlusion manifested ST elevation ≥ 1 mm** (0.1 mV) during dilatation, as compared with 84% of LAD and 92% of RCA occlusions. During circumflex occlusion, four patients (21%) manifested ischemia with only precordial ST depression and nine patients (47%) manifested no ECG changes.

Comment: Balloon dilatation is not prolonged and duration of occlusion affects the presence or absence of ST elevation.

FTT Collaborative Group. Indications for fibrinolytic therapy in suspected acute myocardial infarction: collaborative overview of early mortality and major morbidity results from all randomised trials of more than 1,000 patients, 1994.

Methods: The Fibrinolytic Therapy Trialists (FTT) collaborative group (30) combined data from nine randomized fibrinolytic trials, many of which did **not** require ST elevation for entry (see Appendix C). One-third of patients were from GISSI, which required ST elevation in only one lead.

Findings: When present, ST elevation did not necessarily occur in two consecutive leads. Patients with ST elevation were divided into groups of anterior, inferior, and "other" (primarily lateral or posterolateral) AMI. Thirty-five-day mortality for this "other" group was 13.4% for controls and 10.6% for patients receiving fibrinolytic therapy. In contrast, among patients with ST elevation of inferior AMI, mortality was 8.4% for controls and 7.5% for those who received fibrinolytics. Thus the **mortality benefit for lateral AMI was approximately 28 lives saved per 1,000 treated,** as compared with nine lives saved per 1,000 inferior AMI patients.

Veldkamp RF, et al. Performance of an automated real-time ST segment analysis program to detect coronary occlusion and reperfusion, 1996.

　　Methods: Veldkamp et al. (212) recorded 12-lead ST segments continuously during angioplasty balloon inflation.

　　Findings: **Peak ST elevation > 2 mm** resulted in 19 of 26 (73%) LAD inflations and 15 of 30 (50%) RCA inflations, but in **only 1 of 22 (5%) circumflex inflations.**

　　Comment: Again, the duration of angioplasty balloon occlusion is much shorter than thrombotic occlusion and the applicability is suspect. Nevertheless, it shows that circumflex occlusion is not as readily detectable by the ECG as other coronary occlusion.

Figueras J, et al. Relevance of electrocardiographic findings, heart failure, and infarct size in assessing risk and timing of left ventricular free wall rupture during acute myocardial infarction, 1995.

　　Methods: Figueras et al. (213) studied 227 patients who died of AMI.

　　Findings: LV free wall rupture occurred in 93 patients. Although early myocardial rupture (<1 day post AMI) was associated with high ST elevation in anterior AMI (6.8 ± 4.0 mm), 10% of ruptures were due to lateral AMI and had minimal ST elevation.

O'Keefe JH Jr., et al. Do patients with left circumflex coronary artery-related acute myocardial infarction without ST-segment elevation benefit from reperfusion therapy, 1995. See annotation (206) in Chapter 16.

15

RIGHT VENTRICULAR AMI

KEY POINTS

- Most cases of RV AMI occur CONCURRENT with inferior AMI.
- ALWAYS record a RIGHT-SIDED ECG in inferior AMI to look for RV AMI.
- Right-sided ECG: look for ≥ 1 mm of ST elevation in V2R–V7R, especially V4R. V2R is placed in the same position as V1.
- Left-sided ECG: look for ST elevation in V1.
  - ST elevation may also be present in V2–V5; if so, the magnitude of ST elevation will decline progressively from V2 to V5.
- RV AMI is a frequent cause of hypotension in inferior AMI. It is associated with high mortality if it is not reperfused and also with excellent response to reperfusion therapy.

ANATOMY

The **RV marginal branch** of the RCA supplies the RV (**Fig. 15-1**). The medial RV may also be partially supplied by small branches of the **LAD.**

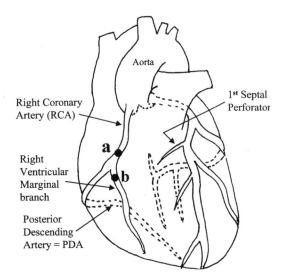

FIGURE 15-1. RCA occlusion in RV AMI. a: RCA occlusion proximal to the RV marginal branch. **b:** Occlusion of the RV marginal branch.

- **RCA occlusion proximal** to the RV marginal branch (**Fig. 15-1a**) causes **concurrent RV AMI and inferior AMI.** This accounts for the **vast majority** of RV AMIs.
- **RV marginal branch occlusion (Fig. 15-1b)** causes **isolated RV AMI,** which is much less common than concurrent RV and inferior AMI. Isolated RV AMI may also occur in the presence of an **old** Q-wave inferior MI; this may happen if the old MI was due to RCA occlusion distal to the RV marginal branch and the new occlusion is proximal to the RV marginal branch.
- Small LAD branches frequently supply the medial RV wall, generally leading to clinically insignificant medial RV infarction during anterior AMI (**204**). Large RV AMI in the presence of LAD occlusion is rare.

RIGHT-SIDED ECGs

Right-sided ECGs are primarily useful in patients with old or acute inferior MI. When performed in all patients, right-sided ECGs lead to many false positives (214) and they appear to be less sensitive for RV AMI concurrent with anterior AMI than with inferior AMI (134,204). In the presence of inferior Q waves without inferior ST elevation, ST elevation in right-sided leads may indicate a new and more proximal RCA occlusion. **ST elevation as high as 0.6 mm in V4R** (measured at 40 ms after the J point and relative to the TP segment) can be seen in normal individuals. **In the context of inferior AMI, ST elevation > 0.5 mm** should be interpreted as **RV AMI (215,216). Q wave**s are a normal finding in right precordial leads.

Right-Sided Lead Placement

Right-sided lead placement is a mirror image of left-sided leads (215) (Fig. 4-1). P,17

- V1R: positioned identically to V2, left sternal border, third intercostal space.
- V2R: positioned identically to V1, right sternal border, third intercostal space.
- V3R: midway between V1 (V2R) and V4R.
- V4R: right midclavicular line, fifth intercostal space.
- V5R: right anterior axillary line in the same horizontal plane as V4R.
- V6R: right midaxillary line in the same horizontal plane as V4R.

ST Elevation in Right-Sided Leads

ST elevation in right-sided leads, especially V4R, is the best ECG evidence of RV AMI (204,207,216,217). It should be measured 40 ms after the J point, relative to the TP segment **(207,218)**. ST elevation in any of **V3R–V7R is very sensitive** for RV AMI; the more of these leads that are involved, the larger the infarct **(204)**. ST elevation in V4R may have poor sensitivity for RV AMI associated with LAD occlusion (134,204). Alternatively, it may be **falsely positive** for RV AMI when there is actually **infarction of the septum**, especially the posterior septum **(217)**.

ECG DIAGNOSIS OF RV AMI

RV AMI and Concurrent Inferior AMI

Left-Sided 12-Lead ECG

Look for ST elevation in **V1** (see Cases 15-1 to 15-3). **ST depression may be present in V5–V6,** reflecting the left lateral reciprocal view of right-sided ST elevation (see Cases 15-2 and 15-4).

ST elevation may also be present in **V2–V5,** especially in a large RV AMI. This ST elevation mimics LV anterior AMI, also called "pseudoanteroseptal AMI" (see Cases 13-3 and 13-6). However, the **ST elevation of RV AMI declines progressively from V2–V5** (138,200,201), whereas LV anterior AMI manifests maximal ST elevation in V2–V4.

Right-Sided ECG

Look for ST elevation in leads **V2R–V7R. V4R** is the best single lead **(207,217)**. ST elevation of < 1 mm in these leads is significant **(216)**. See Cases 15-1, 15-4, and 15-5.

RVH

RV AMI in the presence of **RVH** may manifest extensive anterior ST elevation nearly indistinguishable from a large anterior AMI. Inferior ST elevation and maximal ST elevation in V2 help to distinguish this from anterior LV AMI. See Case 15-6.

Isolated RV AMI (Rare)

Left-Sided 12-Lead ECG

Look for ST elevation in **V1–V2.**

Right-Sided ECG

Look for ST elevation ≥ 1 mm in **V2R–V7R. V4R** is most important. This ST elevation may be associated with inferior Q waves due to old inferior MI with new occlusion proximal to the RV marginal branch. See Case 15-3.

RV AMI and Concurrent Inferoposterior AMI

Left-Sided 12-Lead ECG

Look for ST elevation in **V1** with ST depression in **V2** (219). ST elevation in V1 **may be attenuated, canceled, or replaced** by the ST depression of posterior AMI. Conversely, ST depression of posterior AMI **may be cancelled out or attenuated** by ST elevation of RV AMI (138). See Cases 15-1, 15-2, and 15-4.

Right-Sided ECG

Look for ST elevation in **V3R–V7R,** especially **V4R.** This ST elevation may also be **attenuated, canceled, or replaced** by ST depression of posterior AMI. See Cases 15-1 and 15-4. (See also Case 16-10 of an RV and posterior AMI manifesting ST elevation in V1; Case 7-2 of a large, infero-postero RV AMI; and Case 27-1 of a large inferoposterior AMI with ST depression in V1–V6, under which an RV AMI was hidden.)

RV AMI MORTALITY

RV AMI with concurrent inferior AMI has been well studied **(207,216,218,220,221)**. It is a frequent cause of **hypotension** in inferior AMI, due to decreased RV systolic performance and distention of the RV in a fixed pericardial space, which compromises LV filling. RV AMI with concurrent inferior AMI has a **high short-term mortality and complication rate (207)**, especially if there is no reperfusion **(218,221)**. Preinfarction angina may attenuate this high complication rate (as is likely the case with AMI in other locations as well) **(222)**. If the patient survives to 10 days, then the RV recovers well, with little **excess** long-term mortality or morbidity **(220)**. Short-term complications and mortality are dependent on RV function. Long-term complications and mortality depend on LV function.

MANAGEMENT

Reperfusion Therapy in RV AMI

Record right-sided leads in inferior AMI. **RV AMI with concurrent inferior AMI** is associated with **great benefit from reperfusion therapy,** both angioplasty **(221)** and thrombolytics **(218)**. Isolated RV AMI is rare and is not well studied. We recommend reperfusion therapy, including thrombolytics, for unstable patients with isolated RV AMI.

Treatment of Hypotension Due to RV AMI

Use caution when volume loading for hypotension; excess volume may compromise LV filling due to leftward displacement of the interventricular septum during diastole (223). Administer 500 to 1,000 cc of normal saline for hypotension. **Avoid NTG** in hemodynamically significant RV AMI. If volume loading fails to improve cardiac output, administer dobutamine for inotropic support (105). Consider hemodynamic monitoring.

CASE 15-1

Infero-Posterior RV AMI

History
This patient presented with CP.

ECG 15-1A (Type 1a)
This shows third-degree atrioventricular (AV) block.
- ST elevation: II, III, aVF; and ST depression: aVL, are diagnostic of **inferior AMI.**
- ST elevation: V1, is **suspicious** for RV AMI.
- ST depression: V2, is **suspicious** for posterior AMI.

ECG 15-1B (Type 1a)
A right-sided ECG.
- ST elevation: > 1 mm, V2R–V6R confirms **RV AMI.**

Conclusion
Reperfusion therapy is indicated.

ECG reproduced from unpublished data with permission of K. Wang, M.D.

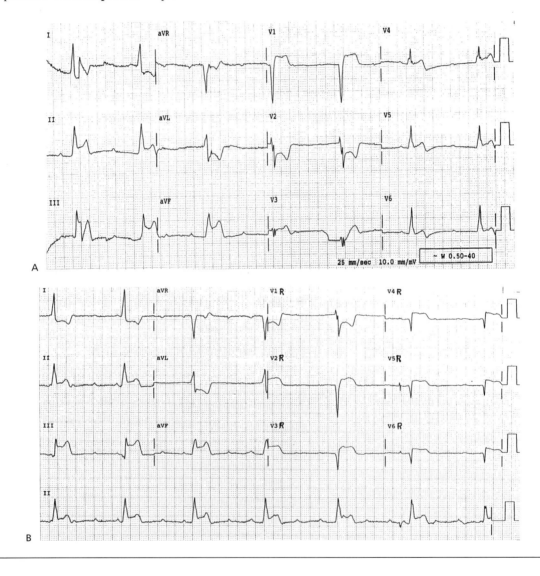

CASE 15-2

RV AMI Indicated by ST Elevation in V1

History

This 40-year-old man presented with CP and BP = 85/55, elevated neck veins, and clear breath sounds. His BP responded to fluids.

ECG 15-2 (Type 1a)
- LVH by voltage; second-degree AV block is also apparent.
- ST elevation: III, aVF; and ST depression: aVL are diagnostic of **inferior AMI.**
- ST elevation: large, V1 is **highly suspicious** for RV AMI.

- ST depression: V4–V6 is **suspicious** for RV AMI, lateral ischemia, or posterior AMI.

Clinical Course

A subsequent right-sided ECG confirmed **RV AMI**, with high ST elevation in V2R–V6R.

Conclusion

Reperfusion therapy is indicated. ST depression in V4–V6 may be reciprocal to right-side ST elevation.

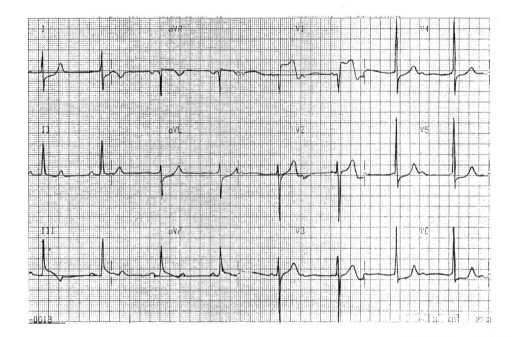

CASE 15-3

Isolated RV AMI in the Context of Previous Inferior MI

History

This 66-year-old man with history of five MIs and coronary artery bypass graft (CABG) (distal RCA and an obtuse marginal) presented with 1.5 hours of typical CP. His prehospital BP = 110 systolic but dropped to 90 after two sublingual NTG, without relief of pain. Breath sounds were clear and his BP responded to fluids.

ECG 15-3 (Type 1b)

- Old inferior Q waves: II, III, aVF, indicate old inferior MI, likely due to previous RCA occlusion. The old infarction alerts us to RCA disease and the likelihood of RV AMI.
- ST elevation: new, decreasing from V1–V3 is diagnostic of **RV AMI.** This is **not** anterior (LV) AMI.

- There is **NO** inferior ST elevation.

Clinical Course

The patient received tPA for presumed anterior AMI. ST elevation quickly and completely resolved to baseline, with a low peak CK of 190 IU/L but a diagnostic MB fraction of 7.6 IU/L. Subsequent angiography revealed a 50% proximal RCA culprit lesion. Convalescent echocardiography revealed an inferoposterior WMA.

Conclusion

Despite proximal RCA occlusion, inferior ST elevation is absent, presumably because of old, complete infarction. Immediate reperfusion therapy is indicated for this patient with an RV STEMI.

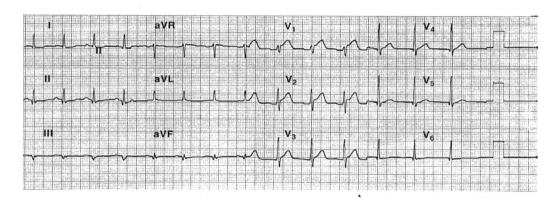

CASE 15-4

Right-Sided ST Elevation of RV AMI Obscured by ST Depression of Posterior AMI (Infero-Posterior RV AMI)

History

This 67-year-old man with a history of MI presented with CP.

ECG 15-4A (Type 1a)

- ST elevation: II, III, aVF; and ST depression: aVL, are diagnostic of **inferior AMI.**
- ST depression: V1–V3 is diagnostic of **posterior AMI. ST depression in V1 hides** what might otherwise be ST elevation of RV AMI.
- ST depression: V4–V6 may be due to posterior AMI, a reciprocal view of the RV, or to lateral LV subendocardial ischemia.

ECG 15-4B (Type 1a)

Right-sided ECG

- **ST elevation:** 1 mm, V4R–V6R supports the diagnosis of **RV AMI.**

Clinical Course

The patient received half dose tPA with successful reperfusion. Immediate angiography confirmed TIMI-3 reperfusion of a tight RCA stenosis proximal to the RV marginal branch. This reoccluded during angiography and was angioplastied and stented.

Conclusion

ST elevation in all right-sided leads would be greater and ST depression in all precordial leads would be less if the ST elevation of RV AMI and ST depression of posterior AMI did not cancel each other out. Reperfusion therapy is indicated.

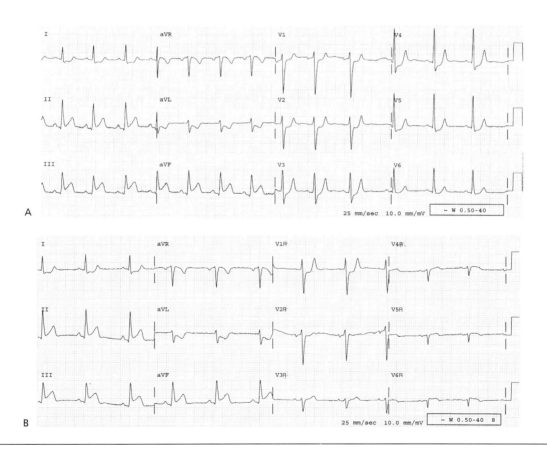

CASE 15-5

Inferior AMI with RV Involvement

History

This patient presented with CP.

ECG 15-5 (Type 1a)

This is a **right-sided ECG. Limb leads are not changed** when recording a right-sided ECG.

- ST elevation: II, III, aVF; and ST depression: aVL, are diagnostic of **inferior AMI.** Limb leads here are the same as in a left-sided ECG that was also recorded.

- Q-waves: III, aVF (Q-waves in right-sided leads are a normal finding)
- ST elevation: precordial leads V1R–V6R, is diagnostic of **RV AMI.**

Conclusion

Reperfusion therapy is indicated.

ECG reproduced from unpublished data with permission of K. Wang, M.D.)

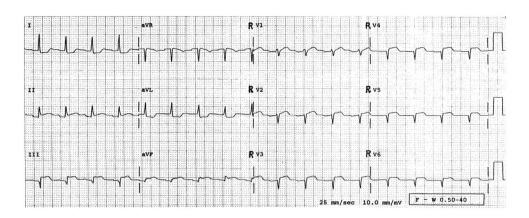

CASE 15-6

Pseudoanteroseptal (RV) AMI with Severe RVH

History
This 77-year-old man was resuscitated from a cardiac arrest.

ECG 15-6 (Type 1a)
- Right axis deviation
- S wave: large, V1
- ST elevation: II, III, aVF, also V1–V6, highest in V2, is diagnostic of **AMI;** location is unclear.

Clinical Course
The patient received tPA, with subsequent resolution of ST elevation and terminal T-wave inversion. Clinicians discovered his history of pulmonary fibrosis with pulmonary HTN. During transfer to a tertiary care center, the patient developed bradycardia, hypotension, and decreased level of consciousness (LOC). He was intubated, externally paced, and started on pressors. There was no pulmonary congestion. Echocardiography revealed RVH with poor function. Angiography revealed subtotal occlusion of a proximal nondominant RCA. Pulmonary capillary wedge pressure was 18 mm Hg (low). Shock progressed to death despite fluids, pressors, and full support.

Conclusion
In the presence of RVH, RV AMI may present with a very high ST score and mimic anterior AMI. Consequences in this context can be devastating.

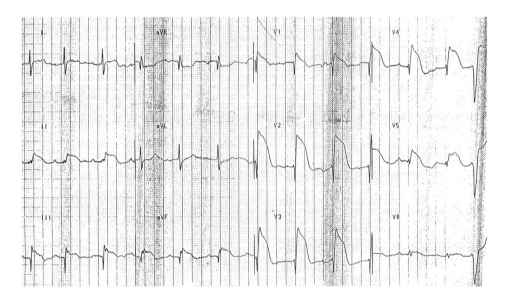

ANNOTATED BIBLIOGRAPHY

Right-Sided ECGs
Andersen HR, et al. The normal right chest electrocardiogram, 1987.

Methods: Andersen et al. (215) recorded ECGs of 109 staff members and patients who were normal with regard to the following: asymptomatic, no history of cardiopulmonary disease, vital signs, height and weight, heart and lung auscultation, chest morphology, chest x-ray, and 12-lead ECG findings. ST elevation was measured at 40 msec after the J point relative to the TP segment.

Findings: There was a wide range of R-wave, S-wave, and secondary R-wave amplitudes. The maximum ST-segment elevation in leads V3R–V7R was +0.8 mm, +0.6 mm, +0.6 mm, +1.0 mm, and +0.9 mm, respectively.

ECG Diagnosis and Clinical Course of RV AMI
Erhardt LR, et al. Single right-sided precordial lead in the diagnosis of right ventricular involvement in inferior myocardial infarction, 1976.

Methods: Erhardt et al. (217) analyzed data from 92 consecutive patients who suffered inferior "transmural" LV AMI **AND** who had right-sided ECGs recorded. AMI was diagnosed by ST elevation, evolution of T-wave inversion, and development of Q waves in II, III, and aVF.

Findings: Of 18 patients who died, nine had ST elevation in V4R. At autopsy, "major" RV involvement was found in seven, and minor in two patients. Of the nine deceased patients without ST elevation in V4R, five had no RV involvement and four had minor RV involvement. Of the 74 survivors, 16 had ST elevation in V4R. Incidence of complications among those with versus without ST elevation in V4R was as follows: hypotension, 50% versus 19%; oliguria, 19% versus 5%; right heart failure, 63% versus 21%; and left heart failure, 94% versus 57%. **Mortality** was 38% (nine of 25 patients) in those with ST elevation in V4R, versus 13% (nine of 67) without. ST elevation in V4R correlated with RV AMI, high mortality, and high incidence of complications in survivors.

Andersen HR, et al. Right ventricular infarction: diagnostic accuracy of electrocardiographic right chest leads V3R to V7R investigated prospectively in 43 consecutive fatal cases from a coronary care unit, 1989.

Methods: Andersen et al. (204) compared ECGs and autopsy findings of 43 consecutive patients who died in CCUs.

Findings: Seven patients did not have MI and 36 had LV AMI, 27 of whom had concurrent RV AMI. Of 12 patients with inferior LV AMI, 11 had concurrent RV AMI. Of 18 patients with anterior LV AMI, 15 had RV AMI. Of six patients with lateral AMI, one had RV AMI. When associated with anterior AMI, the amount of RV involvement was small. Right-sided ECGs were most accurate at identifying RV AMI associated with inferior AMI. **ST elevation ≥ 1 mm in V6R–V7R had a specificity and PPV of 100% for RV AMI, but the highest sensitivity in any one lead was only 41%.** Sensitivity was associated with RV AMI size; accordingly, it was low for RV AMI associated with anterior AMI. When all right-sided leads were involved, RV AMI was always extensive and associated with inferior AMI.

Simon R, et al. Right ventricular involvement in infero-posterior myocardial infarct: clinical significance of ECG diagnosis, 1993.

Methods: Simon et al. (216) retrospectively studied right-sided ECGs from 144 inferior AMI patients.

Findings: RV AMI, as measured by ST elevation ≥ 0.5 mm in right-sided leads, especially **V4R**, was found in 31 patients (22%). These patients had much higher incidence of **biventricular failure, right heart failure, hypotension, cardiogenic shock, and dysrhythmias** than did those without RV AMI.

Zehender M, et al. Right ventricular infarction as an independent predictor of prognosis after acute inferior myocardial infarction, 1993.

Methods: Zehender et al. (207) recorded V4R in 200 consecutive inferior AMI patients. V4R was measured 40 ms after the J point, presumably relative to the TP segment. RV AMI was diagnosed by autopsy, angiography/ventriculography, nuclear imaging, and/or hemodynamic measurements, with a total of 296 such tests. Clinical course was recorded for all patients.

Findings: ST elevation of 1 mm in **V4R** was 88% sensitive and 78% specific for RV AMI. Patients with ST elevation in V4R had **higher in-hospital mortality** (31% versus 6%) and a higher incidence of **major complications** (64% versus 28%) than did those without ST elevation in V4R.

Chou TC, et al. Electrocardiographic diagnosis of right ventricular infarction, 1981.

Methods: Chou et al. (224) analyzed ECGs of 11 patients with concurrent inferior and RV AMI as diagnosed by autopsy in five cases and by hemodynamic data in six cases.

Findings: V1 showed ST elevation in eight patients, two of whom had ST elevation in V1–V3. V1 showed ST depression in three patients (probably due to concurrent posterior AMI), two of whom also had ST depression in V4–V6. Measurement at 40 msec and 80 msec after the J point resulted in significant differences.

Efficacy of Therapy

Zehender M, et al. Eligibility for and benefit of thrombolytic therapy in inferior myocardial infarction: focus on the prognostic importance of right ventricular infarction, 1994.

Methods: Zehender et al. (218) analyzed outcome data from their study cited earlier (207). They compared inferior AMI patients, with and without RV AMI (as indicated by ST elevation in V4R), who received thrombolytics with patients who were deemed ineligible to receive thrombolytics due to presentation more than 6 hours after symptom onset, age of more than 75 years, or contraindications.

Findings: Of 200 patients, 71 underwent thrombolysis. Of 107 patients with RV AMI, 41 underwent thrombolysis and 66 were ineligible. In-hospital mortality for these 107 patients, with and without

thrombolysis, was 10% versus 42%, and the complication rate was 34% versus 54%, respectively. Of 93 patients without RV AMI, 30 received thrombolysis and 63 were ineligible; in-hospital mortality with and without thrombolysis was 7% versus 6%, and the complication rate was 27% versus 29%. **Thrombolysis was far more important to inferior AMI patients with concurrent RV AMI.**

Andersen HR, et al. Prognostic significance of right ventricular infarction diagnosed by ST elevation in right chest leads V3R to V7R, 1989.

Methods: Andersen et al. (220) studied the clinical course of 129 patients **who survived the first 10 days following AMI in any location.**

Findings: Seventy patients had inferior/posterior AMI. Among them, **cumulative percent survival** to a mean of 1.8 years tended to be **better for patients with ST elevation of 1 mm in any of leads V3R–V7R** (n = 25) than it was in patients with inferior/posterior AMI without ST elevation of 1 mm in any of leads V3R–V7R ($n = 45$, $p = .09$). Though not statistically significant, this does demonstrate that those with RV AMI who survive the first 10 days have no worse long-term prognosis than those without RV AMI.

Bowers TR, et al. Effect of reperfusion on biventricular function and survival after right ventricular infarction, 1998.

Methods: Bowers et al. (221) studied 41 RV AMI patients and compared the outcomes of patients who received reperfusion therapy.

Findings: Angioplasty with reperfusion in 33 patients was associated with early recovery of RV function and only 3% mortality. Unsuccessful reperfusion in 12 patients resulted in lack of recovery of RV function and persistent hypotension in 10 of 12 patients (83%), and in death in seven of 12 patients (58%).

Shiraki H, et al. Association between preinfarction angina and a lower risk of right ventricular infarction, 1998.

Methods: Shiraki et al. (222) retrospectively studied 113 patients with first inferior AMI due to RCA occlusion.

Findings: Patients with inferior AMI who had angina 24 to 72 hours prior to infarction (preinfarction angina) were much less likely to suffer RV AMI and had much lower mortality; the mechanism is unknown, but may be partly due to the development of collateral circulation.

Pseudoanteroseptal AMI

Khan ZU, et al. Right ventricular infarction mimicking acute anteroseptal left ventricular infarction, 1996.

Methods: Khan et al. (200) studied four patients whose concurrent inferior and RV AMI mimicked inferior and anteroseptal LV AMI.

Findings: ECGs of all patients showed ST elevation not only in V1, but also in V2–V3. More surprising still was the development of Q waves in V1–V3 without the presence of anterior AMI.

Geft IL, et al. ST elevations in leads V1 to V5 may be caused by right coronary artery occlusion and acute right ventricular infarction, 1984.

Methods: Geft et al. (201) used angiography and scintigraphy to study 69 patients with ST elevation in V1–V5.

Findings: The RCA was occluded, the LAD was open, and the RV was the area of infarct in five patients (7%). In cases of anterior AMI due to LAD occlusion, ST elevation was least in V1 and maximal in V2–V4, whereas in RV AMI, ST elevation was highest in V1–V2 and decreased toward V5. RV AMIs were also associated with inferior ST elevation.

RV AMI Without Inferior AMI

See annotation of Mittal et al. (134) in Chapter 12.

16

POSTERIOR AMI

KEY POINTS

- Isolated posterior STEMI is frequently MISSED and UNDERTREATED. It is missed because of the ABSENCE of ST elevation.
- Posterior AMI may be isolated or concurrent with inferior, RV, and/or lateral AMI.
- See algorithm in Figure 16-4 for reperfusion indications in suspected posterior STEMI.
- When the differential is posterior STEMI versus anterior unstable angina/non-ST-elevation MI (UA/NSTEMI), use posterior leads V7–V9. If inconclusive, echocardiography is very helpful.

SIGNIFICANT ISSUES IN POSTERIOR AMI

From 3.3% to 8.5% of all AMIs, as diagnosed by CK-MB, are **posterior AMIs that present WITHOUT ST elevation** on the 12-lead ECG. The vast majority of these AMIs manifest **ST depression in V1–V4 and/or ST elevation in V7–V9 (145, 206,225,226).**

Precordial ST depression and posterior ST elevation, occurring either singly or concurrently, have never been validated as

criteria for treatment in placebo-controlled thrombolytic trials such as GISSI-1, TIMI, and ISIS-2. However, much ancillary evidence supports the use of thrombolytics in this situation. **The ACC and AHA recommend thrombolytics if the physician can interpret the ECG accurately** (48,105).

ANATOMY

The posterior wall may be supplied by either the **circumflex artery** or the **RCA (Fig. 16-1)**. Occlusion of either artery may affect the posterior wall, regardless of "dominance" (which refers to the arterial supply of the inferior wall). Common branches affected are the obtuse marginal branches and posterolateral branch of the circumflex artery, and posterior branches of the RCA.

- **Circumflex occlusion** (Fig. 16-1a) or occlusion of one of its **obtuse marginal branches** (Fig. 16-1b) accounts for the majority of **isolated posterior AMIs.**
- **RCA** occlusion (Fig. 16-1c) is the most common cause of **concurrent posterior and inferior AMI** because the RCA is usually dominant and branches frequently supply the posterior wall.

GENERAL BACKGROUND

Circumflex Artery Occlusion and Isolated Posterior AMI

Circumflex occlusion is responsible for the **majority** of isolated posterior AMIs. Four studies of 12-lead ECGs documented 201 circumflex occlusions; 40 occurred during AMI **(68)** and 161 occurred during angioplasty balloon occlusion **(69,144,211)**. Findings indicated that **33% manifested no ST deviation, only 36% manifested ST elevation** in inferior and/or lateral leads with or without anterior ST depression, **and 30% manifested only precordial ST depression.** No posterior leads were recorded. This contrasts with angioplasty balloon occlusion of the LAD (anterior AMI) or RCA (inferior AMI), which manifested ST elevation in 70% to 92% of cases **(68,69)**. An additional study of 43 circumflex balloon occlusions (83) demonstrated ST depression with or without ST elevation in V2 and/or V3 in 35 cases (81% sensitivity). Data on the number of patients with ST depression **only** was unavailable.

When circumflex occlusion manifests ST elevation, with or without ST depression, **lateral AMI** may be present, but lateral ST elevation will rarely be pronounced (212). There may also be **inferior AMI** with inferior ST elevation if the circumflex artery is dominant (i.e., a "left dominant" coronary system; see Fig. 13-2).

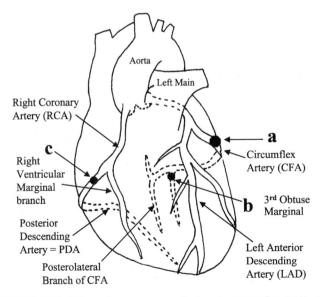

FIGURE 16-1. Sites of coronary occlusion in posterior AMI. A right-dominant system is pictured, in which the RCA supplies the inferior wall. **(a)** Circumflex occlusion. **(b)** Occlusion of one of the obtuse marginal branches of the circumflex. **(c)** RCA occlusion.

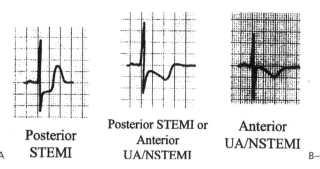

Posterior
STEMI

A

Posterior STEMI or
Anterior
UA/NSTEMI

Anterior
UA/NSTEMI

B–C

FIGURE 16-2. ST depression in posterior AMI versus UA/NSTEMI. Persistent ST depression, maximal in V1–V4 is usually due to posterior injury. This is especially true with an upright T wave. **(a)** If the T wave is inverted and asymmetric **(b)**, it could also be due to anterior UA/NSTEMI. If, as in **(c)**, the QRS returns to baseline before the ST segment downslopes, anterior UA/NSTEMI is likely, especially with a symmetrically inverted T wave.

RCA Occlusion Resulting in Posterior AMI with Concurrent Inferior AMI

RCA occlusion is the most common cause of posterior AMI, almost always in the context of a concurrent inferior AMI that manifests inferior ST elevation (**208**). **Proximal RCA occlusion** may cause RV AMI concurrent with inferior AMI or inferoposterior AMI. This results in **larger AMIs, higher mortality, and more benefit from reperfusion therapy than isolated inferior AMI** (**125,208**).

ECG DIAGNOSIS OF ISOLATED POSTERIOR AMI

ST Depression in Precordial Leads

Some ST elevation in leads V1–V4 manifests in 90% of normal individuals. Thus **any** ST depression may be large **relative to the baseline.**

Persistent ST depression in V1–V4, which may extend to V5–V6, indicates **isolated posterior AMI (Fig. 16-2).** Consider the following:

- **Maximal ST depression ≥ 2 mm in V1–V3** may be as much as 90% specific for posterior AMI (139,140,**144**).
  - **ST depression maximal in V1–V3 but less than 2 mm** is less specific (**71**,144,145).
  - **ST depression in leads V4–V6 ONLY** is less reliable (**144**).
- **T waves** are usually upright but may be asymmetrically inverted (**145**,176,**211**) (Fig. 16-2).
- **ST depression in precordial leads alone, with no ST elevation anywhere on the ECG, is an indication for thrombolytics in the context of high clinical suspicion of AMI** (105).
- **ST depression ≥ 1 mm in V1–V4,** in the right setting, is approximately 65% sensitive for **circumflex occlusion** (**68,69,71,72,83,144,208,211**).
  - **ST depression 0.5 to 1.0 mm** may detect more circumflex occlusions (**71**). Many of those missed can also be detected with **≥ 0.5 mm** of ST elevation on **posterior leads** (**71**).
- **ST depression in V1–V4** may be due to **anterior UA/NSTEMI** (anterior "subendocardial ischemia/infarction").
  - **Persistent** ST depression is more commonly due to **posterior STEMI** (139,140,**144**,145). However, **transient** ST depression in these leads in patients with severe CAD may be a result of **LAD disease,** and it does not respond to thrombolytics.

With associated **deep, symmetrical T-wave inversion, anterior UA/NSTEMI is most likely (Fig. 16-2).**
- ST depression of UA/NSTEMI is usually transient, **rarely** with tall upright T waves, and often < 2 mm.
- **ST depression maximal in lateral precordial leads V4–V6:**
  - May represent posterior AMI, whether isolated or not
  - May just as commonly represent UA/NSTEMI (subendocardial ischemia/infarction) (**144**). (See Case 37-1 for an ambiguous case.)

For examples of posterior AMI, see Cases 16-1 through 16-7. (See also Case 18-8 of isolated posterior AMI with LBBB; Case 18-7 of LBBB and inferoposterior AMI with an isoelectric ST segment that is depressed relative to its baseline; Case 8-4 of isolated posterior AMI with myocardial rupture; and Case 22-7 with ST depression of posterior AMI obscured by ST-T abnormalities of LVH.)

Posterior Chest Leads

Record posterior chest leads V7–V9 for patients with **high** clinical suspicion for AMI but without diagnostic ST elevation. Look for ST elevation in these leads. As shown in Figure 16-3, placement of V7–V9 should be in the fifth intercostal space (at the same level as V6) for all leads, with V7 at the posterior axillary line, V8 just under the tip of the scapula, and V9 at the same level at the paraspinal border. Normal elevation at the J point, relative to the PR segment, is up to 0.5 mm in all three leads (227).

Sensitivity and Specificity

The **sensitivity of posterior ST elevation ≥ 0.5 mm in two consecutive leads is unknown,** but it is likely more sensitive than 1 mm of precordial ST depression (**71**). The **specificity,** however, is **nearly 100% for posterior AMI (71,72). Routine** use of posterior leads is **not** warranted because the vast majority will be normal (**214,228**); however, when the clinical situation is highly suspicious for AMI, posterior leads may make the diagnosis (**72,214**) (Case 16-8).

Beware of Posterior AMI Look-Alikes

Conditions such as reversible ischemia (see Case 8-6), Wolff-Parkinson-White (WPW) (see Case 8-3), RVH (see Case 8-2), and subarachnoid hemorrhage (see Case 8-8) may have ECG manifestations that mimic posterior AMI.

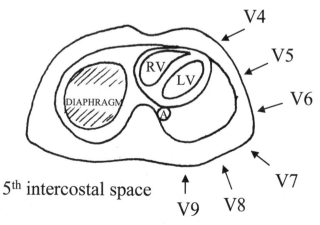

FIGURE 16-3. Placement of posterior leads.

ECG DIAGNOSIS OF CONCURRENT INFERIOR AND POSTERIOR AMI

Inferior ST Elevation Concurrent with ST Depression in V1–V4

Inferoposterior AMI is typically due to **RCA occlusion** and manifests inferior ST elevation with concurrent ST depression in V1–V4 (see Cases 16-9 and 16-10). There may also be **concurrent RV AMI, which may attenuate or cancel out** ST depression of posterior AMI. **Any ST depression in V1–V3** should help confirm suspicions that ST elevation elsewhere (e.g., inferior or lateral) is due to STEMI. (See also Cases 3-3 and 33-2, in which the first ECG of inferoposterior AMI shows ST deviation only in the precordium.)

THE ECG AND REPERFUSION OF POSTERIOR AMI

In STEMI in other locations, the T wave inverts over time or with reperfusion (see Chapter 27). Conversely, **in posterior AMI, the T wave remains upright and enlarges** (176). See Case 16-9. (See also Case 13-4 of reperfusion and reocclusion of a large inferoposterior AMI.)

Nonreperfused Posterior AMI

Look for the development of **tall R waves in V1–V3** (reciprocal to posterior Q waves) and **eventual** development of **tall, wide, upright T waves** (176). This contrasts with the development of deeply inverted T waves in reperfused anterior AMI.

Reperfused Posterior AMI

Look for **precordial** T waves. Whether they are initially upright or asymmetrically inverted, they typically become **tall, wide, and upright** (176). Although this happens in both reperfused and unreperfused AMI, it happens **more quickly with reperfusion.**

MANAGEMENT

See Figure 16-4 for an algorithm of posterior AMI treatment.

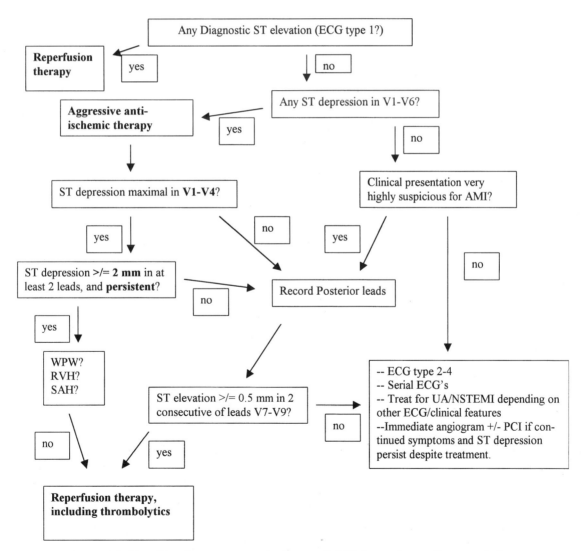

FIGURE 16-4. Algorithm for management of precordial ST depression and/or suspected posterior AMI. In contrast with ST elevation, the efficacy of reperfusion for isolated posterior AMI has never been conclusively proven in randomized placebo-controlled trials. Its efficacy is extrapolated from ancillary evidence.

CASE 16-1

Large Isolated Posterior AMI Manifesting Minimal ST Depression That Is ≥ 2 mm on Comparison with the Previous ECG

History
This 51-year-old woman presented with 1 hour of CP.

ECG 16-1A (Type 2)
- ST depression: < 1 mm, V2–V3.
- When this is compared with ECG 16-1B, a previous ECG, **there is an ST change of > 2 mm.** There is also a new tall R wave: V2. This ECG is highly suggestive of ischemia, especially **posterior STEMI.**

ECG 16-1B
Previous ECG
- J-point elevation: 2 mm.

Clinical Course
The emergency physician and the cardiologist did not appreciate the significance of the ST depression, so this STEMI was unrecognized and the patient was initially treated without reperfusion therapy. Symptoms continued, but clinicians did not record an immediate repeat ECG. She ruled in for a **large posterior AMI** with a peak cTnI of 72 ng/mL and a peak total CK of 3,400 IU/L. Subsequent echocardiography revealed an **akinetic posterior wall** and mild decrease in LV function. Subsequent ECGs showed tall R waves in V1–V3 with tall T waves. Angiography the next day revealed 95% stenosis of the second obtuse marginal, which was angioplastied and stented.

Conclusion
Immediate intensive evaluation is indicated: repeat ECGs, echocardiography, or angiography ± PCI. Posterior leads would have been useful.

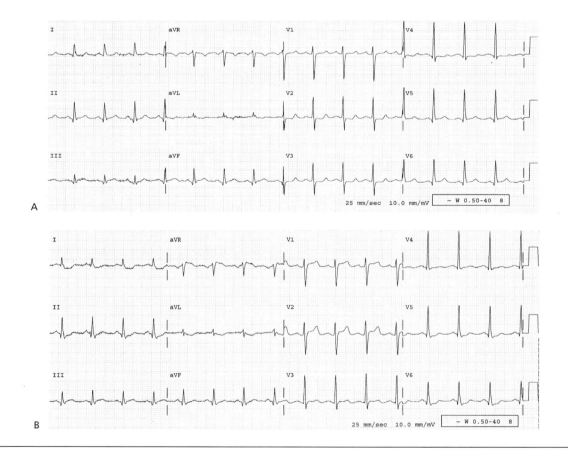

CASE 16-2

Thirty-one-Year-Old Woman with Large Posterior AMI Manifesting Minimal ECG Changes: ST Depression in V1–V3

History

This 31-year-old woman was working the night shift when substernal CP began, which worsened with climbing stairs and was associated with SOB, diaphoresis, vomiting, and arm tingling. She then had a near-syncopal episode. She had experienced 2 weeks of intermittent "heartburn." Paramedics found her with no BP in the upright position. BP in the ED was 120/60.

ECG 16-2A (Type 1b)

At 08:36

- ST depression: V1–V3, 1 mm, with biphasic T wave; and ST elevation: 1 mm V5–V6 and minimal, I aVL. By themselves these changes are minimal and nondiagnostic; together they are **diagnostic of posterior "STEMI."** The 1 mm of ST elevation in V5–V6 meets the ACC/AHA "criteria" for thrombolytics.

Clinical Course

Immediate echocardiography confirmed a posterolateral WMA and the patient was taken for angiography and PCI at

08:49, only 13 minutes later. A 100% proximal circumflex occlusion was opened. The LAD and RCA were completely normal.

ECG 16-2B

Five hours later

- ST segments were normalized.

Clinical Course

Initial cTnI was < 0.1 ng/mL, the 4-hour level was 0.1 ng/mL, and the 8-hour level peaked at 143 ng/mL. Total CK peaked at 6,085 IU/L. Convalescent echocardiography showed anterior, inferior, posterior, and lateral hypokinesis with mildly decreased LV function.

Conclusion

Circumflex artery occlusion may show minimal ECG changes even with a very large myocardial risk area.

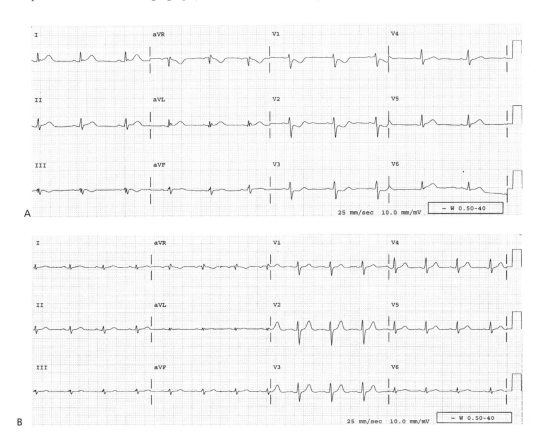

Resuscitated Cardiac Arrest: Isolated Posterior AMI Unrecognized on ECG

History
This 37-year-old man experienced CP and collapsed. Paramedics found him in ventricular fibrillation and defibrillated him successfully. He was unconscious in the ED and intubated. P = 90 and BP = 150/80.

ECG 16-3 (Type 2), recorded 25 minutes after defibrillation
- ST depression: **1 mm,** V1–V3, with upright T waves; tall R waves: V1–V3; no ST elevation. This ECG is **highly suspicious** for posterior AMI.

Clinical Course
No posterior leads were recorded, nor was angiography or PCI performed. The patient ruled in for AMI with a cTnI peak of 15 ng/mL and a CK peak of 850 IU/L. Angiography on day 2 revealed occlusion of the second obtuse marginal branch of the circumflex.

Conclusion
ECG 16-3 is suspicious but nondiagnostic because the ST depression is only 1 mm. **Immediate angiography ± PCI is indicated. With ST elevation on posterior leads (not recorded), thrombolytics would also be indicated.**

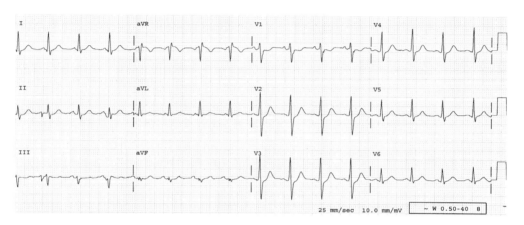

25 mm/sec 10.0 mm/mV ~ W 0.50-40 8

Isolated Posterior AMI

History
This 48-year-old man was resuscitated from a cardiac arrest.

ECG 16-4 (Type 1b)
- ST depression: II, aVF, V2–V4, maximal in V2; upright T waves: V3; R/S ratio > 1; tall R waves in V1–V2; T waves slightly peaked due to hyperkalemia.

This ECG is diagnostic of **posterior AMI.**

Clinical Course
Due to anoxic brain injury, no reperfusion was undertaken. CK peaked at 1,256 IU/L and cTnI peaked at 19.5 ng/mL. Echocardiography confirmed posterior AMI.

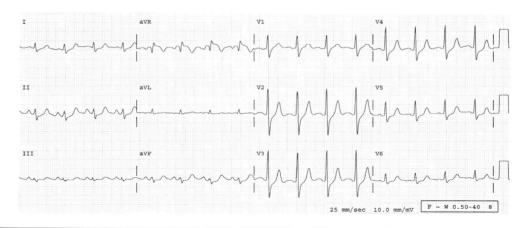

25 mm/sec 10.0 mm/mV F ~ W 0.50-40 8

Isolated Posterior AMI with New RBBB

History

This 56-year-old man with a history of CABG and MI presented diaphoretic, with 45 minutes of crushing CP. He was taking warfarin and was **hemodynamically unstable.** An old ECG showed LVH only, with minimal ST elevation in V1–V3 and no BBB.

ECG 16-5A (Type 2)

- IVCD: QRS = 135 ms.
- ST depression: V2–V6, maximal in V4–V5. This is **highly suspicious** for posterior AMI. **Angiography ± PCI** is indicated.
- ST depression: II, III, aVF; and **ST elevation: minimal,** aVL are **suspicious** for lateral AMI.

Comment

This ECG is highly suggestive of posterior lateral AMI, although ST depression is not maximal in V2–V3. **Immediate angiography ± PCI is indicated** due to a **Type 2 ECG and hemodynamic instability. Posterior leads** would be helpful.

ECG 16-5B (Type 1b)

Fifty-two minutes later; was delayed too long.

- Wider QRS (147 ms); wide S wave: V5–V6; and RR′: V1, indicate new RBBB.
- Wide S waves: II, III, aVF (slow, late, upward electrical forces) indicate left anterior fascicular block (LAFB).
- ST depression: maximal in V2–V3, are diagnostic of **posterior AMI.**

Clinical Course

Reperfusion, including thrombolytics, is indicated. The patient was taken for PCI, which demonstrated patency of the saphenous graft to the LAD before the patient arrested and died. No other coronaries were imaged.

Conclusion

Angiography was delayed due to: (a) management of hemodynamic instability in the ED and CCU rather than in the cath lab; and (b) due to clinicians' reluctance to anticoagulate a patient on warfarin, which is necessary for PCI. The risk of angiography, or even thrombolysis, in a patient on coumadin, is not high. Even with an INR ≥ 4 or prothrombin time (PTT) of more than 24 seconds, the risk of intracranial bleeding with thrombolytics only doubles from an overall rate of 1.45% to 3.00% (see Chapter 34). This is insufficient reason to withhold therapy, especially in a high-risk case, and it is especially not sufficient to withhold PCI. **In an unstable patient, aggressive treatment is worthwhile even in the presence of major contraindications.**

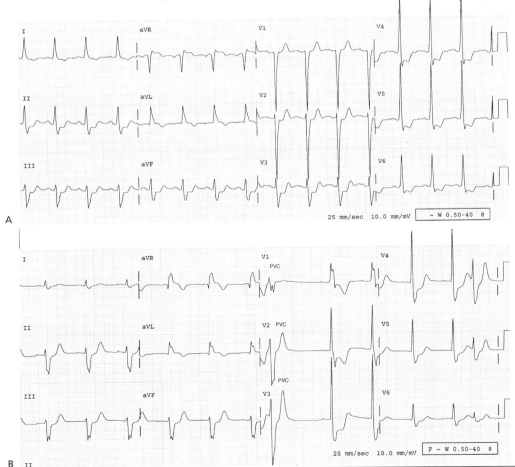

CASE 16-6

Posterior AMI with ST Depression in V4–V6 Only

History

This 57-year-old man with CAD presented with 3 days of intermittent typical left CP at rest. The pain was dull and became constant a few hours prior to presentation. The physical exam, including P and BP, was normal. The patient's **initial ECG was unchanged from a previous ECG,** with Q waves in V1–V4 and chronic T-wave inversions in V2–V4. V5 and V6 were normal, with no ST deviation. **Posterior leads may have helped in this case.** The patient was given aspirin, sublingual NTG, and heparin, but his pain persisted. **Immediate angiography is indicated for refractory typical symptoms.**

ECG 16-6 (Type 2)

One hour later

■ New ST depression: V4–V6.

Clinical Course

Immediate angioplasty opened 100% stenoses of the distal circumflex and the second obtuse marginal arteries. CK peaked at 3,871 IU/L and cTnI peaked at 171 ng/mL.

Conclusion

This large posterior AMI due to circumflex occlusion presented as minimal lateral ST depression only. Angiography and angioplasty were undertaken due to lack of symptom resolution during treatment for UA/NSTEMI.

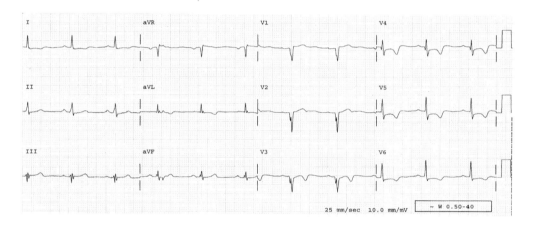

25 mm/sec   10.0 mm/mV   ~ W 0.50-40

CASE 16-7

Isolated Posterior AMI Due to RCA Occlusion, Manifesting ST Depression

History
This 76-year-old man, 4 weeks status post angioplasty and atherectomy of the LAD, presented with acute pulmonary edema, respiratory failure, and shock.

ECG 16-7 (Type 1a)
- Q waves: V3–V6, indicate old anterolateral MI.
- ST depression: deep, V1–V4, maximal in V2–V3, is diagnostic of **posterior AMI.**
- Minimal nondiagnostic Q waves and ST elevation: II, aVF.

Clinical Course
Immediate angiography revealed severe three-vessel disease, with 100% occlusion of a right dominant posterior descending artery (PDA). Angioplasty opened and dilated the PDA lesion and a 95% stenosis of the first right posterolateral branch.

Conclusion
Timely diagnosis enabled balloon pump placement within 30 minutes of presentation and rapid reperfusion. The patient's CK peaked at only 449 IU/L.

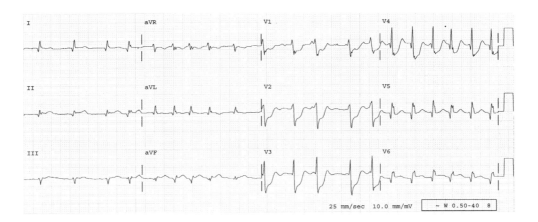

25 mm/sec 10.0 mm/mV ~ W 0.50-40 8

CASE 16-8

Posterior AMI as Diagnosed by Posterior Leads; Thrombolytics Were Given

History

This 56-year-old man presented with 2 hours of substernal CP.

ECG 16-8A (15-lead, Type 1a)

- ST elevation: minimal, aVL, is **suspicious** for lateral AMI.
- ST depression: minimal, II, III, aVF, is also **suspicious** for lateral AMI.
- ST depression: V1–V3, almost 2 mm. T waves are not fully upright. Alone, anterior subendocardial ischemia is likely. In combination with the suspicion of lateral AMI, posterior STEMI is much more likely.
- Three posterior leads, V4R, V8, and V9, show ST eleva-

tion: >1 mm, V8–V9, which is diagnostic of **posterior AMI.**

Clinical Course

Clinicians administered TNK-tPA, with ECG evidence of reperfusion. Nonemergent angiography revealed open arteries, 70% to 90% RCA and circumflex lesions, and a 99% stenosis of the first obtuse marginal branch. Echocardiography revealed minimal posterior hypokinesis. Peak cTnI was 5.4 ng/mL.

Conclusion

Posterior leads facilitated rapid confirmation of posterior STEMI and rapid treatment, resulting in minimal injury.

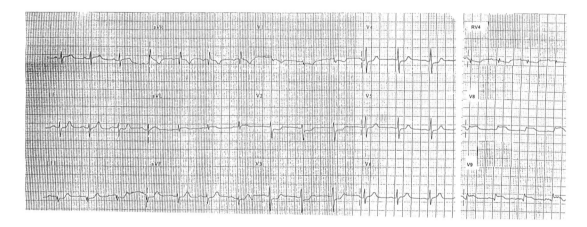

CASE 16-9

Inferoposterior AMI Viewed *Upside Down* as if the Leads Were Posterior: Postreperfusion ECG Shows Typical Enlarged Precordial T Waves

History

This 47-year-old woman presented with CP.

ECG 16-9A (Type 1a)

- ST elevation: II, III, aVF; and ST depression with asymmetric T-wave inversion: V2–V4 are diagnostic of **inferoposterior AMI.**

ECG 16-9B (Type 1a)

V1–V3 only

- This ECG shows V1–V3 from ECG 16-9A **FLIPPED UPSIDE DOWN,** as if taken from posterior leads.
- ST elevation: V2–V3. **This demonstrates how posterior ST elevation manifests as ST depression in precordial leads.**

Clinical Course

Angioplasty opened a 100% occluded dominant RCA 1.5 hours after pain onset. TIMI-3 flow was restored and a stent was placed. CK peaked at 950 IU/L.

ECG 16-9C

Eighteen hours later

- Resolution of ST-segment deviation and T-wave inversion in III and aVF indicate inferior reperfusion. Enlarged upright T waves in V2–V3 indicate posterior reperfusion.

Conclusion

Peaked T waves in V1–V3 are evidence of reperfused posterior STEMI.

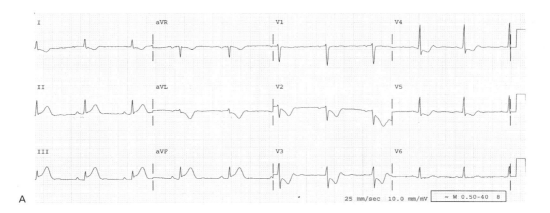

A   25 mm/sec   10.0 mm/mV   ~ W 0.50-40 8

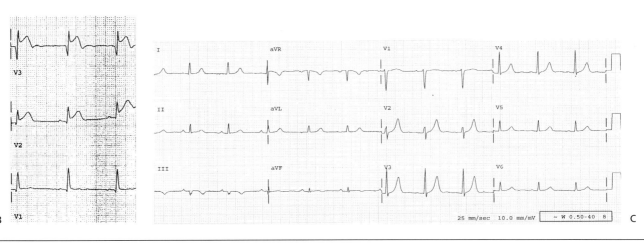

B   25 mm/sec   10.0 mm/mV   ~ W 0.50-40 8   C

CASE 16-10

Large Infero-Posterior RV AMI

History
This 61-year-old man presented with CP.

ECG 16-10 (Type 1a)
- ST elevation: II, III, aVF; and reciprocal depression: aVL, are diagnostic of **inferior AMI**.

- ST elevation: V1, is **highly suspicious** for RV AMI.
- ST depression: V2, is diagnostic of **posterior AMI**.

Conclusion
RV AMI and posterior AMI may cancel each other's effects.

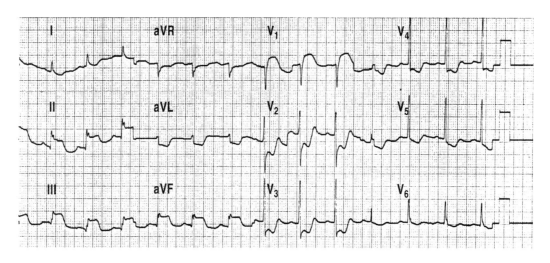

ANNOTATED BIBLIOGRAPHY

Thrombolytics for ST Depression
See annotations and commentary in Chapter 8, especially Langer et al. (167).

Absence of ST Elevation with Circumflex Occlusion
See annotations of Veldcamp et al. (212), Huey et al. (68), and Berry et al. (69) in Chapter 14.

Significance of ST Depression in V1–V4
Three heterogeneous studies strongly indicate that **ST depression ≥ 1 mm (145) or 2 mm (140,144) and maximal in leads V2–V3 is quite specific for posterior AMI.**

Roul G, et al. Isolated ST segment depression from V2 to V4 leads, an early electrocardiographic sign of posterior myocardial infarction, 1991.
   Methods: Roul et al. (145) analyzed data from 328 consecutive AMI patients, as diagnosed by CK-MB.
   Findings: Isolated anterior ST depression in V2–V4, maximal in **V3** (1.8 ± 0.7 mm) **or V4** (2 ± 1 mm) occurred in 28 (8.5%) of 328 patients. **All 28 patients** developed posterior WMAs detected with echocardiography, had CK-MB evidence of AMI and developed posterior Q waves or increased R/S ratio in leads V1 and V2. In all 28 patients the T wave was upright.
   Comment: This study still does not rule out the possibility of isolated anterior ST depression due to anterior subendocardial ischemia because patients with **fully reversible** anterior ischemia would not have ruled in for AMI and would not have been identified for entry into the study. In contrast with this study, Kulkarni et al. (211) (described later) demonstrated that the T wave in posterior AMI was often inverted (Fig. 16-2).

Shah A, et al. Electrocardiographic differentiation of the ST-segment depression of acute myocardial injury due to the left circumflex artery occlusion from that of myocardial ischemia of nonocclusive etiologies, 1997.
   Methods: Shah et al. (144) retrospectively analyzed ECGs of 104 patients with circumflex balloon occlusion during angioplasty. They compared location of ST depression in these patients with that seen during nonocclusive ischemia due to exercise tolerance testing (ETT) of 200 patients. ST depression and elevation were defined as ≥ 0.1 mV for occlusive ischemia. ST depression was defined as ≥ 0.2 mV for nonocclusive ischemia.
   Findings: Of 104 patients with circumflex balloon occlusion, only 36 (35%) had ST elevation at all, with or without ST depression, 31 (30%) had no ST deviation at all, and 37 (36%) had isolated ST depression. Of 200 ETT patients with nonocclusive ischemia, 74 (37%) had ST depression ≥ 0.2 mV in at least one lead (any location) and none had ST elevation. Of these 74 patients, 37 (50%) had precordial ST depression ≥ 0.2 mV and only four (11%) of these 37 patients had maximal depression in V1–V3. The remaining 33 of 37 (90%) had maximal depression in V4–V6. In the balloon occlusion group, 72 of 92 (78%) episodes of precordial ST depression were in V2 or V3.
   Comment: Shah et al. suggest that the specificity of ST depression ≥ 2 mm and maximal in leads V1–V3 for occlusion (posterior STEMI) versus nonocclusive, "subendocardial," ischemia (NSTEMI) was 89%. However, this conclusion is not necessarily justified. It is widely believed that ST depression of exercise testing occurs in either inferior or lateral leads even in the presence of LAD disease that, during acute coronary syndrome (ACS), may result in ST depression in V1–V3.

Bush HS, et al. Twelve-lead electrocardiographic evaluation of ischemia during percutaneous transluminal coronary angioplasty and its correlation with acute reocclusion, 1991.

Methods: Bush et al. (83) analyzed ECG data from 43 circumflex balloon inflations.

Findings: Of 43 balloon inflations, 32 (74%) showed 1 mm ST depression in V2 and 35 (81%) showed ST depression in V2 and/or V3. Thus **ST depression in at least one of leads V2 or V3 was 81% sensitive for circumflex occlusion.** The number of ECGs with ST depression only was not reported.

Boden WE, et al. Electrocardiographic evolution of posterior acute myocardial infarction: importance of early precordial ST-segment depression, 1987.

Methods: Using data from the Multicenter Diltiazem Reinfarction Study, Boden et al. (229) selected 50 (9.2%) of 544 patients with CK-confirmed non–Q-wave AMI whose ECGs manifested isolated ST depression ≥ 1 mm in two consecutive leads from V1–V4.

Findings: ECGs showed R-wave evidence of posterior AMI (R wave ≥ 0.04 sec in V1 and an R:S ratio ≥ 1 in V2) in 23 (46%) of 50 patients. Patients with this evidence of posterior MI had higher mean CK levels and deeper ST depression than patients without this R-wave pattern.

Comment: The development of large R waves after a posterior AMI is analogous to the development of Q waves in other locations; not all STEMI results in Q waves, and not all posterior AMI would be expected to result in R waves. Thus the other 54% of patients with ST depression ≥ 2 mm may have had posterior AMI. This study used no imaging to substantiate the significance of the ECG.

Commentary: Sensitivity of ST Depression

We combined data from four heterogeneous studies referred to earlier, by Shah et al. (144), Huey et al. (68), Berry et al. (69), and Bush et al. (83) and four studies described later, by Matetzky et al. (208), Kulkarni et al. (211), Matetzky et al. (71), and Agarwal et al. (72). Based on this, we estimate that **ST depression is present in approximately 60% to 70% of circumflex occlusions that do not manifest any ST elevation ≥ 1 mm on the 12-lead ECG.** Combining data from the subset of studies in which posterior leads were used (71,72,211), posterior leads detected circumflex occlusion in 56 cases. The number of false negatives is unknown. Of these 56, 37 (66% sensitivity, as compared with posterior leads) manifested ≥ 1 mm of anterior ST depression and 19 (34%) may have manifested some ST depression **< 1 mm**. Several cases showed ST depression during circumflex occlusion that did **NOT** manifest ST elevation on posterior leads (72,211).

Precordial ST Depression "Reciprocal" to Inferior AMI

See Shah (138) annotated in Chapter 13, for a review of literature prior to 1991. See also annotations of Ruddy et al. (139), Edmunds et al. (140), Bates et al. (210), and Wong et al. (141) in Chapter 13.

Posterior Leads

Matetzky S, et al. Significance of ST segment elevations in posterior chest leads (V7–V9) in patients with acute inferior myocardial infarction: application for thrombolytic therapy, 1998.

Methods: Matetzky et al. (208) recorded posterior leads V7–V9 on 87 patients with first inferior AMI who received thrombolytics.

Findings: Of these 87 patients, 46 (53%) had ST elevation ≥ 0.5 mm in two or more of leads V7–V9 (Group A) and 41 (47%) did not have this ST elevation (Group B). Group A had significantly more posterolateral involvement (89% versus 46%, $p < 0.001$) and significantly lower EF (53% versus 60%, $p < 0.003$), as measured by radionuclide ventriculography. Severe WMAs or severe hypokinesis was found in 87% of patients in Group A versus 24% in Group B. Group A had larger infarct areas as measured by CK and a higher incidence of adverse events as defined by reinfarction, heart failure, or death. The circumflex was the IRA in 35% of Group A patients versus 5% in Group B; of 18 circumflex occlusions, 16 (89%) were in Group A. It is important to note that in Group B patients, EF was no better if the IRA was patent at angiography than if it remained occluded (59% versus 61%, $p = 0.4$). In contrast, Group A patients whose IRA was patent had significantly higher EF than did those in whom it was occluded (56% versus 44%, $p < 0.012$). **This implies that reperfusion therapy was more important**

in the group with posterior ST elevation. Of 46 patients with ≥ 0.5 mm ST elevation in two or more of leads V7–V9, 36 (78%) manifested ≥ 1 mm of ST depression in V1–V3. Of 52 patients with ≥ l mm of ST depression in V1–V3, 46 (88%) manifested ≥ 0.5 mm ST elevation in two or more of leads V7–V9.

Kulkarni AU, et al. Clinical use of posterior electrocardiographic leads: a prospective electrocardiographic analysis during coronary occlusion, 1996.

Methods: Kulkarni et al. (211) studied posterior chest leads in 59 consecutive patients who underwent single-vessel angioplasty of the circumflex artery or the RCA.

Findings: Of 38 circumflex dilations, 10 (26%) showed no ECG change. Of the 28 (74%) circumflex dilations that did show ECG changes, nine (32%) resulted in ST depression in varying locations, including anterior, but **no posterior ST elevation.** Nineteen (68%) of the 28 circumflex dilations resulted in posterior ST elevation of 1 mm. In only two (11%) of these 19 cases was there ST elevation in posterior leads **alone**, without either ST depression in anterior leads (five of 19) or ST elevation in inferior leads (12 of 19). Anterior ST depression manifested both with upright T waves and with asymmetrically inverted T waves.

Comment: In only two cases was ST deviation seen only on posterior leads.

Oraii S, et al. Prevalence and outcome of ST-segment elevation in posterior electrocardiographic leads during acute myocardial infarction, 1999.

Methods: Oraii et al. (225) placed **posterior** leads on 210 consecutive patients admitted to the CCU with a diagnosis of AMI.

Findings: Of 210 patients, 19 (9%) had ST elevation ≥ 1 mm in two or more posterior leads. Seven (3.3%) patients had this posterior elevation as an isolated finding and 12 (5.7%) demonstrated it in conjunction with either inferior or lateral ST elevation.

Comment: Critical information is lacking, however, which raises the following questions: Was the diagnosis established by enzymes before the posterior leads were placed? What was the time period from symptom onset to lead placement? Was reperfusion undertaken? How many patients had ST depression?

Posterior Leads Are Important for the High-Risk CP Patient

Agarwal JB, et al. Importance of posterior chest leads in patients with suspected myocardial infarction, but nondiagnostic, routine 12-lead electrocardiogram, 1999.

Methods: Agarwal et al. (72) recorded posterior leads in 58 CP patients with nondiagnostic standard 12-lead ECGs; *nondiagnostic* was defined as no ST elevation > 0.1 mV. ST elevation > 0.1 mV or Q waves > 0.04 seconds in two or more contiguous **posterior** leads was considered positive.

Findings: Of 25 patients who ruled out for AMI, **none had posterior ST elevation or Q waves.** Of 33 patients who ruled in for AMI, **18 (55%) had ST elevation and/or Q waves in the posterior leads; all 18 had circumflex involvement.** The average size of the AMI was large, with a mean peak total CK of 2,703 IU/L. Of these 18 patients, 13 (72%) had ST depression in V1–V4. It is uncertain how many of the patients who ruled out for AMI had ST depression in V1 or V2, leaving unclear the specificity and PPV of ST depression. How many of the 15 AMI patients had undetected posterior AMI (no posterior ST elevation) is unknown, leaving unclear the sensitivity of posterior leads for posterior AMI. **None of the patients who ruled out for AMI had posterior ST elevation or Q waves.** Thus the posterior ST elevation was very **specific** for AMI.

Matetzky S, et al. Acute myocardial infarction with isolated ST-segment elevation in posterior chest leads V7–V9: "Hidden" ST-segment elevations revealing acute posterior infarction, 1999.

Methods: Matetzky et al. (71) studied 33 consecutive patients with ischemic CP suggestive of AMI without ST elevation on a standard ECG but with ≥ 0.5 mm of ST **elevation in posterior leads.**

Findings: Of 33 patients, 30 (91%) had ST elevation in V7–V9 and three (9%) had ST elevation in V8 only. Thirty-two patients had echocardiography performed within 48 hours of presentation and 20 patients had angiography. Cardiac enzymes confirmed AMI in all patients. Echocardiography of all 32 patients revealed posterior WMAs, and seven (22%) had moderate or severe mitral regurgitation. The circumflex was the IRA in all 20 patients who underwent angiography. Of 33 patients total, 20 (61%) **had ST depression ≥ 1 mm in V1–V3**, and 22 (67%) had ST depression in two consecutive leads from V1–V6. Ten (30%) patients had < 1 mm of ST depression on the standard 12-lead ECG, but the number of patients with 0.5 to 1.0 mm ST depression is not reported. **Further, both of the ECGs displayed as examples of "no ST depression" had noticeable ST depression < 1 mm in V1–V3. This raises the question: How many patients had at least some ST depression, even if less than 1 mm?**

Routine Use of 15- or 18-Lead ECGs on All Chest Pain Patients Is Unwarranted

Brady WJ, et al. A comparison of 12- and 15-lead ECGs in ED chest pain patients: impact on diagnosis, therapy, and disposition, 2000.

Methods: Brady et al. (228) prospectively recorded 15-lead ECGs on 595 patients admitted to a CP evaluation unit in June and July of 1996. They compared outcomes, management, and physician perceptions of these patients with a retrospective group of 599 patients admitted to CP units in June and July of 1995 who had only 12-lead ECGs.

Findings: Of 595 patients with 15-lead ECGs, 13 (2.2%) had AMI, as compared with 11 out of 599 patients (1.8%) with 12-lead ECGs. Physicians felt that the 15-lead ECG provided a more complete anatomic picture of the heart, but they also felt that it **did not alter ED diagnosis, ED-based therapy, or hospital disposition of adult CP patients.**

Zalenski RJ, et al. Value of posterior and right ventricular leads in comparison to the standard 12-lead electrocardiogram in evaluation of ST-segment elevation in suspected acute myocardial infarction, 1997.

Methods: Zalenski et al. (214) utilized 18-lead ECGs (12-lead plus V7–V9 and V4R–V6R) on 533 patients with suspected AMI admitted to CCUs. ST elevation was measured at 80 ms after the J point and AMI was diagnosed primarily by CK-MB.

Findings: Of 533 patients, 345 (64.7%, which is very high) ruled in for AMI, of whom 216 (40.5%) had **diagnostic** ST elevation on the 12-lead ECG and 132 received thrombolytics. Regional ST elevation ≥ 1 mm in two consecutive leads of the standard 12-lead ECG was present in 258 patients (48.4%), and an additional 42 (7.9% of all patients, or 12.2% of AMI) had ST elevation on nonstandard leads only; nine of the 42 had ST elevation ≥ 1 mm in V7–V9 only. Only three of 188 patients without AMI had such ST elevation. **For 1,000 AMI patients without ST elevation on the 12-lead ECG, nonstandard leads would detect an additional 200 patients at the expense of 76 false positives.** This calculation was not done for V7–V9 alone, but in this study, the added sensitivity of these leads for AMI was almost offset by the decreased specificity.

Additional Studies

Rich MW, et al. Electrocardiographic diagnosis of remote posterior wall myocardial infarction using unipolar posterior lead V9, 1989.

Methods: Rich et al. (230) studied 27 patients who met thallium criteria for completed posterior AMI.

Findings: **Q wave 0.04 seconds or more in left paraspinal lead V9 was the best single ECG marker for posterior AMI.**

Lim R, et al. Abolition of electrocardiographic pattern of left ventricular aneurysm by posterior myocardial infarction, 1990.

Findings: Lim et al. (231) report a case of **posterior AMI manifesting as normalization,** or relative depression of chronically elevated anterior ST segments in a patient with **ventricular aneurysm** (old MI with persistent ST elevation).

Melendez LJ, et al. Usefulness of three additional electrocardiographic chest leads (V7, V8, V9) in the diagnosis of acute myocardial infarction, 1978.

Methods: Melendez et al. (226) recorded posterior leads on 117 consecutive patients admitted to a CCU.

Findings: Of 117 patients, 46 (39%) had proven AMI. Nine (21%) of these 46 had ST elevation (amount unspecified) and/or abnormal Q waves in posterior leads V7–V9, six of whom also had either inferior or lateral ST elevation. Three patients (7%) had neither ST elevation nor precordial ST depression on the 12-lead ECG.

Therapy of Posterior AMI

O'Keefe JH Jr., et al. Do patients with left circumflex coronary artery-related acute myocardial infarction without ST-segment elevation benefit from reperfusion therapy? 1995.

Methods: O'Keefe et al. (206) prospectively enrolled 120 AMI patients with suspected RCA or circumflex occlusion, as based on inferior ST elevation or anterior ST depression, who underwent thrombolysis or primary angioplasty within 6 hours of symptom onset. AMI was confirmed by CK-MB.

Findings: Immediate and pre-discharge sestamibi scans and angiography revealed 78 (65%) patients with RCA occlusions and ST elevation, 32 (27%) with circumflex occlusions and ST elevation, and 10 (8%) with circumflex occlusion and ST depression only. The area of myocardium at risk (mean, 20% of total) and the area that was salvaged by reperfusion therapy (mean, 50% of area at risk, or 10% of total myocardium) were identical regardless of artery occluded or presence or absence of ST elevation.

Comment: Circumflex occlusions that did not manifest ECG changes would not have been included, so this study does not suggest that all circumflex occlusions have ST changes.

17

RIGHT BUNDLE BRANCH BLOCK AND FASCICULAR BLOCKS

KEY POINTS

- **Right bundle branch block (RBBB) with AMI carries very high mortality and a high incidence of complications.**
- **ST elevation is NOT obscured by RBBB to the trained observer, in most cases.**
- **In contrast to left bundle branch block (LBBB), thrombolytics are NOT indicated for new RBBB as an isolated finding.**
- **Left main coronary artery occlusion is often associated with RBBB.**

RBBB

General Background

RBBB is a conduction abnormality in which specialized conduction ("Purkinje") fibers of the "right bundle" are nonfunctional, resulting in electrical propagation through slow-conducting myocardium (Figs. 17-1 and 17-2). RBBB may be due to infarction or ischemia of the conduction system or to other chronic conditions. It may be transient, intermittent, or both. It may also be rate-related, such that the refractory period of the right bundle may be too long for a fast HR; in this case, the RBBB resolves with a slower HR.

ECG Diagnosis of RBBB

In RBBB with or without AMI (Fig. 17-2), the rightward component of the ECG complex is wide (wide = slow), because of the propagation of depolarization through slow-conducting myocardium. See Cases 17-1 and 17-2.

Criteria for Diagnosis of RBBB

The following criteria **must** be present for the diagnosis of RBBB:

1. **QRS ≥ 120ms.**
   - An incomplete RBBB pattern with QRS <120 ms may be due to true **incomplete RBBB** or to right ventricular hypertrophy (RVH).

2. RBBB **must** manifest a **wide S wave in I, aVL, and/or V6.**
3. **Delayed intrinsicoid deflection** of the latter part of QRS > 40 to 50 ms (the intrinsicoid deflection is the time from the beginning of the QRS to the peak of the R′ wave)
4. **RSR′ in V1, with amplitude and width of R′ > R.**
   - However, a QR pattern may be present instead if the first R wave is replaced by a Q wave. Do not confuse the large R wave with posterior AMI, RVH, or Wolff-Parkinson-White (WPW) syndrome.

Typical Features of RBBB

The following typical features of RBBB are frequently present (see next page):

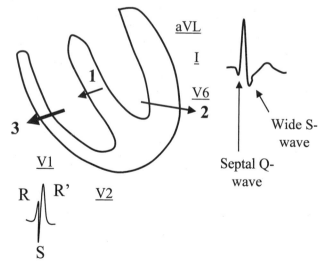

FIGURE 17-1. Sequence of depolarization during RBBB. The septum is rapidly depolarized (narrow complex), left to right, by the functioning left bundle. This manifests a narrow R wave in V1 and a septal Q wave in lateral leads I, aVL, and V6 (*Arrow 1*). The left ventricle (LV) is rapidly depolarized (narrow complex) from right to left by the left bundle. This manifests a narrow S wave in V1 and R waves in I, aVL, and V6 (*Arrow 2*). The right ventricle (RV) is slowly depolarized (wide complex) because depolarization must propagate through myocardium rather than through specialized conducting fibers. This manifests a wide R′ wave in V1 and wide S wave in lateral leads I, aVL, and V6 (*Arrow 3*).

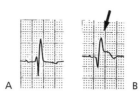

FIGURE 17-2. RBBB without AMI and RBBB with AMI. A: RBBB without AMI as seen in lead V2. Note the RSR'; the end of the QRS is isoelectric (no ST elevation). **B:** RBBB with AMI, as seen in lead V2. As shown here, there may be a Q wave instead of an R wave. The R' ends in an elevated ST segment. (ECG reproduced from unpublished data with permission of K. Wang, M.D.)

- The T wave is generally inverted in leads with an rSR′ or RSR′ (V1 ± V2 ± V3).
- The T wave is typically upright in leads with a prominent S wave (I, aVL, and V4–V6).
- ST segments are not usually deviated, **except for frequent J-point depression (approximately 1 mm) in right precordial leads, especially V1.** Thus, unlike in LBBB, ST deviation, especially ST elevation, is usually due to ischemia.

RBBB WITH AMI

General Background

RBBB is present in approximately 6% of all AMIs (**232**,233). In one study, 13% of AMI patients who received thrombolytics had new RBBB at some time during the first 36 to 72 hours of hospitalization; 52% of these patients had left anterior descending artery (LAD) occlusion (**234**). Although RBBB in AMI is typically a result of the infarction; it may also be preexisting (233,**235–237**).

Mortality of AMI with RBBB was extremely high in the pre-reperfusion era (78,233). **AMI patients with RBBB suffer more complications and higher mortality** than other AMI patients, including patients with LBBB, especially without reperfusion (**232,236,238,242**). Patients with **chronic** LBBB, however, seem to have a higher mortality than those with **chronic** RBBB (**239**). **AMI patients with RBBB are also much less likely to receive reperfusion therapy** than patients with AMI and no BBB (**232**). This is largely because the wide QRS of RBBB makes it difficult for the inexperienced ECG interpreter to distinguish the end of the QRS from the beginning of the ST segment, which is necessary in order to detect ST deviation.

ECG Diagnosis of RBBB with AMI

Because RBBB alone does **NOT** affect the ST segment, for a skilled ECG interpreter, the sensitivity of ST elevation for AMI is presumably the same with RBBB as without RBBB (Fig. 17-2). RBBB obscures interpretation of ST elevation to a lesser extent than LBBB.

Method for Identifying ST Elevation

Training and experience enable the clinician to identify ST elevation in the presence or absence of RBBB with nearly equal facility. We suggest the following steps:

- **Find the lead in which it is easiest to measure QRS duration.** Computer algorithms provide accurate measurement of QRS duration, which is the same in all leads.
- Using this known QRS duration, you can **determine the end of the QRS in any lead,** no matter how distorted the terminal QRS. The end of the QRS is the beginning of the ST segment.
- Because the QRS duration in BBB is long, atrial repolarization is complete at the end of the QRS. Therefore **measure the ST segment deviation at its beginning and relative to the TP segment.**

See Cases 17-3 through 17-6. (See also Case 16-5 of an unstable patient with posterior AMI with concurrent RBBB.)

Ventricular Aneurysm with RBBB May Mimic Acute MI

Ventricular aneurysm (old MI with persistent ST elevation, see Chapter 23) in the presence of RBBB may mimic RBBB with acute MI. Ventricular aneurysm **WITHOUT** RBBB typically manifests a **QS pattern. WITH** RBBB, this may be transformed to a **QR pattern** in leads V1–V3 and persistent ST elevation may be even more readily misdiagnosed as AMI. In these cases, the clinical history and previous ECGs are very important. **If previous ECGs are unavailable for a patient with a clinical history consistent with AMI, assume the MI is acute.** (See Cases 17-7 and 23-8.)

Other pathology may also produce RBBB with ST elevation mimicking AMI. (See Case 17-8 of tricyclic overdose with RBBB and ST elevation.)

Management of RBBB with AMI

Although major clinical trials have determined that thrombolytics are indicated for patients with clinical presentation and ECG manifestations consistent with concurrent AMI and "BBB," most studies do not differentiate between right, left, new, or old BBB (30,102). Current guidelines proposed by the American College of Cardiology/American Heart Association (ACC/AHA) are also vague. ECG findings of "BBB" and "LBBB" are proposed as indications for reperfusion therapy, even in the absence of ST elevation, but RBBB is never specifically mentioned (105). **We believe new RBBB without diagnostic ST deviation is NOT an indication for thrombolytic therapy, but with an appropriate clinical presentation, emergent angiography ± percutaneous coronary intervention (PCI) may be indicated.**

LAFB AND LPFB

Left anterior fascicular block (LAFB) is a conduction abnormality in which a nonfunctional posterior fascicle depolarizes slowly, while a functional anterior fascicle depolarizes rapidly. In left posterior fascicular block (LPFB), the situation is reversed such that the posterior fascicle is nonfunctional and depolarizes slowly and a functional anterior fascicle depolarizes rapidly. LAFB or, less commonly, LPFB, may occur concurrent with RBBB. This is called **bifascicular block** and may obscure diagnosis of AMI.

ECG Diagnosis of LAFB

LAFB typically manifests the following ECG characteristics:

- **Left** axis deviation (usually −60)
- Slightly wide, deep S waves in inferior leads
- Small Q wave in leads I and aVL, small R wave in II, III, aVF
- Normal QRS duration (<100 ms)
- Late intrinsicoid deflection in aVL (>0.045 sec)
- Increased QRS voltage in limb leads
- The peak of the terminal R wave in aVR occurs later than the peak in aVL
- **No ST elevation**

See Case 17-9 of LAFB with anterolateral ST-elevation MI (STEMI).

RBBB and LAFB Often Appear Concomitantly

RBBB and LAFB with AMI is associated with **left main coronary artery occlusion** and is associated with a particularly **high mortality (236).** (See Cases 17-10 and 17-11.)

RBBB and LAFB with AMI May Mimic Ventricular Tachycardia

RBBB may mimic ventricular tachycardia, especially on a single-lead monitor (see Case 17-10).

ECG Diagnosis of LPFB

LPFB typically manifests the following characteristics:

- **Right** axis deviation
- Narrow (fast) Q wave (negative) in inferior leads followed by a slightly wide R wave
- Narrow (fast) R wave in aVL followed by a slightly wide S wave
- **No ST elevation**

CASE 17-1

Simple RBBB

History
This 64-year-old patient presented with CP.

ECG 17-1 (Type 3)
- rSR′ and wide R′: V1; wide S wave: I, aVL, V5–V6; QRS > 120 ms (143 ms); and no elevation beyond the end of the QRS (no ST elevation) are diagnostic of **RBBB.**

Clinical Course
The patient ruled out for AMI by negative cardiac troponin I (cTnI).

Conclusion
It is appropriate that this patient did **NOT** receive thrombolytics.

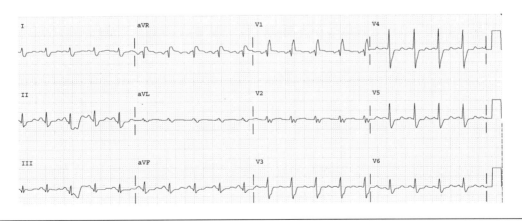

CASE 17-2

RBBB and RVH with NSTEMI; the Wide, Flattened QRS Could Be Misread as ST Elevation

History

This 42-year-old man presented with a history of Ebstein's anomaly, coarctation, and partial anomalous venous return, repaired 29 years prior. He presented with 2 weeks of exertional CP and dyspnea, followed by "indigestion" and left shoulder ache for 4 days, followed by CP at rest.

ECG 17-2 (Type 3)

- Typical **RBBB,** including QRS > 120 ms (**180 ms**): I, II, V6.
- Although V1–V3 **appear** to show ST elevation, there is **none;** close analysis of V1–V3 reveals that 180 ms after the start of the QRS, the ST segment is isoelectric. What appears to be ST elevation is actually a very tall and wide R wave in V1–V3, due to concurrent RVH.
- ST depression: very subtle, <1 mm, V4–V6.
- Q waves and loss of R wave: V1–V4, probable old anterior MI.

Clinical Course

Aspirin, nitroglycerine (NTG), and heparin relieved symptoms. Total CK peaked at 800 IU/L. Serial ECGs were identical. Echocardiography confirmed RVH and subsequent angiography revealed 99% LAD stenosis and 50% right coronary artery (RCA) stenosis. The patient underwent PCI of the LAD.

Conclusion

This difficult and confusing case illustrates the method of measuring ST elevation or its absence by finding the end of the QRS. Although AMI was proven in retrospect by CK, thrombolytics were not indicated. Approximately 50% of patients who do not meet ECG eligibility for reperfusion therapy ultimately prove to have elevated CK-MB, consistent with non-ST-elevation MI (NSTEMI). Therapy for unstable angina (UA)/NSTEMI is indicated. Angiography ± PCI may be indicated.

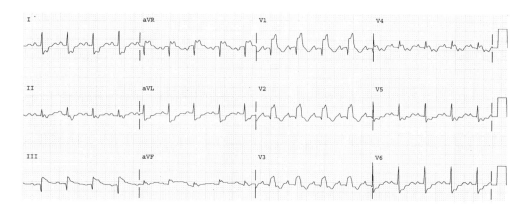

CASE 17-3

RBBB with Anteroseptal AMI

History
This 47-year-old man presented with CP.

ECG 17-3 (Type 1a)
- Wide S waves: I, aVL, V5–V6; RSR′: V1; and QRS > 120 ms (132 ms) are diagnostic of RBBB.

- ST elevation: V1–V4 is diagnostic of **anteroseptal AMI.**

Conclusion
Thrombolytic-eligible AMI may be readily diagnosed in the presence of RBBB.

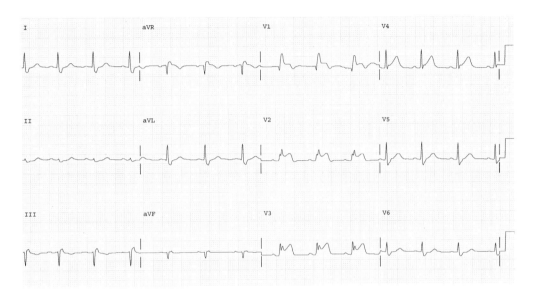

CASE 17-4

RBBB and Anterolateral AMI with Terminal QRS Distortion

History
This 46-year-old presented with CP.

ECG 17-4 (Type 1a)
- QRS > 120 ms, best measured in V1; and rSR′ and tall R′ wave: V1, are diagnostic of RBBB.

- No wide S wave is visible; V5–V6 are artifactual.
- I and aVL hide the S wave behind obvious ST elevation (terminal QRS distortion); and ST elevation: V2–V4, I, aVL, are diagnostic of **anterolateral AMI.**
- Reciprocal ST depression: II, III, aVF.

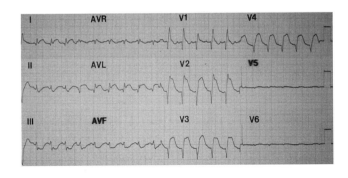

CASE 17-5

RBBB and RVH with Anterolateral AMI

History

This 27-year-old woman with history of repaired Tetralogy of Fallot presented with CP.

ECG 17-5A (Type 3)

ECG from 4 months prior

- Very large RR′: **RBBB** and **RVH,** also **LAFB.**
- Baseline **ST depression:** V1–V3, and absence of Q waves is consistent with RBBB.

ECG 17-5B (Type 1a) at 12:38

- qR pattern (no first R wave): V1–V4; and wide S wave: V5–V6, are diagnostic of **RBBB** with **new or old MI.**
- Very tall and wide R wave: V1–V4, is diagnostic of RVH.
- **ST elevation: V4–V6** (because the QRS duration is 133 ms and there is positive deflection beyond 133 ms in these leads) and **relative** ST elevation: V1–V2 (compared with

chronic ST depression in V1–V3 seen on ECG 17-5A), are diagnostic of **anterolateral AMI.**

Clinical Course

Clinicians administered aspirin and heparin but were uncertain about the ECG. Immediate echocardiography revealed RVH, LVH, and a new anterior-apical-septal wall motion abnormality (WMA). Angiography after this one-hour delay revealed a clot in the left main artery, which extended and occluded the LAD. Angioplasty was too high risk and the patient was started on abciximab. An intra-aortic balloon pump was placed and coronary artery bypass graft (CABG) performed. CK peaked at 2,032 IU/L and cTnI peaked at 97.2 ng/mL at 14 hours.

Conclusion

ST elevation can be found even when the QRS appears very distorted.

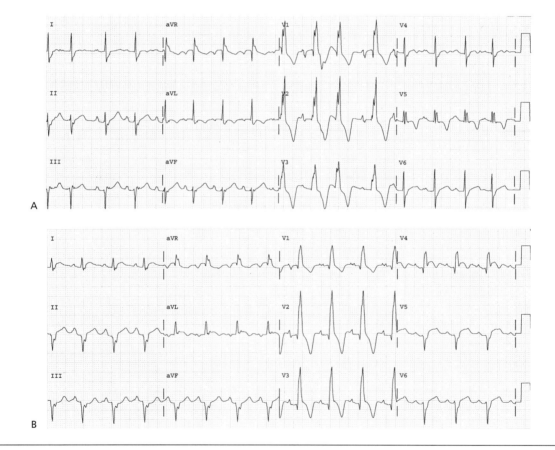

CASE 17-6

RBBB and Anterior AMI, Artifact of Fast Paper Speed

History
This 69-year-old man presented with CP and no past history of MI.

ECG 17-6A (Type 1a)
V1–V6 only
- Very wide QRS is an artifact due to fast paper. The speed written on the bottom is **50 mm/sec (standard is 25 mm).**
- Although this is RBBB, ST elevation in V1–V6 is diagnostic of **anterolateral AMI.** Clinicians were puzzled by the wide QRS and repeated the ECG.

ECG 17-6B (Type 1a)
34 minutes later
- QRS > 120 ms (130 ms), best seen in V5–V6; and wide S wave: I, aVL, V5–V6 are diagnostic of RBBB.

- ST elevation: V1–V5, at least 4 mm in V3.
- **QR pattern:** well-formed Q waves in all precordial leads. Is this QR pattern with ST elevation due to RBBB and ventricular aneurysm (old MI with persistent ST elevation) or due to RBBB and acute MI? **Assume acute MI:** ST elevation > 3 mm, presence of CP, and no history of MI.

Clinical Course
Reperfusion therapy is indicated. Streptokinase (SK) was administered but delayed due to nonrecognition of the artifact. The patient ruled in for a large anterior AMI, with anterior, septal, and apical as well as infero-posterior WMA and moderately severe decreased LV function. Echocardiography one month later revealed dyskinesis and diastolic distortion (aneurysm).

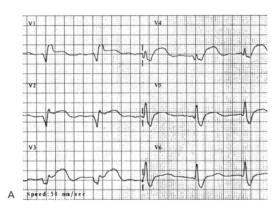

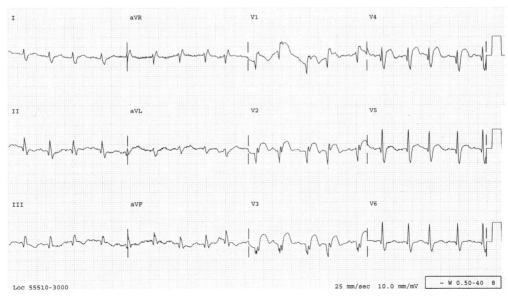

CASE 17-7

RBBB Transformed the QS of Ventricular Aneurysm into a QR Pattern Misinterpreted as AMI: Thrombolytics Were Administered

History

The 69-year-old man from Case 17-5, with history of anterior AMI treated with SK, re-presented 1 month later with tachycardia, hypotension, diaphoresis, and tachypnea but **no CP.**

ECG 17-7 (Type 1c)

■ Irregular fast rhythm (atrial fibrillation) distracts from interpretation of ST segments.

■ Wide S wave: I, aVL, V5–V6; and QRS > 120 ms, best measured in V2, are diagnostic of **RBBB.**

■ ST elevation: V1–V6, I, aVL, is **suspicious** for AMI or ventricular aneurysm.

■ Well-developed Q waves with QR pattern: V1–V2, are consistent with (a) anterior AMI with new Q waves or (b)

old anterior MI with preexisting Q waves (ST elevation reflecting either superimposed AMI or ventricular aneurysm).

■ **Small T waves** are suggestive of aneurysm.

Clinical Course

Clinicians administered thrombolytics. The patient ruled out for AMI. The most recent previous ECG was identical and echocardiography later confirmed ventricular aneurysm.

Conclusion

RBBB can transform ventricular aneurysm morphology into a QR pattern that is suggestive of AMI. Compare with previous ECGs before administering thrombolytics, especially in the context of no CP and a history of anterior AMI.

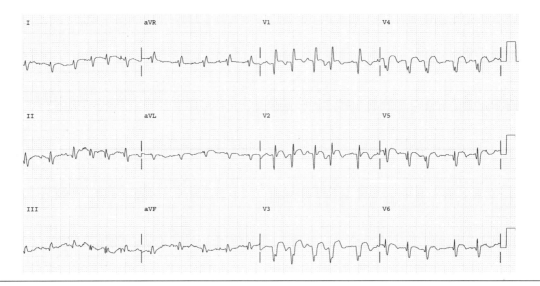

CASE 17-8

Tricyclic Antidepressant Overdose with RBBB and ST Elevation

History

This 23-year-old woman presented with amitryptilene overdose.

ECG 17-8A (Type 1a)

- QRS > 120 ms (148 ms) and other classic morphology are diagnostic of RBBB.
- ST elevation: V1–V2 and aVL. Although diagnostic of AMI, this is a **false positive.**

ECG 17-8B (Type 3)

This ECG was recorded after intravenous (IV) bicarbonate was administered.

- QRS = 120 ms and ST elevation has resolved.

Conclusion

Consider the clinical setting. Non-acute coronary syndrome (ACS) etiologies of conduction delay may result in a Type 1a ECG. Repeat the ECG after appropriate therapy for the clinical condition.

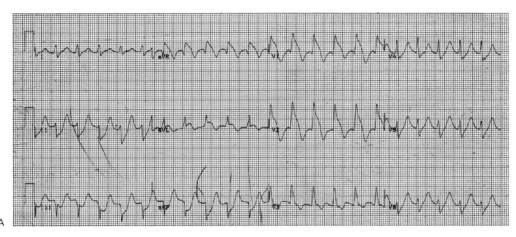

A

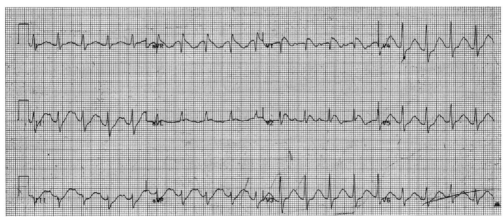

B

CASE 17-9

Anterolateral AMI and LAFB

History

This 54-year-old man presented with 20 minutes of chest tightness.

ECG 17-9 (Type 1b)

- Deep S waves: III, aVF; left axis deviation; and QRS = 110 ms are diagnostic of **LAFB;** Q waves, I, aVL are due to LAFB, **not** MI.
- ST elevation: > 2 mm, V2–V3 and minimal in I and aVL; with reciprocal depression: III are diagnostic of **anterolateral AMI.**

Clinical Course

The patient received tissue plasminogen activator (tPA) within 20 minutes. Two hours later, **ST segments had recovered and LAFB remained.** Over 36 hours, T-wave inversion evolved. CK peaked at 469 IU/L and CK-MB peaked at 24 IU/L at 16 hours. Angiography 3 days later showed TIMI-3 flow and an ulcerated plaque in the LAD with filling defects consistent with thrombus.

Conclusion

LAFB alone does not affect the ST segments, even in leads I and aVL.

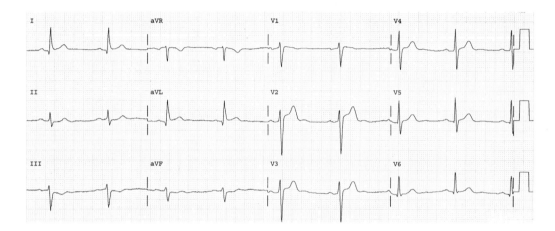

CASE 17-10

Cardiogenic Shock from Left Main Thrombus; ECG with AMI, RBBB, and LAFB

History

This 50-year-old man presented with CP, hypotension, and pulmonary edema.

ECG 17-10 (Type 1a)

■ QRS: wide and distorted, and tall R′ wave are diagnostic of **RBBB.**

■ Late superior forces, as seen in limb leads, are diagnostic of **LAFB.**

■ QR wave: V1–V4.

■ ST elevation: V1 (9 mm), V2 (10 mm), V3 (12 mm), V4 (6 mm), V5 (2 mm), I, aVL; **V4 is easiest to interpret;** the downstroke of the R wave stops and flattens out (elevated ST segment); ST depression: V6, II, III, aVF; total sum of ST elevation and depression = **54 mm.**

■ This ECG is diagnostic of **anterolateral AMI** and suspicious for left main occlusion.

■ If you can imagine any one of those leads on a rhythm monitor, it would be easy to mistake this for ventricular tachycardia.

Clinical Course

Angiography revealed a left main thrombus and CABG was performed.

Conclusion

In such an extensive AMI with very high risk of mortality, the benefit of reperfusion outweighs nearly any risk.

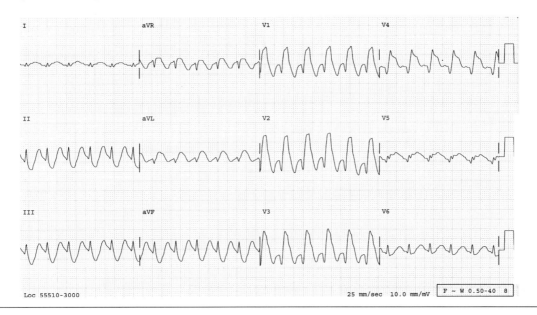

Loc 55510-3000   25 mm/sec   10.0 mm/mV   F ~ W 0.50-40 8

CASE 17-11

Large AMI with RBBB and LAFB, Due to Left Main Occlusion

History

This 60-year-old man presented with CP that began at 08:30. He called 911 and was found with a systolic BP of 60. He was resuscitated from ventricular fibrillation. He arrived in the ED at 09:05, was endotracheally intubated, and resuscitated again from ventricular fibrillation. He was in cardiogenic shock.

ECG 17-11 (Type 1a)

At 09:11

■ Wide S wave: V5–V6; tall R wave: V1; and QRS duration = 160 ms in II and V5 are diagnostic of **RBBB**.

■ Small narrow R wave and wide S wave: II, III, aVF; and left axis deviation are diagnostic of **LAFB**.

■ ST elevation: **V4,** is clearly diagnostic of **anterior AMI.**

Clinical Course

The patient received thrombolytics and was taken for angiography, which showed a patent left main coronary artery with thrombus. He was sent for immediate CABG.

Conclusion

RBBB with a very wide QRS is a sign of a very large AMI, often with left main coronary artery occlusion.

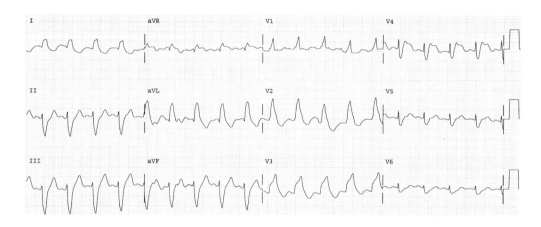

ANNOTATED BIBLIOGRAPHY

Incidence and Mortality of BBB in AMI

Sgarbossa EB, et al. Acute myocardial infarction and complete bundle branch block at hospital admission: clinical characteristics and outcome in the thrombolytic era, 1998.

Methods: Sgarbossa et al. (236) analyzed data from all 26,003 North American patients in GUSTO-I; all were diagnosed with AMI and received thrombolytics (see Appendix C*).*

Findings: BBB was present in 420 patients (1.6%); 131 had LBBB and 289 had RBBB. **RBBB, especially if also associated with LAFB, was associated with both LAD occlusion and anterior infarction (65%) and also with higher 30-day mortality** (21% for RBBB and 23% for RBBB with LAFB versus 11% for AMI and no BBB). The mortality of patients with AMI and LBBB (in which the LAD was the affected artery in only 35%) was only 10%.

Comment: This data underestimates the incidence of BBB in AMI because inclusion in this study required treatment with thrombolytics; patients with BBB are under-enrolled in such trials.

Go AS, et al. Bundle-branch block and in-hospital mortality in acute myocardial infarction, 1998.

Methods: Go et al. (232) analyzed data from 297,832 National Registry of Myocardial Infarction (NRMI) patients (see Appendix C).

Findings: RBBB was concurrent with AMI in 8,354 (6%) patients and was associated with higher in-hospital mortality than AMI with no BBB. **Only 32.0% of patients with RBBB and AMI** for whom reperfusion therapy was clearly indicated actually received it, compared with **66.5% of patients with a clear indication and no BBB.** Patients with RBBB also received **aspirin or beta-blockers less frequently** than patients without any BBB. The odds ratios (ORs) for death in AMI with RBBB and LBBB (versus AMI with no BBB) were 1.64 and 1.34, respectively.

Hod H, et al. Bundle branch block in acute Q-wave inferior wall myocardial infarction. A high-risk subgroup of inferior myocardial infarction patients, 1995.

Methods: Hod et al. (238) retrospectively studied 2,215 patients with inferior Q-wave AMI, as determined by typical CP of 30 minutes or more, new pathologic Q waves in inferior leads, and elevation of creatine kinase (CK)-MB.

Findings: Of 2,215 patients, 85 (3.84%) had RBBB and 23 (1.04%) had LBBB. **RBBB, but NOT LBBB,** was an independent predictor of **in-hospital mortality** (22% versus 13%), **5-year mortality** (33% versus 23%), and **in-hospital complications,** including atrioventricular (AV) block.

Newby KH, et al. Incidence and clinical relevance of the occurrence of bundle-branch block in patients treated with thrombolytic therapy, 1996.

Methods: Newby et al. (234) analyzed data from subgroups of patients enrolled in GUSTO-I, TAMI-9, and their substudies, who had prospectively undergone 36- to 72-hour continuous ST-segment monitoring. BBB was defined as present or persistent if it occurred during or throughout the monitoring period, respectively.

Findings: Of 681 patients in this subgroup, 23.6% had BBB at some point during monitoring; BBB was transient in 18.4% and persistent in 5.3%. AMI with RBBB was found in 13%, AMI with LBBB in 7%, and alternating in 3.5%. LAD occlusion was found in 52% of AMI with RBBB and 43% of AMI with LBBB. Thirty-day mortality was 8.7% in patients who had AMI with BBB versus 3.5% in AMI with no BBB. Mortality was higher in patients with AMI with persistent BBB (19.4%) versus AMI with transient BBB (5.6%). **AMI with persistent LBBB was associated with a 36% mortality, and AMI with persistent RBBB with 12% mortality.**

Roth A, et al. Rapid resolution of new right bundle branch block in acute anterior myocardial infarction patients after thrombolytic therapy, 1993.

Methods: Roth et al. (237) studied 211 consecutive patients with anterior AMI who received thrombolytics.

Findings: Of 211 patients, 8 (3.8%) had AMI with RBBB. Mean time to treatment was 122 minutes. All patients reperfused and had resolution of RBBB within 3 hours. Only one patient required prophylactic pacing. Six patients underwent angiography, all with high-grade LAD stenosis or occlusion.

BBB Without AMI

Freedman RA, et al. Bundle branch block in patients with chronic coronary artery disease: angiographic correlates and prognostic significance, 1987.

Methods: Freedman et al. (239) analyzed data from the 15,609 patients in the Coronary Artery Surgery Study.

Findings: All patients had angiographic evidence of coronary artery disease (CAD) and 522 patients had BBB. **Two-year mortality of patients with RBBB was twice that of patients without any BBB. Mortality of patients with LBBB was five times that of controls.** In patients with chronic BBB and CAD, chronic LBBB was associated with higher long-term mortality than for patients with no BBB or than in patients with chronic RBBB.

Prognosis of RBBB Without AMI

Schneider JF, et al. Newly acquired right bundle-branch block: The Framingham Study, 1980.

Methods: Schneider et al. (240) analyzed data from 18 years of biennial follow-up in the Framingham Study on all 70 patients who developed complete RBBB.

Findings: Although the onset of RBBB was usually unaccompanied by overt clinical events, cardiovascular disease mortality in patients with RBBB was almost three times greater than that of an age-matched sample of the general population.

Hiss RG, et al. Electrocardiographic findings in 122,043 individuals, 1962.

Methods: Hiss et al. (235) studied the ECGs of 122,043 normal males (with **no** history of CAD) entering flight training in the Air Force.

Findings: The incidence of RBBB was 1.8% (231 of 122,043); seven-year follow-up revealed no increased incidence of cardiovascular disease.

18

LEFT BUNDLE BRANCH BLOCK

KEY POINTS

- LBBB is a common reason that appropriate reperfusion therapy is delayed or withheld.
- NEW LBBB and a clinical presentation suggestive of AMI is an indication for reperfusion therapy.
  - Specific ECG indicators of AMI in the presence of LBBB may confirm the diagnosis.
  - Do not let absence of specific indicators dissuade you from reperfusion therapy when clinical suspicion is high.
- Patients with OLD LBBB and (a) increased ST elevation from a previous ECG or on serial ECGs OR (b) with specific ECG indicators of AMI should receive reperfusion therapy.
- Patients with LBBB not known to be old, with symptoms highly suspicious for AMI, may receive thrombolytics if there are no significant contraindications, and there are no alternative diagnostic methods immediately available.
- See Figures 18-5 and 18-6 for treatment algorithms.

GENERAL BACKGROUND

LBBB is a conduction abnormality in which specialized conducting ("Purkinje") fibers of the "left bundle" are nonfunctional, resulting in electrical propagation through slow conducting myocardium (**Fig. 18-1**). LBBB may be due to many disease states, including cardiomyopathy and AMI. Unlike RBBB (see Chapter 17), **LBBB with or without AMI typically manifests ST elevation in the ABSENCE of any ischemia or infarction.** Consequently, the specificity of ST elevation for AMI when there is concurrent LBBB is much less than when there is normal conduction.

LBBB

ECG Diagnosis of LBBB

In LBBB with or without AMI (**Fig. 18-2**), the leftward component of the ECG complex is wide (wide = slow), due to the propagation of depolarization through slow-conducting myocardium.

Criteria for the Diagnosis of LBBB

The following are criteria that **must** be present for the diagnosis of LBBB:

- QRS > 120 ms.
- Lead I: wide, monophasic R wave.
- Any Q wave in leads I, aVL, V5, or V6 is due to the presence of MI (acute or old), not a result of LBBB.
- Delayed intrinsicoid deflection in leads V5–V6 (> 0.04 sec to peak of R).

Note: Important leads in LBBB are I, V1, and V6.

Typical Features of LBBB

The following are typical features of LBBB that are frequently present (opposite page):

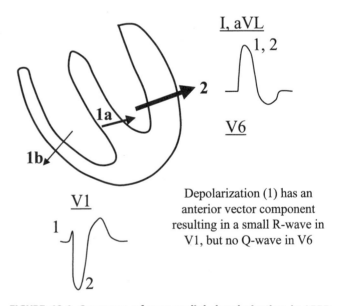

Depolarization (1) has an anterior vector component resulting in a small R-wave in V1, but no Q-wave in V6

FIGURE 18-1. Sequence of myocardial depolarization in LBBB and corresponding ECG manifestations in aVL, V6, and V1. The rapidly depolarized right bundle simultaneously causes depolarization of the septum in a leftward direction **(1a)** and of the RV free wall in a rightward direction **(1b)** (which is not recorded in lead V6 because forces are so small compared with the septum), and some anterior depolarization, which is seen as a small R wave in V1–V3. Because the conducting system is blocked, depolarization must propagate through myocardium and there is slow leftward activation of the LV free wall **(2)**, which is seen as a wide R wave in leads I and V6.

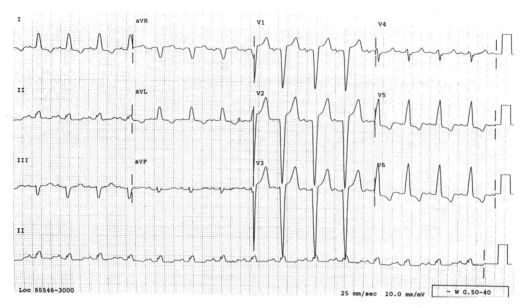

FIGURE 18-2. LBBB. This ECG fulfills the criteria for LBBB listed above. The degree of ST elevation evident in leads V1–V3 is common in uncomplicated LBBB. Although these ST segments are concave upward, this is frequently NOT the case in LBBB. (ECG reproduced from unpublished data with permission of K. Wang, M.D.)

- V1: QS or RS pattern, with large, deep S wave.
- Left axis deviation.
- Discordant ST deviation and T-wave inversion. Uncomplicated LBBB almost always manifests **discordant ST deviation (typically < 5 mm) and discordant T waves,** which means that ST segments and T waves are in the direction **opposite** to the predominance of the QRS complex. The magnitude of the discordance should be proportional to the voltage of the QRS. For example, leads V1–V3 typically manifest a QRS that is predominantly negative, with up to 5 mm (occasionally more) of ST elevation. **When discordance is NOT present, suspect ischemia or infarction.**

LBBB Variations

Incomplete LBBB manifests a QRS duration of 100 to 120 ms; other criteria are identical to those listed earlier for LBBB.

Rate-related BBB may occur if the HR is too fast [usually > 100 beats per minute (bpm)] to allow repolarization of an abnormal conduction system with a prolonged refractory period. In these cases, BBB may resolve with slowing of the HR, thus making the ECG diagnosis easier (see Case 18-1).

Intraventricular conduction delay (IVCD) is a term used to describe a wide QRS complex (100 ms or more) that occurs with no specific morphology (i.e., criteria for LBBB or RBBB are absent).

LBBB WITH AMI

Clinical Factors

The prevalence of AMI (as diagnosed by CK-MB) in patients with ischemic symptoms and LBBB depends on the clinical sit-

uation. Combining five studies (**20,241,242,**242.5,416) of patients at high suspicion for **persistent coronary occlusion**, the mean prevalence of AMI in patients with LBBB was 188 of 448 (42%). In two other studies of patients in chest pain units with a lower suspicion for persistent coronary occlusion (**243, 244**), patients with LBBB had a prevalence of AMI of 49 of 372 (13%). The combined prevalence for all seven studies is 237 of 820 (29%), which is significantly higher than that of patients with ischemic symptoms but without LBBB (16.6% [18,21]).

LBBB is associated with chronic ischemic and nonischemic cardiomyopathy as well as with AMI. A history of congestive heart failure (CHF), dilated cardiomyopathy, low ejection fraction (EF), or a chest film revealing cardiomegaly provides evidence that the LBBB is **not** new. Because LBBB may be present in many patients with nonischemic CP, if the LBBB is not **known** to be new and there are no specific ECG findings of AMI, **it is important to ensure that the patient is experiencing typical and ongoing symptoms** before administering thrombolytics.

LBBB occurs in **6.7% of all AMI** as diagnosed by CK-MB (**232**). LBBB, detected during continuous monitoring for 36 to 72 hours after thrombolytics, may appear at least transiently in up to 10.5% of AMI patients (234). Compared with patients with AMI and neither RBBB nor LBBB, patients with AMI and LBBB are **older** (76 years versus 68 years), more likely to **present without CP** (only 54% LBBB with CP versus 70% with CP in patients without LBBB), and more likely to be **female** (50% versus 41%) (**232**). As diagnosed by CK-MB, **only 8.4% to 16.6% of patients with LBBB and AMI receive any reperfusion therapy,** most commonly because of a "nondiagnostic" ECG (**232,245**). This is in contrast to 32% of patients with AMI and no BBB (and 20% of patients with AMI and **R**BBB) (**232**) who receive reperfusion therapy. Patients with LBBB and

AMI are also much less likely to receive aspirin and beta-blockers than patients with AMI and no BBB (**232**), especially in the absence of CP (**245**). In-hospital mortality of all patients with LBBB and AMI is 22.6% versus 13.1% for patients with AMI and no LBBB (**232**). Overall 30-day mortality was 8.7% in a study of patients with LBBB and AMI who received reperfusion therapy (versus 3.5% for patients with AMI and no BBB), but **new and persistent LBBB with AMI was associated with 36% mortality** (234). **LBBB has been shown to be associated with LAD occlusion** in up to 43% of patients with LBBB and AMI (234).

Many physicians do not even attempt ECG diagnosis of AMI with LBBB because it is frequently taught that it is not possible. The notorious reputation of LBBB for obscuring the diagnosis of AMI is due in large part to the difficulty of diagnosing **previous** MI in the presence of LBBB, because LBBB alters Q-wave patterns. **Acute** MI is also difficult to diagnose in the presence of LBBB because LBBB typically manifests ST segment deviation. ST elevation due to the presence of AMI may be misinterpreted as due to LBBB, and, conversely, the ST elevation of LBBB may be interpreted as due to AMI. Nevertheless, there are many circumstances in which **acute MI can be diagnosed with high specificity** in the presence of LBBB, which we discuss later (**241,246,247**).

Specific ("Sgarbossa") Criteria for AMI with LBBB

Specific criteria depend upon concordance and discordance. **Concordance** refers to the ST and/or T wave being in the same direction as the majority of the QRS. ST and T-wave discordance is the normal condition of LBBB. Although the presence of concordant T waves (positive in leads I, aVL, V5 or V6) is abnormal and may be seen in AMI, it is not very specific (**246**) (see Case 18-2). The following morphologies have **good specificity for LBBB with AMI**, and, although the sensitivity is debated, they have performed nearly as well in some studies as ST elevation for STEMI without LBBB (**241,246,247**). See Cases 18-3 to 18-11.

- **Concordant ST elevation** ≥ 1 mm in one or more leads, which means ST elevation in leads in which the QRS is predominantly positive (**V5, V6, I, aVL, or II**). This is **diagnostic of AMI** and contrasts with LBBB with **no** AMI, as described earlier, which typically manifests **discordant** ST deviation.
- **Concordant ST depression** ≥ 1 mm in one or more leads, which means ST depression in leads in which QRS is predominantly negative (V1, V2, V3, ± V4). This is 90% specific for AMI due to posterior injury.
- **Discordant ST elevation > 5 mm and disproportionate with the QRS voltage** appears to be 85% to 90% specific for AMI. This contrasts with uncomplicated LBBB, in which discordant ST elevation is typically < 5 mm.

Diagnostic Changes from a Previous ECG

AMI superimposed on chronic LBBB may show diagnostic changes (**241**,248). **Obtain a baseline ECG,** if possible. If a

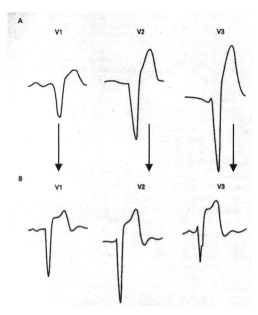

FIGURE 18-3. Serial ECG changes in a patient with LBBB. These changes occurred over 2 hours and are diagnostic of an evolving anterior STEMI, subsequently confirmed. (Reproduced, with permission of BMJ Publishing Group, from Edhouse JA, et al. *J Accid Emerg Med* 1999;16:331–335.)

previous ECG shows LBBB **without** ST segment deviation, **new ST elevation** is diagnostic of AMI. If a previous ECG shows LBBB **with** discordant ST segment deviation, **increased ST elevation** (change compared with previous LBBB) may be as sensitive for AMI as increased ST elevation in patients without LBBB (**249**) (Figs. 18-3 and 18-4). If no

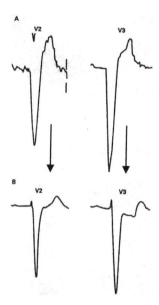

FIGURE 18-4. Serial ECG change in a patient with LBBB. These changes occurred over 15 minutes and are diagnostic of posterior STEMI, subsequently confirmed. (Reproduced, with permission of BMJ Publishing Group, from Edhouse et al., *J Accid Emerg Med* 1999; 16:331–335).

previous ECG is available for comparison, **record serial ECGs or perform continuous ST segment monitoring.** Changes typical of AMI on serial ECGs or continuous monitoring may be diagnostic (**182,241,**250). See Cases 18-7, 18-11, 18-12, and 18-13.

LBBB with Isoelectric ST Segments

If there is LBBB **without** any ST elevation, even on serial ECGs, the significance is uncertain. Even in the right clinical situation, and even with new LBBB, it is uncertain whether this is an indication for thrombolytics. On the other hand, LBBB without ST elevation in V1–V3 may represent **relative ST depression,** especially if changed from previous tracings. Consider that a **posterior AMI** may be lowering the normal ST elevation of a baseline LBBB (see Case 18-7).

MANAGEMENT

A number of major randomized, placebo-controlled trials of thrombolytic therapy combined all BBB together for analysis, whether the BBB was new or old, right or left, and with or without specific criteria for AMI (30,102). This combined group was defined as patients with "suspected AMI and BBB." These clinical trials demonstrated the **benefit of thrombolysis for the BBB group as a whole.** However, a relationship between new LBBB and angiographic occlusion has never been demonstrated.

Specific indicators of AMI with LBBB may not be very sensitive. If physicians rely too heavily on specific ECG criteria for AMI, many patients with LBBB and AMI who need reperfusion therapy but lack these specific criteria may go untreated. Thus many experts argue that **all patients with clinical presentations suspicious for AMI and with LBBB on the ECG should receive reperfusion therapy;** most, however, would **NOT** administer thrombolytics to a patient whose ECG has LBBB **known to be old AND without specific indicators.**

ESSENTIAL CONSIDERATIONS IN THE MANAGEMENT OF SUSPECTED AMI WITH LBBB

- **Clinical suspicion** of AMI
- LBBB **new or old**
- **Specific criteria** for AMI (presence or absence)
- Availability of **angioplasty**
- Thrombolytic **contraindications**

Specific Criteria for AMI with LBBB Are Present

When specific ECG criteria for AMI (see earlier) are present, **reperfusion therapy is indicated.**

New Versus Old LBBB with No Specific Criteria for AMI

See description below and treatment algorithms in Figures 18-5 and 18-6, later.

New LBBB may result from AMI and may not show any specific criteria for AMI. Thus new LBBB, even without specific criteria, suggests AMI and should prompt reperfusion therapy in the right clinical situation. Although old LBBB may very easily hide the ST-segment manifestations of new AMI, if the most recent ECG is available and there is no change from the old LBBB, thrombolytics should not be administered based on that ECG alone. Remember that a **high clinical suspicion,** based on ongoing typical symptoms, age, risk factors, and physical findings (pretest probability), makes it much more likely that LBBB (new or old) represents AMI. The applicability of any ECG criteria for the diagnosis of AMI is clearly dependent on such pretest probability of AMI (**242–244, 246,251–254**).

If LBBB is known to be **new,** even **without specific criteria,** administer reperfusion therapy when the clinical presentation is **suspicious** for AMI.

If LBBB is of **unknown duration** and there are **no specific criteria,** base the reperfusion decision on clinical (pretest) probability. Angiography ± PCI is preferred, but thrombolytics should not be withheld if **clinical suspicion is very high** and there are minor contraindications. If doubt persists and no catheterization (cath) lab is available, record serial ECGs and/or an echocardiogram before administering thrombolytics.

If LBBB is known to be **old** and there are **no specific criteria,** angiography ± PCI is preferred. If a cath lab is not available, the stable patient should only receive thrombolytics if there is a **very high** clinical probability, no contraindications, and no response to anti-ischemic therapy. Thrombolytics are certainly indicated if serial ECGs or other diagnostic modalities confirm AMI.

LBBB and Thrombolysis

Although early large thrombolytic trials indicated that patients with **LBBB and symptoms highly suspicious of AMI should receive thrombolytics** (30,255), clinicians have not followed this recommendation adequately. Consequently, despite higher mortality (30,234,**245**), patients with LBBB have been **substantially undertreated** (25,28,**232,245**). This is due to reluctance to administer a potentially harmful thrombolytic to a patient who might not be suffering AMI (**246**). **Mortality odds,** however, **favor the patient with CP and LBBB who receives thrombolytics** over the patient who does not (30, **252**).

When in doubt, it is generally better to administer reperfusion therapy in patients with CP and LBBB than to withhold it (**252**). **Errors of omission** (not giving thrombolytics when the patient has AMI) **are much more common than errors of commission** (giving thrombolytics when the patient does not

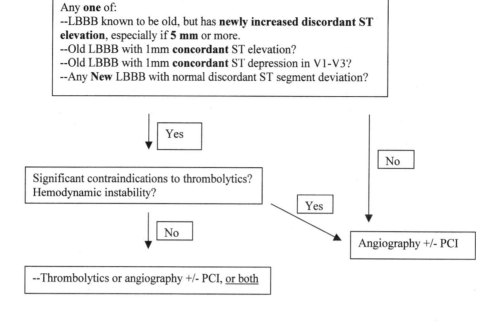

FIGURE 18-5. Guidelines for management of patients with ACS symptoms and LBBB if PCI IS available at your institution.

have AMI), **and these patients are consistently under-treated.**

Management Guidelines

If PCI IS available at your institution, see Figure 18-5.
If PCI is NOT available at your institution, see Figure 18-6.

Management of LBBB Variations

Incomplete LBBB and IVCD

Patients with incomplete LBBB or IVCD should be approached just as if they have LBBB, although there is no guidance from the literature. **ST elevation** should be **at least** as suggestive of AMI as it is in the case of LBBB, and **concordance** is just as important as a diagnostic marker for AMI. See Case 18-5.

Rate-Related BBB

If you suspect that the LBBB is rate-related and the diagnosis of AMI is in doubt, **slow the HR** before initiating reperfusion therapy. **Correct the physiologic causes** of tachycardia, including metabolic abnormalities. If this is unsuccessful, give IV beta-blockers (i.e., metropolol or esmolol) unless contraindicated. See Case 18-1.

Serial ECGs and Echocardiography

Record serial ECGs if the certainty of the diagnosis is not high enough to justify the level of risk for intervention. Although echocardiography may be useful for the detection of WMAs in AMI with LBBB, it is technically difficult due to the abnormal depolarization sequence of LBBB.

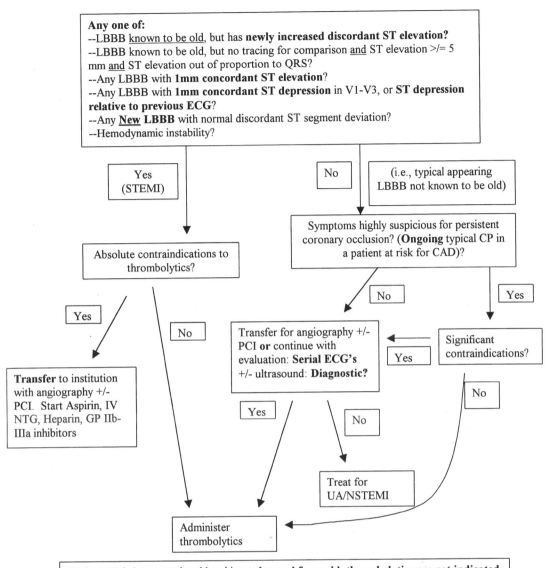

Any one of:
--LBBB <u>known to be old</u>, but has **newly increased discordant ST elevation?**
--LBBB known to be old, but no tracing for comparison <u>and</u> ST elevation >/= 5 mm <u>and</u> ST elevation out of proportion to QRS?
--Any LBBB with **1mm concordant ST elevation**?
--Any LBBB with **1mm concordant ST depression** in V1-V3, or **ST depression relative to previous ECG**?
--Any **New** LBBB with normal discordant ST segment deviation?
--Hemodynamic instability?

Yes (STEMI)

No

(i.e., typical appearing LBBB not known to be old)

Symptoms highly suspicious for persistent coronary occlusion? (**Ongoing** typical CP in a patient at risk for CAD)?

Absolute contraindications to thrombolytics?

No

Yes

Yes

Transfer for angiography +/- PCI **or** continue with evaluation: **Serial ECG's** +/- ultrasound: **Diagnostic?**

Significant contraindications?

Yes

No

Yes

No

No

Transfer to institution with angiography +/- PCI. Start Aspirin, IV NTG, Heparin, GP IIb-IIIa inhibitors

Treat for UA/NSTEMI

Administer thrombolytics

1) If LBBB is known to be old and is **unchanged from old, thrombolytics are not indicated**
2) If there is new or old LBBB and ST segments are **isoelectric** (they are normally discordantly deviated), then the presence of anterior, lateral, or inferior STEMI is unlikely.
3) **Isoelectric ST segments in V1-V3** may represent ST depression relative to the baseline LBBB, and if depressed from a previous ECG, are likely to represent posterior AMI.

FIGURE 18-6. Guidelines for management of patients with ACS symptoms and LBBB if PCI is NOT available at your institution.

CASE 18-1

Rate-Related LBBB

History
This 49-year-old woman presented with 1.5 hours of typical CP.

ECG 18-1 (Type 1c)
- Tall, wide R wave: V6, with a late intrinsicoid deflection; and QRS ≥ 120 ms are diagnostic of **LBBB;** ST-segment deviations are typical of LBBB. However, the patient's HR was 120 bpm.

Clinical Course
No old ECG was available for comparison. Thrombolytics are indicated if there are no significant contraindications.

While the physician was preparing for thrombolysis, the HR decreased and a repeat ECG revealed normal QRS, ST segments, and T waves, with no LBBB. Reperfusion therapy was put on hold. Levels of cTnI were normal, and this was revealed to be **rate-related LBBB.**

Conclusion
In patients with LBBB and tachycardia, attempt to slow the HR with airway management, fluid, or beta-blockers as indicated, and assess accordingly for reperfusion therapy.

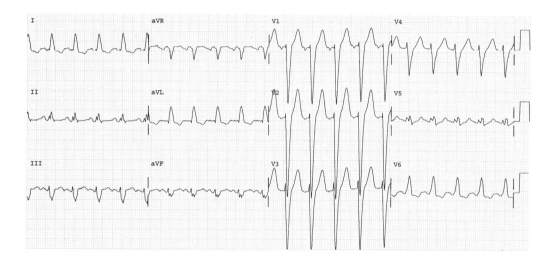

CASE 18-2

LBBB with Nearly Isoelectric ST Segments

History

This 60-year-old man without other risk factors presented with 2 hours of atypical CP.

ECG 18-2 (Type 3)

■ This ECG is diagnostic of **LBBB.** ST segments are nearly isoelectric.

■ Upright concordant T wave: I and V6 are **suspicious** for AMI.

Clinical Course

An old ECG was found later, indicating old LBBB and identical concordant T waves. The patient ruled out for AMI by CK-MB.

Conclusion

The pretest probability of AMI in this patient with atypical CP was not high. Additionally, it is uncertain whether reperfusion therapy is indicated with LBBB and isoelectric ST segments. When there is no change from the previous ECG, reperfusion therapy is not indicated.

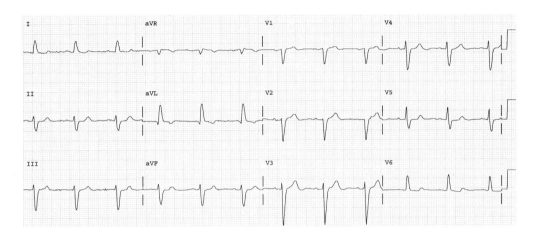

CASE 18-3

LBBB and Anterior AMI

History

This 60-year-old man presented with typical CP.

ECG 18-3 (Type 1a)

■ This ECG is diagnostic of **LBBB** but **discordant ST elevation** in V1–V2 is excessive and **suspicious** for anterior AMI.

■ Concordant ST elevation and T wave: V3, is diagnostic of **anterior AMI** (see handwritten star).

Conclusion

This ECG would be diagnostic of LBBB with anterior AMI even if the patient had presented with less typical symptoms.

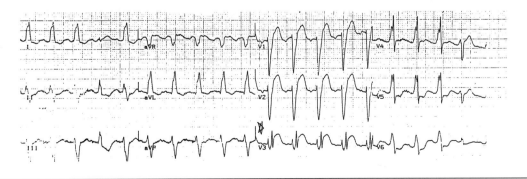

CASE 18-4

LBBB and Anterolateral AMI

History

This 91-year-old man presented with CP. No previous ECG was available.

ECG 18-4A (Type 1a)

Limb leads recorded at **double standard** doubles the millimeters of amplitude and exaggerates the appearance of limb lead voltage. Precordial leads remain 1 mm = 0.1 mV.

- The rhythm appears to change from junctional to sinus rhythm; there are no P waves in V1–V3, but they appear in V4–V6. However, QRS width does not change. Therefore both rhythms appear to be supraventricular, not idioventricular.
- Morphology of classic **LBBB.**
- **QRS: very high voltage, so expect large ST segment deviation;** ST elevation: very high, increases from V1–V4, with up to 10 mm (1.0 mV) in V4. This is **highly**

suspicious for anterior AMI; and clearly **concordant ST elevation: V5, is diagnostic** of **lateral AMI**.

Clinical Course

Clinicians (appropriately) gave thrombolytics. CK-MB and angiography demonstrated a proximal LAD lesion with reperfusion.

ECG 18-4B

Forty-five minutes later, with limb leads at standard voltage and precordial leads at half standard (1 mm = 0.2 mV).

- Decreased ST elevation: 3 mm = 0.6 mV (down from 1.0 mV) after reperfusion.

Conclusion

This ECG is more than 90% specific for AMI and thrombolytics may even be indicated without very typical symptoms.

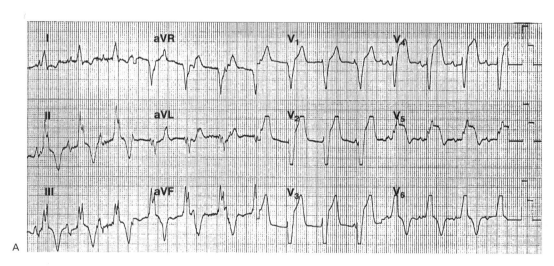

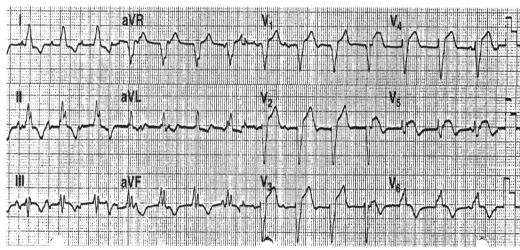

CASE 18-5

New Pulmonary Edema and IVCD: V4 Is Subtly Diagnostic of Anterior AMI

History

This 45-year-old man with no history of cardiac disease presented with new-onset pulmonary edema at 08:30. He had lost consciousness and been intubated, but it is unknown whether or not he experienced CP. BP before and after intubation ranged from 90 to 110 systolic, with a HR of 100 to 130 bpm.

ECG 18-5 (Type 1a)

- Wide QRS: indicative of **IVCD,** misses LBBB criteria because the intrinsicoid deflection V5–V6 < 40 ms. It is unknown whether this is new or old. In the absence of more specific diagnostic and therapeutic guidelines, we will evaluate it like LBBB.
- Discordant ST elevation: V1–V3, with typical LBBB morphology.
- Q waves: I, aVL, V5 **suspicious** for acute or old MI.

- ST elevation: V4, **disproportionate** to the QRS even for LBBB and is **highly specific for anterior AMI.**

Clinical Course

Clinicians missed this diagnostic feature. En route to the intensive care unit (ICU), a passing cardiologist was concerned by the ECG and took the patient for angiography and possible PCI, arriving in the cath lab at 10:00. Despite full support including a balloon pump, the patient died due to 100% mid-LAD occlusion.

Conclusion

In the appropriate clinical setting, this abnormally high ST segment in V4 is highly suspicious for STEMI. Additionally, in the absence of any previous cardiac disease, pulmonary edema with LBBB should strongly suggest AMI. Angiography ± PCI is preferred if available, but **thrombolytics should not be withheld.**

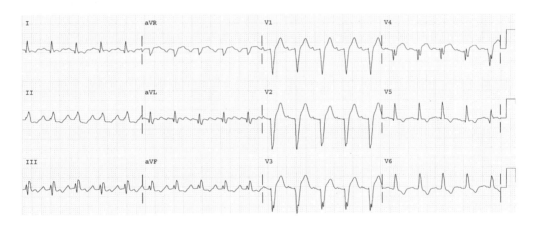

CASE 18-6

LBBB and Inferior AMI

History

This 67-year-old woman presented with 1 hour of typical CP.

ECG 18-6 (Type 1a)

- Abnormal rhythm.
- Q wave and concordant ST elevation: III; and concordant reciprocal ST depression: aVL, are diagnostic of **LBBB and inferior AMI** (T waves remain discordant).

Clinical Course

The patient ruled in for AMI by CK-MB. Reperfusion therapy was not undertaken. Later angiography confirmed distal RCA occlusion and moderately severe decreased LV function with an EF of 25%.

Conclusion

Reperfusion therapy is indicated.

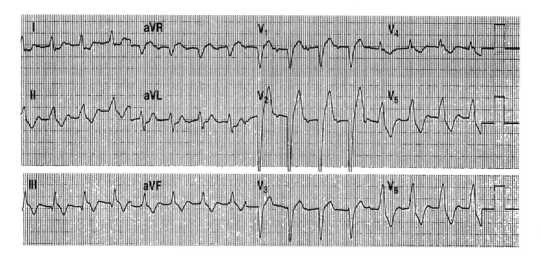

CASE 18-7

LBBB with Inferior Concordant ST Elevation and *RELATIVE* ST Depression in V1–V3

History
This 52-year-old man developed epigastric pain immediately after returning to the ICU from the operating suite. He had undergone CABG to the LAD and to a large dominant RCA with posterior branches.

ECG 18-7A (Type 1a)
- Morphology of classic **LBBB.**
- Concordant ST elevation and T waves: II, III, aVF, are diagnostic of **inferior AMI.**
- Isoelectric ST segments: V1–V3 are **suspicious** for posterior AMI (**relative ST depression**).

ECG 18-7B
Previous ECG, recorded before CABG, V1–V3 only.
- Normal discordant ST segment and T wave of LBBB confirm that the new isoelectric ST segments are due to rela-

tive ST depression, which helps to diagnose **inferoposterior STEMI.**

Clinical Course
Because of clinical constraints, reperfusion therapy was not initiated. CK peaked at 24 hours at 4,157 IU/L and cTnI at 110 ng/mL. The RCA graft was presumably occluded.

Conclusion
This ECG is diagnostic of inferoposterior STEMI. In the absence of contraindications, reperfusion therapy, including thrombolytics, would be indicated.

ECG reproduced from unpublished data with permission of K. Wang, M.D.

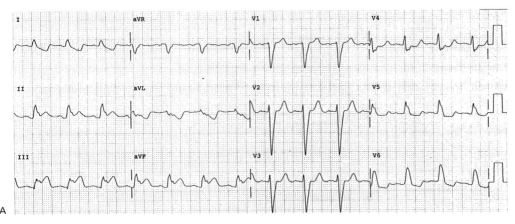
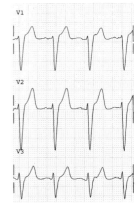

CASE 18-8

LBBB and Posterior AMI

History

This 76-year-old woman presented with 1 hour of typical CP.

ECG 18-8 (Type 1b)

- Morphology of classic **LBBB.**
- Concordant ST depression: V3, is 90% to 95% specific for AMI. V2 is also **suspicious** for AMI because it would normally have discordant ST elevation; instead, the ST segment is isoelectric or slightly depressed.

Clinical Course

Reperfusion therapy, including thrombolytics, was indicated but not administered. The patient was admitted to the CCU with ongoing CP and ruled in for AMI with CK-MB. She developed hypotension and echocardiography revealed a large inferoposterior WMA with 3 to 4+ mitral regurgitation. Subsequent angiography revealed three-vessel disease, with a 99% proximal circumflex lesion. A balloon pump was placed and CABG performed.

Conclusion

ST depression in V1–V3, in the context of LBBB, is approximately 90% specific for AMI and reperfusion therapy is indicated.

ECG reproduced from unpublished data with permission from K. Wang, M.D.

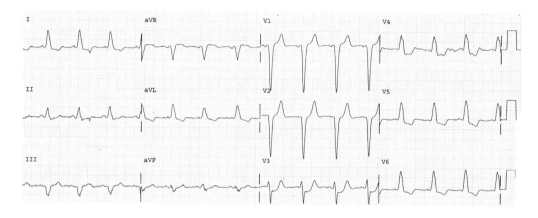

LBBB and Lateral AMI Due to a 100% Occluded First Diagonal Coronary Artery

History

This 61-year-old woman presented with 3 hours of CP.

ECG 18-9 (Type 1a)

- Classic morphology of **LBBB.**
- Concordant ST elevation: I, aVL,V6; and reciprocal ST depression: III, are diagnostic of **lateral AMI.** Q waves are also evident in I, aVL.

- Unusually isoelectric ST segments: V1–V3. Is this relative ST depression?
- Discordant ST elevation: excessive, V5.

Clinical Course

A 100% occluded first diagonal artery was successfully opened and stented.

Conclusion

Reperfusion therapy, including thrombolytics, is indicated.

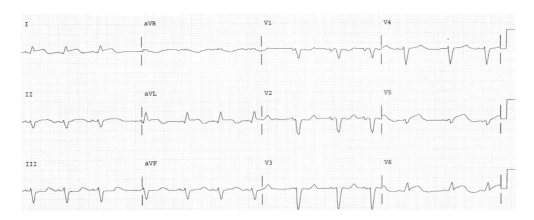

LBBB and Lateral AMI

History

This 71-year-old man presented with 3 hours of severe CP and CHF. He deteriorated rapidly into cardiogenic shock and cardiac arrest.

ECG 18-10 (Type 1a)

- Classic morphology of **LBBB.**
- QRS: very wide (195 ms) and peaked T waves are suspicious for hyperkalemia.

- Concordant ST depression: II, III, aVF; and concordant ST elevation in aVL are diagnostic of **lateral AMI.**

Clinical Course

The patient's potassium level was normal and CK-MB was diagnostic of AMI.

Conclusion

This ECG is diagnostic of lateral AMI, even with less typical symptoms.

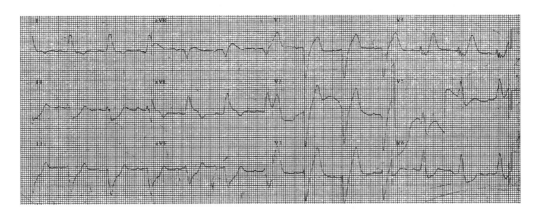

CASE 18-11

Subtle Lateral AMI in the Presence of LBBB

History

This 46-year-old woman with severely decreased LV function presented with sudden dyspnea without CP. She was taking warfarin, had heme + stools, and had mild pulmonary edema. Relative contraindications to thrombolytics include warfarin use and possible gastrointestinal bleed. HR = 100 bpm and BP = 150/100.

ECG 18-11A (Type 1c)

This is an **old ECG.**

- **IVCD:** due to the absence of wide monophasic R wave in V5–V6 and QRS < 120 ms, this ECG is not LBBB.
- Discordant ST segments and T waves are similar to LBBB.

ECG 18-11B (Type 1a), LBBB, at the time of presentation.

- Concordant ST depression: II, III, aVF is **suspicious** for lateral AMI.
- Concordant ST elevation: I, aVL. In comparison with the

discordant ST depression on ECG 18-11A, this is **diagnostic of lateral AMI.**

Clinical Course

Angiography ± PCI was indicated but was not undertaken. The cTnI peaked at 10 ng/mL. Angiography the next day demonstrated occlusion of the lateral branch of the PDA.

Conclusion

Fortunately for the patient, this was a small AMI. Despite its size, it is clearly apparent on the ECG. Even without LBBB or IVCD, a large lateral AMI may not manifest on the ECG due to electrocardiographically silent areas of the myocardium (see Chapter 14). Based on ECG criteria alone, this could be a large AMI. Reperfusion therapy is indicated, but in this case there are significant contraindications to thrombolytics.

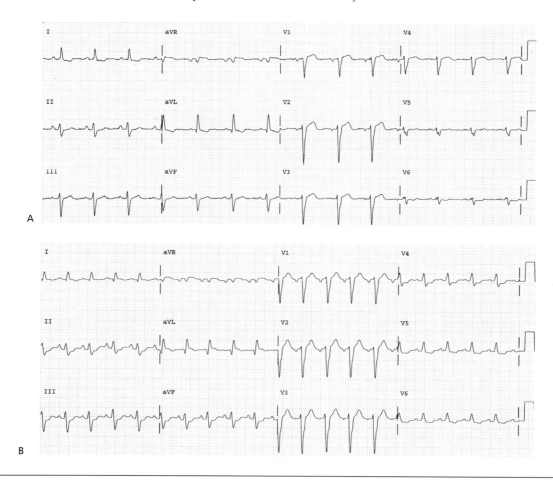

CASE 18-12

LBBB with Developing Inferior AMI and Hyperacute T Waves on Serial ECG

History

This 75-year-old woman presented with epigastric burning and a history of LBBB.

ECG 18-12A (Type 1c)

■ Concordant T waves: I, V5, V6; and large T waves: II, III, aVF are **suspicious** for AMI. Because symptoms are atypical, reperfusion is not immediately indicated, but **serial ECGs are indicated.** No previous ECG was available.

ECG 18-12B (Type 1a)

■ Increased ST elevation and hyperacute T waves: II, III, aVF; and increased reciprocal depression: aVL, are diagnostic of **inferior AMI.**

Clinical Course

Immediate angiography revealed an RCA occlusion that was stented.

Conclusion

This ECG is diagnostic of inferior AMI. Reperfusion, including thrombolytics, is indicated.

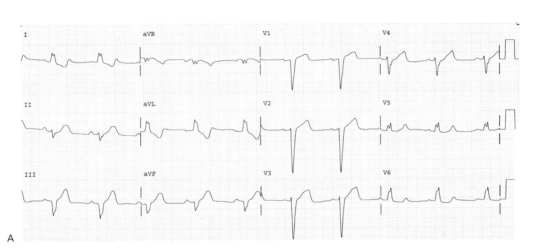

A

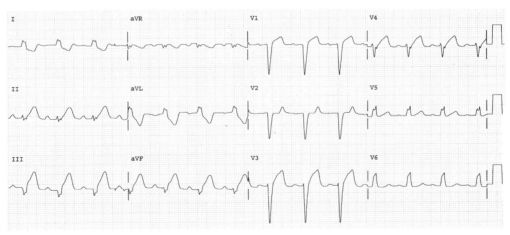

B

CASE 18-13

Initial ECG Shows IVCD Only and Subsequent ECG Shows Obvious AMI

History

This 63-year-old man with a history of MI and angina presented with 45 minutes of typical CP.

ECG 18-13A (Type 1a)
■ Nonspecific **IVCD.**
■ Discordant ST deviation: I, II, III, aVL, aVF is similar to LBBB.
  ■ The precordial leads have unusually low voltage because of a vertical axis. The ECG lacks typical late posterior and lateral forces. This makes it difficult to ascertain

whether the QRS is predominantly positive or negative and thus whether there is concordance or discordance.

ECG 18-13B (Type 1a)
Eighteen minutes later
■ New ST elevation: V1–V3, is diagnostic of **anterior AMI.**

Clinical Course

The patient received tPA and subsequently ruled in for AMI. Angiography revealed proximal LAD stenosis with reperfusion and TIMI-3 flow, as well as a 95% RCA stenosis. Echocardiography demonstrated an EF of 30% and an anterior WMA.

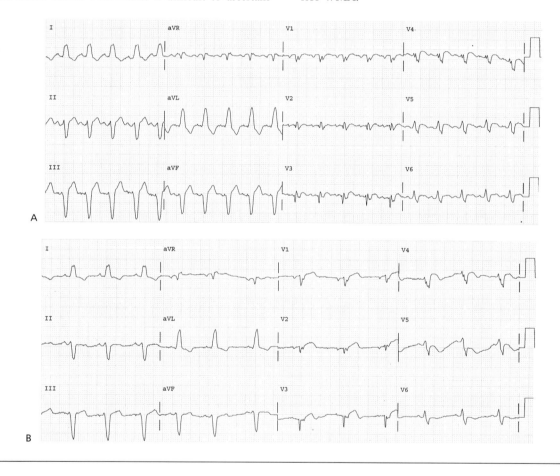

ANNOTATED BIBLIOGRAPHY

Mortality of BBB and AMI

See annotations of Sgarbossa et al. (236), Go et al. (232), Hod et al. (238), and Newby et al. (234) in Chapter 17.

Undertreatment of AMI with LBBB, Especially with No CP

Go AS, et al. Bundle-branch block and in-hospital mortality in acute myocardial infarction, 1998.

Methods: Go et al. (232) analyzed NRMI-I data (see Appendix C) on 297,832 AMI patients.

Findings: There were 19,067 patients with LBBB (6.7% of all AMI). **Only 16.6%** of patients with LBBB and AMI for whom thrombolytic therapy was clearly indicated **received thrombolytics,** compared with **66.5% of patients with a clear indication and no BBB.** Patients with LBBB and AMI also received aspirin or beta-blockers less frequently.

Shlipak MG, et al. Treatment and outcomes of left bundle-branch block patients with myocardial infarction who present without chest pain, 2000.

Methods: Shlipak et al. (245) analyzed NRMI-II data (see Appendix C) on 772,586 AMI patients. Diagnosis of AMI was based on CK-MB.

Findings: There were 29,585 patients with LBBB and AMI, which was 3.8% of all AMI. Mean age of patients with LBBB and AMI was 76.4 years (versus 68 years for all AMI) and, as is frequently the case with elderly patients with AMI, 47% of these LBBB and AMI patients had **no** CP (versus 33% for all AMI from the same database) (52). Of patients with LBBB and AMI without CP, 65% had at least Killip class I heart failure and only 14% had an admitting diagnosis of AMI (versus 25% of patients with LBBB and AMI with CP, for a total of 20% of all patients with LBBB and AMI, with or without CP). Only **8.4%** of patients with LBBB and AMI received acute reperfusion therapy (13.6% of those with CP versus 2.6% of those without CP) and this was seven to 11 times more likely if the admitting diagnosis was AMI versus one of several other diagnoses. In-hospital mortality for patients with LBBB and AMI **without** CP was 27% versus 18% with CP, but this difference was eliminated after adjustment for treatment, including aspirin and other therapies. **Patients with LBBB and AMI who present with CP** are much more likely to receive optimal therapy and more likely to survive.

Melgarejo MA, et al. The incidence, clinical characteristics, and prognostic significance of a left bundle-branch block associated with an acute myocardial infarct, 1999.

Methods: Melgarejo et al. (256) studied 1,239 consecutive AMI patients.

Findings: Of 1,239 patients, 42 (3.3%) had concurrent LBBB. Similar to the NRMI results listed earlier (232,245), only **21% of patients with LBBB and AMI received thrombolytics** (versus 56% with AMI and no LBBB).

Incidence of AMI in the Context of LBBB and Chest Pain

In seven relevant studies (four are annotated later), the numbers of symptomatic patients studied, the number of patients with LBBB, and the percentage of these with AMI, were, respectively: Rude et al.(20): 3,697 with symptoms, 178 with LBBB, 82 (46%) with LBBB and AMI; Edhouse et al. (241): 797 with symptoms, 48 with LBBB, 24 (50%) with LBBB and AMI; Hands et al. (242): 985 with CP, 35 with LBBB, and 20 (58%) with LBBB and AMI; Kudenchuk et al. (416): 3,027 with symptoms, 60 with LBBB, and 22 (37%) with AMI; Cannon et al. (242.5): 1,414 with symptoms, 127 with LBBB, and 40 (32%) with AMI. Kontos et al. (243): 7,725 patients with symptoms, 182 with LBBB, and 24 (13%) with LBBB and AMI; and Li et al. (244): unknown number with symptoms, 190 with LBBB, and 25 (13%) with LBBB and AMI. AMI was diagnosed by CK-MB, which is much less sensitive for detection of AMI than current troponin measurements. The prevalence was lowest in the groups that studied a very large number of patients with a lower overall incidence of AMI [Kontos et al. (243) and Li et al. (244)]. Thus the incidence of AMI among patients with symptoms and LBBB is higher than it is among all patients with ischemic symptoms and **no** LBBB, and positive predictive values (PPVs) of LBBB will be accordingly higher for any given specificity.

Hands ME, et al. Electrocardiographic diagnosis of myocardial infarction in the presence of complete left bundle branch block, 1988.

Methods: Hands et al. (242) prospectively studied 985 CP patients.

Findings: Of 35 patients (36%) with LBBB at presentation, 20 (57%) had AMI and LBBB as diagnosed by CK-MB. Of these 20 patients with LBBB and AMI, 10 had **acute** MI only and 10 had acute MI and old MI. Of the 15 LBBB with no AMI, four had old MI and 11 had never had MI. Thus **the incidence of AMI** (as diagnosed by CK-MB) **in the context of CP and LBBB was 57%**. ECG findings that were highly predictive of acute **or** old MI included: Q waves in at least two of leads I, aVL, V5 and V6; R-wave regression in V1–V4; notching of the upstroke of the S wave in two or more leads V3–V5; and concordance of the ST segment and/or T wave. ST segment concordance had a sensitivity of only 30% for AMI.

Specific ECG Diagnosis of AMI with LBBB

Wackers FJT. The diagnosis of myocardial infarction in the presence of left bundle branch block, 1987.

Methods: Wackers (247) analyzed ECGs of 96 patients with LBBB, including 55 consecutive cardiac care unit (CCU) admissions and 41 consecutive ambulatory patients. Criteria evaluated included Q waves or QRS notching (which are more likely to diagnose previous MI) and ST and T changes likely to detect AMI. Diagnosis of AMI was based upon history, CK-MB, and thallium scintigraphic imaging.

Findings: AMI was diagnosed in 48 patients, old MI in 16, and no MI in 32 (controls). Criteria for QRS abnormalities could not distinguish AMI from controls or prior MI. Presence of ST elevation did distinguish AMI: 2 mm of concordant ST elevation **or** 7 mm of discordant ST elevation was found in **26 of 48 patients with AMI (54%)** but in only **1 of 16 (6%) with old MI** and **1 of 32 (3%) of controls**. This degree of ST elevation was thus 54% sensitive and 97% specific for AMI, which compares favorably with the sensitivity and specificity of ST elevation for AMI without LBBB (18,19). Serial changes were found in 32 of 48 AMI patients, but because the tracings were recorded over days, not hours, the changes are not relevant to reperfusion therapy.

Sgarbossa EB, et al. Electrocardiographic diagnosis of evolving acute myocardial infarction in the presence of left bundle-branch block, 1996.

Methods: Sgarbossa et al. (246) compared ECGs of GUSTO-I patients (see Appendix C) who had LBBB and AMI (as diagnosed by CK-MB) with ECGs of patients with chronic CAD and LBBB but no symptoms. The purpose was to assess the utility of 10 previously published ECG criteria for the diagnosis of LBBB with AMI and to develop independent criteria with maximum sensitivity and at least 90% specificity. They derived a decision rule for the diagnosis of LBBB with AMI from these new criteria and tested it prospectively in a validation sample of 45 patients, 22 with AMI and 23 with UA (Note: The pretest probabilities of AMI and of CAD in this validation sample are 50% and 100%, respectively, which may be high.) The criteria earned points from the decision rule based upon their specificity; specificity > 90% earned five points, specificity of 90% earned three points, and specificity even slightly < 90% earned two points.

Findings: The independent ECG criteria (we refer to these as **Sgarbossa criteria**) for the diagnosis of LBBB with AMI and the odds ratios (ORs) for AMI with versus without each criterion were as follows (points are additive for use in the validation sample):

- ST elevation ≥ 1 mm in any of lateral or inferior leads and concordant with QRS complex (OR 25.2; range, 11.6 to 54.7): five points.
- ST depression ≥ 1 mm in any of leads V1–V3. (OR 6.0; range, 1.9 to 19.3): three points.
- Discordant ST elevation ≥ 5 mm in any lead. (OR 4.3; range, 1.8 to 10.6): two points.

The decision rule was applied to the validation sample. A total of three or more points had a sensitivity of 36%, specificity of 96%, likelihood ratio (LR) for positive result of 9.0, LR for negative result 0.7, PPV of 88%, negative predictive value (NPV) of 61%, and a misclassification rate of 33%.

Comment: Although the decision rule of Sgarbossa et al. gained much attention, several letters pointed out that the method of validation (which purported to show the utility of these criteria) was flawed and that, in fact, the proposed criteria lack adequate sensitivity for AMI in real clinical situations (**251**,257,258). Critics have argued that using the decision rule would lead to **continued underdiagnosis and underutilization of reperfusion therapy for patients with LBBB and AMI** (252,257). An editorial by Wellens (255), therefore, persisted in recommending thrombolytics for patients with CP and LBBB if there are no contraindications. **However**, it is important to remember that **even without BBB, the sensitivity of ST elevation for AMI** (as diagnosed by CK-MB) **is only approximately 45% to 50%** (18,21).

The PPV of a score of 3 in the Sgarbossa criteria is, of course, dependent on the incidence of AMI in patients with symptoms of AMI and LBBB (pretest probability). The 50% pretest probability, on which Sgarbossa's PPV of 88% is based, would probably not be so high in practice.

Commentary on Sgarbossa Criteria

Ackermann RJ, et al. Electrocardiographic diagnosis of acute myocardial infarction in the presence of left bundle-branch block, 1996.

Findings: Ackermann et al. (251) criticize Sgarbossa et al. (246) for assuming an overly high pretest probability (50%) of AMI in patients with CP and LBBB (50%). They argue that, since the prevalence of AMI in all patients with CP is approximately 20%, the prevalence of AMI in patients with both CP and LBBB is lower than 50% and that, consequently, the true PPVs of the Sgarbossa criteria are lower. As mentioned earlier, the prevalence of AMI in patients with CP and LBBB ranges from 13% to 58%, with a mean of 29%.

With a high pretest probability, the criteria have good sensitivity as well as good specificity

Edhouse JA, et al. Suspected myocardial infarction and left bundle branch block: electrocardiographic indicators of acute ischaemia, 1999.

Methods: Edhouse et al. (241) collected data on 797 patients with suspected AMI, and studied those with ECG criteria for LBBB. Sgarbossa criteria (246) were retrospectively applied.

Findings: LBBB was present in 48 patients who presented within 12 hours of symptom onset, 24 of whom had AMI by CK-MB, for a prevalence of 50%. All 24 patients with negative CK-MB had a Sgarbossa score of 0 (specificity and PPV = 100%). Of those with proven AMI, 19/24 had a score of 2 or more (sensitivity = 79% and NPV = 83%), and serial tracings identified two or more (sensitivity = 88% and NPV = 89%).

Comment: This study, along with that of Wackers et al. (247), indicates very good PPV and NPV of Sgarbossa criteria.

Studies Suggesting that the Utility of Specific ECG Criteria for AMI in LBBB is Low

Shlipak MG, et al. Should the electrocardiogram be used to guide therapy for patients with left bundle-branch block and suspected myocardial infarction? 1999.

Methods: Shlipak et al. (252) retrospectively applied the algorithm of Sgarbossa et al. (246) to 83 patients with LBBB who presented with acute CP, acute pulmonary edema, or cardiac arrest. AMI was diagnosed by CK-MB of 7 ng/mL or **cTnI of 1.5 ng/mL** or more.

Comment: These biomarker elevations could be caused by cardiac arrest or pulmonary edema without coronary occlusion.

Findings: **The Sgarbossa criteria were insensitive for myocardial damage** so defined. Results of this study were extrapolated (perhaps inappropriately) to indicate that **for every 1,000 patients with LBBB and clinical presentation suggestive of AMI, 929 would survive without major stroke if all patients received thrombolytics.** This is in contrast to the stroke-free survival of only 918 patients if the Sgarbossa criteria were used to determine therapy.

Comment: This calculation was based on an overly high excess stroke rate of 8.4 per 1,000; the actual overall excess **nonfatal** (disabling or not) stroke rate for tPA is closer to 3.5 per 1,000 if both infarct and hemorrhage are considered (see Chapter 34).

Kontos MC, et al. Can myocardial infarction be rapidly identified in emergency department patients who have left bundle branch block? 2001.

Methods: Kontos et al. (243) evaluated 7,725 patients with ischemic symptoms over 6 years. They reviewed the incidence of LBBB, LBBB and AMI, and predictors of AMI in the presence of LBBB with special attention to new versus old LBBB and to the Sgarbossa criteria.

Findings: LBBB was found in 182 patients; AMI was diagnosed in 24. Presence of one or more of the Sgarbossa criteria had sensitivity of 46%, specificity of 93%, PPV of 50%, and NPV of 92%. New or indeterminate age LBBB had sensitivity of 83%, specificity of 41%, PPV of 18%, and NPV of 94%. Addition of a positive initial CK-MB to Sgarbossa criteria improved sensitivity to 63% with a specificity of 99%, and PPV and NPVs of 88% and 94%. Mean peak total CK and CK-MB were 2,750 IU/L and 212 ng/mL in the group with positive criteria, and 370 IU/L and 32 ng/mL in the group without the criteria, though use of reperfusion therapy is not stated.

Comment: The authors considered the sensitivity of criteria unacceptably low, identifying only 11 of 24 patients with AMI, yet also having a poor PPV. They also were of the opinion that "LBBB not known to be old" performed poorly. They concluded that basing reperfusion on "LBBB not known to be old" **or** on Sgarbossa criteria without the addi-

tion of CK-MB, would result in too many patients, or too few patients, respectively, being treated. These points are just as valid for the use of ST elevation criteria in patients without LBBB.

Li F, et al. Electrocardiographic diagnosis of myocardial infarction in patients with left bundle branch block, 1999.

Methods: Li et al. (244) reviewed the charts of all patients with suspected ischemia and LBBB admitted to their urban teaching hospital from June 1995 to June 1997. Two physicians blinded to patient outcome rated the ECGs for the presence of Sgarbossa criteria.

Findings: Of 190 eligible patients, 25 (13%) had AMI as confirmed by CK-MB. **Sensitivity of Sgarbossa criteria was only 0 to 16%;** thus the NPV was very low. Despite good specificity (93% to 100%), the low incidence of AMI resulted in a low PPV. Only **concordant ST elevation** had a clinically useful likelihood ratio of 16, with a very wide confidence interval. **Patients with new LBBB were five times as likely to have AMI as those with old LBBB.**

Ozment A, et al. An analysis of ECG criteria for acute myocardial infarction in the presence of left bundle branch block (abstract), 1999.

Methods: Ozment et al. (253) evaluated the Sgarbossa criteria in 132 patients with LBBB evaluated for AMI.

Findings: Prevalence of AMI was only 17%. Thirteen of 22 patients who ruled in for AMI met the criteria (similar to ST elevation without LBBB). Twenty-two of 110 patients who ruled out for AMI also met the criteria. The Sgarbossa criteria were 59% sensitive, 80% specific, and had a PPV of 37% and an NPV of 90% **in this population.**

Sokolove PE, et al. Interobserver agreement in the electrocardiographic diagnosis of acute myocardial infarction in the presence of LBBB, 2000.

Methods: Sokolove et al. (254) analyzed a test set of 224 ECGs from patients with LBBB with and without AMI.

Findings: Agreement between emergency physicians and cardiologists was excellent for diagnosing AMI in patients with LBBB using the three Sgarbossa criteria.

Comparison with a Previous ECG, Serial ECGs, or 12-Lead Monitoring

Stark KS, et al. Quantification of ST-segment changes during coronary angioplasty in patients with left bundle branch block, 1991.

Methods: Stark et al. (249) compared changes in ST elevation from baseline ECGs during balloon occlusion of coronary arteries in patients with and without LBBB.

Findings: ST elevation increased by ≥ 1 mm in eight of 10 patients (80%) with LBBB (mean increase 2.6 ±1.7 mm). ST elevation increased by ≥ 1 mm in 15 of 20 (75%) patients without conduction abnormality. This supports the premise that **comparison with a previous ECG is useful and serial ECGs or continuous 12-lead monitoring** may be useful in patients with LBBB and an uncertain diagnosis. It also supports the notion that ST elevation in the presence of LBBB is indeed a reliable marker for coronary occlusion.

Fesmire FM. ECG diagnosis of acute myocardial infarction in the presence of left bundle-branch block in patients undergoing continuous ECG monitoring, 1995.

Findings: Fesmire (182) presents five patients with CP, LBBB, and a final diagnosis of AMI on whom continuous 12-lead ST-segment monitoring was performed in the ED. All demonstrated significant ECG changes indicative of STEMI while monitored.

Mortality of CP and LBBB with and Without Thrombolysis

ISIS-2 Collaborative Group. Randomised trial of intravenous streptokinase, oral aspirin, both, or neither among 17,187 cases of suspected acute myocardial infarction: ISIS-2, 1988.

Methods: The ISIS-2 study (102) included 17,187 patients who entered 417 hospitals within 24 hours of onset of suspected AMI (see Appendix C).

Findings: In patients with "BBB" (old, new, right, or left are unspecified) and suspected but unproven AMI, SK treatment of 419 patients, compared with placebo treatment of 409 patients, led to a 5.2% reduction in 35-day mortality (from 25% to 19.8%).

FTT Collaborative Group. Indications for fibrinolytic therapy in suspected acute myocardial infarction: collaborative overview of early mortality and major morbidity results from all randomised trials of more than 1,000 patients, 1994.

Methods: The FTT Collaborative Group (30) reported the combined results of all nine placebo controlled thrombolytic trials, including ISIS-2, and GISSI-1 (see Appendix C).

Findings: Of 2,146 cases of "BBB" (new, old, right, or left are unspecified), 35-day mortality for the thrombolytic group was 18.7% versus 23.6% for placebo. **The benefit associated with thrombolytic therapy for typical CP with LBBB far outweighs the associated risks.**

Comment: The benefit of thrombolytics for "suspected AMI and BBB" was demonstrated almost 15 years ago. In the intervening years, physicians have come to recognize atypical CP as a symptom of AMI and probably obtain many more ECGs than in the past. Though it has never been shown and would be impossible to prove, "suspected AMI" today may have a more liberal definition in the minds of clinicians than 15 years ago. If so, the pretest probability of AMI is lower and recommendations for thrombolysis for every patient with "suspected AMI" and LBBB would be too liberal. Perhaps this accounts for the low prevalence of AMI in patients with LBBB in Kontos et al. (243), Li et al. (244), and Ozment et al. (253).

A more appropriate indication for reperfusion therapy is for those patients with symptoms suspicious for **persistent coronary occlusion** who have LBBB not known to be old.

19

ARTIFICIAL VENTRICULAR PACING
AND AMI

KEY POINTS

- **Diagnosis of STEMI in the context of artificial ventricular pacing is essentially the same as diagnosis of in the context of LBBB.**

ARTIFICIAL VENTRICULAR PACING

Artificial ventricular pacing alters the ECG because depolarization does not propagate through specialized conducting fibers (Fig. 19-1). As a result, repolarization is also altered, comparable to LBBB. The vast majority of pacing leads are placed in the RV, which makes the subsequent ECG morphology very similar to LBBB. Interpretation of ST segments is similarly difficult and methods for diagnosing AMI in the presence of pacing are therefore believed to be comparable to those with LBBB. However, there is much less published research on paced rhythms than on LBBB. When post-surgical pacing leads are placed in the LV, the resultant ECG morphology is similar to RBBB.

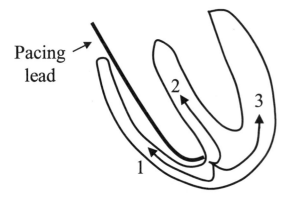

FIGURE 19-1. Depolarization in ventricular paced rhythm. The depolarization wave in artificial ventricular pacing starts at the tip of the pacing lead in the apex of the RV, very close to lead V4. It then slowly propagates away from V4, traveling superior, posterior, and leftward, beginning in the RV **(1)**, then proceeding to the septum **(2)**, then traversing the LV **(3).** As in LBBB, the complex is wide (wide = slow) because it is propagated through slow-conducting myocardium instead of through specialized conducting fibers.

ECG Manifestations of Artificial Pacing

Look for the following ECG features in patients who are artificially paced:

- Pacer spike
- Left axis deviation (QRS axis between 0 and −90)
- Wide QRS complex
- Negative QRS in leads V1–V4, II, III, and aVF (and typically V5–V6)
- Positive QRS in I, aVR, and aVL (and occasionally V5–V6)
- Discordant ST deviation (in the opposite direction from the QRS) and discordant T waves

Depolarization differs from LBBB only in that LBBB always has a positive QRS in leads I, aVL, V5, and V6, and often has a positive QRS in inferior leads II, III, and aVF. Because the QRS is usually negative in all leads except I, aVR, and aVL (and occasionally V5–V6), **discordant ST elevation manifests as a normal finding in most leads.** Interpretation of the ECG in artificially paced rhythms is very similar to that in LBBB. See Case 19-1.

ARTIFICIAL VENTRICULAR PACING AND AMI

ECG Diagnosis of AMI with Artificial Ventricular Pacing

First, look for nonpaced beats on the ECG, which may reveal the native QRS with intrinsic ST changes. If there are no such beats, diagnosis of AMI in the presence of artificial ventricular pacing presents the same basic problems as AMI diagnosis with concurrent LBBB (see Chapter 18). As in LBBB:

- **Concordant ST elevation** (≥ 1 mm) is **highly suspicious** for AMI (Type 1a ECG). In leads with a **positive QRS** (lateral leads I and aVL, and sometimes V5–V6), **ST elevation,** because it is concordant, is diagnostic of **lateral AMI.**
- **Concordant ST depression** is **suspicious** for AMI. In inferior leads with a negative QRS, ST depression is concordant and is **suspicious** for lateral AMI. In leads V1–V3 concordant ST depression is **highly suspicious** for posterior AMI.
- **Excessively high ST segments** (≥ 5 mm or out of proportion to the QRS), even if discordant, are **highly suspicious** for AMI.

See Cases 19-2 through 19-5.

Management

If there is no ST deviation whatsoever, thrombolytics are probably not indicated. However, immediate **angiography ± PCI** may be indicated. Follow the guidelines in Chapter 18 for ECG diagnosis and management of LBBB and suspected AMI. See Figures 18-5 and 18-6 for algorithms.

Remember:

- Clinical presentation (pretest probability) is important.
- Compare with a previous ECG.
- Record serial ECGs as indicated.
- Consider thrombolytic contraindications and availability of angiography and PCI.
- **Undertreatment is more common than overtreatment.**

CASE 19-1

Ventricular Paced Rhythm Lacking Infarction or Ischemia

History

This 60-year-old man presented with CP, history of MI, and many presentations for CP, all with identical ECGs.

ECG 19-1 (Type 1c)

- Pacer spikes; wide QRS; and ST segment and T-wave abnormalities are typical of paced rhythm.
- Discordant ST elevation: II, III, aVF; discordant reciprocal depression: aVL; discordant ST elevation: V1–V5; all T waves discordant. This ST elevation could be due to

AMI, especially if it is increased from a previous ECG. It could also be due to paced rhythm alone.

Clinical Course

The patient ruled out for AMI with negative cTnI.

Conclusion

The ECG in the context of an artificial pacemaker may manifest ST elevation, even with reciprocal depression, that mimics AMI.

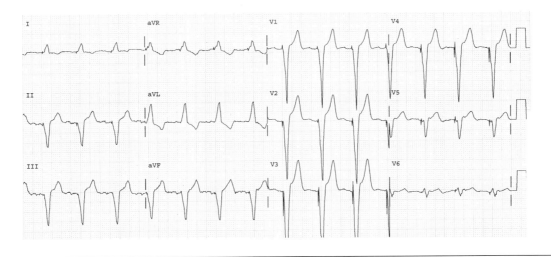

CASE 19-2

ECG Diagnostic of Lateral AMI in the Presence of Ventricular Paced Rhythm

History

This 71-year-old man presented with 3 hours of substernal CP. He had a history of hypertension (HTN) and a pacemaker for sick sinus syndrome.

ECG 19-2 (Type 1a)

- Pacer spikes; wide, predominantly negative QRS: V1–V6, II, III, and aVF; positive QRS: I, aVR, aVL; and normal left QRS axis are characteristic of a paced rhythm.
- Concordant T waves: I, aVL; and concordant ST elevation with hyperacute T waves: I, aVL are diagnostic of **lateral AMI.**

Clinical Course

An old ECG showed discordant ST-T morphology in I and aVL, typical of pacing. A repeat ECG showed increased ST elevation, confirming the diagnosis of AMI. Angioplasty opened a proximal circumflex lesion.

This ECG is reproduced with permission of American Health Consultants: Brady, WJ. Missing the diagnosis of acute MI: challenging presentation, electrocardiographic pearls and outcome-effective management strategies. *Emerg Med Rep* 1997;18:91–102.

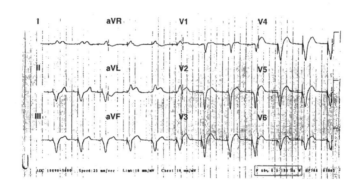

CASE 19-3

Inferoposterior AMI with Atypical Ventricular Paced Rhythm Manifests as Concordant ST Elevation and ST Depression

History

This 76-year-old woman with a ventricular demand (VVI) pacemaker presented with 1 hour of substernal CP and dyspnea.

ECG 19-3 (Type 1a)

- Pacer spikes; and wide, predominantly negative QRS: aVL, V1–V3, are characteristic of a paced rhythm. Positive QRS: II, III, aVF, V4–V6 is a manifestation of atypical axis.
- Concordant ST elevation: II, III, aVF; and reciprocal concordant ST depression: aVL are diagnostic of **inferior AMI.**

- Concordant ST depression: V2–V3, **suspicious** for posterior AMI, supports the diagnosis of AMI.

Clinical Course

The patient received thrombolytics and CP and ECG abnormalities resolved quickly. AMI was confirmed by CK-MB.

Conclusion

AMI **can** be diagnosed in the presence of ventricular paced rhythm.

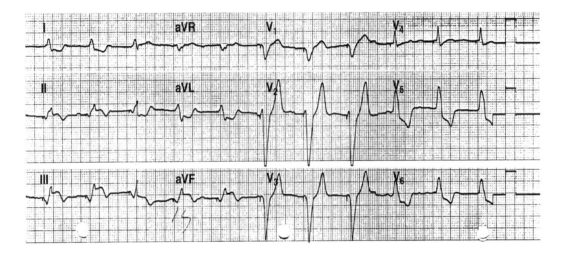

CASE 19-4

AMI and Paced Rhythm Diagnosed by Large Discordant Inferior ST Elevation and Concordant ST Depression

History

This 65-year-old woman with an artificial pacemaker presented with CP.

ECG 19-4A (Type 1a)

- Pacer spikes; wide QRS; negative QRS: II, III, aVF, V1–V5; positive QRS: I, aVR, aVL; and left axis, are characteristic of a paced rhythm with characteristically abnormal conduction.
- Excessive discordant ST elevation: 7 mm, II, III, aVF, is diagnostic of **inferior AMI.**
- Concordant ST depression: 4mm, V2, is diagnostic of **posterior AMI.**

ECG 19-4B (Type 1a), recorded minutes later.

- A faster, irregular supraventricular rhythm inhibits the pacer. **Normal conduction** reveals AMI more clearly.

- ST elevation: II, III, aVF; with reciprocal ST depression: aVL, is diagnostic of **inferior AMI.**
- Deep ST depression: V1–V4, is diagnostic of an obvious **posterior AMI.**
- ST elevation: V5–V6, which had been obscured by the paced rhythm, is diagnostic of **lateral AMI.**

Clinical Course

The patient received thrombolytics. AMI was confirmed by CK-MB.

Conclusion

In some cases, the morphology of STEMI in the presence of pacing is identical to the morphology in the presence of a native supraventricular rhythm and normal conduction.

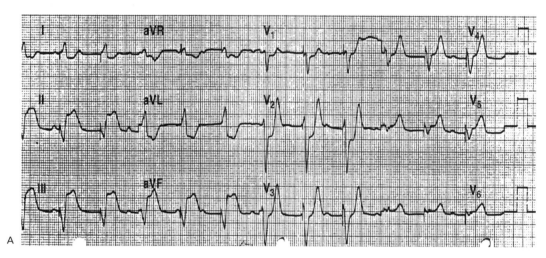

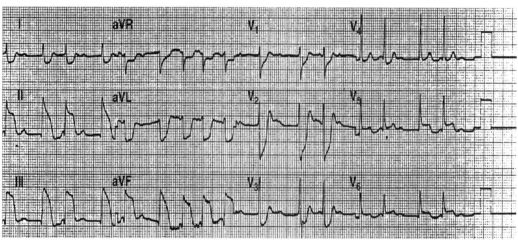

CASE 19-5

Paced Rhythm with Infero-Posterolateral AMI

History

This 72-year-old man with history of MI had a **dual-chamber** pacer due to AV node disease. He presented with typical CP.

ECG 19-5A (Type 3)

This is an old baseline ECG.

- P waves are sensed by the pacer, triggering ventricular pacing.
- Concordant T waves (inverted): V2–V6, due to previous MI.
- Concordant ST depression: 1.5 mm, V4–V6, is **suspicious** for ischemia.

ECG 19-5B (Type 1a)

- New ST depression: concordant in V1–V2, discordant in aVL, is diagnostic of **posterior AMI.**
- New ST elevation: V4–V6, is diagnostic of **lateral AMI.**
- Pseudonormalization of T waves: V2–V5.
- Increased discordant ST elevation: II, III, aVF, is **suspicious** for inferior AMI.

Clinical Course

Angiography revealed an acutely occluded circumflex artery.

Conclusion

Change from a previous ECG revealed AMI despite the presence of a paced rhythm.

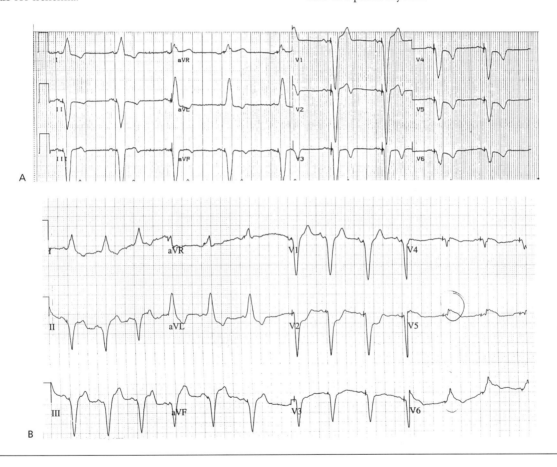

ANNOTATED BIBLIOGRAPHY

Sgarbossa EB, et al. Early electrocardiographic diagnosis of acute myocardial infarction in the presence of ventricular paced rhythm, 1996; Sgarbossa EB. Recent advances in the electrocardiographic diagnosis of myocardial infarction: left bundle branch block and pacing, 1996.

   Methods: Sgarbossa et al. (259,260) analyzed data from GUSTO-1 (86) (see Appendix C).

   Findings: All patients in the study were diagnosed with AMI and included in the GUSTO trial. Many physicians, however, have been reluctant to make this diagnosis and to enter a patient with CP and a paced rhythm into a thrombolytic trial. Consequently, only 32 patients (0.1%) with pacemakers were included in GUSTO-1, which is much lower than the percentage of patients with CP and AMI who have a ventricular pacemaker. We do not know the incidence of (and therefore the pretest probability of) AMI in patients with CP and a pacemaker, and this study provides no helpful data in that regard. Fifteen of these 32 patients were excluded because their rhythms were not generated by the pacer. The ECGs of the 17 remaining AMI patients were matched with 17 patients with pacers, stable CAD, and no CP. The ECG criteria developed by Sgarbossa et al. (246) for LBBB (see annotation in Chapter 18) were then tested on patients and controls. Results, as follows, were similar to those in the LBBB study.

■ **ST elevation ≥ 5 mm in one lead with a predominantly negative QRS** was the only criterion that had statistical significance **and** high specificity (positive likelihood ratio = 4.41).

Additional findings that could be useful but were not statistically significant:

■ ST elevation ≥ 1 mm in leads with predominantly positive QRS (sensitivity, 53%; specificity, 88%).
■ ST depression ≥ 1 mm in one of leads V1–V3 (sensitivity, 29%; specificity, 82%).

Comment: Numbers are so small that conclusions have limited validity.

Kozlowski FH, et al. The electrocardiographic diagnosis of acute myocardial infarction in patients with ventricular paced rhythms, 1998.

Findings: Kozlowski et al. (261) reported two cases of AMI in the presence of ventricular pacing that conform to Sgarbossa's criteria listed earlier (one is presented as Case 19-2).

20

NORMAL VARIANTS:
BENIGN EARLY REPOLARIZATION AND
BENIGN T-WAVE INVERSION

KEY POINTS

- Early repolarization may mimic ST-elevation MI (STEMI) and vice versa.
- Beware especially of diagnosing early repolarization in patients more than 45 years of age.
- Upward concavity is the most common presentation of anterior STEMI.
- If the T wave towers over the R wave in V2 or V3, early repolarization is less likely and STEMI should be strongly considered.

A normal variant is an ECG that has some variation from "normal" that is not associated with pathology. Some baseline ST elevation is present in the precordial leads in most ECGs recorded from adults; such ST elevation is often a result of "early repolarization" (2). Some ECGs show benign T-wave inversion, which is less common than early repolarization. Both may be mistaken for AMI. We discuss early repolarization and two kinds of T-wave inversion that are normal variants.

EARLY REPOLARIZATION

Early repolarization, also called benign early repolarization, is the most common normal variant. It occurs in individuals of any race and gender, but is more common in African-Americans, especially men, and in those less than 50 years of age (1,97,262). Distinguishing early repolarization from AMI can be very difficult and may require comparison with a previous ECG, serial ECGs, or echocardiography. ST elevation in V1–V3 can be seen in up to 90% of normal individuals (2,96). Early repolarization may be combined with benign T-wave inversion (see later).

ECG Diagnosis of Early Repolarization

See Figure 20-1 for examples of early repolarization in leads V1–V3. The following are typical ECG manifestations of early repolarization (151,262,263):

- **ST elevation.**
  - Predominantly present in **precordial leads**; most commonly in lead V3 (80%); and, in order of decreasing frequency: V4 > V2 > V5.

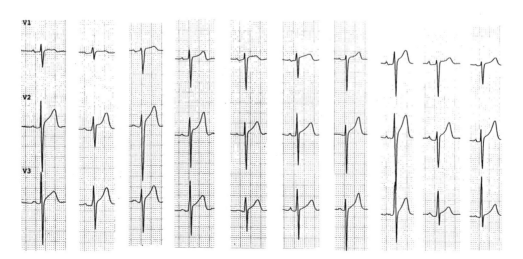

FIGURE 20-1. Examples of early repolarization as seen in leads V1–V3. Notice that in none of these examples does the T wave tower over the R wave and that the ST segment is concave upward in all. (ECG reproduced from unpublished data with permission of K. Wang, M.D.)

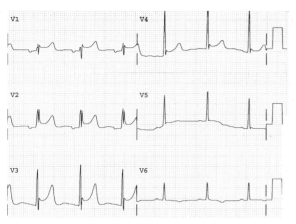

FIGURE 20-2. "Right precordial early repolarization," with a humpback appearance of the ST segment in V2.

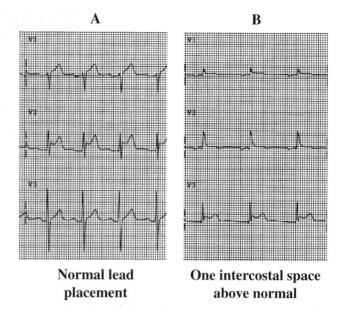

Normal lead placement   **One intercostal space above normal**

FIGURE 20-3. Increased ST elevation due to change of lead position in a patient with CP. A: Baseline early repolarization. **B:** Recorded one interspace higher. Angiography, echocardiography, and serial troponins were normal.

- ■ **ST elevation (continued)**
  - ■ **Upwardly concave** ST segment.
  - ■ "J-point" elevation (elevation of the transition point between the QRS and ST segment).
  - ■ Frequent **"J waves" (notch or slur** on the downstroke of R wave).
  - ■ Up to 5 mm (**262**).
  - ■ ST segment typically < 25% of the height of the T wave in V5–V6 (in contrast to pericarditis or AMI) (**264**).
  - ■ ST segments often drop with exercise or tachycardia (**262**).
- ■ **Tall R waves and early QRS transition** such that the R/S ratio > 1 in V2 or V3 (normal is in V3 or V4); this is also called rightward shift or counterclockwise rotation.
- ■ **Tall, peaked, asymmetric T waves** (steeper downward than upward, see note later); this morphology is **different** from typical hyperacute T waves (**179**).
- ■ **T-wave amplitude in V6 is typically > V1**, in contrast to anterior STEMI (265) (see Case 9-5).
- ■ **NO reciprocal ST depression.**
- ■ Occurs in **younger patients**, usually resolves with age and becomes increasingly unusual as age progresses beyond **45 years** (**179**).
- ■ **Rarely manifests in limb leads without also being in precordial leads.**
  - ■ Very unusual in lateral limb leads (I, aVL).
  - ■ May have ST depression in aVR (50%) (**262**).
- ■ May be confused with, or concurrent with, LVH, as well as with AMI.
- ■ "Right precordial early repolarization" has a typical humpback appearance in V2 (1) (Fig. 20-2).

See Cases 20-1 to 20-4 for examples of early repolarization.

Early Repolarization and AMI

AMI may be misdiagnosed as early repolarization and vice versa (**97**). Change over time is critical (Case 12-4). **Early repolarization may vary from tracings recorded on a previous date,** with ST segments either higher or lower (**262,263**). Such changes may complicate diagnosis significantly (Case 20-5). It is not certain whether such changes are real or are due to change in **lead placement,** which is known to alter the degree of ST elevation (Fig. 20-3). **Serial tracings recorded on the same day should not change significantly** unless the lead placement is changed.

Although nearly all early repolarization exhibits **upward concavity** of ST segments, **31% of anterior AMI patients also manifest upwardly concave ST segments in lead V3;** this compares with 53% that manifest straight ST segments and only 16% that manifest upwardly convex ST segments (87).

It is easy to confuse the tall T waves of early repolarization with hyperacute T waves of early AMI. In our experience, a T wave out of proportion to the R wave in V1–V6 is suggestive of AMI. Early repolarization has well-formed R waves in V2 and V3, at least approaching the height of the T wave. Thus if the T wave towers high over the R wave in V2 or V3, early repolarization is unlikely and STEMI should be strongly considered. **Additionally, hyperacute T waves often, but not always, look wider and "bulkier"** than T waves of early repolarization, partly due to less upward concavity.

Marriott states that, in AMI, the T wave in V1 is of higher amplitude than that in V6, and for early repolarization this is opposite (V6 > V1) (265). According to Collins et al. (**179**), tall T waves of early repolarization **contrast** with hyperacute T waves in a number of ways. **Tall T waves of early repolarization have:**

- ■ J point to T-wave amplitude ratio > 25%.
- ■ T-wave amplitude to QRS amplitude ratio > 75%.
- ■ J-point elevation > 0.3 mV.

See Cases 20-6 through 20-11. (See also Cases 9-2, 9-5, and 12-5, of AMIs that mimic early repolarization.)

NORMAL VARIANTS OF T-WAVE INVERSION

ECG Diagnosis of Normal Variants of T-Wave Inversion

Persistent juvenile pattern is a normal variant that consists of symmetrically inverted T waves and is most common in African-Americans, especially in women. It typically occurs in right precordial leads **V1–V3** (2).

"Benign T-wave inversion" most commonly occurs in young African-American men and trained athletes (2). It is usually seen in combination with ST elevation due to early repolarization. It typically manifests in middle to left precordial leads, especially **V4–V5, associated with ST elevation.** It may be intermittent and is typically an inversion of the terminal part of the T wave (Case 20-11). The **QT_c is short, usually < 400 ms and almost always < 425 ms** (Fig. 20-4).

Benign T-wave inversion resembles Wellens' syndrome (see Chapter 8), which is terminal T-wave inversion seen after an episode of transient STEMI. **Wellens' syndrome** is associated with tight left anterior descending artery (LAD) stenosis and impending anterior AMI, is typically seen in leads **V2–V4,** and **has a longer QTc interval.** The two can only be differentiated with absolute certainty if there are identical ECGs both before and days to weeks afterwards. Benign T-wave inversion may also resemble reversible ischemia. (See Case 21-1 of cocaine-related reversible terminal T-wave inversion.)

MANAGEMENT

To differentiate normal variants from STEMI and unstable angina/non-ST-elevation MI (UA/NSTEMI):

1. Always **compare with a previous ECG,** although early repolarization may infrequently show variation on comparison with previous tracings.
2. **Record serial ECGs.** Remember that **early repolarization should NOT show variation on serial tracings unless lead placement is changed.**
3. Always interpret the ECG within the **clinical context.**
4. Further diagnostic testing may be necessary, including biomarkers and echocardiography.
5. In the right clinical setting and if available, angiography may be necessary.
6. In order that reperfusion is utilized as fully as it should be, it is acceptable if occasional false positives are treated.

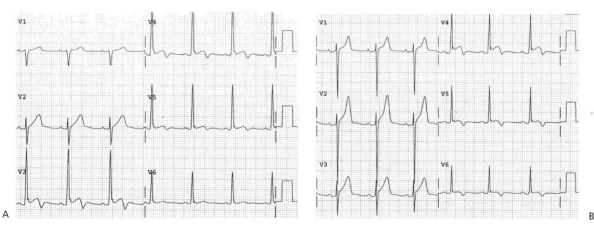

FIGURE 20-4. Examples of benign T-wave inversion. A has a QT_c of 423 ms, and **B** has a QT_c of 377 ms.

CASE 20-1

Typical Early Repolarization

History
This 56-year-old African-American man has a history of hypertension (HTN) and use of atenolol. He presented with an acetabular fracture from a motorcycle collision. He had no chest trauma and no symptoms consistent with AMI.

ECG 20-1 (Type 1c)
- Despite high R-wave voltage, this does not meet criteria for LVH.
- ST elevation: V1–V6; upwardly concave ST segments: V2–V4; tall R waves: V2–V6; and **J waves:** V2–V3 are typical of early repolarization.

Clinical Course
Serial ECGs were all identical and serial cardiac troponin I (cTnI) was normal.

Conclusion
If this patient presented with symptoms of AMI, his ECG would be very confusing.

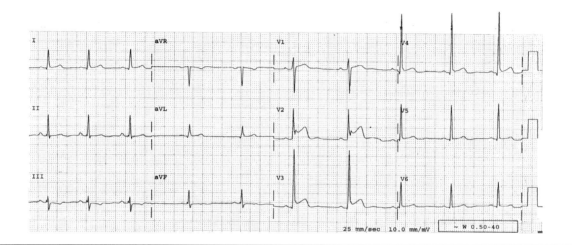

25 mm/sec   10.0 mm/mV   ~ W 0.50–40

CASE 20-2

Atypical Early Repolarization

History

This 47-year-old man presented with typical chest pain (CP).

ECG 20-2 (Type 3)

- ST elevation: V2–V5; **J waves:** V3–V6; tall R waves: V4–V5; and peaked T waves: V3–V5 are typical of early

repolarization. However, the leftward shift is **atypical** of early repolarization.

Clinical Course

The patient was observed and ruled out for AMI by creatine kinase-MB (CK-MB) levels.

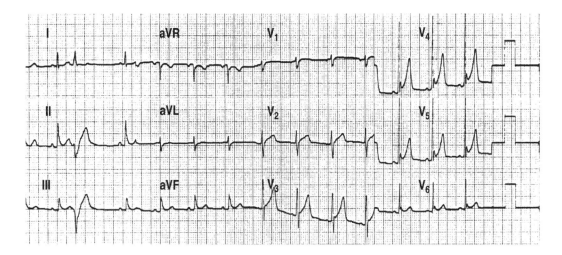

CASE 20-3

Early Repolarization Manifesting in Inferior Leads with NO Reciprocal ST Depression in aVL

History

This 27-year-old man presented on multiple occasions with sharp CP.

ECG 20-3 (Type 1c)

- ST elevation: V2–V6; J waves: V4–V6; asymmetric, peaked T waves: V2–V6; and upwardly convex ST segments: V2–V6, are typical of early repolarization.
- Upwardly concave ST elevation and J waves in II, III, and aVF are **suspicious** for inferior AMI, but there is **no reciprocal depression in aVL.** The ST depression could be

absent due to **cancellation** by ST elevation of a lateral AMI, as indicated by ST elevation in V5–V6.

Clinical Course

This was ultimately shown to be the patient's baseline findings.

Conclusion

Diffuse ST elevation without reciprocal depression in aVL is often early repolarization (or pericarditis) and is not typically due to AMI.

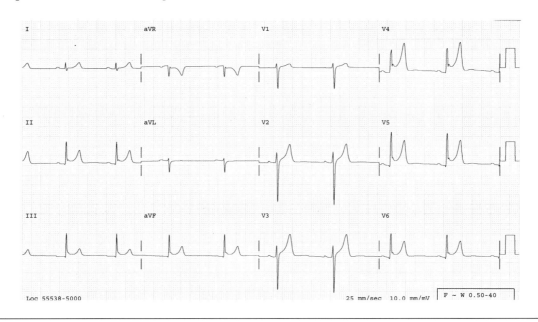

CASE 20-4

Typical Early Repolarization

History

This 50-year-old man presented with epigastric pain and tenderness.

ECG 20-4 (Type 1c)

- ST elevation: V1–V5; upwardly concave ST segments: V2–V5; peaked asymmetric T waves: V2–V4; tall R waves: V4–V5; J-point elevation: V2–V3; and slurred R-wave downstroke: V4–V6, are all typical of early repolarization.
- Also meets criteria for LVH: S (V1) + R (V4) > 45mm.

Clinical Course

CTnI levels were normal, but lipase was diagnostic of pancreatitis.

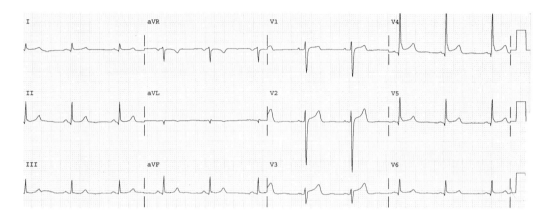

CASE 20-5

Atypical Early Repolarization Shows Increased ST Elevation That Is Identical to STEMI

History

This 49-year-old man with diabetes mellitus (DM) and HTN presented with nausea and abdominal discomfort, but without any CP, jaw, shoulder, or arm pain.

ECG 20-5A (Type 1a versus 1c)

- LVH by voltage.
- ST elevation: V1–V6.
- Distinct J wave: V4; very upwardly concave ST segments; tall, peaked asymmetric T waves: V2–V4; and ST elevation in precordial leads are typical of early repolarization.
- However, ST elevation > 25% of the T-wave height in V4–V6, and small R waves (poor R-wave progression) in V2–V3 are **atypical** of early repolarization and **typical of AMI.**
- ST elevation: V1–V6 is **suspicious** for AMI, especially in V4–V5.

ECG 20-5B (Type 1c)

This is an old ECG from 4 months prior.

- Comparison with this ECG shows that the ST elevation in ECG 20-5A is increased.

Clinical Course

Despite atypical symptoms, this change would normally be considered diagnostic of AMI and reperfusion therapy would be indicated. Because of atypical symptoms, **immediate echocardiography** was ordered and was normal (also without LVH). The patient was observed and ruled out for AMI by creatine kinase-MB (CK-MB).

Conclusion

This is an extremely difficult Type 1c ECG, and it would not be wrong to treat with thrombolytics. **Early repolarization may look very much like AMI, even after comparison with a previous ECG. Echocardiography was critical. Serial ECGs may have been helpful.**

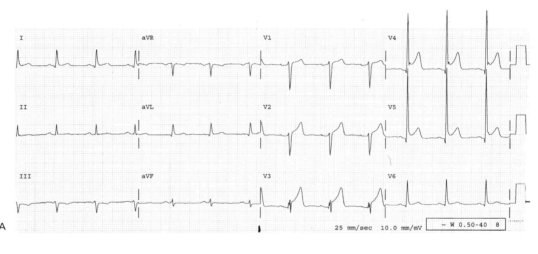

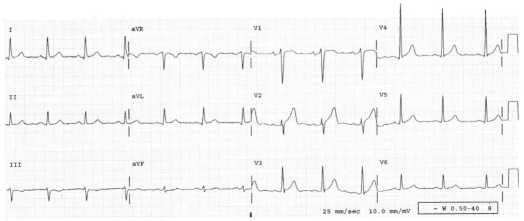

CASE 20-6

Atypical Early Repolarization Mimics AMI

History

This 36-year-old African-American man presented with atypical CP.

ECG 20-6 (Type 1a versus 1c)

■ ST elevation: V1–V4, with upwardly convex ST segments, **appears diagnostic** of AMI.

Clinical Course

In the context of typical symptoms, reperfusion therapy would be indicated. The patient was observed and serial ECGs remained unchanged. Serial cTnI levels were negative and a graded exercise test was normal.

Conclusion

Early repolarization may appear identical to AMI.

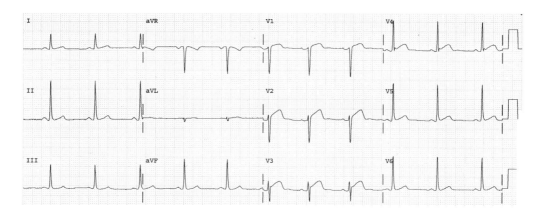

CASE 20-7

CP and Diffuse Early Repolarization Mimics AMI:
The Absence of ST Depression in aVL Makes Inferior AMI Very Unlikely

History
This 42-year-old non-English-speaking man presented with 12 hours of severe CP.

ECG 20-7 (Type 1c)
■ ST elevation: II, III, aVF are **suspicious** for inferior AMI. However, ST depression in aVL is rarely absent in inferior AMI. Concurrent lateral AMI may elevate the ST segment in aVL, canceling out reciprocal changes. Look for ST elevation in V5–V6, which, in this case, is not present.

Clinical Course
Physicians interpreted this ECG as diagnostic of inferior AMI and appropriately sent the patient for angiography, which revealed normal coronary arteries. Serial cTnI levels were normal and serial ECGs remained unchanged over 24 hours.

Conclusion
Widespread early repolarization, with inferior ST elevation, can usually be differentiated from inferior AMI by the absence of reciprocal depression in aVL; however, an **inferolateral** AMI might manifest without this reciprocal depression in aVL.

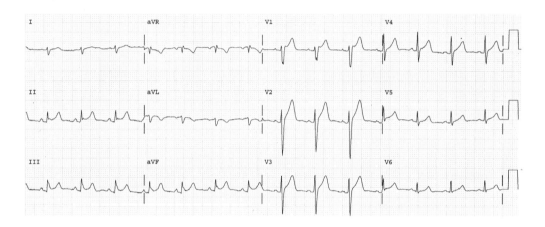

CASE 20-8

Initial ECG Reveals Precordial ST Elevation Due to Early Repolarization Only: Infero-postero-lateral AMI Is Evident Only on a Serial ECG

History
This 55-year-old man presented with typical CP.

ECG 20-8A (Type 1c)
- Upwardly concave ST elevation: V2–V5; J wave: V2; and tall peaked T waves: V2–V5, are typical of early repolarization.

ECG 20-8B (Type 1a)
One hour later
- ST elevation: II, III, aVF with reciprocal ST depression:

aVF is diagnostic of **inferior AMI**.
- ST depression: V1–V3 is diagnostic of **posterior AMI**.
- ST elevation: V5–V6, is much higher than in ECG 20-8A and is diagnostic of **lateral AMI**.

Conclusion
Serial ECGs enabled diagnosis of this large infero-postero-lateral AMI.

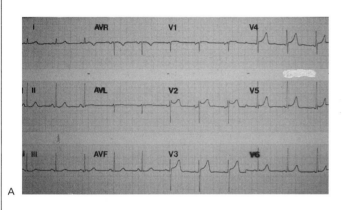

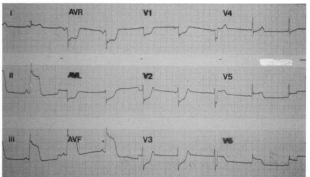

CASE 20-9

Clinicians and the Computer Mistook This AMI for Early Repolarization

History

This 45-year-old man presented with CP.

ECG 20-9 (Type 1a)

- Upwardly concave ST elevation: V1–V6; and peaked T waves: V2–V5, are typical of early repolarization.
- Poor R-wave progression, Q wave in V2, and hyperacute T-wave morphology are diagnostic of **anterior AMI.**

Clinical Course

Clinicians and the computer missed this AMI. A serial ECG recorded 29 minutes later revealed much higher ST segments and thrombolytics were administered.

Conclusion

Although indicated by the first ECG, thrombolysis was delayed by 63 minutes.

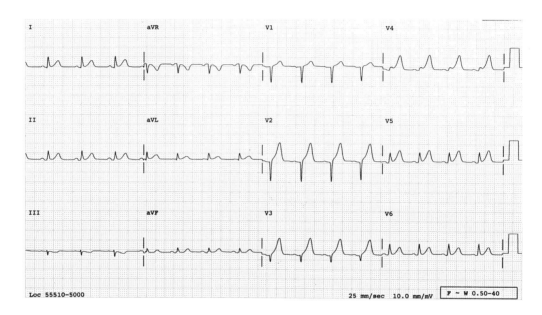

CASE 20-10

T Waves Much Taller Than R Waves Distinguish This AMI from Early Repolarization

History

This 51-year-old man presented with 30 minutes of typical CP after running for a bus.

ECG 20-10A (Type 1a)

- ST elevation: 3 mm, V2–V3; tall T waves: 11 mm in V2, compared with a 3.5-mm R wave; and relatively poor R-wave progression are diagnostic of anterior STEMI.

Clinical Course

The patient received tissue plasminogen activator (tPA) and a repeat ECG was recorded 30 minutes later.

ECG 20-10B

- ST resolution. Except for the tiny Q wave in V2, this ECG viewed in isolation readily mimics early repolarization.

Clinical Course

CK peaked at 2,500 IU/L and cTnI peaked at 130 ng/mL. Due to successful reperfusion and lack of spontaneous or provokeable ischemia, angiography was not performed.

Conclusion

Poor R-wave progression and hyperacute T waves make this ECG diagnostic for STEMI.

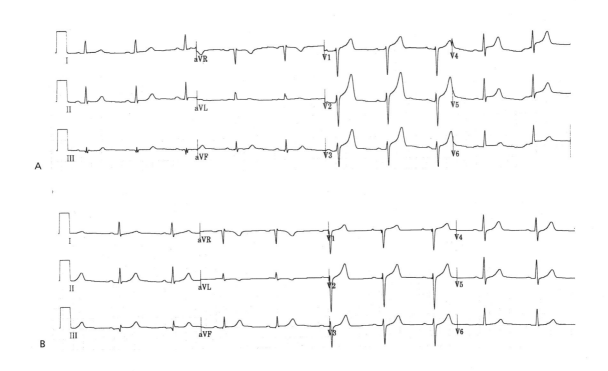

CASE 20-11

Presentation and ECG Consistent with Benign T-Wave Inversion

History

This 42-year-old African-American man presented with atypical CP.

ECG 20-11 (Type 3)

- Terminal T-wave inversion: V3–V5.
- QT_c = 378 ms

Clinical Course

The differential diagnosis includes: anterior AMI with reper-

fusion or "Wellens' syndrome;" benign T-wave inversion; and reversible ischemia, which is often cocaine related. Clinicians suspected benign T-wave inversion due to the clinical presentation, short QT_c, and classic morphology. Serial ECGs were unchanged and serial cTnI levels were normal.

Conclusion

Reperfusion therapy is not indicated. An identical ECG years earlier would be necessary to prove that this ECG does not represent a more remote non–Q-wave MI.

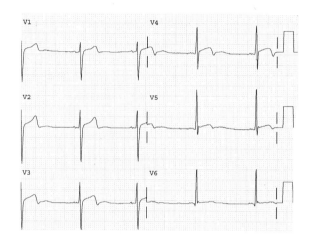

ANNOTATED BIBLIOGRAPHY

Mehta MC, et al. Early repolarization on scalar electrocardiogram, 1995.

> *Methods:* Mehta et al. (262) analyzed 60,000 ECGs over 5 years and selected 600 from patients with no heart disease and that met previous criteria for early repolarization. These ECGs were compared with ECGs of 600 age-, sex-, and race-matched controls.
>
> *Findings:* ECGs with early repolarization were typically from patients less than 50 years of age (the incidence and degree of ST elevation declined with advancing age), had a short and depressed PR interval, had a slightly **asymmetric** T wave, and showed ST normalization with exercise.

Ginzton LE, et al. The differential diagnosis of acute pericarditis from the normal variant: new electrocardiographic criteria, 1982.

> *Methods:* Ginzton et al. (264) compared ECGs of 19 patients with acute pericarditis with ECGs of 20 patients with typical early repolarization.
>
> *Findings:* Early repolarization almost always manifested with the **ST segment in V6 < 25% the height of the T wave.** This feature is most useful for differentiating normal variant from lateral AMI and pericarditis.

Kambara H, et al. Long-term evaluation of early repolarization syndrome (normal variant RS-T segment elevation), 1976.

> *Methods:* Kambara et al. (263) analyzed the ECGs of 65 patients with early repolarization, with a maximal follow-up of 26 years.
>
> *Findings:* Early repolarization showed the following characteristics: (a) upwardly concave elevation of the RS-T segment with distinct J waves, or with slurred R-wave downstroke and/or distinct J point, located predominantly and most distinctly in precordial leads; (b) rightward QRS shift; and (c) persistence for many years. Tall R and T waves in the precordial leads were less commonly found.

Hollander JE, et al. Variations in the electrocardiograms of young adults: are revised criteria for thrombolysis needed? 1994.

> *Methods:* Hollander et al. (97) had two physicians each read ECGs from 414 young subjects with no heart disease.
>
> *Findings:* Physicians diagnosed STEMI in approximately 7% of cases, with **very poor interrater reliability.** The incidence of early repolarization mimicking AMI was much higher in African-Americans and Hispanics than in whites.

Collins MS, et al. Hyperacute T wave criteria using computer ECG analysis, 1990.

> *Methods:* Collins et al. (179) utilized computer analysis of ECGs with ST elevation to develop criteria for differentiation of hyperacute T waves from the tall, peaked T waves of early repolarization.
>
> *Findings:* Hyperacute T waves correlated with (a) J point to T-wave amplitude ratio > 25%; (b) T-wave amplitude to QRS amplitude ratio > 75%; (c) J-point elevation > 0.3 mV; and (d) age > 45 years.

Wasserburger RH, et al. The normal RS-T segment elevation variant, 1961.

> *Methods:* Wasserburger et al. (151) analyzed characteristics of RS-T segment elevation in ECGs of 48 veterans with no clinical evidence of organic heart disease.
>
> *Findings:* The characteristics included those listed earlier in studies by Mehta et al. (262) and Kambara et al. (263). Postexercise ECG recordings in 24 patients indicated that ST segments promptly returned to baseline in 14 patients, with T-wave inversion in nine patients. ECG recordings post-hyperventilation demonstrated T-wave inversion in 17 of 27 patients.

Early Repolarization and Cocaine CP

See annotations (266–270) and, especially, Gitter et al. (271) and Hollander et al. (272) in Chapter 21.

21

COCAINE-ASSOCIATED CHEST PAIN

KEY POINTS

- **AMI is unusual among patients with cocaine-associated chest pain (CACP).**
- **ST elevation is common among patients with CACP and may mimic STEMI.**
- **Thrombolytic therapy should be used very judiciously in this population, only when the ST elevation is unmistakable for AMI and other medical therapies have failed.**
- **Patients with suspected AMI should be asked specifically about cocaine use.**
- **Angiography ± percutaneous coronary intervention (PCI) is preferred.**

GENERAL BACKGROUND

Cocaine use produces centrally and peripherally mediated sympathetic stimulation that results in HTN and tachycardia and, subsequently, increased myocardial oxygen demand. Cocaine use also results in coronary vasoconstriction, plaque rupture, thrombus formation, platelet aggregation, and accelerated atherosclerosis in chronic users (**11,273**). Although acute and chronic use of cocaine increases risk for AMI, the incidence of AMI among patients with CACP is low, from 1% to 6% (**269,274**). Incidence is particularly low if the cocaine use was more than 3 hours before onset of pain (**275**), and the incidence of adverse events is lower still (**267,268,271,276,277**). Acute coronary syndrome (ACS) does **not** cause the vast majority of CACP due to coronary atherosclerosis. Rather, CACP is mostly due to reversible coronary spasm or small-vessel spasm that often has no objective correlate (i.e., it does not result in biomarker leakage, change in baseline ECG, or adverse outcomes) (Case 21-1). Such spasm may, however, result in AMI (Case 21-2). The source of the pain is often not ischemic (as determined by normal sestamibi scanning) and may originate from noncardiac tissue such as the chest wall (**267,278**).

The incidence of AMI in CACP is particularly low, but not negligible, when the patient's age is 30 years or less (**269**). (See Cases 21-3 and 5-3, of young women whose CACP was associated with AMI and significant coronary disease.) However, many patients with CACP but without AMI show ST elevation that exceeds thrombolytic "criteria." These **young patients** have a high incidence of **ST elevation due to early repolarization or LVH** (**97,267–272,**279). **Thus thrombolytics should be administered only very cautiously** to any patient of age less

than 30 years of age who has CACP and whose ECG manifests ST elevation, especially if the ST elevation is in V1–V4.

ECG Diagnosis of CACP

There is no specific ECG morphology of cocaine-induced ischemia. However, as mentioned earlier, false positives are often due to early repolarization or LVH (see Chapters 20 and 22). Record serial ECGs. See Case 21-4. (See also Case 10-8, of cocaine use, CP, pulmonary edema, and ST elevation; and Case 22-12, of LVH versus AMI in a cocaine user.)

MANAGEMENT

Thrombolytics are **not** contraindicated in the **appropriate context of CACP.** However, the incidence of false-positive ECGs in CACP is very high. **For patients with an ECG suggestive of ischemia (Type 1 or 2) (11):**

- Give aspirin.
- Give nitroglycerine (NTG), sublingual ± intravenous (IV).
- Use IV diltiazem, 0.3 mg/kg (**11**).
- Use IV lorazepam, 1 to 4 mg, especially for anxiety, tachycardia, and/or HTN (**273**).
- Use IV metoprolol or esmolol if BP remains > 150 systolic, or pulse remains > 100.
    - Avoid nonselective beta-blockers (e.g., propranolol; see discussion later).
- **Repeat the ECG.** If it is unchanged, consider **angiography ± PCI.** If your facility has no catheterization (cath) lab and the ECG shows unmistakable ST elevation, administer thrombolytics. If doubt persists, record **serial ECGs and/or an echocardiogram,** if available, to inform the reperfusion decision.

NTG and calcium channel antagonists counteract coronary vasoconstriction (**11**). Avoid nonselective beta-blockers, especially propranolol (280) and labetolol, because they leave the vasoconstricting alpha-adrenergic effect of cocaine unopposed by the vasodilating effects of beta-2 stimulation. Selective beta-blockers are probably safe but are not proven (**11**).

Further evaluation should be cautious, as it is for other patients with CP, and is beyond the scope of this book. It may include additional serial ECGs, serial troponin, exercise stress testing, radionuclide imaging, or angiography. Clinical parameters (symptoms, risk factors, and ECG characteristics), with the exception of age of less than 30 years, have proven poor at distinguishing those with AMI from those without AMI (as diagnosed by CK) (**266,267,269**).

CASE 21-1

CACP with ECG Showing LVH and ST Elevation with Reversible Terminal T-Wave Inversion: cTnI Was Normal

History
This 43-year-old man presented with 2 days of CP while binging on crack cocaine.

ECG 21-1A (Type 1c)
V1–V6
- LVH by voltage.
- ST elevation: 2 mm: V2–V4, is consistent with STEMI but more typical of pure LVH.

Clinical Course
The patient signed out against medical advice (AMA) and returned 2 hours later with continued CP.

ECG 21-1B (Type 1d)
V1–V6 only
- ST elevation with terminal T-wave inversion: V3.

Comment
Is this reperfusion of STEMI with injury (Wellens' syndrome), or is it fully reversible ischemia manifested as T-wave inversion? Worsening symptoms and an initial ECG not classic for STEMI suggest the latter.

Clinical Course
Reperfusion therapy is not indicated. Clinicians initiated anti-ischemic therapy. Symptoms resolved and the ECG reverted to the morphology of ECG 21-1A within 4 hours.

Comment
These upright T waves represent resolution of reversible ischemia, **not** pseudonormalization due to reocclusion of STEMI.

Clinical Course
Total CK peaked at 771 IU/L but serial cTnI were normal and convalescent echocardiography showed only LVH. Follow-up ECGs were identical to ECG 21-1A. The patient had an identical admission 6 months later.

Conclusion
Cocaine use may produce completely reversible ischemia. Baseline ST elevation can be confusing.

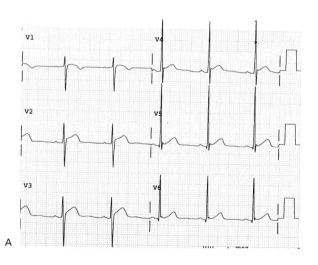

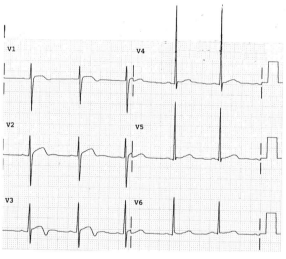

CASE 21-2

CACP and ST Elevation (That Turns Out to Be Baseline) with Resulting Positive cTnI but Completely Normal Coronary Arteries: Small NSTEMI Due to Coronary Spasm

History

This 45-year-old man presented with 2 days of pleuritic left chest and axillary pain.

ECG 21-2 (Type 1c versus 1a)

At 23:18

■ ST elevation: V1–V5 is **highly suspicious** for AMI.

Clinical Course

Serial ECGs over 7 hours were identical. Thrombolytics were not given and cTnI returned at 6.0 ng/mL. Angiography the next day showed normal coronary arteries but left ventriculography revealed LVH and severe anteroapical hypokinesis and an ejection fraction (EF) of 48%. Urine was positive for cocaine metabolites. Subsequent ECGs developed T-wave inversion in V3–V6 within 12 hours, with no Q waves, and no change in R waves. Convalescent echocardiography was normal. ST segments never changed and were identically elevated 2 years later, suggesting that the ST elevation was baseline.

Conclusion

Normal coronary arteries confirm that myocardial damage (positive cTnI, positive echocardiogram, and ECG development) was due to cocaine use with probable coronary spasm versus transient thrombosis. Transient STEMI is very unlikely, given the identical ST elevation at follow-up and the lack of angiographic evidence of occlusive thrombus. Myocarditis is also possible.

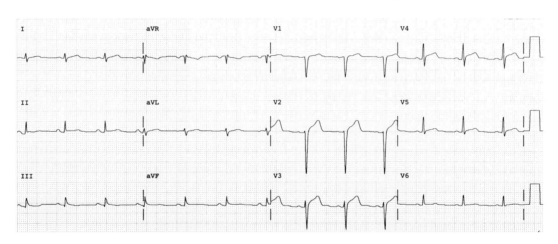

CASE 21-3

Thirty-six-Year-Old Woman with Very Atypical CACP and an ECG Subtly Suspicious for Lateral AMI: This Was Missed and She Ruled In for AMI

History
This 36-year-old woman complained of sharp, pleuritic CP after crack cocaine use. Her pain resolved after administration of an antacid and viscous xylocaine in the emergency department (ED).

ECG 21-3A (Type 3, but suggestive)
At 0 hours
- ST elevation: 1 mm, V1–V4, is consistent with early repolarization.
- ST elevation: < 1 mm, I, aVL; and reciprocal depression: III. This ECG is **very subtle,** but **suspicious** for lateral

AMI. Medical therapy and serial ECGs are indicated, with angiography ± PCI if pain and ECG abnormalities persist.

Clinical Course
The patient remained pain-free, no immediate repeat ECG was recorded, and she was discharged. Her cTnI returned at 7.8 ng/mL and she was called back.

ECG 21-3B (Type 3)
At 12 hours
- **T-wave inversion: aVL,** V5–V6.

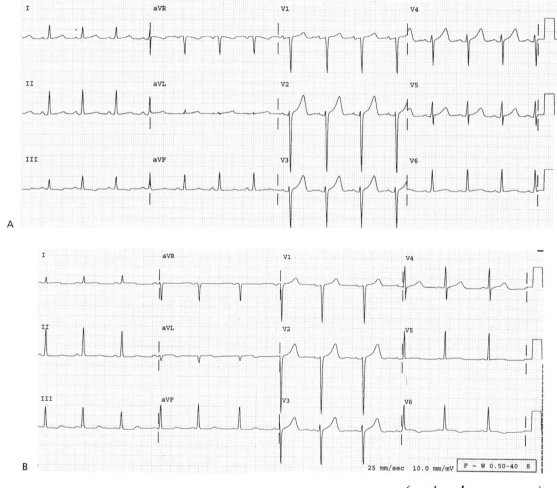

(continued on next page)

CASE 21-3

Thirty-six-Year-Old Woman with Very Atypical CACP and an ECG Subtly Suspicious for Lateral AMI *(continued)*

ECG 21-3C (Type 2)
At 40 hours
■ T-wave inversion: deeper, aVL, V5–V6.

Clinical Course
The patient refused treatment and left the hospital AMA. She returned later with CP after smoking more crack cocaine.

ECG 21-3D
At 68 hours
■ **Pseudonormalization of lateral T waves,** suggestive of **reocclusion/reinfarction.**

Clinical Course
The patient was started on aspirin, heparin, and NTG; her symptoms improved; the ST elevation resolved; and T waves

again inverted. Angiography revealed a 99% first diagonal ostial lesion, which was stented, an 80% mid-circumflex stenosis, an 85% second obtuse marginal stenosis, and 90% first posterolateral stenosis. The mid-right coronary artery (RCA) and mid-LAD each had 40% lesions. Convalescent EF was normal.

Conclusion
Patients with CACP may have significant coronary disease. In this case, CACP was associated with AMI and suspicious ST elevation was missed. Immediate reperfusion was not indicated due to cocaine use, atypical pain, age, symptom resolution, and minimal ECG findings. **Observe closely, record serial ECGs, and consider angiography if available.** In this case, thrombolytics are not indicated in the absence of further ECG evolution of STEMI.

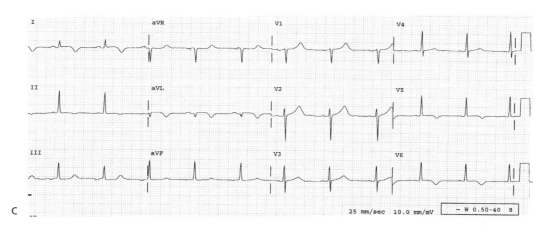

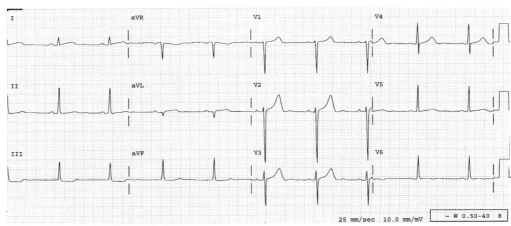

CASE 21-4

CACP and ECG with Large ST Elevation and Minor Change from Previous Tracing, Normal Coronary Arteries

History
This 29-year-old man presented with severe CP after smoking crack cocaine. He had presented identically 10 days prior.

ECG 21-4A and ECG 21-4B (Type 1a versus 1c)
V1–V3 only
- These ECGs are subtly different; upward convexity of ST segments is greater in ECG 21-3A (the earlier ECG).

Clinical Course
The computer read "Acute Infarct" for ECG 21-4A. The

patient was treated with anti-ischemic therapy, had normal serial cTnI levels, and had normal coronary arteries.

Conclusion
Patients with CACP without coronary artery disease (CAD) may have ECGs diagnostic for STEMI, and the ECG may subtly change over time. Thrombolytic therapy is only indicated if symptoms are refractory to medical therapy AND the ECG is classic for STEMI or echocardiography confirms wall motion abnormality (WMA). Angiography ± PCI is preferable.

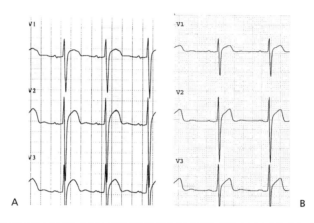

ANNOTATED BIBLIOGRAPHY

Management of Cocaine-Associated Myocardial Ischemia
Braunwald E. ACC/AHA guidelines for the management of patients with unstable angina and non–ST-segment elevation myocardial infarction, 2000; Hollander JE. Current concepts: the management of cocaine-associated myocardial ischemia, 1995.
Findings: Braunwald et al. (11) and Hollander (273) review the toxicity and management of cocaine-induced myocardial ischemia.

Hollander JE, et al. Complications from the use of thrombolytic agents in patients with cocaine-associated chest pain, 1996.
Methods: Dual case report.
Findings: Hollander et al. (281) report two patients with CACP and diagnostic ST elevation. Both patients received thrombolytics and suffered bleeding complications, including one intracranial hemorrhage (ICH). Both patients ruled out for AMI and showed ST elevation persistent beyond resolution of CP.

Incidence of AMI and Timing of Onset After Cocaine Use
Mittleman MA, et al. Triggering of myocardial infarction by cocaine, 2000.
Methods: Mittleman et al. (275) interviewed 3,946 AMI patients and included questions about frequency of cocaine use and use within the 3 hours before CP onset.
Findings: Thirty-eight patients had used cocaine within 1 year; nine, within 60 minutes of symptoms; and two, within 60 to 180 min-

utes. The relative risk (RR) of AMI **during the first hour** after cocaine use was 23.7 (confidence interval [CI]: 8.5 to 66.3) and decreased to 4 (CI: 0.5 to 32) by 3 hours after use.

Hollander JE, et al. Cocaine-induced myocardial infarction: an analysis and review of the literature, 1992.
Findings: Hollander et al. (282) reviewed clinical literature for case reports of cocaine-associated AMI through February 1991. They identified 91 cases, with a mean age of 32.8 years (range, 18 to 52 years). Although **67% had pain onset within 3 hours of cocaine use,** the range was up to 4 days. ECG findings were not reported. Nasal cocaine use occurred in 48%, and 58% had neither HTN nor tachycardia. Of 54 patients who underwent cardiac catheterization, 31% had atherosclerosis and an additional 24% had thrombotic occlusion but no "significant" coronary disease. All 11 patients who received ergonovine had a negative response.

Prospective Studies of ECGs and Outcome in CACP
Feldman JA, et al. Acute cardiac ischemia in patients with cocaine-associated complaints: results of a multicenter trial, 2000.
Methods: Feldman et al. (274) analyzed data from a prospective study of 10,689 patients with symptoms suggestive of cardiac ischemia; the study also prospectively collected data on cocaine use (283).
Findings: Of 293 patients who reported cocaine use or had positive toxicologic screening, 94% had CP and 65% had dyspnea. Only two of these 293 (0.7%) had AMI and four others were thought to have ischemia. ECGs received no comment.

Hollander JE, et al. Prospective multicenter evaluation of cocaine-associated chest pain, 1994.

> **Methods:** Hollander et al. (269) conducted a prospective multicenter observational study of patients with CACP.
>
> **Findings:** Of 246 patients, 14 (5.7%) ruled in for AMI based on elevated CK-MB; the only two patients who died arrived in cardiac arrest. Mean age was 36.5 years in patients with AMI (range, 33 to 44 years) and 33 years in patients without AMI (range, 26 to 38 years). **No patient under the age of 33 years had AMI.** Of the 14 AMI patients, 12 smoked cigarettes and 13 used cocaine regularly, with a 5-year mean duration of use. For all patients (with or without AMI), CP was substernal in 73%, began a median of 1 hour after cocaine use, and lasted a median of 120 minutes. The ECG was 36% sensitive and 90% specific for AMI (but the method of interpretation was not specified). Of 242 patients, **76 (31%) had ST elevation > 1 mm due to early repolarization,** 12 patients had arrhythmias, and four developed congestive heart failure (CHF). No clinical parameter differentiated patients with and without AMI.

Kontos MC, et al. Myocardial perfusion imaging with technetium-99m sestamibi in patients with cocaine-associated chest pain, 1999.

> **Methods:** Kontos et al. (267) studied 241 episodes of CACP in 218 patients. Low- to moderate-risk patients (*n* = 216) were promptly injected with technetium-99m sestamibi and scanned 60 to 90 minutes later, whereas 25 "high-risk" patients were admitted without scans. AMI was diagnosed by CK-MB.
>
> **Findings:** Mean age was 36 ± 8 years. ST elevation due to early repolarization was present in 20%; an additional 13% had LVH on the ECG. AMI was confirmed in six patients; four of these six, and five others, had significant coronary artery disease (CAD) at angiography. Of 216 scans, five were positive (two with AMI); of 211 patients with negative scans, none had cardiac events at 30 days. Clinical characteristics did not differentiate patients with or without ischemic etiology of CP. Age was 40 ± 8 years in the AMI group and 36 ± 8 years in the group without AMI. The incidence of AMI among these patients with CACP was 2.8%. The vast majority of patients with CACP not only rule out for AMI, but do not have cardiac ischemia as the etiology of CP.

Feldman BA, et al. The evaluation of cocaine-induced chest pain with acute myocardial perfusion imaging, 1999.

> **Methods:** Feldman et al. (278) performed myocardial perfusion scanning on 14 consecutive patients who presented to the ED with unexplained but persistent CP, nondiagnostic ECGs, and cocaine use within 3 days.
>
> **Findings:** Of 14 patients, 12 had CP at the time of tracer injection. Four patients were admitted and AMI ruled out with biomarkers. Four patients had abnormal scans; of these, two were persistently abnormal at follow-up, indicating a chronic condition unrelated to the episode of CACP. The other two had neither repeat scans nor subsequent hospitalizations for cardiac ischemia.

Hollander JE, et al. Cocaine-associated chest pain: one year follow-up, 1995.

> **Methods:** Hollander et al. (276) performed a 1-year follow-up study of 203 patients who presented with CACP.
>
> **Findings:** Mortality data were obtained on all patients and additional clinical data were obtained on 185 (91%). Nonfatal AMI occurred in 1%. There were no reported deaths or AMI in patients who reported having ceased cocaine use.

Retrospective Studies on ECGs and Outcome in CACP

Gitter MJ, et al. Cocaine and chest pain: clinical features and outcome of patients hospitalized to rule out myocardial infarction, 1992.

> **Methods:** Gitter et al. (271) reported 101 patients **hospitalized** for CACP.
>
> **Findings:** Symptoms mimicked AMI; 43% of patients had ST elevation meeting the criteria for thrombolytic treatment (1 mm in two consecutive leads), but AMI was ruled out in all patients. ST elevation was interpreted as myocardial injury in 8%, early repolarization in 32%, LVH in 16%, normal in 32%, and "other" in 12%.

Hollander JE, et al. "Abnormal" electrocardiograms in patients with cocaine-associated chest pain are due to "normal" variants, 1994.

> **Methods:** Hollander et al. (272) compared ECGs of 56 patients with CACP to age-, sex-, and race-matched normal controls.
>
> **Findings:** Incidence of ECG abnormalities of patients with CACP and controls was equal. Specifically, **early repolarization accounted for the majority of abnormal ECGs in patients with CACP due to its high incidence in this age group (18 to 35 years).**

Zimmerman JL, et al. Cocaine-associated chest pain, 1991.

> **Methods:** Zimmerman et al. (268) reviewed records of 48 cocaine abusers admitted with CP.
>
> **Findings:** ECGs of 18 patients (37%) showed abnormal ST elevation. T-wave inversions in 20 patients (41%) often persisted on serial ECGs. Three patients ruled in for AMI by CK-MB (6%). None suffered complications.

Tokarski GF, et al. An evaluation of cocaine-induced chest pain, 1990.

> **Methods:** Tokarski et al. (277) studied 42 consecutive patients admitted with CP and cocaine use within 6 hours of presentation.
>
> **Findings:** CK and CK-MB were elevated in eight of 42 patients (19%), but only two had the typical evolutionary CK pattern consistent with AMI. Mean total CK elevation was 214 IU/L, with a maximum of 367 IU/L. Mean CK-MB elevation was 8 ng/mL with a maximum of 16 ng/mL. No patient had either single or serial Type 1 or Type 2 ECGs, and none suffered complications.

Amin M, et al. Acute myocardial infarction and chest pain syndromes after cocaine use, 1990.

> **Methods:** Amin et al. (266) studied 70 patients hospitalized with CACP.
>
> **Findings:** AMI was confirmed by CK-MB in 22 patients (31%) and excluded in 48 (69%). Coronary risk factors did not differentiate the two groups. The ECG was abnormal in 20 of 22 patients with AMI and in 19 of 48 without AMI. Total CK levels, but not CK-MB levels, were elevated in 65% of patients who ruled out for AMI. Four of eight patients with AMI who had angiography performed had significant coronary stenoses. Onset of AMI pain occurred as late as 18 hours after cocaine use.

Hollander JE, et al. Cocaine-associated myocardial infarction: mortality and complications, 1995.

> **Methods:** Hollander et al. (284) identified 136 cases of cocaine-associated AMI in 130 patients by retrospective cohort review of records from 29 hospitals; some patients may have been duplicated from another paper by Hollander et al. (282).
>
> **Findings:** The initial ECG was diagnostic of AMI in 44% and of ischemia in another 18% of patients. Neither ischemia nor infarction was apparent on ECGs of 38%. Complications occurred 64 times in 49 patients, including CHF in nine patients, ventricular tachycardia in 23, supraventricular tachycardia in six, and bradydysrhythmias in 26. Angiography of 52 patients demonstrated significant CAD in 66%.

McLaurin M, et al. Cardiac troponin I and T concentrations in patients with cocaine-associated chest pain, 1996.

> **Methods:** McLaurin et al. (279) studied 19 patients admitted with CACP.
>
> **Findings:** Sixteen patients had abnormal ECGs and 14 patients had elevated total CK levels, three of whom had elevated CK-MB. However, none developed elevated cTnI or cTnT.

Weber JE, et al. Cocaine-associated chest pain: How common is myocardial infarction? 2000.

> **Methods:** Weber et al. (270) reviewed 250 patients admitted with discharge diagnoses for CP and cocaine use. Because all such patients were admitted for 23 hours at the authors' institution, they are confident that their review missed none.
>
> **Findings:** CK-MB confirmed AMI in 15 patients (6%), nine with Type 1 ECGs and four with Type 2 ECGs. Only 67 (27%) had Type 4 (normal) ECGs and 158 (63%) had Type 3 ECGs, including 125 (50%) with ST elevation of early repolarization. Seven patients had complications, none beyond 12 hours post-ED arrival.

22

LEFT VENTRICULAR HYPERTROPHY

KEY POINTS

- ST elevation due to LVH may mimic STEMI or hide the ST elevation of simultaneous AMI.
- ST deviation due to LVH is generally DISCORDANT (opposite) to the QRS.
- Do not ascribe ST elevation to LVH unless voltage criteria for LVH are present.
- ECG morphology can be affected by the loading conditions of severe HTN.

GENERAL BACKGROUND

The ECG morphology of LVH is commonly associated with "inadvertent" thrombolytic administration for AMI (see Chapter 3) (285) and is one of the most common reasons for false-positive ST elevation (106,286). Anatomic LVH may be present in the absence of ECG criteria for LVH, but in order to ascribe ST elevation to LVH, the ECG MUST meet the criteria. Criteria for LVH can be found in many textbooks, and the ECG computer algorithms perform this function well; see Table 22-1 for a summary of LVH criteria (2). In distinguishing LVH from ischemia or infarction, certain rules outlined later are important, but recognition of morphology is also very important. Furthermore, loading conditions of the left ventricle (LV) (i.e., severe HTN) can affect the ECG morphology. ST segments may be either upwardly concave or convex, but as always, convexity is more likely to be AMI.

TABLE 22.1. LVH DIAGNOSTIC CRITERIA

LVH is considered to be present if **one or more** of the following voltage criteria are present. **All are applicable ONLY** if the QRS duration is < 120 ms.

Limb Leads
R-wave in lead I + S-wave in lead III > 25 mm
R-wave in aVL > 11 mm
R-wave in aVF > 20 mm
S-wave in aVR > 14 mm

Precordial Leads
R-wave in V5 or V6 > 26 mm
R-wave in V5 or V6 + S-wave in V1 > 35 mm
Largest R-wave + largest S-wave in precordial leads > 45 mm

ECG DIAGNOSIS OF LVH

The ECG Should Meet LVH Criteria

High QRS voltage is the most common criterion for LVH. Not all ECGs manifesting LVH criteria have secondary ST or T-wave abnormalities, but **nearly all ECGs manifesting ST/T abnormalities due to AMI will also meet LVH criteria;** these are the difficult ECGs (2) (see Cases 22-1 to 22-3). No matter how similar ST/T abnormalities are to those of LVH, **if the ECG does not meet LVH criteria (usually high voltage), BEWARE** of attributing the ST/T abnormalities to LVH. (See Case 22-4 for an exception to this rule.)

Are the ST-T Abnormalities Secondary to LVH?

Discordant ST Elevation

ST elevation due to LVH is generally discordant. As in LBBB, ST elevation that is **concordant** with the predominance of the QRS is **highly suspicious for AMI.**

ST Elevation in Leads V2–V3 That Is Due to LVH

- Is discordant with the main QRS (usually a deep S wave).
- Is usually upwardly concave but may be upwardly convex.
- Is proportional to the depth of the S wave.
- Is usually ≤ 3 mm.
- Is nearly always accompanied by ST/T abnormalities in lateral precordial leads V4–V6 (see later).
- May have many different morphologies (Fig. 22-1a).

ST Elevation in Lead III Due to LVH

- Is discordant with a predominantly negative QRS.
- Is usually upwardly concave, but may be upwardly convex.
- Will also manifest reciprocal depression in aVL, as in AMI.

ST Elevation in aVL

- ST elevation in aVL is **unlikely to be due to LVH,** unless it is discordant to a predominantly negative QRS, which is unusual in this lead.
- ST elevation in V4–V6 or in I and/or aVL can only be due to LVH if the QRS is predominantly negative in these leads, which is **very unusual.**

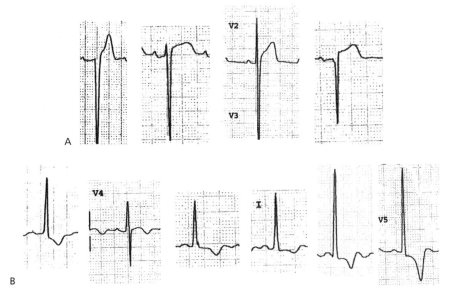

FIGURE 22-1. Morphologies of LVH. A: ST elevation in V2. **B:** ST depression in lateral leads.

ST Depression in V2

ST depression in V2 **is not due to LVH.** It is due to posterior AMI or possibly anterior UA/NSTEMI.

ST Depression in V3

ST depression in V3 is **very unusual in LVH.** Flat or deep ST depression in V3 is due to posterior AMI or UA/NSTEMI. Shallow, down-sloping ST depression in V3 may be due to LVH if it is discordant to a predominantly positive QRS (i.e., if there is a tall R wave), which is unusual in LVH. Otherwise, this down-sloping ST depression is most likely to be due to posterior AMI or anterior UA/NSTEMI.

ST Depression in V4–V6 That Is Due to LVH

(This was formerly called "**LVH with strain.**")

- Is not an indication for thrombolytics (as is the case with **any** ST depression in V4–V6).
- Is discordant with the main QRS deflection.
- Is down-sloping, not flat.
- Is proportional in degree to the height of the R wave.
- May show similar morphology in limb leads I and aVL, or in II, III, aVF.

ST Depression in V4–V6 Suggestive of Ischemia

In the presence of LVH, ST depression in V4–V6 is suggestive of ischemia if it is **either**:

- Flat, not downsloping.
- Deep and disproportionate to the QRS (R wave).

See Figure 22-1b for typical morphologies of lateral ST depression due to LVH.

Q Waves

A **QS pattern** or Qr with very small R wave in V1–V2 may be due to LVH. A QR pattern with a well-formed R wave is not due to LVH alone; it is due to either acute or old MI.

T Waves in V4–V6 Due to LVH

- May be upright or inverted.
- If discordant with the main QRS deflection, may be **large;** if concordant, they are **small.**
- Are proportional in size to the QRS.

Summary of LVH Features Suggestive of Ischemia or Infarction

There is little literature that addresses the differentiation of ST elevation due to AMI from ST elevation of LVH. We believe that visual recognition of LVH by an experienced observer is important, but it has not been formally studied. By studying the ECG examples, you will be better able to recognize and differentiate LVH from AMI. There are no systematic studies of these criteria, but it is our experience that the following **features of LVH suggest ischemia or infarction;** items 1 to 3 are observations that have also been made by Chou (2).

1. Discordant ST depression or T-wave inversion that is disproportionate to R-wave height.
2. ST depression in leads in which the predominant QRS deflection is negative (e.g., V1–V3) (**concordant ST depression**).
3. T-wave inversion in V1–V2.
4. **Concordant ST elevation.**
5. **ST elevation disproportionate to S-wave depth in V1–V3.**
6. Flat ST depression (as opposed to down-sloping).

See Cases 22-1 through 22-12. (See also Case 8-5 of acute ischemia misinterpreted as LVH; Case 9-8 of STEMI and LVH with hyperacute T waves; Cases 21-1 and 21-4 of LVH and CACP; and Case 26-5 of pulmonary edema with LVH and ST elevation but normal coronary arteries.)

MANAGEMENT

Adjunctive diagnostic measures may be necessary to differentiate LVH from STEMI.

- Treatment of HTN with **NTG and/or beta-blockers** may relieve symptoms and may even resolve suspicious ST elevation.
- **Compare with a previous ECG.**
- **Record serial ECGs.**
- Perform echocardiography.
- As with other pseudoinfarction patterns, in the appropriate clinical setting, angiography may be necessary to distinguish LVH from AMI.

CASE 22-1

CP and ST Elevation Due to LVH

History
This 50-year-old man with history of severe HTN presented with typical CP. BP = 180/110.

ECG 22-1 (Type 1c)
- QS: V2–V3, is suggestive of old MI with ST elevation but is actually due to LVH.
- Large ST deviation in V3–V4 due to LVH is proportional to a very high QRS voltage.

Clinical Course
Clinicians suspected LVH and administered aspirin, meto-

prolol, and IV NTG; the patient's pain resolved, with BP = 140/90. The ECG did not change. Coronary arteries and cTnI were normal.

Conclusion
ST elevation of LVH may mimic ST elevation of STEMI. Angina may be due to LVH and HTN without coronary occlusion.

Reproduced from unpublished data with permission of K. Wang, M.D.

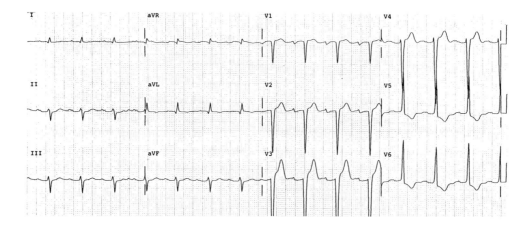

CASE 22-2

CHF and New ST Elevation, All Due to LVH and Stress

History

This 34-year-old man with history of severe HTN and medical noncompliance presented with vague symptoms. He denied CP or shortness of breath (SOB), but he had clinical CHF with mild hypoxia and cardiomegaly on a chest film. BP = 220/150, potassium = 2.6 mEq/L, and creatinine = 3.1 mg/dL.

ECG 22-2A (Type 1a versus 1c)

- LVH by voltage.
- ST elevation: V1–V4, is **suspicious** for anterior AMI.
- ST depression: I, aVL, V6, with T-wave inversion, are typical of LVH but ischemia cannot be ruled out.

ECG 22-2B

ECG recorded 6 weeks prior.

- Comparison with this ECG indicates a change in ST elevation, which makes ECG 22-2A **highly suspicious** for anterior AMI.

Clinical Course

In the context of CP, such new ST elevation with upward convexity is an indication for reperfusion therapy **if ECG findings are persistent after correction of severe HTN.** This patient was initially treated with furosemide and nitroprusside. Because serial ECGs showed no improvement (nor did they show evolution), echocardiography was performed and revealed severe concentric LVH with **no** wall motion abnormality (WMA). Thus reperfusion was not undertaken. All cTnI levels were normal. BP lowered gradually over 24 hours to 150/90. A sestamibi stress test was normal. All subsequent ECGs had the same ST elevation and T-wave inversion.

Conclusion

LVH, especially with stress, may manifest ST elevation indistinguishable from STEMI. The clinical presentation is critical. Echocardiography may be very useful.

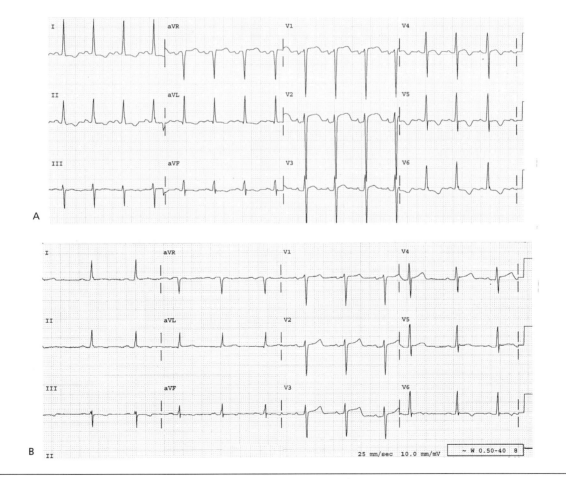

25 mm/sec   10.0 mm/mV   ~ W 0.50-40   8

CASE 22-3

Baseline ECG Shows LVH but Without Anatomic LVH: ST Elevation Meets Thrombolytic "Criteria"

History

This 40-year-old athletic man presented with atypical CP.

ECG 22-3 (Type 1c)

■ Meets criteria for LVH.

Clinical Course

Immediate echocardiography revealed no WMA, no

anatomic LVH, and normal cTnI. ECG findings were unchanged on serial ECGs.

Conclusion

ECGs of young athletes may be falsely positive for anatomic LVH and may mimic STEMI.

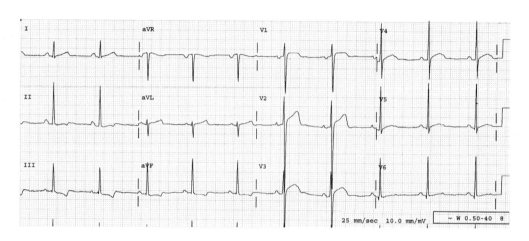

CASE 22-4

CP with ST Elevation Due to LVH but Without Meeting LVH Criteria: ST Segments May Be Upwardly Concave or Convex at Different Points in Time

History
This 50-year-old man presented with CP on two separate occasions.

ECG 22-4A (Type 1c)
His first presentation
- **Does not quite meet LVH criteria.**
- ST elevation: discordant in V2–V4, and upwardly convex in V2–V3, is **highly suspicious for AMI**.

ECG 22-4B (Type 1c)
His second presentation, 1 month later, recorded at **half standard** voltage in precordial leads, V1–V6 only.

- Similar to ECG 22-4A, except that the ST elevation is now upwardly concave in V2–V4 **and** this ECG **does** meet LVH criteria in aVL (not shown).

Clinical Course
The patient **received thrombolytics both times,** and both times ruled out for AMI. Echocardiography confirmed LVH.

Conclusion
ST elevation of LVH is easily mistaken for ST elevation of AMI. Morphology may change, especially under different BP loading conditions. Consider comparison with old ECGs, serial ECGs, and echocardiography.

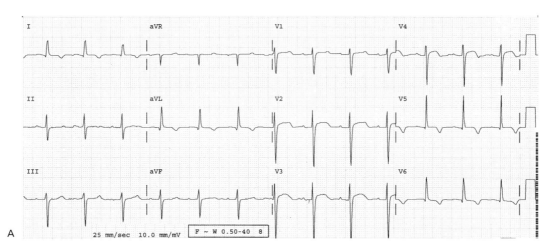

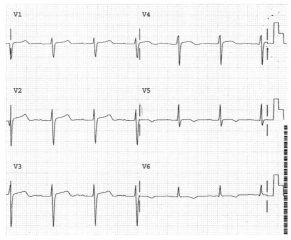

CASE 22-5

ST Elevation Due to LVH; Patient Given Thrombolytics

History

This 58-year-old man presented with typical CP. BP was normal.

ECG 22-5 (Type 1c)

■ Meets LVH criteria.
■ ST elevation: III, V2–V3, was interpreted as due to AMI, but is typical of LVH.

Clinical Course

The patient received thrombolytics (not inappropriately) but angiography and CK-MB were normal.

Conclusion

ST elevation of LVH may mimic STEMI.

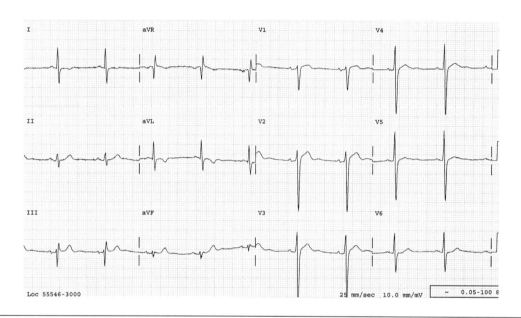

Loc 55546-3000   25 mm/sec 10.0 mm/mV   ~ 0.05-100 8

CASE 22-6

LVH with AMI Due to Occlusion of a "Wraparound" LAD Manifests in Precordial Lead V4 and in Inferior Leads

History

This 43-year-old woman presented with 1 hour of CP unrelieved by three sublingual NTG; see Case 10-10 for her prehospital rhythm strip, which shows high ST elevation. Prehospital systolic BP was 250 mm Hg and was 260/130 in the ED. There was no pulmonary congestion.

ECG 22-6 (Type 1a)
- Meets LVH criteria.
- ST elevation: II, III, aVF, V1–V4. LVH should manifest in V4 as a discordant ST-T complex, as it does in V5–V6. This **concordant** ST elevation suggests **anterior as well as inferior AMI.**

Clinical Course

The patient's BP was controlled with nitroprusside, IV NTG, and metoprolol, and a serial ECG confirmed ST elevation. She was taken to the cath lab. A "wraparound" LAD supplying anterior and inferior walls was occluded just distal to the first diagonal artery; it was successfully angioplastied. After correction of ischemia, the patient's BP was 130/70 on metoprolol only.

Conclusion

Concordance is a clue that the ST elevation is due to AMI.

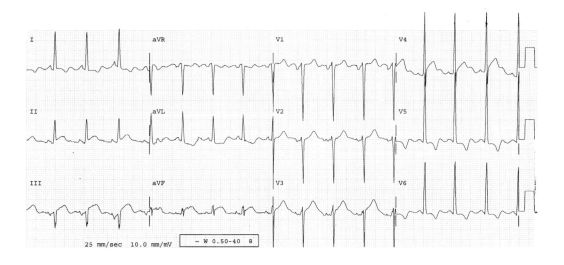

25 mm/sec 10.0 mm/mV   ~ W 0.50-40 8

CASE 22-7

"Primary" ST Depression of Ischemia, Especially V3, Misinterpreted as "Secondary" ST/T Abnormalities of LVH

History

This 72-year-old man with history of single-vessel CABG to the RCA was resuscitated after suffering a cardiac arrest while walking up a hill. He was transported from a facility without a cath lab. On presentation he was hemodynamically stable, intubated, and unconscious. A head computed tomography (CT) was normal.

ECG 22-7 (Type 2, consider Type 1b due to posterior AMI)

Two and one-half hours after cardiac arrest.

- LVH by voltage, with ST-T abnormalities in V4–V6, possibly due to LVH.
- **V3 is not typical of LVH.** V3 should not have ST depression unless the R wave is prominent. Also, the ST depression is **flat,** not downsloping, as it would be in LVH.

Clinical Course

Clinicians read the ECG as "LVH only." The patient underwent angiography 4 hours after the initial cardiac arrest, revealing multivessel disease (70% left main stenosis, patent saphenous vein graft to the RCA, 80% LAD stenosis, 60% stenosis of a large co-dominant circumflex, 70% first diagonal stenosis, and 80% stenosis at ostium of the obtuse marginal). Angioplasty was not performed; the patient underwent three-vessel CABG to the LAD, obtuse marginal, and first diagonal arteries. CK peaked at 2,693 IU/L. No echocardiogram was performed. **Subsequent ECGs revealed deepening T waves in V3–V5, suggesting anterior AMI.** One week later **all ST depression was resolved.**

Conclusion

Immediate angiography ± PCI is indicated, if available, in such a case.

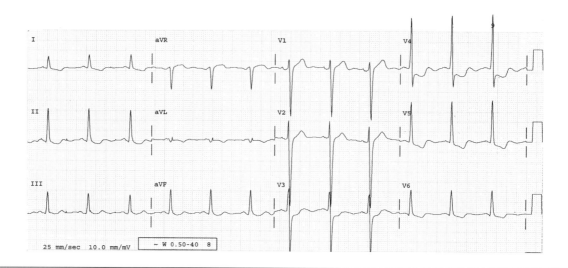

25 mm/sec   10.0 mm/mV   ~ W 0.50-40   8

CASE 22-8

Concordant ST Elevation in V4 Differentiates Anterior AMI from LVH

History
This 77-year-old man presented with 2 hours of typical CP.

ECG 22-8 (Type 1a)
■ Obvious LVH by voltage.
■ ST elevation: V1–V3, **discordant** to deep S waves is possibly due to LVH only, but, at 3 mm, is **suspicious** for anterior AMI. **If this ST elevation in V1–V3 was the only finding, appropriate actions would be as follows:** compare with a previous ECG; perform immediate echocardiography to look for new anterior WMA; send for immediate angiography ± PCI; **or** administer thrombolytics if none of the preceding are available and there are no contraindications. **However, note lead V4:** ST elevation **concordant** to the R wave is **seldom due to LVH.** This is diagnostic of **anterior AMI.** Without V4, leads V1–V3 would be nondiagnostic; with V4, they are diagnostic of anterior AMI (Type 1a).

Clinical Course
The patient was sent for angiography and an occluded LAD was opened.

Conclusion
Concordant ST elevation may be the key to differentiating LVH from AMI.

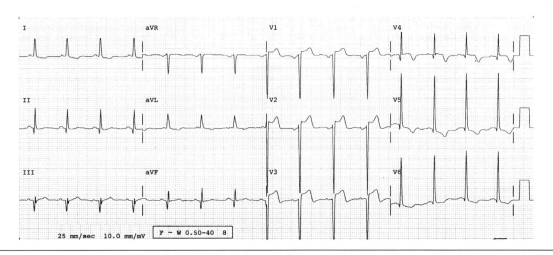

25 mm/sec   10.0 mm/mV   F ~ W 0.50-40 8

CASE 22-9

ECG with LVH and ST Elevation with T-wave Inversion in V4–V5 Due to Early Repolarization with Benign T-wave Inversion and Metabolic Derangement

History
This 35-year-old man presented with typical AMI symptoms but had metabolic derangements, including a glucose > 1,500 mg/dL.

ECG 22-9 (Type 1a vs. 1c vs. 1d)
- Meets LVH criteria. Any ST elevation should be **discordant.**
- QTc = 375 msec.
- Out of context, the concordant ST elevation in V3–V5 is suspicious for AMI vs. early repolarization with benign T-wave inversion.

Clinical Course
The patient ruled out for AMI and the ECG normalized after correction of metabolic abnormalities. However, ECGs two to four years later were identical, confirming benign T-wave inversion.

Conclusion
While transient STEMI due to transient coronary occlusion was not absolutely ruled out, it was very unlikely. A wide variety of ECG abnormalities may result from severe metabolic abnormalities, including acidosis, hyperkalemia, hypoxia, and possibly hyperglycemia. Correct these and repeat the ECG before administering thrombolytics.

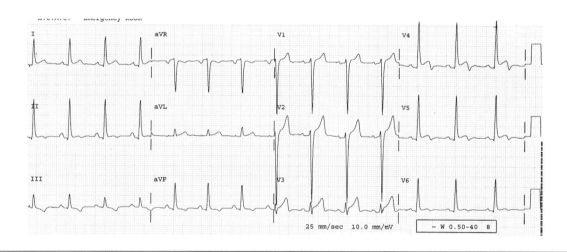

25 mm/sec   10.0 mm/mV   ~ W 0.50-40   8

CASE 22-10

Hypertrophic Cardiomyopathy Mimics Inferior AMI

History
This 55-year-old man presented with CP and a history of hypertrophic cardiomyopathy.

ECG 22-10 (Type 1c)
This is a "half standard" ECG (1 mm = 0.2 mV in precordial leads).
- LVH by voltage.
- ST elevation: III; and reciprocal depression: aVL, are **suspicious** for inferior AMI.

Clinical Course
Biomarkers were negative. Echocardiography was consistent with hypertrophic cardiomyopathy and had no WMA.

Conclusion
It is impossible to know from this ECG alone that this is not an inferior AMI in the context of LVH. **Obtain a previous ECG for patients with CP and known hypertrophic cardiomyopathy, which can mimic AMI.**

Reproduced from unpublished data with permission from K. Wang, M.D.

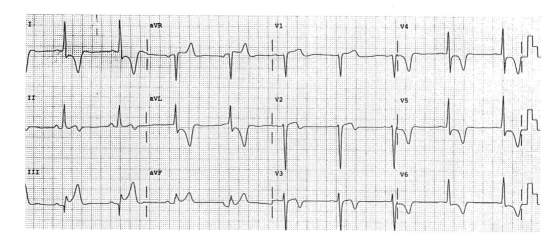

CASE 22-11

Baseline LVH with ST Elevation

History

This 44-year-old man with a history of severe untreated HTN presented with acute hemorrhagic stroke. BP = 194/95.

ECG 22-11 (Type 1c or 1d)

- Unchanged from a previous ECG.
- Very high voltage of LVH; Qr waves: V1–V2, deep but proportional; and discordant negative ST/T waves: V4–V6, are all consistent with LVH.

- ST elevation: > 2 mm, V1–V2; **concordant** ST elevation: 1 mm, V3.

Clinical Course

Repeat ECGs were unchanged and cTnI was normal. The patient underwent rehabilitation for stroke as well as medical therapy for BP control.

Conclusion

LVH can mimic AMI.

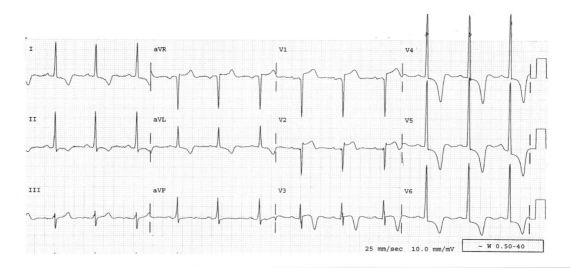

25 mm/sec   10.0 mm/mV   ~ W 0.50-40

CASE 22-12

LVH, Changed from a Previous Tracing, Mimics AMI

History
This 35-year-old man presented with sharp and tender anterior CP. BP = 180/100.

ECG 22-12A (Type 1c)
V1–V6 only
- LVH by voltage.
- ST elevation: V2–V5, is indicative of LVH, or **suspicious** for anterior AMI, or both.
- J-point elevation and J wave: V2.

ECG 22-12B (Type 1c)
This is from 2 months prior, V1–V6 only.
- Shows features typical of both LVH and early repolarization (see Chapter 20).

- Comparison reveals that, on ECG 22-12A, the ST segments in V2–V4 remain elevated 3 to 4 mm, but now have **less upward concavity** than ECG 22-12A. The computer read this as "acute infarct."

Clinical Course
Reperfusion may be appropriate in this case. However, because of very atypical symptoms, serial ECGs were recorded and all remained the same. Serial cTnI levels were normal. Urine was positive for cocaine. ECGs up to 1 year all showed upward concavity.

Conclusion
Transient ischemia producing the ST convexity remains a possibility.

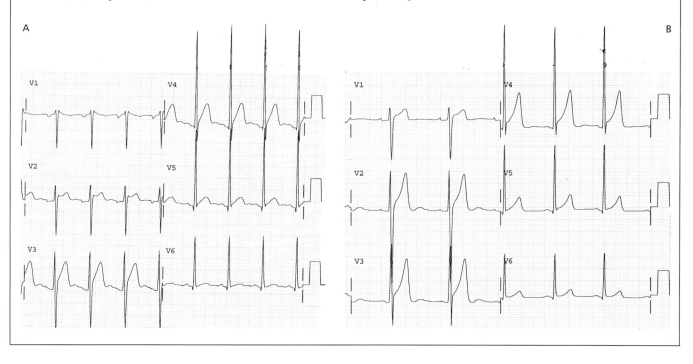

ANNOTATED BIBLIOGRAPHY

Larsen GC, et al. Electrocardiographic left ventricular hypertrophy in patients with suspected acute cardiac ischemia: its influence on diagnosis, triage, and short-term prognosis, 1994.
> **Methods:** Larsen et al. (286) prospectively gathered data on 5,773 patients who presented with cardiorespiratory complaints. Cardiologists later analyzed their ECGs for LVH and the presence of "primary" (a result of cardiac ischemia) and "secondary" (a result of LVH) ST-T abnormalities. They compared these ECG manifestations with presenting complaints and final diagnosis.
> **Findings:** Patients with LVH (with or without secondary ST-T abnormalities) more commonly suffered dyspnea, less commonly had CP, and were four times as likely to have CHF. They were one-third as likely as those without LVH, and only one-fourth as likely as those with primary ST-T changes to have cardiac ischemia as the etiology of their symptoms and signs. Most important, for more than 70% of those with LVH and secondary ST-T changes, these ST-T changes had been misread as primary. Unfortunately, no data are presented to help differentiate primary from secondary ST-T abnormalities in patients who meet LVH criteria.

Khoury NE, et al. "Inadvertent" thrombolytic administration in patients without myocardial infarction: clinical features and outcome, 1996.
> **Methods:** Khoury et al. (285) analyzed ECGs of 609 AMI patients who received thrombolytics. They compared findings of patients with versus without CK-MB confirmation of AMI.
> **Findings:** Thirty-five patients had negative CK-MB, nine (25%) of whom had LVH. Of patients who did rule in for AMI, 7% had LVH. Thus patients with LVH were more than three times as likely to receive "inadvertent" thrombolytics.

Myers G. QRS-T patterns in multiple precordial leads that may be mistaken for myocardial infarction, 1950.

    Methods: Myers (287) studied the pseudoinfarction patterns of LVH in a small series.

    Findings: ST elevation of AMI was likely to be superimposed on the ST elevation of LVH if (a) there was a loss of the normal upward concavity associated with LVH and (b) the ST elevation was high. ST elevation in V1–V3 was more likely due to LVH when the patient was taking digitalis. (ST elevation reached 8 mm in one such patient with LVH.)

Khan IA, et al. Persistent ST segment elevation: a new ECG finding in hypertrophic cardiomyopathy, 1999.

    Findings: Khan et al. (288) report a case of hypertrophic cardiomyopathy with ST elevation that was electrocardiographically indistinguishable from AMI in all respects.

Selzer A, et al. Reliability of electrocardiographic diagnosis of left ventricular hypertrophy, 1958.

    Methods: Selzer et al. (289) conducted a necropsy study of 108 patients who met ECG criteria for LVH.

    Findings: When findings of flattened and inverted T waves and ST depression in leads with the highest deflections were added to voltage criteria, ECG specificity for identification of anatomic LVH increased.

Otto LA, et al. Evaluation of ST segment elevation criteria for the prehospital electrocardiographic diagnosis of acute myocardial infarction, 1994.

    Methods: Otto et al. (106) examined prehospital 12-lead ECGs of 418 CP patients.

    Findings: ST elevation $\geq$ 1 mm was found in ECGs of 123 patients. Sixty-three patients did not have AMI, of whom 21 (33%) had ST elevation due to LVH.

23

"VENTRICULAR ANEURYSM:" PERSISTENT ST ELEVATION AFTER PREVIOUS MI

KEY POINTS

- QS waves with ST elevation ≤ 3 mm and without tall T waves in leads V1–V3 suggest the presence of anterior ventricular aneurysm.
- In inferior ventricular aneurysm, QR waves may be present.
- Ventricular aneurysm may be mistaken for STEMI.
- Previous history and ECGs, as well as immediate echocardiography, may help to differentiate ventricular aneurysm from AMI.

GENERAL BACKGROUND

ST elevation may persist indefinitely after STEMI. This occurs in **up to 60% of anterior MI,** but it is much less common after inferior MI **(95)**. Patients with persistent ST elevation after previous MI may present with CP, be misdiagnosed with **acute** MI, and receive "inadvertent" thrombolytic therapy (37,**290**) (see Chapter 3). Autopsy studies (292–296) have long established an association of persistent ST elevation after previous MI with **anatomic** left ventricular aneurysm, which is visible on autopsy as myocardial wall thinning and bulging. As measured by ventriculography or visualized with echocardiography, **anatomic** aneurysm has been described as showing **diastolic** distortion and myocardial wall thinning **(297,298)**. Because of this association with anatomic features, the morphology of persistent ST elevation after MI has been (and still is) known as "left ventricular aneurysm" or, simply, "ventricular aneurysm." More recent use of imaging modalities, however, has demonstrated that, in old MI, persistent ST elevation may also be associated with **systolic** dyskinesis, akinesis, or a large area of myocardial necrosis, even in the **absence** of anatomic ventricular aneurysm (Case 23-1) **(95,299). We refer specifically to the ECG morphology of persistent ST elevation of old MI as "ventricular aneurysm,"** whether or not anatomic aneurysm is present.

The presence or absence of **anatomic** aneurysm is only important for the reperfusion decision if echocardiography is used to differentiate ST elevation of **acute** MI from that of old MI with persistent ST elevation. If you suspect that ST elevation is due to old MI and you see the **diastolic** distortion and myocardial wall thinning of anatomic aneurysm on an echocardiogram, this strongly supports a diagnosis of **persistent ST elevation of old MI,** with a high positive predictive value (PPV). If you see **systolic** dyskinesis, akinesis, or hypokinesis, however, these may be associated with **either** acute MI or old MI with persistent ST elevation **(95,299)**. Although systolic dyskinesis suggests a nonacute MI, a finding of akinesis or hypokinesis is not discriminatory.

Clinical Presentation

Patients with ventricular aneurysm often present with dyspnea and pulmonary edema due to poor LV function. They may also present with primary ventricular tachycardia or fibrillation due to scarred myocardium (see Case 26-8).

ECG DIAGNOSIS OF VENTRICULAR ANEURYSM

ST elevation of ventricular aneurysm can mimic AMI and lead to "inadvertent" thrombolysis (see Cases 23-2 and 23-3); findings that aid in differentiating the two entities include the following:

ST Elevation of Ventricular Aneurysm (Old MI)

- Most common in leads **V1–V3.**
- Usually ≤ **3 mm** and almost always is ≤ 4 mm.
- **Relatively static on serial ECGs and unchanged from previous ECGs** unless there is **new** occlusion of the infarct-related artery (IRA) **OR** there are **significant changes in HR or BP.**
- May occur simultaneously with LVH (see Case 23-4).

Additional features include the following:

- T waves are **flattened or inverted, NOT tall or peaked.**
- Q waves are **deep and well formed.**
  - **Anterior** wall ventricular aneurysm:

- QS pattern (no R wave or possibly minimal R wave) in V1–V3.
  - QR pattern, instead of QS, is likely in V4 (see Case 23-5).
- **Inferior** wall ventricular aneurysm:
  - QR pattern is common (see Case 23-6). Differentiation from **acute** inferior MI with well-developed Q waves is difficult (see Case 11-4).
  - QS pattern is probably less common (see Case 35-3).
  - Reciprocal ST depression in aVL may occur, as with AMI (see Cases 23-7 and 7-5, of patients with inferior aneurysm treated with thrombolytics).

ST Elevation of Acute MI

- Nearly always has some preservation of the R wave (R wave or QR pattern), unless the AMI is very late in its course (subacute).
- If a Q wave is present, it is much more likely to be **narrow or shallow.**
- T wave remains **tall and/or peaked,** unless the MI is subacute.
- QR pattern with ST elevation may be due to ventricular aneurysm if found in inferior leads, but in the absence of other information such as a previous ECG, it should be assumed to be due to AMI.
- QS pattern in V1–V3 may be transformed into QR pattern by RBBB (or, in aVL, by LAFB) (see Case 23-8).
- Normalization of chronic ST elevation of ventricular aneurysm may indicate posterior AMI (231).

See Table 23-1 for frequency of ECG findings from four studies of patients with LV aneurysm (292–295). Data in some cases is incomplete and does not include findings from Cokki-

nos et al. **(300)** (see Annotated Bibliography). (See also: Case 26-8; Case 33-1; Case 35-1, of a patient with lateral AMI superimposed on anterior ventricular aneurysm; and Case 33-7.)

MANAGEMENT

Administration of thrombolytics in the **absence** of STEMI is always undesirable, but patients with ventricular aneurysm are at additional risk because **anatomic aneurysm** may harbor a thrombus that could embolize as a result of thrombolysis; this is probably rare (301,302).

Adjunctive Diagnostic Studies

Adjunctive diagnostic measures may be necessary in order to rule out AMI.

- Compare with a **previous ECG.** ST elevation new since the previous ECG is likely to represent AMI. It is important to note that a new infarct in the area of the old infarct (area with deep Q or QS waves) receives less benefit from reperfusion than does an AMI in a new location.
- **Record serial ECGs.**
- **Perform echocardiography.** Look for diastolic distortion and myocardial wall thinning of the relevant myocardial wall, as an indication of **anatomic aneurysm;** this supports the ECG diagnosis of ventricular aneurysm. Conversely, systolic dyskinesis, akinesis, or hypokinesis supports the diagnosis of AMI. However, there is great interobserver variability in echocardiography. One echocardiographer's "dyskinesis" may be another's "akinesis."

TABLE 23.1. ECGs OF PATIENTS WITH VENTRICULAR ANEURYSM, COMPILED FROM FOUR CASE SERIES (DATA WERE INCOMPLETE)

	Number	ANY R-wave in V2 or V3	SOME T-wave inversion	ST elevation < 3 mm
Anterior aneurysm	36	3/20 (two of the three have a tiny R after Q)	14/21	33/36
Inferior aneurysm	8	6/7	7/7	8/8

CASE 23-1

Persistent ST Elevation Mimics AMI, but Echocardiography Does Not Reveal Anatomic Ventricular Aneurysm

History
This 83-year-old woman presented with very typical CP and dyspnea.

ECG 23-1 (Type 1c)
- Left anterior fascicular block (LAFB), with left axis deviation and late forces toward aVL
- Deep, wide QS and ST elevation: V2–V3; low and/or inverted T waves: V2–V6. Ventricular aneurysm is probable and **AMI is possible.**

Clinical Course
Immediate echocardiography revealed no aneurysm but indicated a WMA in the apex, probable LV enlargement, and probable LV thrombus. Previous records arrived with old ECGs that confirmed previous MI with persistent ST elevation. Serial ECGs remained unchanged and biomarkers were negative.

Conclusion
Persistent ST elevation can be present even WITHOUT anatomic ventricular aneurysm.

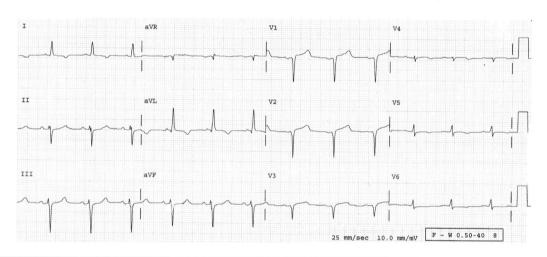

25 mm/sec   10.0 mm/mV   F ~ W 0.50-40 8

CASE 23-2

Patient with Ventricular Aneurysm and CP (No AMI) "Inadvertently" Given Thrombolytics

History
This 71-year-old woman presented with CP.

ECG 23-2 (Type 1c)
■ ST elevation and deep Q waves in anterior leads, with ST elevation of only 1 mm and T waves are normal. This ECG is **highly suspicious** for ventricular aneurysm.

Clinical Course
Thrombolytics were administered but biomarkers were negative, and review of a previous ECG revealed no change.

Conclusion
Ventricular aneurysm can lead to false-positive ST elevation.

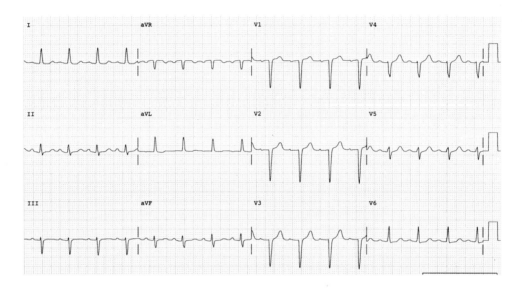

CASE 23-3

Patient with Persistent ST Elevation and CP (No AMI) Given Thrombolytics

History
This 58-year-old woman presented with CP.

ECG 23-3 (Type 1c)
- ST elevation: up to 2 mm, V3–V4; deep Q waves: V3–V4, suggest ventricular aneurysm. T waves are nor-

mal. This ECG is highly suggestive of ventricular aneurysm.

Clinical Course
The patient received thrombolytics, not inappropriately. Biomarkers were negative and review of a previous ECG revealed no change.

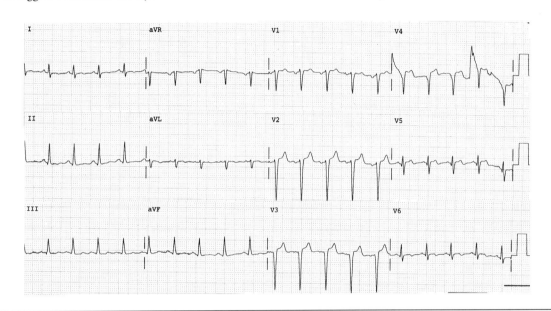

CASE 23-4

Ventricular Aneurysm

History
This 80-year-old man with a history of MI presented with CP.

ECG 23-4 (Type 1c)
- LVH by voltage: aVL.
- Deep QS waves and ST elevation up to 2 mm: V1–V5, are diagnostic of ventricular aneurysm. Although QS waves in V1–V3 can result from LVH alone, QS waves in V4–V5 are not to be expected as a result of LVH.

Clinical Course
The patient had a normal CK-MB. Echocardiography revealed anterior aneurysm, lateral akinesis, and inferior hypokinesis, with moderately severe decreased LV function and **no LVH.** Thus the ECG findings were old.

ECG reproduced from unpublished data with permission of K. Wang, M.D.

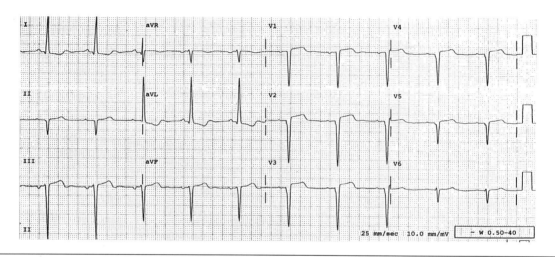

CASE 23-5

CP and ECG Findings Are Consistent with AMI but Old Records and ECGs Confirm Ventricular Aneurysm

History

This 72-year-old woman with a history of CAD complained of 4 hours of CP radiating to her jaw. She experienced some relief after three sublingual NTG tablets.

ECG 23-5 (Type 1c)
- Well-formed QS waves: V1–V3; ST elevation: 3 mm, V1–V3 suggest ventricular aneurysm.
- **ST elevation and QR wave: V4,** are **highly suspicious** for AMI.

Clinical Course

Identical old ECGs and old records confirmed the diagnosis of a large, thin-walled anterior ventricular aneurysm. Biomarkers were negative.

Conclusion

Without old records and ECGs, this would be indistinguishable from acute STEMI.

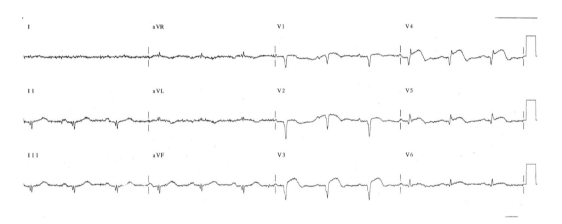

CASE 23-6

Inferior Ventricular Aneurysm with QR Morphology

History

This 77-year-old woman presented with pulmonary edema but no CP.

ECG 23-6 (Type 1c)

- LVH by voltage.
- ST elevation: III, aVF; and reciprocal depression: aVL, only 1 mm.
- Inferior QR waves are typical of inferior ventricular aneurysm.
- ST depression: V5–V6, consistent with LVH.
- A right-sided ECG was not available, although it was indicated in this case. The ECG differential diagnosis includes subacute inferior AMI (Q waves beginning) versus infe-

rior ventricular aneurysm versus old inferior MI with superimposed **acute** MI. Lack of CP is evidence against AMI.

Clinical Course

Thrombolytics were given, biomarkers were negative, and echocardiography confirmed ventricular aneurysm.

Conclusion

Comparison with a previous ECG is critical. Alternatively, immediate echocardiography may be very useful. Without CP and with ECG possibility of ventricular aneurysm, thrombolytics may not be indicated. Angiography ± PCI is indicated if available.

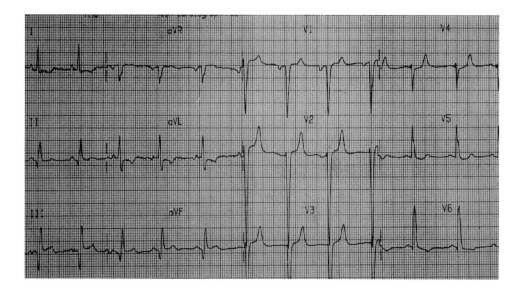

CASE 23-7

Cardiac Arrest and Inferoposterior Aneurysm Mistaken for AMI

History

This 84-year-old woman had sudden back and leg pain. Paramedics found her with mottled and pulseless legs. She then suffered a cardiac arrest and was cardioverted. The initial postresuscitation ECG showed atrial fibrillation with a rapid ventricular response and inferior ST elevation with anterolateral ST depression. The rate was slowed with diltiazem. She was transferred to a tertiary care center with a working diagnosis of aortic dissection. On arrival she was hemodynamically stable with bilateral absence of lower-extremity perfusion.

ECG 23-7 (Type 1c)

- Qr (tiny R) waves with ST elevation: III, aVF; and reciprocal depression: aVL.
- QS waves: V1–V3, probable old anterior MI.
- ST depression: V1–V4, consistent with posterior AMI (or

aneurysm?). This is possibly acute MI, but highly suggestive of inferoposterior aneurysm.

Clinical Course

Clinicians presumed acute MI. Because the surgeons' prognosis for aortoiliac surgery was grim, partly due to concurrent AMI, the family was reluctant to consent to surgery. Ultimately, an aortic bifurcation clot was removed, and the patient survived. All cTnI were negative. Later echocardiography showed an inferoposterior aneurysm.

Conclusion

Surgery was delayed, with potentially fatal effects, because physicians did not recognize this aneurysm morphology and diagnosed **acute** MI. ECG morphology recognition, in conjunction with an immediate echocardiogram demonstrating aneurysm, would have facilitated earlier surgical intervention.

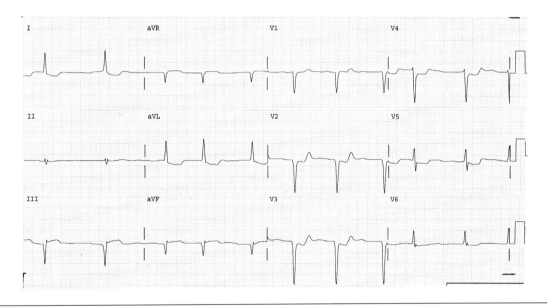

CASE 23-8

RBBB Transforms QS—into a QR Pattern, Obscuring Diagnosis of Aneurysm

History

This 79-year-old man presented with dyspnea. He stated that he had presented with SOB 1 month earlier and had a **painless** MI.

ECG 23-8A (Type 1c)

- RBBB.
- ST elevation: V2–V3; and **QR** pattern: V2–V3, so clinicians did not suspect ventricular aneurysm.

Clinical Course

Thrombolytics were administered without complications. Biomarkers were negative. The patient returned 5 days later to another physician, again with dyspnea. The ECG obtained at this time was identical to ECG 23-8 and **thrombolytics were administered again,** with no complications.

ECG 23-8B (Type 1c)

Forty minutes after thrombolytics, V1–V3 only.

- Spontaneous conversion out of RBBB (intermittent RBBB).
- Deep QS pattern is now obvious: ventricular aneurysm pattern is obvious.

Clinical Course

AMI biomarkers were again negative.

Conclusion

RBBB may transform a QS pattern into a QR pattern.

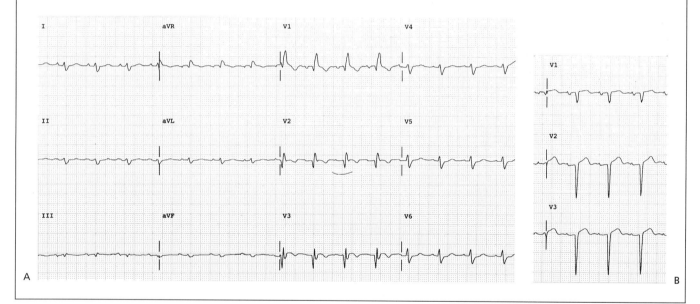

ANNOTATED BIBLIOGRAPHY

Several case series of ventricular aneurysm were published before 1970 (292–296). Virtually all were clinical-pathologic correlations without comparison or control groups. These studies described the findings of ventricular aneurysm, and, if the ECG was addressed, correlated the ECG with the pathologic or imaging studies, with the goal of being able to diagnose ventricular aneurysm. Because the intent of these studies was not to differentiate acute MI from old MI with persistent ST elevation, no data to aid in that task were analyzed, although some can be extracted with close reading. Additional studies used cineangiographic diagnosis of ventricular aneurysm and then correlated the diagnosis with the ECG (303) or echocardiographic (297,298) findings, but none attempted to compare ECG findings of AMI with those of ventricular aneurysm.

Some studies describe or display the ECGs from their case series (293–295);

Moyer et al. (292) reviewed 16 previous cases and added 11 of their own. We summarize the ECG findings from these four studies (292–295) in Table 23-1. (Note that the data in some cases is incomplete.)

Cokkinos DV, et al. Left ventricular aneurysm: analysis of electrocardiographic features and post-resection changes, 1971.

> **Methods:** Cokkinos et al. (300) performed aneurysmectomies on 26 patients and compared the pre- and postoperative ECGs.
>
> **Findings:** ECG findings enabled localization of the aneurysm in all 26 cases. Twenty-one had abnormal Q waves in ≥ two leads, with a mean of 4.4 leads. Mean ST elevation was 3.1 mm, and 23 ECGs had ≤ 4 mm of ST elevation. Fourteen had a QRS duration of ≥ 100 ms. Interestingly, many of these ECG abnormalities significantly improved after aneurysmectomy.

Mills RM, et al. Natural history of ST segment elevation after acute myocardial infarction, 1975.

Methods: Mills et al. (95) examined ECGs of 23 anterior AMI patients and 22 inferior AMI patients to determine the natural history of ST elevation. They also examined the ECGs of 65 patients with angiographically proven CAD and ventriculography-proven ventricular dysfunction (defined as severe hypokinesis, akinesis, or dyskinesis, but not differentiated into diastolic or systolic); they then compared these 65 ECGs with ECGs of patients with angiographically proven CAD (but not necessarily a history of MI) and **no** ventricular dysfunction.

Findings: ST elevation resolved within 2 weeks in 95% of inferior AMIs but in only 40% of anterior AMIs. ST elevation persisting more than 2 weeks after AMI did not resolve. Of 65 patients with CAD and advanced anterior and apical asynergy, 40 (62%) had persistent ST elevation. Of 30 patients with CAD (with or without history of MI is not stated) and normal ventriculograms, only one (3%) had persistent ST elevation.

Arvan S, et al. Persistent ST-segment elevation and left ventricular wall abnormalities: a two-dimensional echocardiographic study, 1984.

Methods: Arvan et al. (299) used echocardiography to study 23 patients with previous anterior MI and persistent ST elevation.

Findings: Of 23 patients, 22 had systolic dyskinesis and 10 **also** had **anatomic** ventricular aneurysm (diastolic wall thinning or bulging). Of 15 patients with chronic anterior MI **without** persistent ST elevation, 13 had **akinesis** (**not** dyskinesis). Of 15 patients with anterior **subacute** MI **without** ST elevation, 10 demonstrated dyskinesis; nine of these subsequently developed chronic ST elevation. In contrast, of five patients with akinesis, none went on to develop ST elevation. Additionally, the patients with dyskinesis (who later developed ST elevation) had an infarct size that was an average of approximately two and a half times as large, as measured by CK. **Authors concluded that dyskinesis is associated with a larger MI and is associated with and precedes the appearance of chronic ST elevation.**

Miller DH, et al. Relationship of prior myocardial infarction to false-positive electrocardiographic diagnosis of acute injury in patients with chest pain, 1987.

Methods: Miller et al. (290) studied the ECGs of 100 consecutive CP patients admitted to a cardiac care unit (CCU) for suspected AMI.

Findings: Of 36 patients with ST elevation, 31 (84%) had AMI proven by CK-MB. Of 10 patients with ST elevation and a history of a previous Q-wave MI, only five "ruled in" for AMI, whereas 21 of 21 without such history "ruled in." In all five patients with previous MI who were also suffering AMI, the leads with ST elevation were the same leads that manifested the previous Q waves. **Differentiating old MI from AMI in the same location is difficult, and previous Q-wave MI lowers the PPV of ST elevation in that same lead.**

Bhatnagar SK. Observations of the relationship between left ventricular aneurysm and ST segment elevation in patients with a first acute anterior Q-wave myocardial infarction, 1994.

Methods: Bhatnagar (304) recorded echocardiograms and ECGs of 78 survivors of first anterior Q-wave AMI on Day 14 after onset.

Findings: Of 78 patients, 19 had ventricular aneurysm. There was no significant difference between the mean persistent ST elevation in V2 for those with or without aneurysm, but the sum of ST elevation in leads V1–V6 was higher in those with aneurysm. Mean ST elevation in V2 in all patients was 3.5 mm.

Comment: Unfortunately, this does not address the level of ST elevation with chronic ventricular aneurysm.

Visser CA, et al. Echocardiographic-cineangiographic correlation in detecting left ventricular aneurysm: a prospective study of 422 patients, 1982.

Methods: In the pre-reperfusion era, Visser et al. (297) compared 2-D echocardiography to cineangiography in 422 patients for diagnosis of ventricular aneurysm, which was defined as a "well-demarcated bulge in the contour of the left ventricular wall during both diastole and systole, demonstrating dyskinesia or akinesia." Unfortunately, they did not correlate anatomic findings with ECG findings.

Findings: Echocardiographic detection of ventricular aneurysm compared to cineangiography was 93% sensitive and 94% specific.

Visser CA, et al. Incidence, timing and prognostic value of left ventricular aneurysm formation after myocardial infarction: a prospective, serial echocardiographic study of 158 patients, 1986.

Methods: Visser et al. (298) performed serial echocardiography on 158 patients with first AMI, to study wall motion and aneurysm formation (as defined by abnormal bulge in both systole and diastole).

Findings: Of 158 patients, 35 developed ventricular aneurysm; these included 29 of 90 anterior AMI patients and six of 68 inferior AMI patients. Aneurysm formation within 5 days of AMI was seen in 15 anterior AMI patients, with an 80% 1-year mortality. No new aneurysm developed after 3 months.

PERICARDITIS AND MYOCARDITIS

GENERAL BACKGROUND

Patients with pericarditis may present with CP and ST elevation on the ECG. As a result, it is commonly confused with AMI. History and physical exam may be useful to differentiate pericarditis from AMI. Pericarditis may be associated with **symptoms of infection** such as fever. It may also be **positional or pleuritic;** in particular, it may be worse in the supine position and relieved by sitting forward. Lastly, auscultation may reveal a **pericardial friction rub,** although this is frequently intermittent or absent.

Symptoms and signs may also be identical to AMI, which leaves the diagnosis largely dependent on skilled ECG interpretation. Inflammation that extends to the myocardium (**myocarditis or myopericarditis**) may be particularly difficult to distinguish clinically and electrocardiographically from AMI. These patients may have elevated troponin and may have WMAs on echocardiograms. They are often distinguished by such clinical characteristics as young age, fever, and prolonged course (**305**). In a series of 45 patients with typical history for AMI but with normal coronary arteries, 35 had myocarditis by nuclear indium scanning; 17 of these 35 were diffuse and 18 were focal (**306**).

ECG DIAGNOSIS OF PERICARDITIS

The following are ECG findings characteristic of pericarditis (**81,307**). See Cases 24-1 to 24-3.

Diffuse ST Elevation

- **Leftward/anterior/inferior** ST axis, in the direction of leads II and V5.
- ST elevation is typically greatest in **II and V5,** also I and V6.
- **Upwardly concave** ST segment.
- There may also be ST elevation in **V4 (greatest)** >V3 > V2 >**V1;** aVF, III, aVL (least).
- ST elevation in V6 usually > **25% the height of the T wave,** in contrast to early repolarization and AMI, both of which usually have tall T waves (264).
- ST elevation usually ≤ 5 mm (1).

ST Depression in aVR

- There is **never ST elevation in aVR, only ST depression.** Remember that ST depression in aVR also occurs in inferior AMI.
- ST segments in V1, III, aVL may also be minimally depressed.

PR-Segment Depression

Some PR depression is a normal ECG finding and is due to atrial repolarization (see Chapter 6) (**81**). However, PR depression may also occur with pericarditis, typically with PR elevation in aVR. In pericarditis:

- PR depression > 0.8 mm, relative to the TP segment, is very specific but not sensitive (**81**).
- PR depression is most common in II, aVF, and V4–V6.
- **PR elevation > 0.5 mm in aVR strongly suggests pericarditis (307).** Because aVR manifests findings in the opposite direction of other leads, PR depression manifests in aVR as PR elevation, and occurs in 80% of pericarditis cases. There is (almost) never PR depression in aVR.

Additional ECG Characteristics

T-wave inversion may develop in pericarditis, similar to AMI. However, in pericarditis, T-wave inversion occurs **after ST normalization (307).** It shows **neither evolution of Q waves nor loss of R wave,** although pericardial effusion may diffusely lower the voltage and is easily detected by bedside echocardiography. Pericarditis may also manifest electrical alternans (QRS alternates high to low voltage from beat to beat), or if there is pericardial effusion, it may result in low QRS voltage.

It is our observation that the **QT$_c$ is significantly shorter in pericarditis than in AMI**.

ECG Stages of Pericarditis

There are typically **four stages of evolution** of the ECG in pericarditis, as follows: (a) ST elevation; (b) return of the ST junction to baseline and decrease in T-wave amplitude; (c) T-wave inversion; and (d) resolution of the ECG (**307**). See Case 24-3.

Reciprocal Changes

Because pericarditis is typically spread diffusely around the epicardium, it manifests as diffuse ST elevation, with **no reciprocal ST depression.** An exception is **localized pericarditis,** which may manifest localized ST elevation with reciprocal changes. For example, pericarditis localized to the inferior wall may mimic inferior AMI, with ST elevation in II, III, and aVF, and ST depression in aVL. Clinical findings are critical for differentiation of localized pericarditis from AMI (see Cases 24-4 and 24-5). If the localized pericarditis affects the myocardium (myocarditis), the ECG may be indistinguishable from AMI and echocardiography **may show a regional WMA** (see Case 24-6).

Hyperacute T Waves

Hyperacute T waves favor the diagnosis of AMI (see Case 24-7). Although they do occur in pericarditis, they are rare (see Case 24-8) (1).

PERICARDITIS AND AMI

AMI May Mimic Pericarditis

AMI with diffuse ST elevation may mimic pericarditis.

Anteroinferior AMI

Anteroinferior AMI results from infarction of a "wraparound" LAD that supplies both the anterior and inferior walls. This manifests **diffuse** ST elevation, but **if there is reciprocal ST depression in aVL, it is highly supportive** of AMI. ST eleva- tion of anteroinferior AMI is maximal in leads V2–V3 and III, whereas the ST elevation of pericarditis is maximal in V5–V6 and II. An AMI of this large size often causes **hemodynamic instability** (see Case 24-7).

Inferolateral AMI

Inferolateral AMI may masquerade as pericarditis. There is typically ST elevation in II, III, aVF, and I and/or aVL, V5–V6. However, **ST elevation of lateral infarct may cancel out reciprocal depression in aVL.** Look for maximal inferior ST elevation in lead III. Maximal ST elevation in lead II is typical of both pericarditis and inferolateral AMI due to circumflex occlusion (131). (See: Case 7-3 of inferolateral AMI with minimal reciprocal depression in aVL, misdiagnosed as pericarditis; and Case 14-3 of a lateral AMI, misread by the computer as "pericarditis" but immediately recognized by clinicians and appropriately reperfused.)

Antero-Infero-Lateral AMI

Antero-infero-lateral AMI typically manifests ST elevation in V2–V6, I, II, III, aVF, and aVL. An AMI of this large size typically leads to hemodynamic instability. ECG 24-8 mimics antero-infero-lateral AMI.

MANAGEMENT

If in doubt about the ECG interpretation, record serial ECGs. The evolution of ECG changes in pericarditis is **much slower** than that in AMI. **Listen frequently for a pericardial friction rub. Echocardiography** will show no WMA in pericarditis, unless myopericarditis (less common) is present and causing myocardial dysfunction (see Case 24-4). Although the presence of **pericardial fluid** is very helpful for confirming pericarditis, its absence does not rule out pericarditis.

Reperfusion Therapy

Although the most feared complication of thrombolysis in a patient with pericarditis is **hemopericardium,** this is both uncommon and treatable (**305,309–314**), but can result in death (**315,316**). Because of the risks of AMI, clinical factors and adjunctive diagnostic modalities may be necessary before ruling out reperfusion therapy (see Cases 24-8 and 24-9).

CASE 24-1

Classic Pericarditis

ECG 24-1 (Type 1c)

■ Diffuse ST elevation with no reciprocal depression; maximal limb lead ST elevation: lead II; PR segment depression, greatest in lead II; and ST depression and PR elevation in aVR are characteristics of classic pericarditis.

Reproduced from unpublished data with permission of K. Wang, M.D.

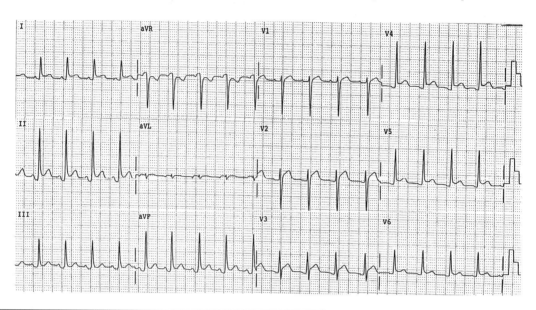

CASE 24-2

Pericarditis with Pronounced ST Elevation

History

This 40-year-old woman presented with nonspecific CP and a normal physical exam.

ECG 24-2 (Type 1c)

■ ST elevation: I, II, III, aVF, V1–V6, with no reciprocal depression; maximal limb lead ST elevation: II; and PR depression: V2–V6, II, III, aVF are typical of pericarditis. If this were an infero-antero-lateral AMI, the patient would likely be unstable.

■ Septal Q waves: V3–V4, are suspicious for AMI.

Clinical Course

The patient was admitted. CTnI levels were all normal.

Conclusion

Immediate echocardiography is indicated to help exclude ischemia.

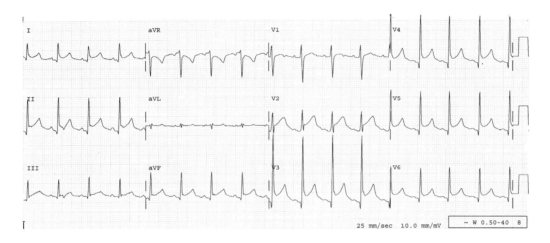

CASE 24-3

Stage 2 Pericarditis

History

This 45-year-old woman presented with severe atypical CP. Her previous ECGs had isoelectric ST segments.

ECG 24-3 (Type 1c)

■ Diffuse ST elevation, II > III, with no reciprocal depres-

sion; and decreased T-wave amplitude with minimal inversion: III and V4, are typical of stage 2 pericarditis.

Clinical Course

Immediate echocardiography revealed no WMA and biomarkers were negative, confirming that this does not represent AMI. This is a typical ECG example of stage 2 pericarditis.

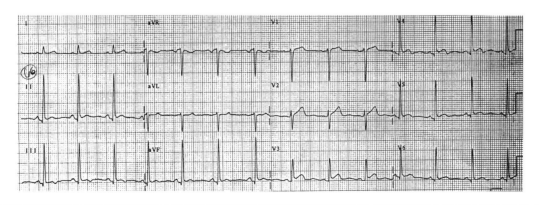

CASE 24-4

Inferior Localized Pericarditis with Inferior ST Elevation and Reciprocal Depression in aVL Superimposed on Early Repolarization

History

This 52-year-old man presented with 12 hours of burning CP, which worsened significantly with supine position and deep inspiration.

ECG 24-4 (Type 1c)

- Diffuse ST elevation is typical of pericarditis.
- Precordial leads: early transition, tall R waves, distinct J wave, and ST elevation in V6 < 25% the height of the T wave are consistent with early repolarization.

- Limb leads with reciprocal ST depression in aVL are **very suspicious** for inferior AMI, although ST elevation maximal in lead II is consistent with pericarditis.

Clinical Course

The clinical presentation was suggestive of pericarditis. Emergent echocardiography revealed normal inferior wall motion, confirming localized pericarditis.

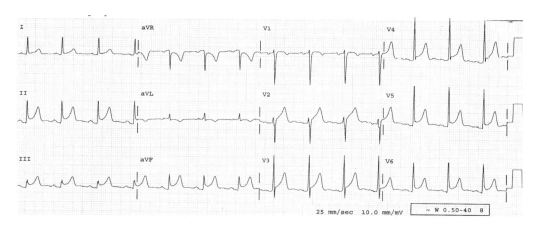

25 mm/sec   10.0 mm/mV   ~ W 0.50-40 8

CASE 24-5

Localized Pericarditis Mimics Inferior AMI

History

This 27-year-old man presented with classic pain of pericarditis.

ECG 24-5 (Type 1a versus 1c)

■ ST elevation: II, III, and aVF; and minimal reciprocal ST depression: aVL, are **very suspicious** for inferior AMI. In a patient with risk factors and typical symptoms, this would be diagnostic of inferior AMI.

Clinical Course

The emergency physician performed bedside echocardiography, which revealed pericardial effusion. Thrombolytics were withheld pending formal echocardiography, which subsequently revealed no WMA.

Conclusion

Reciprocal depression in aVL may occur in localized pericarditis. Bedside echocardiography, as well as formal echocardiography, may be useful.

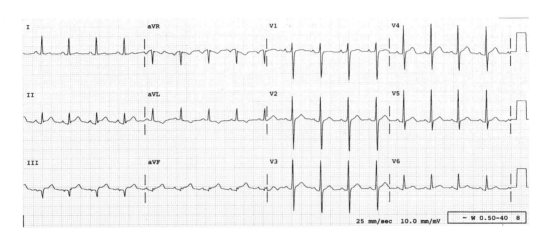

25 mm/sec   10.0 mm/mV   ~ W 0.50-40 8

CASE 24-6

Infero-Postero-Lateral Myocarditis Mimics AMI on the ECG and on an Echocardiogram

History
This 20-year-old man presented with continuous severe, nonpleuritic, "bandlike" pain across his entire chest. He had presented the day before with CP and fever, was diagnosed with pneumonia, and was treated with antibiotics.

ECG 24-6 (Type 1a versus 1c)
- ST elevation: V5–V6 and in II, III, aVF and minimal in I, aVL, could be due to simultaneous inferolateral AMI or to pericarditis.
- ST depression: V2–V3 is diagnostic of **posterior myocardial injury.**

Clinical Course
Echocardiography revealed an infero-postero-lateral WMA. Due to atypical symptoms and his young age, the patient was taken to the cath lab and his angiogram was normal. His CK peaked at 1,974 IU/L and cTnI peaked at 37 ng/mL. A sputum culture grew *S. pneumoniae* and he was diagnosed with myopericarditis.

Conclusion
Pain, ECG and echocardiographic findings of myopericarditis may mimic AMI exactly. In the context of atypical situations, including young age, fever, and lengthy, continuous symptoms, perform angiography ± PCI, if necessary.

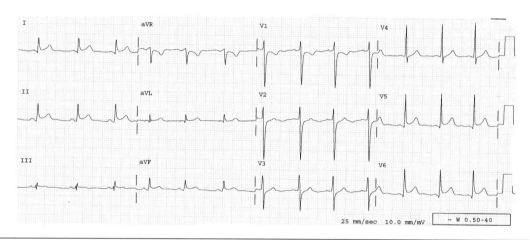

25 mm/sec   10.0 mm/mV   ~ W 0.50-40

CASE 24-7

Large Antero-Inferior AMI Easily Misdiagnosed as Pericarditis: aVL is the Clue

History

This 48-year-old woman presented with 1 hour of CP that she described as identical to pain experienced previously with pericarditis.

ECG 24-7 (Type 1a)

- The computer read this ECG as "pericarditis." However, ST elevation: II, III, and aVF; and **reciprocal ST depression: aVL,** are highly suspicious for **inferior AMI.** There are also hyperacute T waves: III, aVF, V2–V3.

Clinical Course

The patient was admitted with a diagnosis of pericarditis. Clinicians noticed the ST depression in aVL 2.5 hours later, and a repeat ECG revealed evolution of the AMI. The patient was taken to the cath lab and underwent successful angioplasty of a distally occluded "wraparound" LAD. A left ventriculogram showed acute apical dyskinesis.

Conclusion

A very large AMI may mimic pericarditis on the ECG.

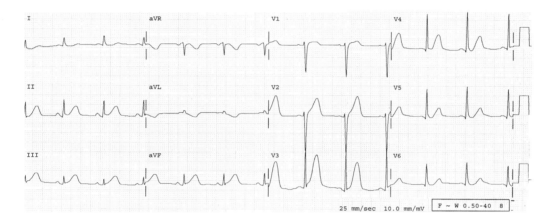

25 mm/sec   10.0 mm/mV   F ~ W 0.50-40 8

CASE 24-8

Thrombolytics Given in a Case of Pericarditis with an Extremely Difficult ECG

History
This 48-year-old man presented with 2 days of positional, pleuritic CP. He was hemodynamically stable.

ECG 24-8 (Type 1a versus 1c)
■ Diffuse ST elevation: characteristic of pericarditis with relative sparing of inferior leads, but **suspicious** for antero-infero-lateral AMI.
■ ST elevation is as high in V2 as in lateral leads, and there

is more ST elevation in the precordial leads than in the limb leads, both of which are unusual for pericarditis.
■ T wave appears hyperacute in V2, **suspicious** for AMI.

Clinical Course
The cardiologist diagnosed AMI and administered streptokinase (SK). Subsequently, he reconsidered and ordered an echocardiogram, which indicated no WMA. The infusion was stopped. The final diagnosis was pericarditis.

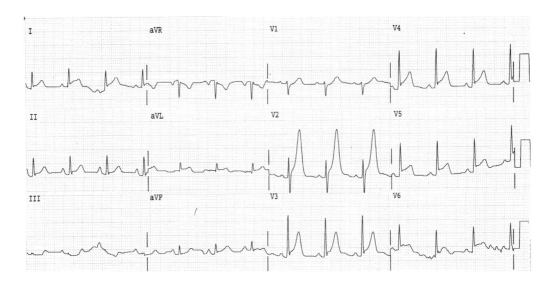

CASE 24-9

Clinical Symptoms Typical of Pericarditis and an ECG Very Worrisome for AMI

History

This 33-year-old man presented with constant sharp CP that worsened while supine and improved when sitting forward. There was no friction rub.

ECG 24-9 (Type 1a versus 1c)

■ Diffuse ST elevation: V1–V6, I, aVL, and minimal in II, aVF, is suggestive of pericarditis.

■ Reciprocal depression: III is **suspicious** for anterolateral AMI.

■ With early repolarization, which is also on the differential

diagnosis, the ST segment in V6 is generally less than 25% the height of the T wave.

Clinical Course

Immediate echocardiography was normal and serial cTnI levels were normal.

Conclusion

The ECG of pericarditis may mimic AMI. Clinical factors and adjunctive diagnostic modalities may be necessary to be sure that reperfusion therapy is not indicated.

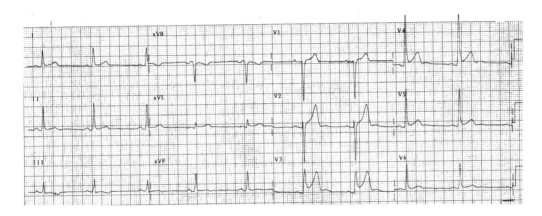

ANNOTATED BIBLIOGRAPHY

ECG Diagnosis of Pericarditis

Charles MA, et al. Atrial injury current in pericarditis, 1973.
Findings: Charles et al. (81) report five cases of pericarditis with PR-segment depression in all leads except aVR, which manifested PR elevation. They also review pre-1993 literature, which indicates that normal PR-segment depression does not exceed 0.8 mm.

Spodick DH. The electrocardiogram in acute pericarditis: distributions of morphologic and axial changes in stages, 1974.
Methods: Spodick (307) analyzed serial ECGs of 50 patients with pericarditis for ST, PR, and T-wave vectors over time.
Findings: All 50 patients had ECG findings of pericarditis, with 82% showing PR segment shifts that manifested as depression in most leads, with a right-posterior-superior PR vector. ST elevation in precordial leads increased from V1–V6, with the frontal plane vectors ranging from 0° to 90° in all cases (corresponding to leads I–aVF); the majority were from 30° to 60° (corresponding to maximum ST elevation in lead II).

Myocarditis as Pseudoinfarction

Sarda L, et al. Myocarditis in patients with clinical presentation of myocardial infarction and normal coronary arteries, 2001.
Methods: Sarda et al. (306) studied 45 consecutive patients admitted with (a) a diagnosis of AMI made by CP of 30 minutes or more, ischemic ECG abnormalities, and either elevation of CK-MB or cTnI and (b) normal coronary arteries by angiogram. They excluded patients with a clinical or ECG diagnosis of myocarditis, and those with pericarditis were obviously excluded by absence of biomarkers. Myocardial indium-111 antimyosin antibody/rest thallium 201 imaging allowed noninvasive detection of myocarditis.
Findings: Over a 31-month period, 1,280 patients were admitted for AMI; 45 (3.5%) had normal coronaries. ST elevation was present in 29 of 45, and thrombolytics or immediate angiography was performed in 18 of 45. Imaging revealed that 35 had myocarditis, 17 diffuse, and 18 focal. ST elevation correlated with regional wall motion and focal myocarditis.

Thrombolysis for Presumed AMI in Patients with Pericarditis Carries Little Excess Hazard

Millaire A, et al. Outcome after thrombolytic therapy of nine cases of myopericarditis misdiagnosed as myocardial infarction, 1995.
Findings: Millaire et al. (305) report nine patients with myopericarditis who received thrombolytics and heparin for presumed AMI. No severe complications occurred. One patient developed a pericardial effusion without tamponade. None developed hemopericardium. ECGs are not shown, but ST elevation is described as inferior and lateral in six cases, lateral in only two cases, and inferior in only one case. There is **no mention of ST depression,** which should be present in aVL for a diagnosis of **inferior AMI.**

Juneja R, et al. Intrapericardial streptokinase in purulent pericarditis, 1999.
Findings: Juneja et al. (309) report six cases of children with purulent pericarditis who were intentionally treated with intrapericardial SK.

Although one child developed intrapericardial hemorrhage, this child also had a submitral pseudoaneurysm that required surgery.

Comment: When pericarditis is present and severe, thrombolytics do not present an especially high risk for tamponade.

Huang CH, et al. Thrombolytic therapy complicated hyperacute cardiac tamponade in a patient with purulent pericarditis, 1996.

Findings: Huang et al. (311) report the case of an acutely ill-appearing 55-year-old febrile diabetic man with CP and ST elevation of 8 mm in V2. The patient received tPA and developed tamponade. Pericardiocentesis returned serosanguinous fluid diagnostic for purulent pericarditis. The patient ultimately did well.

Heymann TD, et al. Cardiac tamponade after thrombolysis, 1994.

Findings: Heymann et al. (317) report a case of hemopericardium with tamponade in a patient with recurrent pericarditis who received SK for suspected AMI. The ECG is not shown but is described as showing "widespread ST elevation" without ST depression.

Kahn JK. Inadvertent thrombolytic therapy for cardiovascular diseases masquerading as acute coronary thrombosis, 1993.

Findings: Kahn (310) reports one case each of pericarditis and myocarditis misdiagnosed as inferior AMI and given thrombolytics. Neither ECG manifested the reciprocal ST depression in aVL that is important for the diagnosis of AMI, and neither patient suffered adverse events.

Tilley WS, et al. Inadvertent administration of streptokinase to patients with pericarditis, 1986.

Findings: Tilley et al. (312) report two cases of pericarditis misdiagnosed as inferior AMI and given thrombolytics. Neither patient's ECG manifested the necessary reciprocal ST depression in aVL and neither patient suffered adverse events.

Ferguson DW, et al. Clinical pitfalls in the noninvasive thrombolytic approach to presumed acute myocardial infarction, 1986.

Findings: Ferguson et al. (313) report a case of myopericarditis misdiagnosed as inferior AMI and given thrombolytics. The ECG did not manifest the necessary reciprocal ST depression in aVL and the patient suffered no adverse events.

Blankenship JC, et al. Cardiovascular complications of thrombolytic therapy in patients with a mistaken diagnosis of acute myocardial infarction, 1989.

Findings: Blankenship et al. (314) report a case of pericarditis misdiagnosed as AMI and given thrombolytics. The ECG is atypical for AMI. Hemopericardium developed but was managed without adverse consequences.

Eriksen UH, et al. Fatal haemostatic complications due to thrombolytic therapy in patients falsely diagnosed as acute myocardial infarction, 1992.

Findings: Eriksen et al. (315) report a case of pericarditis misdiagnosed as AMI and given thrombolytics. The ECG was not diagnostic of AMI. The patient suffered lethal cardiac tamponade.

Barrington WW, et al. Cardiac tamponade following treatment with tissue plasminogen activator: an atypical hemodynamic response to pericardiocentesis, 1991.

Findings: Barrington et al. (316) report a patient who received tPA for suspected AMI and developed cardiac tamponade. Surgery revealed hemorrhagic pericarditis to be the source of 1.5 to 3.0 mm of ST elevation in leads V1–V6. The patient ultimately died as an indirect result of thrombolysis.

Khoury NE, et al. "Inadvertent" thrombolytic administration in patients without myocardial infarction: clinical features and outcome, 1996.

Methods: Khoury et al. (285) studied 609 consecutive patients treated with thrombolytics.

Findings: Thirty-five patients ruled out for AMI, three of whom had pericarditis and one of whom died. Cause of death is not reported and the ECGs are not shown.

25

HYPERKALEMIA

KEY POINTS

- Hyperkalemia may manifest ST elevation that mimics AMI.
- Look for prolonged QRS and peaked, tented T waves.
- ST elevation in the absence of QRS prolongation is NOT due to hyperkalemia.
- If there is any question, obtain serum potassium before committing to reperfusion therapy.

ECG DIAGNOSIS OF HYPERKALEMIA

Although hyperkalemia can usually be recognized by typical ECG manifestations, it may also occasionally be nearly indistinguishable from AMI. In addition to the clinical finding of elevated potassium, look for:

- **Diffuse, "tented" T waves** (narrow-based, very peaked), typically most prominent in **precordial leads V2–V5.**
- **Short QT interval,** when no QRS prolongation.

These findings may progress to intraventricular conduction delay (IVCD) with prolonged PR and QRS intervals, decreased P-wave amplitude or loss of P wave, ST-segment changes that simulate AMI, and cardiac arrhythmias. **In our experience, if ST elevation is due to hyperkalemia, the QRS will always be PROLONGED.**

The tented T waves of hyperkalemia contrast with **hyperacute T waves of AMI,** which are **localized, bulky, and wide, without much upward concavity** (176–178). Hyperacute T waves may be symmetric or asymmetric, peaked or blunted, and are typically associated with a prolonged QT interval (see Chapter 9).

Cases 25-1 through 25-4 were selected because they present diagnostic dilemmas. We have not selected the most typical, classic ECGs of hyperkalemia, which manifest peaked T waves, unless they also manifest ST elevation suggestive of STEMI.

CASE 25-1

Hyperkalemia Mimics Infarction

History

This 47-year-old man presented with DM and crushing chest CP.

ECG 25-1 (Type 1c)

- Peaked T waves, especially in V3–V6; prolonged QRS (125 ms); indistinct P waves; and prolonged PR segment are typical of hyperkalemia.
- ST elevation: V2–V3, is **suspicious** for AMI.

Clinical Course

The patient nearly received thrombolytics. Serum potassium was 9.0 mEq/L, pH was 6.97, and glucose was 700 mg/dL. The ECG recorded immediately after administration of calcium, bicarbonate, and insulin was nearly normal, and serial cTnI were normal.

Conclusion

The final diagnosis was diabetic ketoacidosis (DKA), with neither ACS nor AMI.

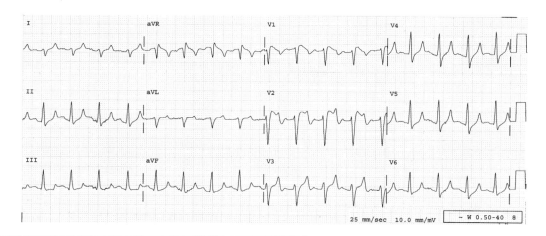

CASE 25-2

DKA Mimics Infarction

History

This 38-year-old diabetic man presented with nausea, vomiting, polyuria, and polydipsia. He had neither CP, abdominal pain, nor dyspnea.

ECG 25-2 (Type 1c)

- Peaked, tented T waves, especially in V3–V6; and prolonged QRS (119 ms) are typical of hyperkalemia.

- ST elevation: V2–V3, is **suspicious** for AMI.

Clinical Course

The patient's ECG normalized after he was treated for hyperkalemia.

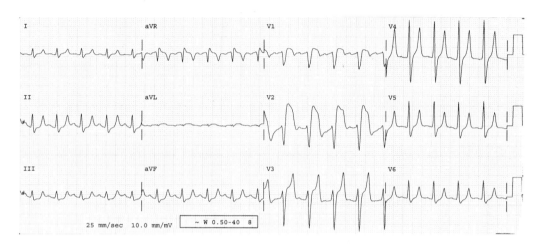

CASE 25-3

ECG Pseudoinfarction (New Atypical LBBB) Due to Hyperkalemia

History

This 76-year-old man with end-stage renal disease, who was regularly dialyzed, presented with weakness and malaise.

ECG 25-3 (Type 1c)

- ST elevation: V1–V3. Note also the very wide QRS (231 ms). The morphology is similar to a wide LBBB.

Clinical Course

The patient's serum potassium was 8.4 mEq/L. His ECG normalized 45 minutes later, following treatment of hyperkalemia.

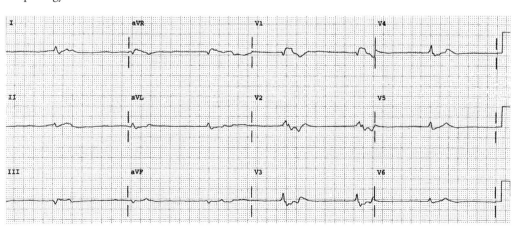

CASE 25-4

Hyperkalemia Mimics Inferior AMI

History

This 77-year-old man with a history of CHF, HTN, and atrial fibrillation, who was taking atenolol, diltiazem, digoxin, lisinopril, and furosemide, presented with dyspnea, bradycardia, hypotension, and waning mental status (shock). There was no improvement with atropine. The patient was intubated and paced transcutaneously with capture.

ECG 25-4 (Type 1c)

■ Possible idioventricular rhythm: bradycardia, no P waves, wide QRS (139 ms).
■ Low voltage, no peaked T waves.
■ ST elevation: II, III, reciprocal depression in aVL; and ST depression: V2–V6.

■ This ECG is not typical for hyperkalemia and is **suspicious** for inferoposterior AMI.

Clinical Course

The patient was treated with pressors. Potassium was returned at 8.0 mEq/L. After treatment with calcium, bicarbonate, glucose, and insulin, and hemodialysis for acute renal failure, the ECG normalized. Echocardiography revealed no WMA and serial cTnI were normal.

Conclusion

Hyperkalemia can produce various pseudoinfarction patterns.

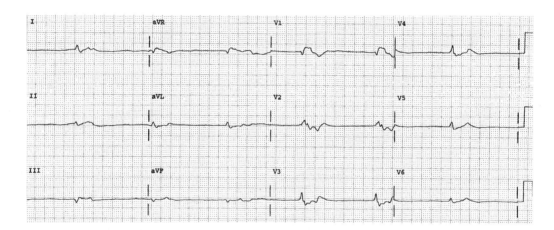

26

DYSPNEA, PULMONARY EDEMA, AND CARDIAC ARREST

KEY POINTS

- AMI often presents as dyspnea with or without chest pain (CP).
- When patients present with pulmonary edema and a suspicious ECG, treat the hemodynamic, physiologic, and metabolic abnormalities promptly and repeat the ECG before making the reperfusion decision.
- Suspect AMI even when dyspnea is explained by other etiologies.
- Altered mental status with ST elevation MI (STEMI) after resuscitated cardiac arrest is rarely due to intracranial bleed. In the absence of a preceding headache or significant trauma, do not delay thrombolytics.

DYSPNEA, PULMONARY EDEMA, AND THE ECG

General Background

It is beyond the scope of this book to discuss the pathophysiology and presentation of dyspnea, acute congestive heart failure (CHF), and pulmonary edema. We wish only to clarify the difficulties of interpretation of ST elevation in these clinical contexts and the subsequent implications for reperfusion therapy.

AMI often presents as dyspnea with or without CP (so-called anginal equivalent). In fact, the majority of AMI patients who present without CP (33% of all AMI) present with dyspnea (52). AMI may also present as **pulmonary edema** (see Cases 26-1 and 26-2). Furthermore, AMI may occur **concurrently** with dyspnea of other etiologies, especially underlying pulmonary disease. **In the presence of ST elevation, suspect AMI even when the dyspnea is explained by other clinical data** (see Cases 26-3 and 26-4). As with other atypical symptoms suggestive of AMI, always record an ECG in patients with dyspnea and risk factors for coronary artery disease (CAD).

Conversely, cardiogenic pulmonary edema is frequently the result of acute myocardial dysfunction that is not due to coronary occlusion, with ST elevation that simulates AMI. Thrombolytic "criteria" may be present, even in the absence of coronary occlusion, because many patients with pulmonary edema have cardiomyopathies with preexisting LVH, LBBB, or other intra-

ventricular conduction delay (IVCD) (see Case 26-5). Myocardial stunning from severe stress may result in ST elevation (Cases 26-6 and 26-7). Secondary ischemia may be present due to severe hypertension (HTN), tachycardia, anemia, or hypoxia.

Management

In patients with pulmonary edema and ST elevation, **treat the hemodynamic and metabolic abnormalities promptly and repeat the ECG** before making the reperfusion decision.

- Treat hypoxia and respiratory distress; endotracheal intubation may be necessary. **Avoid nasotracheal intubation if thrombolytic administration is a possibility.**
- Sedate, usually with a benzodiazepine, after intubation.
- Treat severe HTN with intravenous (IV) nitroglycerine (NTG).
- Treat pulmonary edema with high-dose NTG and a loop diuretic.
- Administer aspirin and an antithrombotic.
- Consider esmolol if not contraindicated by atrioventricular (AV) block, active wheezing, cardiogenic shock, or hypotension.
- Repeat the ECG immediately after stabilization.
- Treat **cardiogenic shock** (shock/hypotension with pulmonary edema) with angiography ± percutaneous coronary intervention (PCI), if available; consider hemodynamic monitoring and intraaortic balloon pump.

CARDIAC ARREST

AMI may present as resuscitated cardiac arrest, especially after ventricular tachycardia or fibrillation, and, less commonly, after bradyasystolic arrest. Any of these conditions may have nonischemic etiologies, but there may be confusing ST elevation due to conduction abnormalities, ventricular aneurysm, LBBB, or LVH.

Cardiac Arrest Without AMI

Consider primary ventricular fibrillation without AMI as the cause of cardiac arrest when there is

- A history of MI with subsequent poor ventricular function.
- A history of cardiomyopathy and low ejection fraction (EF).

- A history of previous malignant ventricular dysrhythmia.
- An absence of symptoms, especially CP or dyspnea, prior to arrest.
- LBBB (see Chapter 18), LVH (see Chapter 22) or ventricular aneurysm (see Case 26-8, Chapter 23, and Case 23-7).

Management

If the ECG shows unequivocal AMI, immediate reperfusion therapy is indicated. Even when the ECG is unequivocal, patients with **altered mental status** due to cardiac arrest are often **undertreated,** or experience treatment delays, due to concern for intracranial hemorrhage (ICH) (28). ICH only very rarely results in cardiac arrest due to ventricular fibrillation or ventricular tachycardia, and it is even more rare for a patient with primary ICH to have an unequivocally diagnostic (Type 1a or Type 1b) ECG. In this rare event, the prognosis is grim no matter what the management. Such a cardiac arrest should be assumed to be of cardiac etiology and altered mental status should be assumed to be due to hypoxia while in arrest. **Do not delay thrombolysis unnecessar-** ily to perform computed tomography (CT) of the head unless there is clear evidence, from history or physical exam, of significant head trauma during a fall after arrest. If there is significant suspicion of head trauma or spontaneous ICH, the patient should undergo a head CT. If the **head CT is positive, both angiography ± PCI and thrombolytic therapy are contraindicated** due to the need for procedural anticoagulation.

If the ECG manifests morphology of LBBB or ventricular aneurysm, obtain previous medical records and ECGs. With a history of cardiomyopathy, low EF, presence of an intraventricular cardioverter defibrillator or antidysrhythmic medications, consider a nonischemic cause of arrest. Previous echocardiography reports may also provide evidence of cardiomyopathy. **Keep in mind that these patients may also, of course, have coronary occlusion.** Emergency echocardiography may be very helpful by detecting a new regional wall motion abnormality (WMA) or by demonstrating ventricular aneurysm, although myocardial stunning can lead to false positives (150) (see Chapter 23). When the **diagnosis is in question, angiography ± PCI is preferred if available.**

CASE 26-1

Flash Pulmonary Edema and New LBBB Due to Coronary Occlusion

History

This 85-year-old man with no past medical history presented with sudden severe dyspnea but no CP. Physical exam revealed severe respiratory distress, pulmonary edema, BP = 180/90, and P = 110 to 145, in atrial fibrillation. He was intubated and given nitrates and diuretics.

ECG 26-1 (Type 1b versus 2)
- New LBBB and atrial fibrillation.
- ST depression: **concordant** in V3, and discordant but very deep in V4–V6, is **suspicious** for posterior STEMI and diagnostic of **ischemia.**

Clinical Course

Symptoms and ECG findings persisted despite medical therapy, but no immediate reperfusion therapy was undertaken. Cardiac troponin I (cTnI) returned at 10.4 ng/mL and angiography the following day revealed severe three-vessel disease, including 95% left anterior descending artery (LAD) stenosis, with flow, which was opened with angioplasty, and 100% right coronary artery (RCA) occlusion with collateral flow.

Conclusion

Reperfusion therapy is indicated for ischemic symptoms and new LBBB that persist despite anti-ischemic therapy, and, in this case, in spite of therapy for pulmonary edema and HTN. Fortunately, in this case, the outcome was acceptable without it.

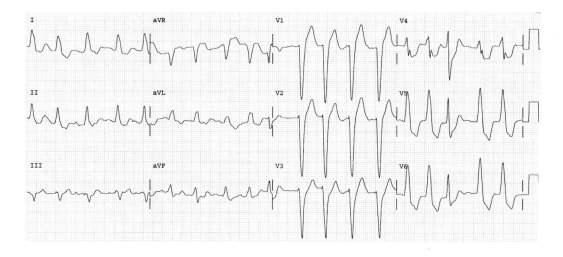

CASE 26-2

CP, Acute Pulmonary Edema, and Shock in a Patient with No Significant Past Medical History and a Nondiagnostic ECG: Immediate Angiography Is Indicated

History

This 71-year-old man with no past medical history complained of CP and severe dyspnea. He was intubated for severe pulmonary edema. An initial BP was moderately elevated at 160/110. NTG, furosemide, and sedation were administered. BP fell to 48/25 and recovered with pressors.

ECG 26-2 (Type 3)

■ QRS = 113 ms, with minimal ST elevation: V1–V3, indicates incomplete LBBB.

Clinical Course

This patient does not meet ECG criteria for thrombolytics. ED bedside echocardiogram revealed global severe hypokinesis. Heparin and aspirin were given, and immediate angiography revealed "severe stenosis" of the left main coronary artery. An intra-aortic balloon pump (IABP) was placed and the patient underwent immediate coronary artery bypass graft (CABG). CTnI were minimally elevated. The patient recovered fully.

Conclusion

Pulmonary edema with or without shock may be due to AMI/ischemia even with a nondiagnostic ECG.

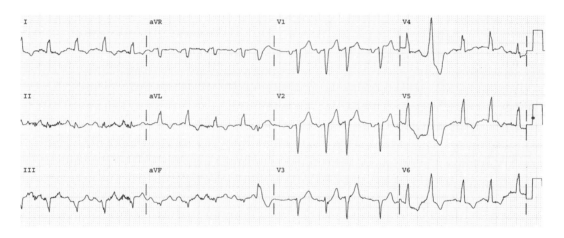

CASE 26-3

Apparent Severe Chronic Obstructive Pulmonary Disease (COPD) Exacerbation: Intubated, Unequivocal Anterior STEMI and Thrombolysis

History

This 72-year-old man with severe COPD presented with a typical exacerbation that was severe enough to require intubation. He did not complain of CP. He was intubated and his respiratory failure was stabilized.

ECG 26-3 (Type 1a)

■ ST elevation: V1–V3, is highly **suspicious** for AMI, and, in V4 is diagnostic of **anterior AMI.** Tall T waves, presence of R waves, and lack of Q waves suggest that coronary occlusion is very recent.

Clinical Course

Thrombolytics were administered. The LAD successfully reperfused. Creatine kinase-MB (CK-MB) levels were diagnostic of AMI.

Conclusion

Although dyspnea is often the only presenting symptom of AMI, when it is otherwise explained, the diagnosis must depend on an UNEQUIVOCAL (Type 1a) ECG. Time of onset may be difficult to ascertain without CP, but the ECG may be useful in determining acuteness (see Chapter 33).

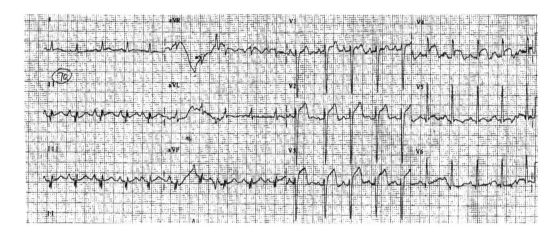

CASE 26-4

Fever, Cough, and Respiratory Failure Distract Clinicians from the ECG: New IVCD and Concordant ST Elevation of Inferior AMI

History
This 80-year-old man with 3 days of upper respiratory symptoms developed fever and severe dyspnea. He was in severe respiratory distress, with oxygen saturation = 68% on room air, with BP = 160/74, P = 133, and T = 103° F. He was intubated and the chest x-ray showed neither pulmonary edema nor infiltrate.

ECG 26-4 (Type 1c)
After stabilization revealed sinus tachycardia.

- QRS duration > 120 ms indicates new IVCD (not LBBB because intrinsicoid deflection is < 40 ms).
- **Concordant** ST elevation: subtle, II, III, aVF; with **concordant** reciprocal depression: aVL, are **suspicious** for inferior AMI.

Clinical Course
Reperfusion, preferably immediate angiography ± PCI, is indicated if there is no ECG resolution after stabilization. If unavailable, immediate echocardiography would be helpful to look for inferior WMA. However, clinicians overlooked the ECG findings. An influenza screen returned positive and the patient developed pulmonary edema. CK peaked at 1,024 IU/L, with a cTnI of 27 ng/mL. A repeat ECG showed **deep inferior Q waves and ST-segment resolution.** Echocardiography revealed anterior-apical and inferoposterior WMAs with severely decreased left ventricular (LV) function. When symptoms recurred 16 hours later, the patient underwent angiography, which revealed severe three-vessel disease. Angioplasty was performed and the patient eventually recovered.

Conclusion
The ECG may reveal an AMI when it is least expected.

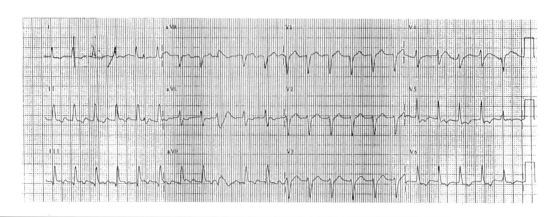

CASE 26-5

Pulmonary Edema and ST Elevation Due to LVH

History

This 45-year-old man with HTN presented with pulmonary edema and no CP. BP = 210/100 and P = 140.

ECG 26-5 (Type 1c)

■ LVH by voltage.

■ ST elevation: 2 mm, V2–V4, is consistent with LVH but **could be** STEMI.

Clinical Course

The patient was intubated and treated with NTG. CK-MB was negative. Echocardiography revealed concentric LVH without WMA and coronary arteries were normal.

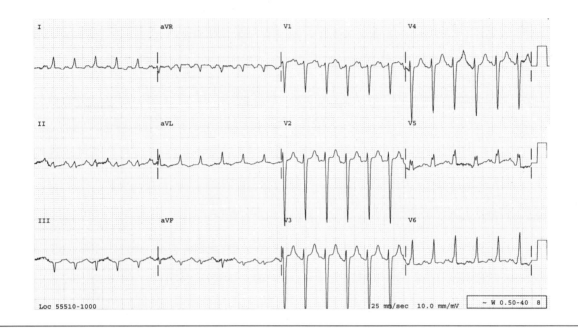

CASE 26-6

ST Elevation and IVCD Associated with Severe HTN and Pulmonary Edema

History

This 74-year-old man presented with sudden severe dyspnea. On exam, he was in severe distress, BP = 240/140, P = 126, and pulmonary edema. Bedside ED echocardiography showed overall poor LV function, but exam quality was inadequate for assessment for a WMA.

ECG 26-6 (Type 1a versus 1c)

■ QRS duration = 116 ms; ST elevation: 2 mm, V1–V3.

Clinical Course

Comparison with an old ECG revealed that these findings were new. The patient was orotracheally intubated and treated aggressively with IV NTG for HTN and pulmonary edema, resulting in a BP = 150/90 and P = 110. ST segments were normalized on a repeat ECG only 19 minutes later. Angiography revealed no significant coronary disease and serial troponins were negative.

Conclusion

Severe respiratory distress with severe HTN may be associated with ST elevation that may resolve after stabilization. Reperfusion therapy is indicated for persistent ECG changes. Echocardiography would be helpful. Given the uncertainty, angiography ± PCI is a more prudent strategy of reperfusion. This permits both diagnosis and therapy, as well as hemodynamic monitoring and placement of intra-aortic balloon pump, if necessary.

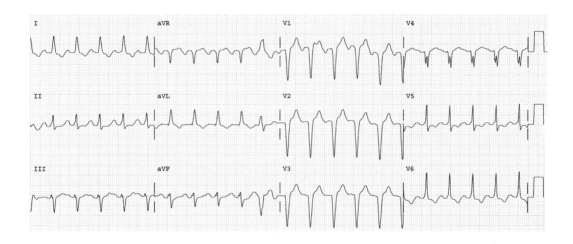

CASE 26-7

COPD and Respiratory Failure with Diagnostic ECG but No Coronary Occlusion

History

This 54-year-old man with COPD called 911 for dyspnea and CP. He presented to a small hospital in respiratory failure with severe acute respiratory acidosis. Attempted nasotracheal intubation resulted in significant bleeding. Orotracheal intubation was successful.

ECG 26-7A (Type 1a)

V1–V6 only

- ST elevation: V1–V3, up to 5 mm in V3, is diagnostic of **anterior AMI.**

Clinical Course

Thrombolytics would be indicated except for the nasal bleeding. The patient was transferred to tertiary care center. His vital signs were stable on arrival. He was sedated and paralyzed.

ECG 26-7B (Type 1c)

V1–V6 only

- ST elevation: resolved in V3, but persistent in V1–V2.

Clinical Course

The patient was taken immediately for PCI. Angiography revealed normal coronary arteries but a ventriculogram revealed severely depressed LV function. Cardiac troponin I (cTnI) peaked at 10 ng/mL. The patient fully recovered with therapy for COPD. Convalescent echocardiography demonstrated an EF that was near normal.

Conclusion

"**Myocardial stunning**" from critical illness can mimic AMI on the ECG and on ventriculography and echocardiography. It is believed to be due to extreme sympathetic overload with vasospasm and may be fully reversible.

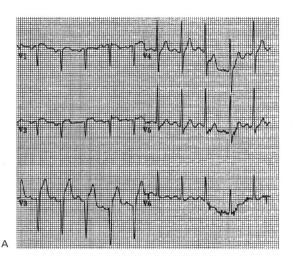

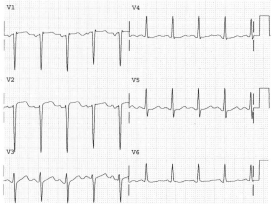

CASE 26-8

Ventricular Fibrillation with ST Elevation Mimics AMI but Is Due to Ventricular Aneurysm

History

This 72-year-old man's wife witnessed his collapse and reported that he had not complained of CP. He was resuscitated and transported.

ECG 26-8 (Type 1c)

- ST elevation: V1–V4, and minimal: V5, **suspicious** for AMI.
- QR pattern with ST elevation: V4; Qr wave with ST elevation: V3; deep QS wave: V1, V2 suggest ventricular aneurysm.

- Although the presentation and ECG suggest ventricular aneurysm, **acute STEMI is possible.**

Clinical Course

Reperfusion therapy was not undertaken. Biomarkers were negative.

Conclusion

The patient's clinical presentation was not highly suggestive of AMI and the ECG was typical of ventricular aneurysm. Thrombolytics are not indicated in a case such as this, although angiography ± PCI may be indicated.

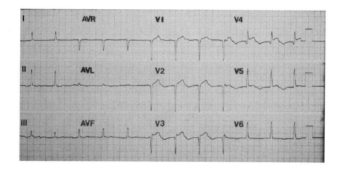

27

REPERFUSION AND REOCCLUSION

KEY POINTS

- **Strongly consider rescue angioplasty if there is no ECG evidence of reperfusion by 60 minutes after thrombolytic administration, particularly if there is a large amount of myocardium at risk.**
  - **ECG evidence of reperfusion: (a) 50% resolution or more of ST segments, without reelevation OR (b) Terminal T-wave inversion.**
- **If relief of CP is unaccompanied by any ST resolution or T-wave inversion, it is NOT diagnostic of reperfusion.**

GENERAL BACKGROUND

Arterial Patency and Microvascular Circulation

Reperfusion therapy is guided by the ongoing assessment of myocardial reperfusion. This depends on two factors: (a) **reperfusion** of the epicardial infarct related artery (IRA); and (b) reperfusion of the **microvascular circulation,** which may be damaged by ischemia and reperfusion (the "no-reflow" phenomenon) and result in impeded capillary flow.

Hemodynamic status and **age** are the best clinical prognostic indicators for AMI outcome. The best ECG indicator for AMI outcome is **ST resolution** or the lack thereof **(318–322)**. The **best overall predictor** of failed myocardial reperfusion is a finding of **< 50% recovery of ST segments from maximal elevation.** However, the ECG cannot determine whether the cause of failed reperfusion is persistent arterial occlusion or microvascular damage. Angiography is necessary to assess and grade IRA patency and microvascular circulation and to guide subsequent therapy. **Rescue PCI,** which we define as PCI undertaken within 6 hours of the start of thrombolytic therapy **(323)**, should be strongly considered when clinicians have determined that thrombolytic reperfusion has failed **(324)**. This is especially true for a **large AMI,** as indicated by anterior location, high ST elevation, or ST deviation in numerous leads. A patent IRA with inadequate flow may be due to residual stenosis or abnormal microvascular circulation and may be treated with **vasodilators, antiplatelet, and antithrombotic agents ± PCI.**

TIMI Grading of IRA Patency

IRA patency can only be definitively assessed by angiography. Angiographic assessments are then systematized by TIMI grading, as follows (325):

- TIMI-0 = no flow.
- TIMI-1 = penetration of contrast without perfusion. These patients have persistent ST elevation and a poor prognosis and must be identified for rescue PCI.
- TIMI-2 = partial reperfusion. These patients may have resolution of ST elevation and a prognosis intermediate between TIMI 0/1 and TIMI 3 flow.
- TIMI-3 = complete reperfusion. These patients usually (but not always) show ST resolution. TIMI-3 flow after reperfusion is associated with lower mortality and lower incidence of CHF **(326,**327), but its prognostic value **may not be independent of resolution of ST elevation (318)**.

By outcome measures, a flow grade **of less than TIMI-3 indicates failed reperfusion** (26,328). After reperfusion therapy for AMI, TIMI-3 flow is associated with a 30- to 42-day mortality of 3.6%, in contrast to TIMI-2 flow (6.6% mortality) and TIMI-0/1 flow (9.5% mortality) (327).

TIMI Frame Count

The TIMI frame count (TFC) further systematizes TIMI flow categorization. The TFC is the measure of the exact number of cineangiographic frames required for contrast to reach a defined distal segment of the IRA. (See the background discussion under "Angiographic Reperfusion Grades" in the annotated bibliography of this chapter.)

TIMI Myocardial Perfusion Grading of Microvasculature

TIMI flow and TFC are impacted by both the severity of the underlying stenosis and thrombus and by the microvasculature. Intact microvasculature is most accurately assessed by the appearance on an angiogram of diffuse and faint highlighting of the myocardium by contrast, known as "myocardial blush." These assessments are systematized with TIMI myocardial perfusion grading (TMP), which is based on a scale from 0 to 3 as follows **(319,326,329)**:

- TMP grade 0 = no microvascular perfusion
- TMP grade 1 = no clearance of contrast
- TMP grade 2 = slow clearance of contrast
- TMP grade 3 = normal clearance

An open coronary artery may have brisk TIMI-3 flow but have a TMP grade of 0 or 1 (**326**); patients with these findings show persistent ST elevation (**318,319,329**). **TMP grade 3 is associated with a good prognosis, independent of TIMI flow.**

ECG DIAGNOSIS OF REPERFUSION

ST Segments in Reperfusion

With a **reperfused IRA AND intact microcirculation,** ST segments usually fall **rapidly** and are near baseline **within 3 hours** of reperfusion (see Case 27-1). Approximately 80% of cases with IRA reperfusion manifest 50% ST recovery within 90 minutes. Most of the remaining 20% likely have microvascular injury with resultant poor capillary flow; their prognosis is as poor as patients with poor flow in the IRA (**318,319,329**). This contrasts with a **nonreperfused IRA,** in which ST segments fall **gradually and plateau,** with or without persistent elevation. ST resolution without IRA reperfusion is a result of **myocardial cell death,** and occurs as early as 6 to 12 hours after occlusion (**330**).

ST resolution is an accurate predictor of reperfusion, especially in patients whose ECGs show ST elevation > 4 mm (**331**). During or shortly before reperfusion, ST segments often continue to rise before resolving, frequently with an increase in CP (**156,157,332,333,334**). Some patients experience "**cyclic reperfusion,**" in which there is reperfusion and subsequent reocclusion. This may occur with or without therapy. Cyclic reperfusion occurs in 25% to 30% of AMI before reperfusion therapy and can be detected with ST-segment monitoring (**335**).

T Waves in Reperfusion

In **reperfused AMI, terminal T-wave inversion** often occurs **rapidly** (within 90 minutes) in the leads that manifested the greatest ST elevation on presentation, and before full ST resolution (**156,157**). This contrasts with **nonreperfused AMI, 90% of which show gradual T-wave inversion** (over 48 to 72 hours), with a depth < 3 mm (**94**) (Fig. 8-3). If there is some **myocardial injury,** as measured by elevated troponin, expect terminal T-wave inversion to **develop into deep and symmetric T-wave inversion over the first 48 hours** after the onset of AMI (**94**) (see Case 27-2). Accordingly, early T-wave inversion (less than 24 hours) is associated with greater IRA patency, better perfusion grade, and a more benign in-hospital course than later inversion (**336**). In some patients with very early reperfusion and very little or no myocardial cell death, as measured by troponin, there may be no T-wave inversion, very late inversion, or reversible inversion (**94**).

Q-wave and R-wave changes are **not** accurate markers of AMI reperfusion (**337**).

Reperfusion Monitoring

Monitoring for reperfusion may include observation of 5 elements, as follows: (1) ST resolution, or "recovery"; (2) terminal T-wave inversion; (3) resolution of CP; (4) reperfusion arrhythmias; and (5) biochemical markers.

1. ST Resolution

ST-segment resolution, or "recovery," is the best marker for reperfusion (see Cases 27-1 and 27-2). ST segments may be monitored continuously or with static ECGs every 5 minutes from the time of thrombolytic administration. **If ST elevation is > 4 mm and there is NEITHER ≥ 50% recovery at 60 minutes NOR terminal T-wave inversion, TIMI-3 flow is unlikely. Strongly consider rescue PCI.**

Continuous ST-segment monitoring is the best method for monitoring ST-segment changes (**156,159,338,339**) (see Case 27-3). Commercial products are available. Select one lead with the greatest ST elevation, plot the ST-segment elevation continuously, and observe for peaks and troughs. By convention, ST elevation is measured on continuous monitors at 80 ms after the J point. See Table 27-1.

- **ST recovery ≥ 50% from MAXIMAL** ST elevation (peak level attained) within 60 minutes and without re-elevation is a very good predictor of reperfusion. These patients do not need early angiography or rescue PCI. ST recovery of ≥ 50% or more has a positive predictive value (PPV) for patency (TIMI-2 or -3 flow) of 87%.
- **ST recovery < 50%, consider rescue PCI.** The negative predictive value (NPV) for occlusion (lack of recovery) is 71% (i.e., 71% of patients who do not show ST recovery ≥ 50% have closed arteries and 29% have TIMI 2–3 flow). These patients **are** candidates for rescue PCI. Most important, **ST recovery < 50% with no terminal T-wave inversion indicates a TIMI flow of 0–2 with a PPV of 86%.** TIMI-3 flow is true successful reperfusion. Of patients with persistent ST elevation (< 50% recovery), 14% have TIMI-3 flow but presumably continue to have ST elevation due to microvascular injury.
- The higher the maximal or initial ST elevation, the more accurate the patency prediction (**331**).

Although **static ECGs** are inferior to continuous ST-segment monitoring (**339**), if continuous monitoring is unavailable, recording **static ECGs every 5 minutes** from the time of thrombolytic administration is a reasonable substitute (**158**). Use the single lead with the highest ST elevation and measure resolution from the maximal height. ST resolution > 50% at 60 minutes after treatment is a good indicator of reperfusion (**158**). Complete ST resolution ensures reperfusion but occurs infrequently by 60 minutes after treatment (**339**).

2. Terminal T-Wave Inversion

See also Chapter 8.

Terminal T-wave inversion within the first 90 minutes is a specific marker of reperfusion and is approximately 60% sensitive (**156,157,158**). If leads with ST elevation develop terminal T-wave inversion within 60 minutes of thrombolysis, reperfusion is highly

TABLE 27.1. UTILITY OF "OCCLUSION" FOR PREDICTING TIMI-0 TO -2 FLOW (NOT -3)ᵃ

Sensitivity	Specificity	PPV	NPV ("probably not occluded")
45%	94%	86%	67%

ᵃ*Occluded* refers to < 50% decrease in ST elevation, or increase, or reocclusion. *Probably not occluded* refers to ≥ 50% decrease of ST elevation with no reelevation.

likely. Because T-wave inversion usually indicates some myocardial injury, rapid ST resolution without any T-wave inversion may be evidence that reperfusion occurred before myocardial cell death; in such cases, biomarkers may not be elevated. Terminal T-wave inversion usually occurs before full resolution of the ST segment.

Deep, symmetric T-wave inversion (> 3 mm) indicates reperfusion that is **less recent** than reperfusion indicated by terminal T-wave inversion (see Case 27-2). Terminal T-wave inversion undergoes further development into symmetric T-wave inversion (**94**). Deep, symmetric T-wave inversion need not be preceded by ST elevation, although there is usually no development of Q waves without ST elevation. Symmetric T-wave inversion is generally present after full resolution of the ST segment.

T waves also eventually invert in persistently occluded vessels. T-wave inversion in the presence of deep Q waves, especially QS waves, may be a manifestation either of reperfusion late in the course of AMI or of a **well-developed, nonreperfused AMI** (**94**,340). These inverted T waves are usually < 3 mm, in contrast with inverted T waves of reperfused AMI, which are > 3 mm (**94**). Such T-wave inversion may be evident at presentation if the patient presents late after onset (see Case 33-3).

With posterior AMI, if the T wave is upright before reperfusion and there is ST recovery, reperfusion usually results in precordial T waves (especially V2) becoming fully upright and taller and wider than before AMI onset. This is a reciprocal view of posterior inverted T waves. Reocclusion in this case is unlikely to result in T-wave inversion. If the T wave is asymmetrically inverted before reperfusion, reperfusion usually results in T waves pseudonormalizing (turning upright) and becoming taller and wider than before the onset of AMI; reocclusion generally results in reinversion of T waves (see Case 27-1; see also Cases 13-4 and 16-9).

3. Relief of CP

Two studies showed that **complete relief of CP,** often with an initial transient **increase** in pain, had a good PPV, with an 84% (**339**) to 96% (156) chance of reperfusion. However, relief of CP with neither any recovery of ST segments nor terminal T-wave inversion is unlikely to represent reperfusion. If CP resolves, record serial ECGs; pursue rescue angioplasty if there is no ECG evidence of reperfusion.

With **spontaneous relief of CP,** do not abort reperfusion unless accompanied by some amount of ST recovery:

- With increased, unchanged, or < 25% ST elevation resolution, continue reperfusion therapy.
- With 25% to 50% resolution, or terminal T-wave inversion, record serial ECGs or continuous monitoring and look for ≥ 50% ST resolution.
- With 50% to 100% resolution, reperfusion therapy may be suspended, pending further assessment, especially continuous ST monitoring.

Relief of CP has a poor NPV, in that persistent pain did not necessarily imply persistent occlusion (**159,339**).

4. Reperfusion Arrhythmias

Occurrence of accelerated idioventricular rhythm (AIVR) indicates reperfusion with 97% specificity but only 45% sensitivity (**166,335**). A sudden burst of ventricular tachycardia may also indicate reperfusion.

5. Biochemical Markers of Reperfusion

Biochemical markers may also be useful in assessing reperfusion; see Chapter 29 for details.

See Cases 27-1 to 27-3 for examples of reperfusion. (See also Cases 6-4, 12-3, 16-9, 20-10, and 32-1.)

Management

A meta-analysis of randomized trials showed that rescue angioplasty performed in patients with failed reperfusion results in a decreased incidence of CHF, death, and recurrent MI, without significant adverse effects (**324**). These trials were performed **without** the latest technology and with prolonged time intervals from thrombolysis to rescue. In this age of GPIIb–IIIa inhibitors and stenting, **we highly recommend rapid rescue PCI for failed reperfusion** as evidenced by the previously mentioned ECG indicators or by persistent clinical instability. If TIMI-3 flow is present but TMP grade is low, treatment with vasodilators, antiplatelet, and antithrombotic agents is particularly important.

REOCCLUSION

Once reperfusion is achieved, monitor ST segments for reocclusion. Symptoms are **not** reliable indicators of reocclusion and many recurrent AMIs are asymptomatic (69,**89**). If continuous monitoring is unavailable, **record frequent static ECGs every 30 to 60 minutes until stability is ensured.** At a minimum, record hourly ECGs for several hours after reperfusion.

ECG Manifestations of Reocclusion

Each AMI has an "ischemic fingerprint," such that reocclusion of the same vessel at the same location reproduces the same ECG findings (83,**190**). Thus reocclusion manifests the reverse of reperfusion on the ECG, as follows:

- **Initial rapid "pseudonormalization" of T waves,** in which inverted T waves turn upright.
- **Subsequent re-elevation of ST segments.**

Caution: **post-infarction regional pericarditis (PIRP)** may mimic reocclusion (see Chapter 28) (**94**). This is characterized by **gradual** pseudonormalization of T waves or persistent upright T waves in the leads that had the greatest ST elevation at presentation. There is also **gradual ST re-elevation,** over 24 to 72 hours. PIRP lacks the typical diffuse ST elevation of nonspecific pericarditis.

See Case 27-3, of reocclusion. (See also Case 8-12, of pseudonormalization of symmetrically inverted T waves; Case 13-4, of an inferoposterior AMI with reperfusion and reocclusion; and Case 3-3, of reocclusion a week after reperfusion.)

Management

Reocclusion after thrombolysis mandates either repeat thrombolysis or, preferably, rescue angiography ± PCI (340.5).

CASE 27-1

Complete ST-Segment Recovery Indicating Rapid TIMI-3 Reperfusion

History
This 45-year-old male smoker with history of single-vessel CABG 4 years earlier presented with 1.5 hours of severe left-sided CP that was unrelieved by 4 sublingual NTG tablets.

ECG 27-1A (Type 1a)
- ST elevation: II, III, aVF; with ST depression: aVL, V1–V6, are diagnostic of **inferoposterior AMI.**

Clinical Course
A right-sided ECG revealed 3 mm ST elevation in V3R–V6R, diagnostic of extensive **infero-postero-right ventricular (RV) AMI.** ST depression in V4–V6 may be re-ciprocal to right-sided ST elevation. The patient received tPA within 10 minutes of ECG 27-3A.

ECG 27-1B (Type 2)
Twenty minutes after tPA bolus
- Complete resolution of ST elevation and depression.
- Shallow symmetric T-wave inversion: II, III, aVF, consistent with reperfusion. Notice the large upright T waves in V2, indicative of posterior reperfusion.

Clinical Course
Peak cTnI was 2.7 ng/mL, which indicates minimal injury.

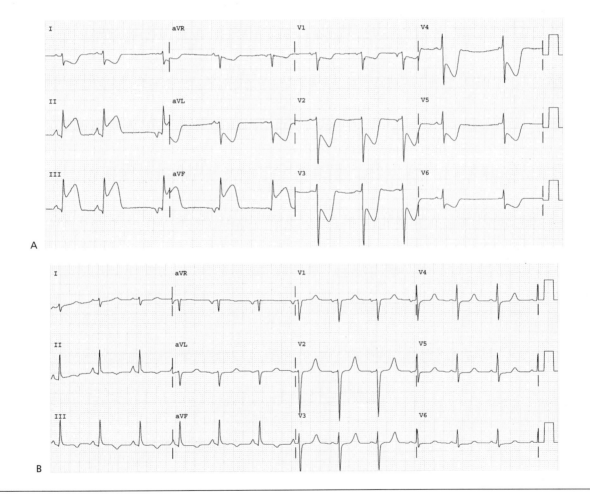

CASE 27-2

Reperfusion Demonstrated by Terminal T-Wave Inversion, Despite Increased ST Elevation

History
This 69-year-old man presented with CP.

ECG 27-2A (Type 1a)
- ST elevation: II, III, AVF, maximum of 2 mm in II; and ST depression: aVL, V2–V3, are diagnostic of **inferoposterior AMI.** The ST score (summed ST elevation and depression) is 7. Clinicians administered tPA immediately.

ECG 27-2B (Type 1d)
Thirty-two minutes after tPA
- ST score has increased to 9 to 10. It is **unclear** whether the ST segment is now rising or falling, because these are static ECGs.

- Terminal T-wave inversion: II, III, aVF, is highly specific for reperfusion; newly upright T wave: V2, and newly inverted T wave: V3, indicate posterior reperfusion.

ECG 27-2C (Type 2)
Ninety minutes after tPA
- ST resolution is complete, and symmetrically inverted T waves in II, III, aVF, and V3–V5 indicate that reperfusion is less acute. Notice the upright T wave in V2.

Conclusion
These ECGs demonstrate reperfusion.

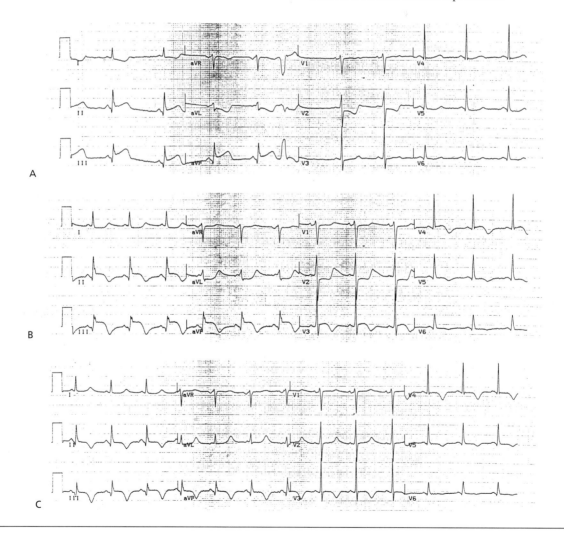

CASE 27-3

Continuous ST Monitoring Reveals Reperfusion and Subsequent Reocclusion

History

This 47-year-old man presented with CP that started at 16:30. He received tPA at 17:40 and was transferred to the cardiac care unit (CCU) on two-lead continuous ST monitoring of II and aVF, starting at 17:49. Lead aVF was monitored due to greatest initial ST elevation (9.7 mm), as measured 80 ms after the J point, which is the convention with continuous monitors.

ECG 27-3A

At 17:49, 9 minutes after tPA, shows II and aVF only.
- ST elevation: 4.2 mm in aVF.

ECG 27-3B

At 19:02, shows II and aVF only. CP was completely resolved.
- ST segments are nearly isoelectric.

ECG 27-3C

At 19:45, shows II and aVF only. At 125 minutes after tPA, the alarm sounded for recurrent ST elevation. The patient experienced recurrent CP.
- ST elevation: 4.9 mm, aVF.

ECG 27-3D

- Graphs of time versus ST elevation for leads II and aVF shown in ECGs 27-3A through 27-3C. This illustrates the dramatic ST resolution and subsequent reelevation.

Clinical Course

Rescue angioplasty opened a 100% occluded RCA.

Conclusion

Continuous monitoring clearly shows reperfusion and reocclusion.

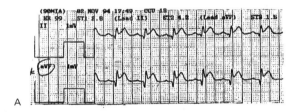

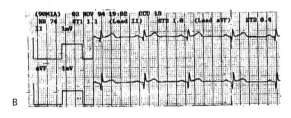

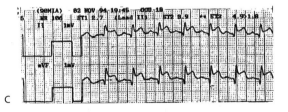

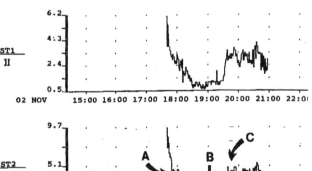

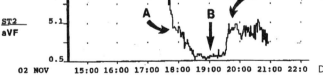

ANNOTATED BIBLIOGRAPHY

Reperfusion: General Background

Krucoff MW, et al. Continuously updated 12-lead ST-segment recovery analysis for myocardial infarct artery patency assessment and its correlation with multiple simultaneous early angiographic observations, 1993.

Methods: Krucoff et al. (341) performed angiography and continuous ST-segment monitoring in 22 AMI patients.

Findings: Forty-four episodes of arterial patency and multiple ST trend transitions in 11 of 22 patients after thrombolysis suggested cyclic changes in coronary flow before catheterization.

Comment: These authors and others (158,159) have shown repeatedly that ST recovery must be measured from **maximal** ST elevation for accurate assessment of reperfusion. Peak ST elevation may occur in the absence of or any time after thrombolytic therapy. Static ECGs are less effective than continuous monitoring because ST segments may rise from baseline before actual reperfusion and fall again (or vice versa) to nearly the same level without detection.

Angiographic Reperfusion Grades, Persistent ST Elevation, and Prognosis

Background: **TIMI flow grade** is a measurement of reperfusion of a coronary vessel, and **TMP flow grade** is a measurement of myocardial microvascular perfusion. TFC is the measure of the exact number of cineangiographic frames required for contrast to reach a defined distal segment of the IRA. TFC is especially helpful to further categorize TIMI-2 and TIMI-3 flow. Normal mean TFCs are 36.2 ± 2.6 for the LAD, 20.4 ± 3.0 for the RCA, and 22.2 ± 4.1 for the circumflex artery (342). To standardize TFC for all arteries, the TFC of the LAD is divided by 1.7 to give a "corrected" TFC (CTFC) (342). At 90 minutes after thrombolysis for STEMI in all locations. a CTFC of 0 to 13 is above normal blood flow and is associated with 0 mortality. A CTFC of 14 to 40 is associated with mortality of 2.7%, and a CTFC of more than 40 is associated with mortality of 6.4% (343). Of patients with TIMI-3 flow, a CTFC $\leq$ 20 versus one > 20 is associated with complication rates of 7.9% versus 15.5%, respectively (343).

Van't Hof, et al. Clinical value of 12-lead electrocardiogram after successful reperfusion therapy for acute myocardial infarction, 1998.

Methods: Van't Hof et al. (320) studied ST resolution in 403 AMI patients with TIMI-3 flow after primary angioplasty.

Findings: ST segments normalized in 51% of patients (ST < 0.1 mV). Partial normalization (30% to 70% of initial height) was associated with a relative risk (RR) of death of 3.6 (confidence interval [CI] = 1.6 to 8.3) compared with full normalization (< 30% of initial height). Absence of resolution or increased ST elevation was associated with a RR of death of 8.7 (range, 3.7 to 20.1).

Van't Hof AW, et al. Angiographic assessment of myocardial reperfusion in patients treated with primary angioplasty for acute myocardial infarction: myocardial blush grade, 1998.

Methods: Van't Hof et al. (329) studied myocardial blush during primary angioplasty in 777 AMI patients.

Findings: Angioplasty resulted in TIMI-3 flow in 89% of patients and in TIMI-0, -1, or -2 flow in 11%. Patients with TMP grades 3, 2, and 0/1 had (a) CK infarct sizes of 757 IU/L, 1,143 IU/L, and 1,623 IU/L; (b) EFs of 50%, 46%, and 39%; and (c) mortality (after a mean follow-up of 1.9 ± 1.7 years) of 3%, 6%, and 23%, respectively. TMP grade predicted mortality independently of Killip class, TIMI grade flow, EF, and other clinical variables. TMP grade was the best predictor of 3-year mortality, with rates of 3%, 15%, and 37% for patients with grades 3 (19% of patients), 2, and 0/1, respectively. Among TMP grade 3 patients, ST elevation normalized in 65% and ST elevation decreased in an additional 28%.

Gibson CM, et al. Relationship of TIMI myocardial perfusion grade to mortality after administration of thrombolytic drugs, 2000.

Methods: Gibson et al. (326) studied 762 patients in the TIMI-10B trial, in which 854 patients with AMI were randomized to tenecteplase tissue plasminogen activator (TNK-tPA) or standard alteplase and underwent angiography at 90 minutes post-thrombolytic administration.

Findings: TMP grade 3 myocardial perfusion was independently associated with low 30-day mortality of 2.0%, as compared with 3.5% for patients with TIMI-3 flow. The decreased risk was additive to the low risk of TIMI-3 flow, such that mortality was a mere 0.73% (1 of 137) for patients with TIMI-3 flow **and** TMP grade 3 perfusion compared with a 10.9% mortality (14 of 129) for those with both TIMI 0-2 **and** TMP 0/1 grading. Mortality was approximately the same for patients with (a) both TIMI 0-2 flow and TMP grade 3 perfusion, presumably through collaterals; and (b) both TIMI-3 flow and TMP 0/1 perfusion.

ST Recovery and Prognosis

ST recovery can be a good prognostic indicator, even in the presence of an occluded vessel. Lack of ST recovery portends a poor prognosis, even with an open artery.

Claeys MJ. Determinants and prognostic implications of persistent ST-segment elevation after primary angioplasty for acute myocardial infarction: importance of microvascular reperfusion injury on clinical outcome, 1999.

Methods: Claeys et al. (319) studied 91 AMI patients with reperfusion after angioplasty.

Findings: Of 91 patients, 75 had TIMI-3 and 16 had TIMI-2 flow. Persistent ST elevation, defined as ST $\geq$ 50% of the initial height, was observed in 33 (36%) patients and was associated with high 1-year mortality (15% versus 2%) and high total major adverse cardiac event rate (45% versus 15%). **Persistent ST elevation was the most important independent determinant of major adverse cardiac event rate,** with an adjusted RR of 3.4, and both were attributed to impaired microvascular circulation.

Shah A, et al. Prognostic implications of TIMI flow grade in the infarct-related artery compared with continuous 12-lead ST-segment resolution analysis: reexamining the "gold standard" for myocardial reperfusion treatment, 2000.

Methods: Shah et al. (318) identified 258 AMI patients who underwent thrombolysis and then angiography in the TIMI-7 and GUSTO-1 trials (see Appendix C). Patients were stratified according to TIMI 0-3 reperfusion and by ST resolution $\geq$ 50% versus < 50%.

Findings: **ST resolution WAS an independent predictor of the combined clinical outcome of death or CHF but TIMI flow grade was NOT.** ST resolution among patients with TIMI grade 0–1 flow identified a group with a relatively benign clinical course.

Dissman R, et al. Early assessment of outcome by ST-segment analysis after thrombolytic therapy in acute myocardial infarction, 1994.

Methods: Dissman et al. (321) studied CK levels and EFs in 77 AMI patients to correlate ST resolution and infarct size.

Findings: The enzyme-determined infarct size and the resulting EF correlated closely with complete (> 70%), partial (30% to 70%), or no ST (< 30%) resolution at 3 hours after thrombolysis. EFs were 58%, 53%, and 43% for patients with complete, partial, or no resolution, respectively.

Schroder R, et al. Extent of early ST-segment elevation resolution: a strong predictor of outcome in patients with acute myocardial infarction and a sensitive measure to compare thrombolytic regimens, 1995.

Methods: Schroder et al. (322) analyzed ECGs, CK levels, and mortality data of 1,909 AMI patients randomized to reteplase or streptokinase (SK).

Findings: In 1,398 patients who presented 6 hours or more from AMI onset, 35-day mortality rates for complete ($\geq$ 70%), partial (30% to 70%), or no (< 30%) ST resolution by 3 hours after thrombolytic administration were 2.5%, 4.3%, and 17.5%, respectively.

Saran RK, et al. Reduction in ST-segment elevation after thrombolysis predicts either coronary reperfusion or preservation of left ventricular function, 1990.

Methods: Saran et al. (344) studied ST-segment changes and angiographic findings in 45 patients. (See more detailed annotation later.)

Findings: LV function was well preserved if the ST segment had fallen by ≥ 25% at 3 hours.

Continuous ECG Monitoring for Prediction of Reperfusion

Note: It is important to remember when evaluating the following studies that 15% of IRAs are open **without any treatment** (including aspirin and heparin) by 6 to 8 hours after coronary occlusion (345).

Krucoff MW, et al. Continuous 12-lead ST-segment recovery analysis in the TAMI 7 study. Performance of a noninvasive method for real-time detection of failed myocardial reperfusion, 1993.

Methods: Krucoff et al. (159) tested a method of 12-lead continuous ST-segment recovery in a blinded, prospective, and angiographically correlated study of 144 TAMI-7 patients who received thrombolytics in early AMI. Summated ST elevation was plotted against time by PC-based software and read by experienced cardiologists. The ST segment was plotted and assessed for peaks, troughs, and general trend. The ST score at the moment of angiography was compared with the peak elevation attained. Patency was predicted based on ST recovery, defined as a 50% drop from the maximum summated ST elevation, and continued downward trend. Occlusion was predicted by (a) persistent ST elevation, (b) reelevation after recovery or a downward trend, or (c) increased ST elevation. The study was considered indeterminate if no definite peaks or troughs and corresponding trends could be discerned.

Findings: There were 144 ST-segment analyses. Of 35 angiograms performed during definite (re-)elevation periods (indicating **occlusion**), 25 IRAs were angiographically occluded. Of 91 angiograms during definite recovery periods (indicating **reperfusion**), 81 IRAs were angiographically patent. Of 18 indeterminate analyses, 14 were angiographically patent. If the indeterminate group is considered to be "probably not occluded," then the IRA was patent in 95 of 109 cases (87%) so predicted and occluded in 25 of 35 cases (71%) so predicted. Of 35 patients whose ST recovery analysis determined IRAs to be "occluded" (based on persistent or recurrent ST elevation), only five had TIMI-3 flow. In 109 patients, analysis determined "probably not occluded" ("indeterminate" or "patent"), and 73 of these had TIMI-3 flow, 22 had TIMI-2 flow, and 14 had TIMI-0 or 1 flow. Thus **"occluded" had a PPV for TIMI 0-2 flow of 86% and "probably not occluded" had a sensitivity of 94% and a PPV of 67% for TIMI-3 flow and of 87% for TIMI-2 or -3 flow.**

Comment: Postthrombolytic TIMI-3 flow is associated with a much better outcome than even TIMI-2 flow (26,328). Therefore the ability to distinguish TIMI-3 flow from TIMI-0 to -2 flow on the ECG is important.

Klootwijk P, et al. Non-invasive prediction of reperfusion and coronary artery patency by continuous ST segment monitoring in the GUSTO-I trial, 1996.

Methods: Klootwijk et al. (331) studied ECGs of 373 GUSTO-1 patients (see Appendix C) using continuous 12-lead ST-segment recovery analysis.

Findings: The predictive values for reperfusion or persistent occlusion were not as good as in the study of Krucoff et al. described earlier (159). Angiograms were performed significantly later (between 90 and 180 minutes) in this study. Thus the predictive accuracy would be expected to be lower because ST segments in areas of persistent infarction decline over time, due to myocardial cell death. A decrease of ≥ 50% from peak and no persistent reelevation before angiography was used as a prediction of "patent." Accuracy was very high (79% to 100%) in patients with high ST elevation (> 4 mm). In 116 patients with a peak ST elevation ≥ 4 mm, a prediction of "patent" had a PPV of 79% and NPV of 75%.

Doevendans PA, et al. Electrocardiographic diagnosis of reperfusion during thrombolytic therapy in acute myocardial infarction, 1995.

Methods: Doevendans et al. (156) performed continuous ST-segment monitoring of 61 AMI patients for 60 minutes after thrombolytic therapy.

Findings: **Reperfusion was associated with rapid ST resolution, often after a transient elevation.** Of 44 patients with reperfusion, 42 showed ≥ 25% decrease in ST elevation from maximal height (sensitivity 95%), but only one of 17 patients without reperfusion showed this amount of normalization (specificity 94%). Using a 50% decrease in ST elevation as a cutoff, sensitivity was 85% (38 of 44 patients) and specificity was, again, 94%. **Relief of CP** was also a very sensitive sign of reperfusion; 25 of 26 patients with reperfusion had relief within 1 hour. Eighteen patients experienced relief after a transient, often marked, increase in pain. **Terminal T-wave inversion was very specific for reperfusion;** 28 of 44 patients with reperfusion had terminal T-wave inversion, whereas only one of 17 without reperfusion had terminal T-wave inversion. **AIVR was a specific but insensitive marker of reperfusion;** 16 of 42 in the reperfused group demonstrated AIVR versus one of 17 in the nonreperfused group. Other "reperfusion arrhythmias" were uncommon and of little prognostic utility. CK-MB peaked earlier in the reperfused group.

Veldkamp RF, et al. Comparison of continuous ST-segment recovery analysis with methods using static electrocardiograms for noninvasive patency assessment during acute myocardial infarction, 1994.

Methods: Veldkamp et al. (346) analyzed ECGs and clinical data from 82 patients in the preceding study by Krucoff et al. (159) to compare continuous ST recovery analysis with five static methods.

Findings: Static methods such as those used by Saran et al. (344), Hackworthy et al. (347), and Clemmensen et al. (348) had comparable accuracies to continuous ST recovery analysis; see the following section on static ECGs.

Hohnloser SH, et al. Assessment of coronary artery patency after thrombolytic therapy: accurate prediction using the combined analysis of three noninvasive markers, 1991.

Methods: Hohnloser et al. (338) used Holter monitoring and angiography in a prospective study of 82 patients undergoing thrombolysis for first MI.

Findings: Of 82 patients, 63 had TIMI-2 or -3 reperfusion. A 50% reduction in ST elevation measured 60 to 90 minutes after thrombolysis had a PPV of 97% and an NPV of 43% for reperfusion. **CK peak of less than 12 hours was an accurate marker of reperfusion.**

Frequent Static ECGs

Shah PK, et al. Angiographic validation of bedside markers of reperfusion, 1993.

Methods: Shah et al. (158) obtained static ECGs every 5 to 10 minutes after thrombolytic therapy in 82 AMI patients, for up to 3 hours, until angiography.

Findings: Their findings were very similar to those of Doevendans et al. (156) described earlier. Angiography demonstrated that 69 of 82 patients had a patent IRA with TIMI-3 flow and that these patients consistently manifested a **rapid, progressive decrease in both CP and ST elevation.** Pain resolved in 24 ± 23 minutes (maximum 50 minutes) and decreased ST elevation ≥ 50% occurred within 16 ± 14 minutes (maximum 41 minutes) after restoration of TIMI-3 flow. **Terminal T-wave inversion and AIVR were also specific but insensitive markers of reperfusion.** This study demonstrates the importance of frequent static ECGs and the insensitivity of using only two static ECGs to detect reperfusion. In 58% of patients, ST segments were unstable, rising and falling, before final resolution.

Infrequent Static ECGs

Califf RM, et al. Failure of simple clinical measurements to predict perfusion status after intravenous thrombolysis, 1988.

Methods: Califf et al. (339) performed angiography on 386 TAMI patients at 60 and 90 minutes after administration of tPA. They recorded a baseline ECG and another at 90 minutes after tPA, before the 90-minute coronary injection.

Findings: **They found no sensitive AND specific marker of reperfusion using infrequent static ECGs.** Complete resolution of ST segment and T-wave changes was associated with a 96% IRA patency rate at 90 minutes after tPA, but this occurred in only 6% of patients. Only 38% of patients had "partial resolution" of ST segments, 84% of whom showed reperfusion. Complete resolution of CP occurred in 29%, of whom 84% had reperfusion of the IRA. Unchanged or worsened CP occurred in 20%, of whom 60% showed reperfusion. Patent IRAs were demonstrated in 56% of patients with neither symptom nor ST resolution and 63% of patients with no change in ST segments showed reperfusion. Although arrhythmias occurred frequently during the first 90 minutes of therapy, none were associated with a higher patency rate.

Saran RK, et al. Reduction in ST-segment elevation after thrombolysis predicts either coronary reperfusion or preservation of left ventricular function, 1990.

Methods: Saran et al. (344) performed angiography on 45 AMI patients by 3 hours after administration of anistreplase.

Findings: Using the lead with the greatest ST elevation on **static ECGs,** ST recovery ≥ 25% at 3 hours was nonspecific. ST segments had fallen by ≥ 25% in 30 of 31 patients with TIMI-2 or -3 reperfusion, but also in eight of 14 patients who had only TIMI-0 or -1 flow. Thus if the ST segment fell by ≥ 25%, the specificity was only 43%; that is, many IRAs remained occluded. **Three hours after thrombolytic therapy is too late for ST recovery** to be a meaningful indication of reperfusion because ST segments fall, even in persistently infarcted myocardium, though more gradually. It is **also too late to make a decision for rescue PCI.** If the ST segment fell by < 25%, persistent occlusion was likely, with a PPV of 86%. Importantly, **the global EF was well maintained** in patients whose **ST segments fell > 25% and whose arteries were occluded.** Saran et al. concluded that a reduction in ST elevation > 25% within 3 hours of thrombolysis indicates either a patent IRA or preservation of LV function.

Clemmensen P, et al. Changes in standard electrocardiographic ST-segment elevation predictive of successful reperfusion in acute myocardial infarction, 1990.

Methods: Clemmensen et al. (348) studied 53 patients up to 8 hours post SK administration. They calculated the ST score as the sum of ST elevation in 11 leads, based on static ECGs obtained within 5 minutes of angiography.

Findings: Angiography demonstrated reperfusion (TIMI-2 or -3 flow) in 33 of 53 patients. A decrease ≥ 20% in ST elevation was 88% sensitive and 80% specific for reperfusion, with a PPV of 88% and an NPV of 80%. Clemmensen et al. concluded that a **decrease of only 20% in the ST score following thrombolytic therapy is a useful and noninvasive predictor of reperfusion status in patients with evolving AMI.**

Comment: The use of angiographic patency assessment up to 8 hours after treatment diminishes the value of this data.

T-Wave Inversion and Prognosis
See also Doevendans et al. (156) earlier.

Oliva PB, et al. Electrocardiographic diagnosis of postinfarction regional pericarditis: ancillary observations regarding the effect of reperfusion on the rapidity and amplitude of T-wave inversion after acute myocardial infarction, 1993.

Methods: Oliva et al. (94) studied 200 AMI patients to assess serial T-wave changes as prognostic indicators.

Findings: Ninety percent of patients with reperfusion demonstrated a maximum T-wave negativity ≥ 3 mm in the lead that initially showed the greatest ST elevation within 48 hours of CP onset. Seventy-six percent of patients with no reperfusion demonstrated a maximum T-wave negativity ≤ 2 mm within 72 hours. Oliva et al. conclude that **rapid evolution and deepening of the T wave may be useful noninvasive markers of reperfusion.**

Matetzky S, et al. Early T wave inversion after thrombolytic therapy predicts better coronary perfusion: clinical and angiographic study, 1994.

Methods: Matetzky (336) et al. performed admission and predischarge angiography and radionuclide ventriculography on 94 consecutive AMI patients who received tPA.

Findings: **Early T-wave inversion (less than 24 hours) was associated with greater IRA patency, better perfusion grade, and a more benign in-hospital course.** Additionally, although the number of patients with normal EFs (>55%) at presentation was similar, 71% of

patients with early T-wave inversion had a normal EF at discharge, versus 44% of patients without early T-wave inversion.

Increased Pain and ST Elevation After Thrombolytic Therapy
Dissman R, et al. Sudden increase of the ST-segment elevation at a time of reperfusion predicts extensive infarcts in patients with intravenous thrombolysis, 1993.

Methods: Dissman et al. (332) measured ST elevation and CK every 15 minutes after thrombolytic administration in 61 AMI patients.

Findings: Eight patients showed increased ST elevation immediately after reperfusion. This was associated with an enzymatically very large AMI, a very early enzyme peak, and much worse LV EF (39% ± 14% versus 58% ± 11%, $p < 0.0005$). Six patients also experienced very clearly intensified CP at the time of the ST elevation. The study by Doevendans et al. (156) described earlier and a study by Wehrens et al. (157) both found a similar increase in CP after treatment and before ECG evidence of reperfusion.

Reciprocal Depression and Reperfusion
Shah A, et al. Comparative prognostic significance of simultaneous versus independent resolution of ST-segment depression relative to ST-segment elevation during acute myocardial infarction, 1997.

Methods: Shah et al. (143) performed continuous ST-segment monitoring of 413 AMI patients who received thrombolytics; 261 patients met technical criteria for blinded analysis of ST depression resolution patterns.

Findings: In-hospital mortality was 13% among patients whose reciprocal ST depression persisted after resolution of ST elevation versus 1% mortality for patients whose ST elevation **and** ST depression resolved simultaneously.

Reperfusion Arrhythmias
Although there is little literature to support malignant reperfusion ventricular arrhythmias, many interventionalists and clinicians who treat AMI are certain that runs of ventricular tachycardia are directly related to opening the IRA, especially in large infarcts that are reperfused very early.

Gorgels AP, et al. Usefulness of the accelerated idioventricular rhythm as a marker for myocardial necrosis and reperfusion during thrombolytic therapy in acute myocardial infarction, 1988; Goldberg S, et al. Limitation of infarct size with thrombolytic agents: electrocardiographic indexes, 1983; and Miller FC, et al. Ventricular arrhythmias during reperfusion, 1986.

Methods: Gorgels et al. (349) and Goldberg et al. (350) were among the first to describe "reperfusion arrhythmias." Gorgels et al. prospectively studied 87 patients admitted with ischemic CP, and Goldberg et al. studied 44 AMI patients who underwent angiography. Miller et al. (351) conducted Holter monitoring of 52 patients.

Findings: Gorgels et al. found AIVR in 27 of 70 AMI patients with reperfusion. Goldberg et al. found some type of reperfusion arrhythmia, most commonly AIVR, in 20 of 27 AMI patients with reperfusion. Miller et al. found no significant relationship of either AIVR or ventricular tachycardia with reperfusion or persistent occlusion.

Hohnloser SH, et al. Assessment of coronary artery patency after thrombolytic therapy: accurate prediction using the combined analysis of three noninvasive markers, 1991.

Methods: Hohnloser et al. (338) prospectively studied 82 first AMI patients treated with thrombolytics.

Findings: AIVR was associated with reperfusion only in inferior AMI.

Shah PK, et al. Angiographic validation of bedside markers of reperfusion, 1993.

Findings: Shah et al. (158) (described earlier) found that 49% of patients with reperfusion developed AIVR.

Gore JM, et al. Arrhythmias in the assessment of coronary artery reperfusion following thrombolytic therapy, 1988.

Methods: Gore et al. (352) performed angiography within 8 hours of symptom onset in 67 AMI patients treated with thrombolytics.

Findings: Fifty-six patients had total IRA occlusion, 25 of whom reperfused within 90 minutes of treatment. Arrhythmias (including AIVR) were not significantly associated with reperfusion.

Gressin V, et al. Holter recording of ventricular arrhythmias during intravenous thrombolysis for acute myocardial infarction, 1992.
> *Methods:* Gressin et al. (353) performed 24-hour Holter monitoring of 40 AMI patients treated with thrombolytics.
> *Findings:* Increased incidence of AIVR was associated with IRA patency.

Clements IP. The electrocardiogram in acute myocardial infarction, 1998.
> *Findings:* Clements (335) cites a thesis by Veldkamp, who combined analysis from six studies (317 patients) and found that early AIVR predicted patency with a specificity of 97% but a sensitivity of only 45%.

Vectorcardiography
Dellborg M, et al. Dynamic QRS complex and ST-segment vectorcardiographic monitoring can identify vessel patency in patients with acute myocardial infarction treated with reperfusion therapy, 1991.
> *Findings:* Dellborg et al. (354) identified 15 of 16 patients with reperfusion and five of six with persistent occlusion using vectorcardiographic analysis of ST vectors. Further detail is beyond the scope of this book. See Clements (335) for an excellent discussion of alternative electrocardiographic methods such as vectorcardiography and precordial mapping. See also von Essen et al. (355) and Badir et al. (356) for vectorcardiographic analyses of reperfusion.

Rescue PCI
Ross AM, et al. Rescue angioplasty after failed thrombolysis: technical and clinical outcomes in a large thrombolysis trial, 1998.
> *Methods:* Ross et al. (323) analyzed GUSTO-1 (see Appendix C) data on rescue angioplasty, defined as angioplasty undertaken within 6 hours of the start of thrombolytic therapy. They compared 198 patients selected nonrandomly for rescue angioplasty, 226 patients with failed thrombolysis who were managed conservatively, and 1,058 patients with successful thrombolysis.
> *Findings:* Patients with rescue angioplasty had more impaired LV function before intervention. Rescue was successful in 88.4% of occluded arteries, resulting in TIMI-3 flow in 68%. Successful rescue angioplasty was associated with **better LV function and lower mortality** than conservative management of occluded arteries. Neither bleeding complications (8.6% versus 6.8%) nor the need for CABG (1.0% versus 0.4%) differed significantly between the two groups.

Ellis SG, et al. Randomized comparison of rescue angioplasty with conservative management of patients with early failure of thrombolysis for acute anterior myocardial infarction, 1994.
> *Methods:* Ellis et al. (357) randomized 151 patients with first anterior AMI and failed thrombolysis, as determined by angiography done within 8 hours after treatment, to angioplasty or to conservative management.
> *Findings:* Angioplasty performed at a mean of 4.5 ± 1.9 hours after thrombolytic therapy was successful in 72 of 78 (92%) patients. Outcomes in the angioplasty versus conservatively managed groups, respectively, were death in 5% versus 10% ($p = 0.18$), severe heart failure in 1% versus 7% ($p = 0.11$), and either death or severe heart failure in 6% versus 17% ($p = 0.05$). LV function at rest did not differ.

McKendall GR, et al. Value of rescue percutaneous transluminal coronary angioplasty following unsuccessful thrombolytic therapy in patients with acute myocardial infarction, 1995.
> *Methods:* McKendall et al. (358) studied 133 patients enrolled in TIMI Phase I Open Label and Phase II trials; 100 had received no rescue angioplasty and 33 patients had undergone rescue angioplasty by protocol (not by physician choice) if the 90-minute angiogram revealed persistent IRA occlusion.
> *Findings:* Time to angioplasty from symptom onset or from thrombolytic treatment is not stated but appears to be **90 to 120 minutes.** The two groups had similar baseline features. Rescue was technically successful in 26 of 33 patients (82%). Mortality at 21 days was

12% in the rescue group and 7% in the no-rescue group (p = NS). Failed rescue was associated with a mortality of 33%. Mean LV EF was the same in both groups.

CORAMI Study Group. Outcome of attempted rescue coronary angioplasty after failed thrombolysis for acute myocardial infarction, 1994.
> *Methods:* The CORAMI Study Group (359) evaluated short- and mid-term outcomes of 299 consecutive AMI patients who received thrombolytics less than 6 hours after symptom onset and underwent angiography at 90 minutes after thrombolytics.
> *Findings:* Of 299 patients, 87 (29%) had failed thrombolysis (TIMI-0 to -1 flow), of whom 72 underwent rescue angioplasty **within 8 hours of symptom onset.** Seven patients (10%) were in cardiogenic shock at the time of angiography. Technical success (TIMI-3 flow) was achieved in 65 patients (90%) at a mean of 300 ± 101 minutes after thrombolytic therapy. Nine patients (12%) had access site hematoma. Three patients (4%) died, two of 65 successful rescues and one of seven failed rescues.

Gibson C, et al. Rescue angioplasty in the Thrombolysis in Myocardial Infarction (TIMI) 4 trial, 1997.
> *Methods:* Gibson et al. (360) studied 95 AMI patients with failed thrombolysis (TIMI 0-1 flow) in the TIMI-4 trial.
> *Findings:* Fifty-eight patients underwent rescue angioplasty **120 minutes** after thrombolytic therapy and 37 had no rescue angioplasty. Rescue and nonrescue groups had similar baseline characteristics. Fifty-two of 58 procedures were successful. In-hospital adverse outcomes, including death, recurrent AMI, severe CHF, cardiogenic shock, and EF of less than 40%, occurred in 35% of rescue cases (29% of successful rescues and 83% of failed rescues, $p = 0.01$), and also in 35% of nonrescue cases (p = NS).

Miller JM, et al. Effectiveness of early coronary angioplasty and abciximab for failed thrombolysis (reteplase or alteplase) during acute myocardial infarction (results from the GUSTO-III trial), 1999.
> *Methods:* Miller et al (361) prospectively studied 392 patients entered into the GUSTO-III trial (reteplase versus tPA for STEMI) (362) who underwent rescue angioplasty in a nonrandomized fashion; 83 patients received abciximab and 309 did not.
> *Findings:* When adjusted for baseline differences, patients who received abciximab had significantly lower mortality. Incidence of severe bleeding (without ICH) with versus without the use of abciximab during angioplasty was 3.5% versus 1.0% ($p = 0.08$).

Ellis SG, et al. Review of immediate angioplasty after fibrinolytic therapy for acute myocardial infarction, 2000.
> *Methods:* Ellis et al. (324) performed a meta-analysis of nine heterogeneous randomized trials of rescue angioplasty (1,456 patients).
> *Findings:* Rescue angioplasty decreased the incidence of CHF, death, and recurrent MI.

In summary, although the value of rescue PCI makes intuitive and scientific sense, the available studies are too small and the methodology inadequate for definite conclusions. All the studies had a minimum delay of 2 hours and a mean delay of 4 to 5 hours between thrombolytic therapy and balloon inflation. None used up-to-date technique, including stents, abciximab, and/or clopidogrel. **We recommend rescue PCI for large infarctions with no ECG evidence of reperfusion at 1 hour after thrombolytic therapy** unless and until there are studies that take these factors into account and demonstrate **lack of efficacy.**

Reocclusion
Langer A, et al. Prognostic significance of ST-segment shift early after resolution of ST elevation in patients with myocardial infarction treated with thrombolytic therapy: the GUSTO-I ST Segment Monitoring Substudy, 1998.
> *Methods:* Langer et al. (363) performed ST-segment monitoring within 30 minutes of thrombolytic therapy in 734 AMI patients.
> *Findings:* "ST-segment shift," defined as elevation ≥ 1 mm in the 6 to 24 hours after reperfusion, was correlated with 7.8% mortality at 30 days and 10.3% mortality at 1 year versus 2.3% and 5.7% mortality, respectively, for patients without ST shift.

Ohman EM, et al. Consequences of reocclusion after successful reperfusion therapy in acute myocardial infarction, 1991.

Methods: Ohman et al. (89) studied 810 AMI patients who had angiography performed 90 minutes after thrombolytic therapy.

Findings: Reperfusion occurred acutely in 735 patients, 645 of whom (88%) underwent angiography 7 days later. IRA **RE**occlusion occurred in 91 patients (14%) and was symptomatic in 53. Reocclusion was associated with greater in-hospital mortality (11% versus 4.5%), a more complicated hospital course, and initial angiographic findings, including RCA stenosis, a greater degree of stenosis, and lower TIMI flow grade.

Dissman R, et al. Early recurrence of ST-segment elevation in patients with initial reperfusion during thrombolytic therapy: impact on in-hospital reinfarction and long-term vessel patency, 1994.

Methods: Dissman et al. (364) performed 24-hour Holter monitoring on 81 AMI patients.

Findings: ST resolution within the first 4 hours occurred in 67 patients (83%), 31 of whom (46%, Group 1a) did have subsequent ST reelevations and 36 of whom (54%, Group 1b) did not. Group 1a had a much greater incidence of CK-MB-confirmed reinfarction (26% versus 6%) and angiographic occlusion at follow-up (40% versus 17%) than Group 1b.

Veldkamp RF, et al. Performance of an automated real-time ST-segment analysis program to detect coronary occlusion and reperfusion, 1996.

Methods: Veldkamp et al. (212) used an automated real-time ST-segment analysis program to detect reocclusion during 78 balloon occlusions in 31 patients.

Findings: The program detected balloon reocclusion and reperfusion within seconds of all occlusions that caused a peak ST elevation of ≥ 0.2 mV.

Krucoff MW, et al. Stability of multilead ST-segment "fingerprints" over time after percutaneous transluminal coronary angioplasty and its usefulness in detecting reocclusion, 1988.

Methods: Krucoff et al. (190) analyzed multilead ST-segment recordings performed during angioplasty in 39 patients.

Findings: Similar to Bush et al. (83) described earlier, within 1 hour, balloon occlusion during repeat angioplasty resulted in an identical "ischemic fingerprint" 90% of the time. AMI of the same vessel within 24 hours of the balloon inflation resulted in this ischemic fingerprint 87% of the time. Thus **reocclusion reliably produces the initial ECG pattern of infarction.** Monitoring for reocclusion can be done using continuous ST-segment monitoring.

28

MYOCARDIAL RUPTURE AND POSTINFARCTION REGIONAL PERICARDITIS

KEY POINTS

- Myocardial rupture occurs in 1% to 3.5% of AMI patients and is often preceded by post-infarction regional pericarditis (PIRP).
- PIRP is indicated by persistently positive (upright) T waves 48 hours after onset of AMI.
- PIRP is very likely if there is premature, gradual reversal of inverted T waves to positive deflections by 48 to 72 hours after AMI onset; this contrasts with the rapid reversal of reocclusion.
- Any patient in shock may have tamponade, usually due to myocardial rupture.
- Bedside echocardiography can easily confirm myocardial rupture.

GENERAL BACKGROUND

At least 10% of all deaths from AMI are due to myocardial rupture (365). Although commonly perceived to be a sudden event, myocardial rupture is often due to an infiltrating intramural hemorrhage and a slow tear that occurs over 24 hours or more (366). Myocardial rupture may therefore be better characterized as myocardial leakage that causes hemopericardium and death due to pericardial tamponade. Myocardial rupture is associated with **late thrombolysis** (12 to 24 hours after symptom onset), and **delayed hospital admission** (more than 24 hours after onset of symptoms) (367,368). Myocardial rupture may involve the septum and lead to acute ventricular septal defect. Although myocardial rupture occurs most commonly among inpatients, it may also occur at presentation to a medical facility for cardiogenic shock, CP, dyspnea, or other symptoms suggestive of AMI.

Myocardial rupture may be preceded by PIRP in up to 94% of cases (366). PIRP may occur when necrosis extends from the subendocardium to the subepicardium (transmural infarction), causing inflammation. PIRP is diagnosable from the ECG with high sensitivity and specificity (94,366). Transmural necrosis and inflammation may result in myocardial rupture or leakage. Obviously, **thrombolytic therapy may be hazardous** in patients with myocardial rupture. Myocardial rupture is eas-

ily confirmed by detection of pericardial fluid with brief, limited bedside echocardiography, which may be performed by clinicians with limited training (369). Note, however, that pericardial fluid may also be due to hemorrhagic PIRP without rupture (370). **If diagnosed immediately, myocardial rupture is treatable with emergency surgery (369,371,372).** Myocardial rupture at hospital presentation is sufficiently rare that routine echocardiography for AMI patients should only be performed if it can be done within minutes. This is only possible if the clinician has immediate access to a sonogram located in the patient care area.

Septal rupture may also result from transmural infarction.

ECG DIAGNOSIS OF PIRP

Atypical T-Wave Development in PIRP

Two patterns of atypical T-wave development occur during PIRP, before free wall rupture (FWR) (94). These patterns contrast notably with typical T-wave development during the course of AMI. **In PIRP,** leads showing ST elevation of AMI will also show:

1. **Persistently positive (upright) T waves** 48 hours after AMI onset; this is **diagnostic** of PIRP.
2. **Premature, gradual reversal of inverted T waves to positive (upright) deflections** by 48 to 72 hours after AMI onset; this is 77% specific for PIRP. Although small AMIs with early reperfusion may also manifest with gradual reversal of inverted T waves, such a small AMI is less likely to have Q waves or significant diminution of R waves.

These two atypical patterns contrast with **typical T-wave development of AMI with NO PIRP.** ECG leads with ST elevation of AMI show **gradual 1- to 3-mm inversion** of T waves over 48 to 72 hours in nonreperfused AMI or **rapid and deep (> 3-mm) inversion** of T waves over 24 hours in reperfused AMI (94).

ST Segments in PIRP

ST segments reelevate in 40% of cases of PIRP. Additionally, PIRP does **not** manifest with diffuse ST elevation, as does viral pericarditis.

Summary

If the T wave flips upright and/or the ST segment reelevates, is it PIRP or reocclusion?

PIRP

- The T wave **gradually** becomes upright, typically beginning **more than 48 hours** after the onset of AMI.
- If the ST segment reelevates, it does so **more slowly** than in reocclusion.
- Pleuritic CP similar to viral pericarditis.
- **Pericardial friction rub** is possible.

Reocclusion

- ST and T wave changes are **rapid.**
- Associated with symptoms of ischemia.

See Case 28-1 for an example of PIRP without rupture, Cases 8-4 and 28-2 for examples of myocardial rupture without evidence of PIRP, and Case 28-3 for an example of septal rupture with PIRP.

MANAGEMENT

ECG evidence of PIRP, as well as clinical suspicion, should prompt vigilance for myocardial rupture, which can then be diagnosed by bedside echocardiography.

CASE 28-1

PIRP

History

This 57-year-old man called 911 for worsening CP of 36 hours duration. The pain was pleuritic and localized to the apex. Cardiac monitoring showed new atrial fibrillation with a HR = 150 and BP = 110/70. ED bedside echocardiography revealed a 1-cm pericardial effusion but no tamponade. No rub or murmur was documented.

ECG 28-1A (Type 1d)

At presentation (Day 1): atrial fibrillation with rapid ventricular response

- ST elevation (4 to 5 mm), QS waves, and T-wave inversion: V1–V4 (T-wave inversion also in V5 and V6), are diagnostic of **anterior AMI** of more than 12 hours duration.

Clinical Course

The patient's HR was controlled with esmolol. He was taken for angioplasty, which revealed two-vessel disease and a subtotal mid-LAD occlusion, which was stented. Initial cTnI was 58.7 ng/mL, with a total CK of only 321 IU/L. These biomarker levels are consistent with **prolonged occlusion**. After reperfusion, cTnI rose to 421 ng/mL.

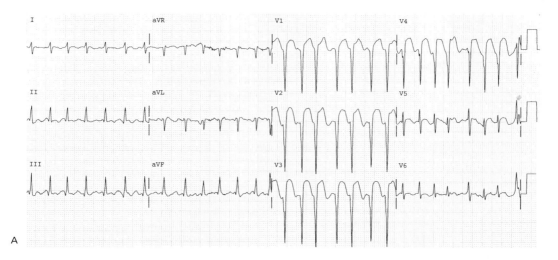

(continued on next page)

CASE 28-1

PIRP *(continued)*

Hemodynamics remained stable, but CP persisted.

ECG 28-1B
Day 2, supraventricular tachycardia, with continued CP, V1–V3 only

- ST-segment resolution > 70%; T waves remain inverted. Echocardiography confirmed a 1-cm pericardial effusion, with anterior, septal, and apical akinesis, EF of 25%, and moderately severe aortic stenosis.

ECG 28-1C
Day 3, continued CP, V1–V6 only

- T waves with deeper inversion. Echocardiography demonstrated improving EF (35%) and decreasing effusion. CTnI levels were decreasing.

ECG 28-1D
Day 4, **increased CP,** quality not documented, V1–V3 only

- **Do symptoms represent recurrent ischemia, rupture, or PIRP?**

- ST segments reelevated, T waves only minimally inverted.

Clinical Course
No friction rub was documented. Immediate echocardiography showed still-improving wall motion, an EF of 40%, and decreasing effusion. CTnI continued to decrease. The diagnosis was PIRP without rupture. For the next week, signs, symptoms, and clinical course improved. An ECG on Day 10 manifested only minimal ST elevation with T waves again inverted. There was never evidence of rupture. The patient ultimately underwent aortic valve repair and CABG.

Conclusion
With the prolonged symptoms, pleuritic pain, and pericardial fluid, this patient may have already developed PIRP before admission. The initial differential diagnosis should include myocardial rupture. ST reelevation, especially with increased pain, could represent reocclusion or myocardial rupture. Echocardiography ruled out these alternative diagnoses.

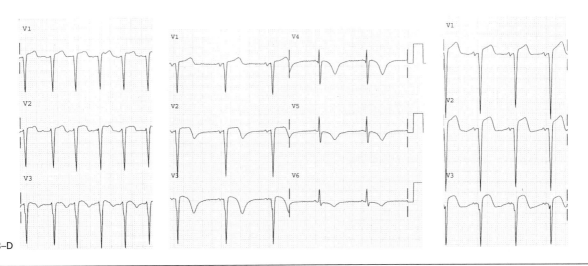

B–D

CASE 28-2

RBBB and Left Anterior Fascicular Block (LAFB) with a Type 1a AMI and Pericardial Fluid Detected by Brief, Limited Bedside Echocardiography

ECG 28-2 (Type 1a)

- QR: V1; and wide S wave: V5–V6, indicate RBBB.
- Late, superior forces in limb leads indicate LAFB (see Chapter 17).
- ST elevation: V1–V5, aVL; and ST depression: II, III, aVF, diagnostic of **anterolateral AMI.**

- PIRP is not evident on this ECG.

Clinical Course

A brief, routine, bedside echocardiogram detected a large amount of pericardial fluid. The patient died of myocardial rupture despite emergent surgical intervention.

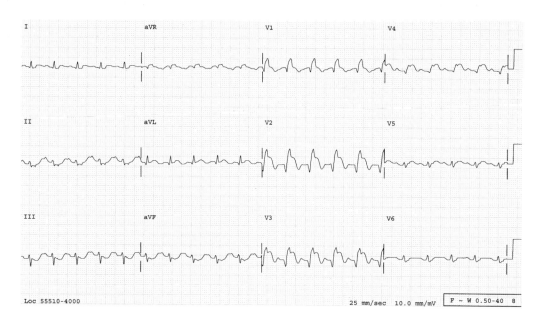

Loc 55510-4000   25 mm/sec   10.0 mm/mV   F ~ W 0.50-40 8

CASE 28-3

A Patient with 3 Days of Symptoms and an ECG Highly Suggestive of PIRP, Diagnosed with Ventricular Septal Rupture

History
This 57-year-old man with no previous cardiac history presented after 3 days of decreasing CP and increasing dyspnea. Physical exam revealed pulmonary edema and a new systolic murmur.

ECG 28-3 (Type 1c)
- ST elevation: 4 mm, V2–V5; and deep, wide, well-formed QS waves: V2–V5, I, and aVL are diagnostic of **anterolateral MI.** The QS waves and the prolonged duration of symptoms suggest **completed** AMI.
- Upright T waves.

Clinical Course
The differential diagnosis includes AMI with late presentation, reocclusion, and subacute MI with PIRP. Uncomplicated subacute MI should have some T-wave inversion after 3 days. There was no abrupt increase in discomfort to suggest reocclusion, although it remains possible. Thus **PIRP is the likely ECG diagnosis.** Echocardiography revealed dyskinesis of the entire septum and apex and a ventricular septal defect. The patient was stabilized with medical treatment and later underwent successful surgical repair.

Conclusion
Rupture may occur through the septum as well as through the free wall.

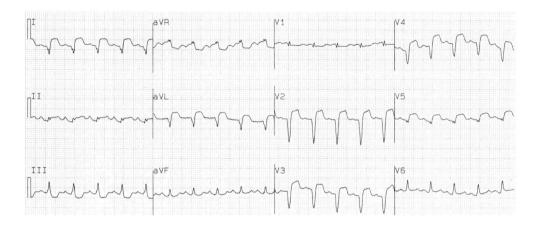

ANNOTATED BIBLIOGRAPHY

The ECG in Myocardial Rupture
Oliva PB, et al. Electrocardiographic diagnosis of PIRP: ancillary observations regarding the effect of reperfusion on the rapidity and amplitude of T-wave inversion after acute myocardial infarction, 1993.

Methods: Oliva et al. (94) studied 200 consecutive AMI patients and compared ECG evolution with development of PIRP as diagnosed by typical clinical signs and symptoms, including pleuritic-positional chest, left shoulder, or scapular pain or friction rub, with no reelevation of CK-MB.

Findings: Of 200 patients, **43 (21.5%) developed PIRP, all of whom displayed one of two types of unusual T-wave evolution (100% sensitivity).** Type I consisted of persistently positive T waves at 48 to 72 hours or more after infarction and occurred in 29 (67%) of cases of PIRP. Specificity for PIRP was 100%. Type II consisted of premature, gradual reversal of inverted T waves to positive deflections of 48 to 72 hours or more after AMI onset in 12 (33%) cases of PIRP. Patients who received cardiopulmonary resuscitation (CPR) or experienced reinfarction or very small infarcts due to thrombolysis also displayed Type II T-wave evolution. Specificity of Type II for PIRP was 77%. Widespread ST elevation of diffuse pericarditis was seen in only two patients (5%) with PIRP. The authors conclude that **premature "reconcordance" of the T wave after AMI** is a **sensitive, fairly specific, and easily recognizable sign of PIRP** and that reperfusion is associated with accelerated T-wave evolution and deepening.

Oliva PB, et al. Cardiac rupture, a clinically predictable complication of acute myocardial infarction: report of 70 cases with clinicopathologic correlations, 1993.

Methods: Oliva et al. (366) compared the clinical and ECG features of 70 AMI patients with myocardial rupture to findings from 100 AMI patients without rupture.

Findings: Patients with rupture had a significantly greater incidence of PIRP and persistent vomiting, restlessness, and agitation; 80% had at least two symptoms versus 3% of AMI patients without rupture. **Deviation from the normal pattern of T-wave evolution occurred in 94% of patients with rupture** and in only 34% of patients without rupture. Midlateral wall rupture secondary to infero-postero-lateral infarction from circumflex occlusion was most common (34%).

Comment: Although reasonably specific for PIRP, this deviation from normal T-wave evolution does not have a high PPV because of the relatively low incidence of rupture.

Detection and Management of Myocardial Rupture
Plummer D, et al. Emergency department two-dimensional echocardiography in the diagnosis of nontraumatic cardiac rupture, 1994.

Findings: Plummer et al. (369) report ED presentations of six patients with myocardial rupture. All patients presented with CP, all ECGs were diagnostic of AMI, and four patients were eligible for thrombolysis (five patients if a pure posterior AMI with only ST depression is included). **Brief, routine, emergency physician-performed bedside echocardiography, using a limited single-window examination, is standard procedure** on critically ill patients (including thrombolytic patients) in the authors' ED. Echocardiographic visualization of pericardial fluid enabled immediate diagnosis of myocardial rupture in six patients, all of whom underwent immediate surgical repair. Three survived surgery, and two were long-term survivors.

Guron CW, et al. Echocardiography allows early detection and long-term survival after infarct free wall rupture, 1998.

> *Findings:* Guron et al. (373) report a patient who suffered postinfarction myocardial rupture in hospital. It was diagnosed with echocardiography and surgically repaired, and the patient was alive 3 years later.

Purcaro A, et al. Diagnostic criteria and management of subacute ventricular free wall rupture complicating acute myocardial infarction, 1997.

> *Methods:* Purcaro et al. (372) prospectively performed echocardiography in every patient who exhibited rapid clinical and/or hemodynamic compromise in the context of AMI.

> *Findings:* They diagnosed 28 cases of subacute myocardial FWR, frequently based on echocardiographic identification of hemopericardium and associated signs of cardiac tamponade. Four patients died awaiting surgery, but 16 of 24 survived surgical repair.

Figueras J, et al. Medical management of selected patients with left ventricular free wall rupture during acute myocardial infarction, 1997.

> *Findings:* Figueras et al. (371) report outcomes of 81 patients with myocardial FWR. Forty-seven patients died within 2 hours without surgery. Fifteen patients underwent surgery, two of whom survived. Nineteen others survived the initial hypotension and were managed conservatively by BP control with beta-adrenergic blocking agents; 15 of these patients survived.

Incidence of Myocardial Rupture

Maggioni AP, et al. Age-related increase in mortality among patients with first myocardial infarctions treated with thrombolysis, 1993.

> *Methods:* Maggioni et al. (365) analyzed data from the GISSI-2 study (98) of 9,720 patients with first MI (see Appendix C). This included autopsy findings from 158 (20%) of the 772 patients who died in the hospital.

> *Findings:* Myocardial rupture was found in six of 31 (19%) autopsies in patients less than 60 years of age, 25 of 43 (58%) aged 61 to 70 years, and 72 of 84 (86%) more than 70 years of age, for a total of 103 cases (1.1% of AMI).

> *Comment:* Even if none of the unautopsied deaths (80%) involved rupture (which is unlikely), **at least 1.1% of AMI and 13% of all deaths** in this study were associated with myocardial rupture.

Honan MB, et al. Cardiac rupture, mortality and the timing of thrombolytic therapy: a meta-analysis, 1990.

> *Methods:* Honan et al. (367) performed a meta-analysis of four thrombolytic trials with a total of 1,638 patients.

> *Findings:* Fifty-eight patients had myocardial rupture, which yields an incidence of 3.5%. Rupture was associated with absence of thrombolytics and strongly associated with late administration of thrombolytics. The 7-hour treatment odds ratio (OR) was 0.4 compared with no thrombolytics and the 17-hour treatment OR was 3.21 compared with no thrombolytics.

Becker RC, et al. Cardiac rupture associated with thrombolytic therapy: impact of time to treatment in the LATE study, 1995.

> *Methods:* Becker et al. (374) analyzed data from 5,711 patients in the LATE trial (169) (see Appendix C).

> *Findings:* Of 5,711 patients, 53 (0.93%) had myocardial rupture that was associated with coronary thrombolysis. However, late treatment, from 12 to 24 hours from symptom onset, was **NOT** significantly associated with increased incidence of rupture.

Kleiman NS, et al. Mechanisms of early death despite thrombolytic therapy: experience from the TIMI Phase II (TIMI II), 1992.

> *Methods:* Kleiman et al. (375) analyzed data from 3,339 TIMI-II patients (376).

> *Findings:* Of 63 patients who died less than 18 hours after symptom onset, 10 (16%) suffered myocardial rupture.

Kleiman NS, et al. Mortality within 24 hours of thrombolysis for myocardial infarction: the importance of early reperfusion, 1994.

> *Methods:* Kleiman et al. (377) analyzed mortality data from 41,021 patients in the GUSTO trial (see Appendix C).

> *Findings:* Of 2,851 deaths in the first 30 days, 1,125 occurred less than 24 hours after symptom onset, of which 106 (9.4%) were due to pericardial tamponade.

Becker RC, et al. A composite view of cardiac rupture in the United States NRMI, 1996.

> *Methods:* Becker et al. (378) analyzed National Registry of Myocardial Infarction (NRMI) data (see Appendix C).

> *Findings:* Of all cases of AMI, 0.76% died from myocardial rupture. The overall mortality for patients not treated with thrombolytics was 12.9%, of which 6.1% were due to rupture. This contrasts with overall mortality of 5.9% for those treated with thrombolytics, of which 12.1% were due to rupture. Thus among those who received thrombolytics, approximately the same percentage suffered fatal cardiac rupture (0.79%) as among those who did not receive them (0.71%). Death from rupture occurred earlier in patients treated with thrombolytics, clustering at 24 hours.

Becker RC, et al. Fatal cardiac rupture among patients treated with thrombolytic agents and adjunctive thrombin antagonists: observation from the TIMI-9 Study, 1999.

> *Methods:* Becker et al. (379) studied 3,759 AMI patients treated with thrombolytics in TIMI-9.

> *Findings:* Myocardial rupture occurred in 65 patients (1.7%) and was fatal in all cases. Rupture was independently associated with an age of more than 70 years, female sex, and prior history of angina, but not with type of anticoagulation (heparin versus hirudin).

Additional Considerations

Figueras J, et al. Relevance of delayed hospital admission on development of cardiac rupture during acute myocardial infarction: study in 225 patients with free wall, septal or papillary muscle rupture, 1998.

> *Methods:* Figueras et al. (368) compared 225 AMI patients with FWR, septal rupture (SR), or papillary muscle rupture (PMR) to 1,012 patients with no rupture.

> *Findings:* Ninety-eight patients had FWR, 100 had SR, and 27 had PMR. Delayed hospital admission (24 hours or more), undue in-hospital physical activity, and recurrence of ischemia correlated very strongly with FWR, SR, and PMR.

Figueras J, et al. Relevance of electrocardiographic findings, heart failure, and infarct size in assessing risk and timing of left ventricular free wall rupture during acute myocardial infarction, 1995.

> *Methods:* Figueras et al. (213) analyzed clinical and ECG features of 227 AMI deaths versus 150 survivors of first AMI.

> *Findings:* LV FWR occurred in 93 patients more than 50 years of age. In early rupture, mean ST elevation was 6.8 mm ± 4.0 mm and mean systolic BP was 155 mm Hg versus 4.0 mm ± 2.7 mm ST elevation and 135 mm Hg systolic BP for late or no rupture. Lateral AMI resulted in 10% of ruptures, and had minimal ST elevation.

29

BIOMARKERS IN THE REPERFUSION DECISION

FRED S. APPLE AND STEPHEN W. SMITH

KEY POINTS

- Elevated biomarkers alone are not an indication for reperfusion therapy.
- Elevated biomarkers may aid in the interpretation of an equivocal ECG (Type 1c, with ST elevation of uncertain etiology).
- Biomarkers are not usually elevated until at least 4 hours after the onset of AMI.
- A rapid rise in biomarkers after therapy is strong evidence of successful reperfusion.
- Admission troponin level may reflect the total ischemic time. If elevated, substantial time may have elapsed since coronary occlusion.

GENERAL BACKGROUND

Although measurement of biomarkers is essential in the evaluation of acute coronary syndrome (ACS) (12,380), the use of biomarkers has a limited role in reperfusion therapy; therefore our discussion is brief.

Biochemical Markers in the Detection of AMI

Measurement of myocardial proteins in blood, including myoglobin, CK, CK-MB, cTnI, and cardiac troponin T (cTnT), can aid in assessment of myocardial damage due to prolonged ischemia. AMI is diagnosed when blood levels of these sensitive and specific biomarkers are increased above the reference range in the clinical setting of acute ischemia (12,380). The biomarkers reflect myocardial damage but not its mechanism. CTnI and cTnT are the preferred biomarkers for myocardial damage because they have absolute myocardial tissue specificity (12,380,381). If unavailable, the best alternative is CK-MB, as measured by the mass assay (12). Measurement of total CK is not recommended for the routine diagnosis of AMI and markers such as lactate dehydrogenase (LD) and LD isoenzymes are no longer useful.

To measure troponins in most patients, **obtain blood at presentation, at 6 to 9 hours, and at 12 to 24 hours if the earlier samples are negative and the clinical index of suspicion is high** (12,380). An increased value for cardiac troponins should be defined as a measurement exceeding the 99th percentile of a refer-

ence control group. Since there are several commercially available troponin assays, reference values must be determined by studies using each specific assay (382). Additionally, due to the lack of standardization, there may be a large difference in absolute concentrations or levels among assays from different manufacturers. It is important to choose the right assay (380).

Because **troponins may remain elevated for 5 to 10 days** after AMI onset, exercise care in attributing increased cardiac troponin levels to acute events. Any patient with troponins elevated above the reference range, by new definition, has sustained an MI (12). It has been convincingly shown that the **risk of short- and long-term ischemic cardiac events (AMI and death) is related to the magnitude of cardiac troponin increase** (13,14,383–386). The prognosis for these patients is worse than that in patients without increased levels of biomarkers, whether this increase is associated with STEMI or NSTEMI.

Unstable angina (UA) and non-ST-elevation MI (NSTEMI) are closely related pathologies that differ primarily in whether ischemia is severe enough to cause myocardial necrosis (11). New definitions use increased cardiac biomarkers for the diagnosis of NSTEMI, while acute coronary syndrome (ACS) patients with normal troponins will be diagnosed with UA (11). Elevated cardiac troponin levels also identify a high-risk subgroup of patients with ACS who benefit from treatment with platelet glycoprotein (GP) IIb-IIIa receptor inhibitors such as abciximab, eptifibatide, or tirofiban, or with one of the low-molecular-weight heparins, such as enoxaparin (384,385).

Biochemical Markers in the Initial Reperfusion Decision

Although cardiac biomarkers are sensitive and specific indicators of AMI, they are not elevated immediately after coronary occlusion. Therefore, **they do not serve alone as an indication for reperfusion therapy** (383,387–389). Reperfusion is only indicated for symptoms of ACS in conjunction with a **Type 1 ECG** (see Chapter 3). However, **biomarkers may be useful in equivocal (Type 1c) ECGs** (11,12). Patients with Type 1c ECGs may or may not have acute coronary occlusion, and additional information is necessary for the reperfusion decision. Though an elevated cardiac biomarker is not to be expected until several hours after the onset of coronary occlusion, **when the significance of ST elevation is in doubt, it is more likely to represent AMI if in the presence of an elevated biomarker.** ST elevation due to

AMI in the presence of a positive biomarker signifies that the AMI has been in progress for at least several hours to days, possibly too long for administration of thrombolytics. A minimally elevated troponin may be seen within 4 hours of onset of occlusion, but a very high troponin level is unlikely to represent early AMI. If NSTEMI temporally precedes coronary occlusion, elevated biomarkers may be present. In any case, an elevated biomarker increases the probability that an equivocal ECG represents STEMI and, thus, may sway the decision toward reperfusion.

Biomarkers in the Assessment of Reperfusion Status

Biomarkers may help to identify patients with failed reperfusion, for whom rescue percutaneous coronary intervention (PCI) would be of benefit (13,390,391). Rapid assays ("near patient" or "bedside" testing) using monoclonal antibodies specific to myocardial proteins such as CK-MB, myoglobin, cTnI, and cTnT, are now available for quantitation in serum, plasma, and whole blood within 20 minutes, 24 hours per day. These assays may aid the assessment of reperfusion success or failure within 2 hours of thrombolytic therapy. The appearance of myocardial proteins in the blood following release from injured myocardium depends on infarct reperfusion. Myoglobin, CK-MB, cTnI, and cTnT demonstrate similar kinetics after successful reperfusion, as demonstrated by TIMI-3 flow at angiography within 120 minutes after giving thrombolytic agents (391). **Early and successful reperfusion** results in an **earlier increase** above the upper reference range and an **earlier and higher peak** after reperfusion.

Several criteria have been studied to determine the presence or absence of reperfusion 60 to 90 minutes following initiation of thrombolytic therapy (390–392). These include (a) **rate of biomarker appearance** (slope of time versus concentration graph); (b) **ratio of biomarker concentration** at a specific time point to its baseline value; and (c) **absolute change** in biomarker concentration from time = 0 minutes until time = 60 or 90 minutes.

Sensitivity and Specificity of Biomarkers for Reperfusion Status

Table 29-1 shows the sensitivities and specificities of four biomarkers. It is important to note, however, that the studies on which Table 29-1 data are based comprise small total sample sizes (fewer than 100 patients per study) and limited angiography data at limited time periods after initiation of thrombolytic therapy for each TIMI flow grade group 0 to 3 (391,392).

See Case 29-1 for an example of biomarkers as indicators of reperfusion. (See also Case 11-2, in which an initially positive troponin-aided ECG interpretation and a rapid rise of troponin

levels suggested reperfusion; and Case 33-8, in which low acuity suggested by deep T-wave inversions was confirmed by a high cTnI at presentation [Type 1d ECG], consistent with either an AMI of long duration [subacute AMI], or an AMI with spontaneous reperfusion.)

Biomarkers in the Assessment of Infarct Size

Biomarkers may be useful in assessing infarct size when there is **NO** reperfusion. However, if there is reperfusion, there is great variability in the amount of protein washout, which makes this assessment impossible.

Biomarkers in Assessment of Infarct Duration

With no reperfusion, total CK, CK-MB, and cardiac troponins typically increase above the normal reference limit 2 to 8 hours after the onset of symptoms. CK and CK-MB peak at 18 to 30 hours and return to the normal reference limit within 2 to 3 days. Troponins peak from 24 to 48 hours and return to the normal reference limit at 3 to 5 days (cTnI) or 4 to 10 days (cTnT). Myoglobin peaks at about 12 hours and returns to the normal reference limit at 24 hours. The minimal recommended timing for ordering of biomarkers would be at presentation, at 2 to 4 hours, and at 6 to 9 hours after presentation, using cTnI or cTnT as the preferred marker. CK-MB mass is recommended if troponin is not available, but measuring both markers at once is not necessary. Additional orders at 12 to 24 hours may be necessary if the earlier samples are negative and the clinical index of suspicion is high. An early marker like myoglobin is recommended only if very early triage (less than 4 hours after presentation) is part of a protocol.

Reperfusion results in earlier peak levels. CK peak at less than 12 hours is an accurate marker of reperfusion (but too late to be of aid in deciding on rescue angioplasty) (338).

MANAGEMENT

Monitor cTnI or cTnT at the initiation of thrombolytic therapy and again 90 minutes later for the most accurate assessment of reperfusion success or failure. Cardiac biomarkers are not currently acceptable criteria for initiation of thrombolytic therapy. However, an increased cardiac biomarker in the setting of ST elevation adds confidence that the ST elevation is due to AMI and that the myocardial ischemia, whether due to constant or intermittent coronary occlusion, has been ongoing for more than 4 hours. Although preliminary data show that the laboratory can assist clinicians in the evaluation of reperfusion success, larger prospective studies are needed.

TABLE 29.1. SENSITIVITIES AND SPECIFICITIES OF FOUR BIOMARKERS OF REPERFUSION

Marker	Sensitivity	Specificity	Guideline
CK-MB	92%	100%	2.5-fold increase at 90 minutes
Myoglobin	95%	100%	>3.0-fold increase at 90 minutes
cTnI	82%	100%	90-minute concentration/baseline concentration > 6.0
cTnT	92%	100%	Increase at 60 minutes ≥ 0.5 μg/mL

CASE 29-1

Reperfusion of AMI Demonstrated by Rapid Increase in Levels of cTnI

History

This 65-year-old man presented to the ED with severe CP.

Clinical Course

His ECG (Type 1a, not shown) showed new, diagnostic ST elevation indicating acute coronary occlusion. Clinicians administered tPA within 60 minutes. Angiography performed 90 minutes after the tPA bolus documented TIMI-3 flow. ST elevation decreased significantly with pain resolution. The patient's cardiac biomarkers are listed in Table 29-2.

Conclusion

At 90 minutes, the patient's biomarker levels were many times higher than the initial (undetectable) level; this rise demonstrates reperfusion. The initially normal biomarker levels at time 0, during AMI without reperfusion, are typical. Cardiac biomarkers generally do not increase above the upper reference limit until 4 to 8 hours after the onset of coronary occlusion.

TABLE 29.2. BIOMARKER LEVELS

Marker and upper reference limit	Time in minutes from tPA administration				
	0	20	40	60	90
CK-MB (5 ng/mL)	<1.0	<1.0	1.6	5.9	8.0
cTnI (0.6 ng/mL)	<0.1	0.6	1.9	3.9	8.5

30

ECHOCARDIOGRAPHY IN THE REPERFUSION DECISION

KEY POINTS

■ A high-quality echocardiographic examination, if done immediately, may help interpret a Type 1c ECG by detecting or ruling out a new wall motion abnormality (WMA) or by diagnosing ventricular aneurysm.

■ Immediate, goal-oriented, bedside echocardiography may be performed by clinicians with little training and may be useful on a routine basis to detect pericardial fluid due to myocardial rupture.

GENERAL BACKGROUND

Inadequate coronary blood flow leads to ischemic myocardium and abnormal contraction, or regional WMA, which is detectable with echocardiography. A WMA may manifest as hypokinesis (decreased wall motion), akinesis (no wall motion), dyskinesis (bulging), or aneurysmal diastolic distortion. The presence of a WMA cannot distinguish AMI from old MI. However, when the ECG differential diagnosis is AMI versus "old MI with persistent ST elevation," the presence of diastolic distortion with myocardial wall thinning and dyskinesis (ventricular aneurysm) strongly supports a diagnosis of old MI (see Chapter 23).

The presence of a **new regional WMA** supports the diagnosis of myocardial ischemia and, in conjunction with **new ST elevation** in the corresponding ECG location, **strongly suggests STEMI.** A new WMA in conjunction with an equivocal (Type 1c) ECG, in the right clinical setting, is an indication for reperfusion therapy.

Normal wall motion rules out a large risk area, but echocardiography is insensitive for small risk areas, so normal wall motion in the presence of a diagnostic ECG does not absolutely rule out a small STEMI. Nonetheless, in the presence of an equivocal ECG (Type 1c), normal wall motion on an echocardiogram of good quality, detected by a skilled technician and interpreter, would provide evidence against AMI and be a good reason to withhold thrombolytics.

ECHOCARDIOGRAPHY AND THE ECG

Uses of the Echocardiogram in the Evaluation of Ischemic Symptoms

Echocardiography aids in the evaluation of ischemic symptoms and in the reperfusion decision in situations with the following ECG findings:

1. **Nonspecific ST elevation (Type 1c ECG) consistent with AMI.** Is this AMI or is this LVH, early repolarization, pericarditis, or ventricular aneurysm? Is reperfusion therapy indicated?
   a. If there is a **new** WMA, the patient is a candidate for reperfusion. (See Case 7-3 of an inferolateral AMI misdiagnosed as pericarditis until echocardiography revealed a WMA. See also Case 12-4.)
   b. If wall motion is **normal,** it makes AMI of a large risk area highly unlikely. See the **following cases,** in which **echocardiography ruled out large AMI by demonstrating normal wall motion:** Case 10-8, of ECG changes and pulmonary edema subsequent to cocaine use; Case 14-8; Case 20-5 of dynamic early repolarization; Case 22-2 of LVH; and Cases 24-4 and 24-8 of pericarditis.

2. **Precordial ST depression that is consistent with either posterior STEMI or anterior UA/NSTEMI but posterior chest leads are nondiagnostic.**
   a. If there is a new posterior WMA, the patient is a candidate for reperfusion therapy (see Case 16-2).
   b. If there is a new anterior WMA, the patient has anterior UA/NSTEMI and is not a thrombolytic candidate.

3. **When the ECG is nonspecific for any kind of ACS (a Type 3 or Type 4 ECG).** The patient is **not** eligible for thrombolytics, but angiography ± PCI may be indicated. Are the patient's symptoms due to ischemia?
   a. **A new WMA** supports the diagnosis of acute ischemia but may also represent infarction at any time since the last echocardiogram.
   b. **Absence of a new WMA** excludes a large AMI but may not exclude ischemia in a small risk area or brief ischemia that has resolved **(393).**

4. **When ST elevation and QS waves are present, and the differential diagnosis is AMI versus ventricular aneurysm** (old MI with persistent ST elevation).

a. Presence of diastolic distortion and myocardial wall thinning supports a diagnosis of ventricular aneurysm and the ST elevation is very likely to be old.

b. Akinesis or hypokinesis without dyskinesis, however, does not necessarily imply that the ECG findings are new. An old MI with persistent ST elevation may be associated with systolic dyskinesis, akinesis, or hypokinesis without aneurysm (95,299).

Limits of Echocardiography

Echocardiography cannot:

■ Distinguish between STEMI and UA/NSTEMI. Either may have a WMA.

■ Determine the time course of AMI. If the ECG is unequivocally diagnostic of AMI (Type 1a), echocardiography provides no useful information for the reperfusion decision and delays therapy unnecessarily (see Case 33-7).

Stress Echocardiography

■ A normal stress echocardiogram in a patient who "rules out" for AMI with negative biomarkers makes it much less likely that CP is due to ischemia and is a useful marker of good long-term prognosis **(394)**. Further management of patients with Type 3 and 4 ECGs is beyond the scope of this book.

LIMITED BEDSIDE ECHOCARDIOGRAPHY

Bedside echocardiography can be performed in seconds to minutes by clinicians with limited training. It is particularly useful for **detection of pericardial fluid,** which may be due to **myocardial rupture** (369) or **hemopericardium** due to thrombolytic complications (see Cases 8-4 and 28-1). **All patients in cardiogenic shock should be screened for tamponade** (395).

If pericarditis is on the ECG differential diagnosis, the presence of pericardial fluid supports its diagnosis, with a high PPV. However, pericarditis commonly occurs without pericardial fluid, so the NPV is low. Additionally, AMI with PIRP with or without myocardial rupture may present with pericardial fluid.

A WMA and/or globally poor LV function may **sometimes** be obvious to even the nonspecialist echocardiographer. However, certainty requires substantial training and experience.

ANNOTATED BIBLIOGRAPHY

Echocardiography in the Detection of Myocardial Rupture

Plummer D, et al. Emergency department two-dimensional echocardiography in the diagnosis of nontraumatic cardiac rupture, 1994. See Chapter 28 for annotation.

False-Positive WMA

Sharkey SW. Reversible myocardial contraction abnormalities in patients with an acute noncardiac illness, 1998.

Findings: Sharkey (150) reports 19 patients with noncardiac illness who had deep precordial T-wave inversion and apical WMA mimicking anterior AMI, but without infarction. Six patients had central nervous system (CNS) injury, three were septic, three had respiratory failure, two had overdosed, and five had metabolic abnormalities.

Echocardiography in Patients with CP and Type 3 or 4 ECGs

Sabia P, et al. Value of regional wall motion abnormality in the emergency room diagnosis of acute myocardial infarction: a prospective study using two-dimensional echocardiography, 1991.

Methods: Sabia et al. (396) performed two-dimensional echocardiography on 180 ED patients with CP. The emergency physician was not informed of the findings.

Findings: Of 180 patients, 140 were admitted. Of these 140, 30 had enzyme-confirmed AMI. Of these 30, only nine had Type 1 ST elevation. Of the 29 AMI patients with technically adequate echocardiograms, 27 had a WMA. Each of the 13 AMI patients with in-hospital complications had a WMA.

Kontos MC, et al. Early echocardiography can predict cardiac events in emergency department patients with chest pain, 1998.

Methods: Kontos et al. (397) performed echocardiography on 260 ED patients with symptoms of cardiac ischemia.

Findings: Presence of a WMA or EF < 40% was a more sensitive predictor of cardiac events such as AMI (*n* = 23) or revascularization (*n* = 22) than ST elevation, ST depression, or T-wave inversion (91% versus 40%). However, specificity of these findings as a predictor of cardiac events was lower (75% versus 94%).

Kontos MC, et al. Comparison between 2-dimensional echocardiography and myocardial perfusion imaging in the emergency department in patients with possible myocardial ischemia, 1998.

Methods: Kontos et al. (398) studied echocardiograms and sestamibi perfusion imaging in 185 ED CP patients with Type 3 and 4 ECGs (diagnostic for neither AMI nor ACS).

Findings: Both modalities identified all 10 patients who had AMI or who needed angioplasty.

Colon PJ. Utility of stress echocardiography in the triage of patients with atypical chest pain from the emergency department, 1998.

Methods: Colon et al. (394) performed stress echocardiography on 108 ED patients with CP and Type 3 ECGs (diagnostic of neither AMI nor ACS).

Findings: All patients with a negative test had cardiac event-free survival at 1 year.

Mohler ER, et al. Clinical utility of troponin T levels and echocardiography in the emergency department, 1998.

Methods: Mohler et al. (393) prospectively evaluated echocardiography and serial cTnT levels in 100 patients admitted to the hospital with chest discomfort.

Findings: Fifteen of 18 AMI patients and only nine of 37 patients with UA had a new WMA evident on the echocardiogram.

Comment: It is clear that the absence of a WMA **does not rule out** ischemic cardiac origin of CP.

31

PREHOSPITAL THROMBOLYTICS AND PREHOSPITAL ECGs

DEBORAH L. ZVOSEC AND STEPHEN W. SMITH

KEY POINTS

- Prehospital ECGs decrease door-to-needle-time (DTNT).
- Prehospital rhythm strips may provide valuable ST-segment data.
- Consider prehospital thrombolytics if transport times are more than 30 minutes.
- Suspected AMI patients with overt heart failure or shock should be transported to a facility with capacity for percutaneous coronary intervention (PCI).

PREHOSPITAL THROMBOLYTICS

Although timely reperfusion therapy of AMI leads to significant reductions in mortality and myocardial injury, data on the benefits of prehospital thrombolysis is somewhat equivocal. Clinical trials of prehospital thrombolysis have shown reductions in time to treatment ranging from 33 minutes (399) to 125 minutes (400), depending on the setting. Statistically significant **mortality benefits** have been demonstrated in some trials (400, 401,402), but not in others (399,403,404,405). Therefore, as of 1994, the American College of Emergency Physicians (ACEP) did not endorse routine use of prehospital thrombolytics in nonrural areas (404). A recent meta-analysis of 6,434 patients in rural and nonrural areas randomized to prehospital thrombolytics versus in-hospital thrombolytics showed statistically significant mortality benefit from prehospital thrombolytics (406).

Benefits of prehospital thrombolysis are undisputed in areas where transport times are long (400,401,402,404,407,408). Prehospital thrombolytics and ECGs are feasible, accurate, and safe when their use is properly supervised (399,401,402, 409–411). **Newer bolus thrombolytics,** such as reteplase (rPA) and tenecteplase (TNK-tPA), may make prehospital thrombolysis easier than before (362,412) (see Chapter 36).

- **Recommendation: Consider instituting prehospital bolus thrombolytics if transport times are more than 30 to 60 minutes.** Prehospital providers must transmit ECGs to a base physician for interpretation.
- Suspected AMI patients with overt heart failure with or without shock should be transported to a nearby hospital with balloon pump and revascularization (PCI) capabilities, if available (413).

PREHOSPITAL ECGs

Prehospital 12-Lead ECGs with or Without Thrombolysis

A prehospital 12-lead ECG facilitates a more rapid DTNT (399,408,414,415) and is associated with decreased mortality (414). **Reciprocal changes** on prehospital ECGs, as on any ECG, greatly improve the specificity of ST elevation for AMI (106). Use of a prehospital ECG in combination with a serially obtained hospital ECG may identify evolving ST segments, T and Q waves, and may increase the sensitivity of the ECG for myocardial ischemia (see also Chapter 10) (416). **The use of prehospital 12-lead ECGs, with transmission to the receiving emergency physician, is recommended.**

Prehospital 12-Lead ECGs with Predictive Instruments

Prehospital 12-lead ECGs with "acute cardiac ischemia time insensitive predictive instruments" (ACI-TIPI) are available. These predictive instruments integrate ECG data with data on patient history and presentation, and compute the probability of acute ischemia. Use of such predictive instruments in the emergency department (ED) (283,417) and prehospital (418) may aid in triage, significantly reduce the number of unnecessary admissions, and help to identify high-risk patients. Predictive instruments have also been developed to predict risks and benefits of thrombolytic therapy (419), but there are no data yet on their impact on treatment times and mortality. **Computer algorithms are quite specific for ST elevation MI (STEMI),** with a high positive predictive value (PPV); however, they are **insensitive** (41–47). Thus paramedic administration of thrombolytics based on algorithm diagnosis of STEMI may be appropriate, but many patients with STEMI cannot be treated until their ECGs are interpreted by an experienced base physician.

Standard Rhythm Monitoring

Standard rhythm monitoring may also reduce time to treatment. ST elevation and depression can be detected in unipolar monitor leads **MCL$_2$** and **MCL$_3$** (equivalent to V2 and V3) and **lead III (83)**. This strategy is less costly than prehospital 12- lead ECGs and may be implemented by prehospital providers who are not yet equipped with 12-lead ECGs (see also Chapter 10). With monitor leads:

- ST depression in leads MCL$_2$ and/or MCL$_3$ may indicate posterior AMI.
- ST elevation in leads MCL$_2$ and/or MCL$_3$ may indicate anterior AMI (see Case 12-3).

- Hyperacute T waves in MCL₂ and/or MCL₃ may indicate anterior AMI (see Case 31-1).
- ST elevation in lead III may indicate inferior AMI (see Case 31-2).
- ST depression in lead III may be a clue to anterior or lateral AMI (see Cases 12-3, 31-1, and 31-3).

Although the specificity of monitor leads as read by paramedics appears to be low, they are useful for screening for ST elevation (106) (Cases 31-1 and 31-2). See Chapter 10 for more cases with prehospital rhythm strips.

NOTE: The **main obstacle to timely thrombolytic therapy is patient delay in calling 911.** Patients with evolving AMI typically wait 1.5 to 2 hours before seeking emergency medical care (58). Educational programs in Switzerland and Sweden improved the median time delay to seeking treatment (420,421), but such a campaign in the United States did not (422). (See annotations in Chapter 32.)

CASE 31-1

ST Depression in a Prehospital Rhythm Strip Provides a Clue to Transient STEMI

History
This 46-year-old man with a history of hypertension (HTN) was smoking a cigarette when he had sudden onset of severe crushing substernal CP with SOB. He called 911. Paramedics found him with BP = 204/palp and P = 94.

ECG 31-1A
Prehospital rhythm strip of lead III at 09:07
- ST depression, 3 to 4 mm

ECG 31-1B
At 09:10, a prehospital rhythm strip of lead MCL-III
- Hyperacute T waves.

Clinical Course
Oxygen, aspirin, and sublingual nitroglycerine (NTG) were administered prehospital and the pain resolved. The patient was transported emergently to the critical care area of the ED. Clinicians recorded a 12-lead ECG and physical exam detected a II/VI systolic murmur.

ECG 31-1C (Type 3)
At 09:27
- ST depression: minimal, II, III, aVF, V4–V6.
- Terminal T-wave inversion: minimal, V1–V2, with Q wave in V2.

Clinical Course
The patient was treated for unstable angina/non-ST elevation MI (UA/NSTEMI) with heparin, NTG, and tirofiban. Initial cTnI drawn at presentation returned at 0.5 ng/mL and was 8.9 ng/mL 4 hours later, at which time echocardiography revealed concentric LVH, an anterior wall motion abnormality (WMA), and severe aortic stenosis. Angiography the following day confirmed 70% proximal left anterior descending (LAD) culprit lesion. The patient underwent successful CABG and valve replacement.

Conclusion
Prehospital rhythm strips may provide important clues about CP etiology.

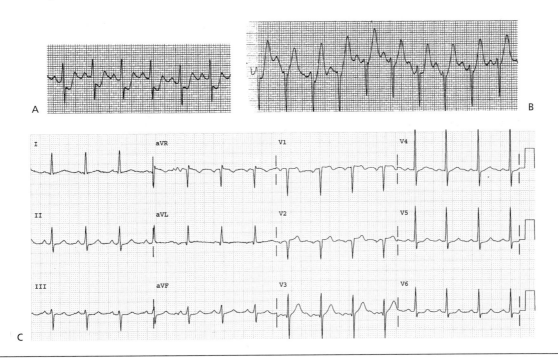

CASE 31-2

Prehospital Rhythm Strips Strongly Suggestive of Inferior AMI

History
This 46-year-old man with CP called 911.

ECG 31-2
Prehospital rhythm strips of lead II
■ High ST elevation.

Clinical Course
Having been taught to recognize such ST elevation, paramedics brought the patient directly to the critical care area. Clinicians recorded a 12-lead ECG within 3 minutes of arrival, which was diagnostic of **inferoposterior AMI.** A right-sided ECG also indicated **right ventricular (RV) AMI.** The patient was sent for PCI in less than 15 minutes.

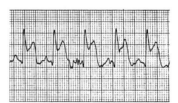

CASE 31-3

ST Depression in Prehospital Rhythm Strip Lead III Alerts to Possible Transient STEMI

History
This 48-year-old man with CP called 911.

ECG 31-3A
Prehospital rhythm strip of lead III
■ ST depression in lead III may result from anterolateral or lateral AMI. The patient received one sublingual NTG.

ECG 31-3B
Prehospital rhythm strip of lead III
■ ST depression has resolved.

Clinical Course
A 12-lead ECG recorded (not shown) in the ED was normal. The patient was treated for ACS. Based on transient ST depression, he was taken to the catheterization (cath) lab, where a 95% circumflex lesion was dilated.

Conclusion
The transient inferior ST depression is likely due to transient total circumflex occlusion. The ST depression was probably **reciprocal to unmonitored ST elevation in aVL** due to high lateral transient STEMI. Subsequent to NTG, the circumflex artery spontaneously reperfused.

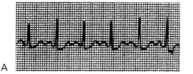

A

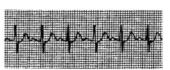

B

ANNOTATED BIBLIOGRAPHY

Morrison, et al. Mortality and prehospital thrombolysis for acute myocardial infarction: a meta-analysis, 2000.

Methods: Morrison et al. (406) performed a meta-analysis of randomized trials of prehospital versus in-hospital thrombolysis. Six studies and three follow-up studies met inclusion criteria after an exhaustive literature search. Four trials are described in the following annotations (399,400,403,405).

Findings: Data from 6,434 patients were pooled. The odds ratio (OR) for all-cause hospital mortality among patients with prehospital versus in-hospital thrombolysis was 0.83, with a confidence interval (CI) of 0.70 to 0.98. Data were insufficient to show a statistically significant difference in 1- or 2-year mortality. Mean time to thrombolysis was 104 minutes for the prehospital group and 162 minutes for the in-hospital group ($p = 0.007$).

Comment: This is a long time to thrombolytic treatment. It is not surprising that prehospital thrombolytics are beneficial when treatment intervals are this long. In areas with short transport times, particularly urban areas, prehospital thrombolytics may not be cost-effective. The benefit of prehospital ECGs was not studied.

Equivocal Evidence of Benefits of Prehospital Thrombolysis

European Myocardial Infarction Project (EMIP) Group. Prehospital thrombolytic therapy in patients with suspected acute myocardial infarction, 1993.

Methods: The EMIP (403) was a 163-center, double-blind, placebo-controlled study of 5,469 AMI patients, 87% of whom showed ST elevation; 2,750 patients were randomized to receive prehospital anistreplase and then placebo on arrival at the hospital (Group 1) and 2,719 patients were randomized to receive placebo prehospital and anistreplase on arrival (Group 2). All mobile emergency units had a doctor, a 12-lead ECG, and resuscitation equipment on board, including a defibrillator.

Findings: Median time from symptom onset to treatment for Group 1 was 130 minutes versus 190 minutes for Group 2. Overall 30-day mortality was not significantly different (9.9% versus 11.1%, $p = 0.08$) but mortality from cardiac causes was significantly lower in Group 1 (8.3% versus 9.8%, $p = 0.049$). For patients with the longest delay (90 minutes or more) between prehospital and in-hospital injections, there was a significant 42% reduction in overall 30-day mortality for Group 1 (7.3% versus 13.4%, $p = 0.047$), but not for Group 2.

Weaver WD, et al. Prehospital-initiated versus hospital-initiated thrombolytic therapy: The Myocardial Infarction Triage and Intervention Trial (MITI), 1993.

Methods: The MITI Trial (399) was a randomized, controlled multicenter study of 360 patients, conducted in the Seattle metro area. An ED physician reviewed ECGs and clinical findings transmitted from the ambulance.

Findings: Prehospital thrombolysis decreased the time from symptom onset to treatment from 110 minutes to 77 minutes. There were no significant differences between prehospital and hospital groups in the composite score (death, stroke, serious bleeding, and infarct size), ejection fraction (EF), or infarct size. **Treatment given within 70 minutes of symptom onset, regardless of prehospital or hospital administration, was associated with lower mortality (1.2% versus 8.7%, $p = 0.04$). Prehospital identification of thrombolytic candidates also reduced IN-hospital treatment times.** DTNTs for patients not included in the study averaged 60 minutes as compared with 20 minutes for study patients who received in-hospital thrombolytics.

Brouwer MA, et al. Influence of early prehospital thrombolysis on mortality and event-free survival, 1996.

Methods: Brouwer et al. (405) reported long term follow-up of 360 patients from the MITI trial (399) (described above).

Findings: Greater long-term mortality was positively associated with increased age, history of congestive heart failure (CHF), and history of coronary artery bypass graft (CABG), but **not** with time to treatment.

Prehospital Thrombolytics in Rural Areas

Benefits of prehospital thrombolytics are most evident in areas with high transport times.

Rawles JM, et al. Quantification of the benefit of earlier thrombolytic therapy: five-year results of the Grampian Region Early Anistreplase Trial (GREAT), 1997.

Methods: GREAT was a randomized, double-blind trial of home versus hospital anistreplase in 311 patients in rural Scotland (423–425).

Findings: Median time to home thrombolysis was 101 minutes and median time to hospital treatment was 240 minutes. The median time difference between home and hospital injections was 130 minutes. Of this 139-minute time difference, **a median time of 87 minutes was estimated to be due to hospital delay** (425). Of 311 cases, 37 patients received the injection within 1 hour of symptom onset and 189 patients within 2 hours. **No patients** in the hospital group received the injection within 1 hour of symptom onset, and only two received it within 2 hours of symptom onset (423). **By 3 months after trial entry there was a 49% relative reduction of deaths from all causes and a 50% reduction in cardiac mortality in the home thrombolysis group.** Survivors of home treatment also had significantly fewer Q-wave infarcts and better left ventricular (LV) function (423). **Benefits were most pronounced** if thrombolytics were given **2 hours or less** after symptom onset (423). Five-year follow-up by Rawles (400) revealed 25% mortality in the home-treated group versus 36% mortality in the hospital group (11% absolute difference). **Extrapolating from these data, improving treatment time by 1 hour due to prehospital therapy would save 43 lives per 1,000.**

Prehospital ECGs

See also annotations of Kudenchuk et al. (46) (Chapter 3) and Massel et al. (41) (Chapter 6) for analysis of computer algorithms.

Weaver WD, et al. Prehospital-initiated versus hospital-initiated thrombolytic therapy: The Myocardial Infarction Triage and Intervention Trial (MITI), 1993.

Methods: See preceding annotation of Weaver et al. (399).

Findings: Patients randomized to the in-hospital treatment group received thrombolytics in an average time of 20 minutes, which is an average of 40 minutes faster than concurrent, nonstudy patients at the same hospitals.

Kereiakes DJ, et al. Relative importance of emergency medical system transport and the prehospital electrocardiogram on reducing hospital time delay to therapy for acute myocardial infarction; a preliminary report from the Cincinnati Heart Project, 1992.

Methods: Kereiakes et al. (408) studied 134 patients transported to hospital by private automobile, local ambulance, and specialized emergency medical service (EMS) units with and without prehospital ECGs transmitted from the field.

Findings: Time to treatment was reduced significantly only in patients transported in an EMS unit **from which an ECG was transmitted.** Specialized EMS transport without ECG transmission did **not** reduce hospital time to treatment when compared with local ambulance or self-transport.

Foster DB, et al. Prehospital recognition of AMI using independent nurse/paramedic 12-lead ECG evaluation: impact on in-hospital times to thrombolysis in a rural community hospital, 1994.

Methods: Foster et al. (415) studied 155 CP patients. Patients were seen first by hospital-based nurses or paramedic Advanced Life Support (ALS) providers who utilized a prehospital ECG and protocol to diagnose AMI and assess thrombolytic indications. They radioed data to the ED and initiated a protocol to prepare potential candidates. An ED physician made the final reperfusion decision after the patient arrived at the hospital.

Findings: Providers diagnosed 17 of 21 patients with AMI, with no false positives. For the 14 patients who received thrombolytics, **average in-hospital DTNTs were 22 ± 13.8 minutes,** compared with a historical control group average of 51 ± 50 minutes for patients with no prehospital ECG.

Otto LA, et al. Evaluation of ST segment elevation criteria for the prehospital electrocardiographic diagnosis of acute myocardial infarction, 1994.

Methods: Otto et al. (106) retrospectively examined prehospital ECGs from 428 stable adult chest pain (CP) patients. They used six predetermined criteria for AMI diagnosis regarding the amount and location of ST elevation (1 or 2 mm, limb or precordial leads) and the presence of reciprocal ST depression.

Findings: Of 123 patients with ≥ 1 mm of ST elevation, 60 patients ruled in by creatine kinase-MB (CK-MB) for AMI. Presence of this criterion with the simultaneous presence of reciprocal changes had a PPV of 94% and included 18 of the 21 AMI patients who had ST elevation **and received thrombolytics within 5 hours of hospital arrival (sensitivity, 86%).**

Kudenchuk PJ, et al. Utility of the prehospital electrocardiogram in diagnosing acute coronary syndromes, 1998.

Methods: Kudenchuk et al. (416) analyzed data from the MITI trial (399) described earlier.

Findings: Compared with identification of ST elevation on a single ECG, **identification of ST-segment changes between a prehospital and hospital ECG improved the sensitivity of acute coronary syndrome (ACS) diagnosis from 34% to 46%.**

Canto JG, et al. The prehospital electrocardiogram in acute myocardial infarction: is its full potential being realized? 1997.

Methods: Canto et al. (414) analyzed NRMI-2 data (see Appendix C) on 66,995 AMI patients.

Findings: Excluding in-hospital AMI, transferred-in referrals, and self-transported patients, 3,768 patients had prehospital ECGs. These patients had: (a) longer time from symptom onset to hospital arrival (91 versus 152 min.); (b) shorter time to initiation of thrombolysis (40 versus 30 minutes) or angioplasty (115 versus 92 minutes); and (c) lower in-hospital mortality (12% versus 8%) than patients without prehospital ECGs.

Having a **prehospital ECG was an independent predictor of lower mortality** with an OR of 0.83 (CI: 0.71 to 0.96). Patients with a prehospital ECG were also **more likely to receive thrombolytics and to undergo primary angioplasty, coronary arteriography, or CABG.**

Thrombolytic Predictive Instruments

Selker HP, et al. Patient-specific predictions of outcomes in myocardial infarction for real-time emergency use: a thrombolytic predictive instrument, 1997.

Methods: Selker et al. (419) assimilated clinical and ECG data on 4,911 AMI patients in three major clinical trials and registries to develop a predictive instrument.

Findings: The predictive model generates probabilities of 30-day and 1-year mortality and rate of cardiac arrest with and without thrombolysis as well as thrombolytic complications such as intracerebral hemorrhage (ICH) and major bleeding. The instrument is designed for incorporation into an ECG upon detection of significant ST-segment elevation. Predictions are then computed and printed on the ECG header.

Comment: The predictive instrument is intended for both prehospital use with supervision of emergency physicians and also for use in the ED. No data are yet available on clinical trials of these prehospital thrombolytic predictive instruments.

Presentation Delay

See annotations in Chapter 32 (420–422) and Chapter 3 (58).

32

SHORTENING DOOR-TO-NEEDLE TIME AND DOOR-TO-BALLOON TIME

DEBORAH L. ZVOSEC AND STEPHEN W. SMITH

KEY POINTS

- Institutional protocols and systems are necessary to decrease time to reperfusion.

GENERAL BACKGROUND

Time to reperfusion therapy is critical in AMI (31). It may be broken down into numerous components, starting with the onset of symptoms, up until administration of a thrombolytic drug or PCI. Here we discuss how institutional protocols may decrease time to treatment, with focus on door-to-needle-time (DTNT) and door-to-balloon time (DTBT). A short DTNT is strongly associated with preserved myocardium and decreased mortality (58,399,424, 426). A DTBT of < 60 minutes has been shown to be strongly associated with decreased mortality (427,428). Cases 32-1 and 32-2 show what speed in systems, diagnostics, and therapy can do.

AMI Symptom Onset to Clot Lysis with Thrombolytics

The sequence of events from onset of AMI symptoms until clot lysis can be broken down into the following five steps. **DTNT involves three steps: door to data, data to decision, and decision to drug (429).**

1. Symptom onset until seeking care.
   - Step 1 cannot be controlled directly. Untargeted community education campaigns have not been consistently effective (420–422). Targeted education of people with known coronary artery disease (CAD) may be more effective.
2. Seeking care until arrival at the door (of a health care facility).
   - Transport time is critical.
   - Consider use of prehospital 12-lead ECGs and prehospital thrombolysis. Prehospital gathering of data impacts the subsequent door-to-data time (see Chapter 31).
   - See recommendations below for improving prehospital care.
3. **Door to data** (history and physical, but especially the ECG).
   - May be decreased (improved) by education of prehospital providers (see later).
   - May be decreased by use of prehospital ECGs and protocols (see Chapter 31) (399,408,415).
   - May be decreased by protocols for in-hospital ECGs ("stat ECGs") (430).
   - May be decreased by prompt comparison with previous ECGs (73,408).
   - See recommendations below for improvement of DTNT.
4. **Data to decision** (to treat).
   - Requires skilled ECG interpretation.
   - Requires protocols and confidence in choice of therapy (thrombolysis versus PCI) (431).
   - See recommendations below for improvement of DTNT.
5. **Decision to drug** (administration of thrombolytic).
   - See recommendations below for improvement of DTNT.
6. Administration of thrombolytic until clot lysis.
   - Should be monitored (see Chapter 27).

Steps 3 to 5 comprise DTNT. See recommendations below on reducing DTNT (430,432–434,435). **The standard of care for DTNT is less than 30 minutes (429),** but may take up to 45 minutes if the diagnosis is difficult and Step 4 is prolonged (38,432).

AMI Symptom Onset to PCI (Balloon Time)

The sequence of events from onset of AMI until balloon inflation of angioplasty is:

1. Symptom onset until seeking care.
   - See Step 1, above.
2. Seeking care until arrival at a health care facility.
   - See Step 2, above.
3. **Door to data.**
   - See Step 3, above.
4. **Data to decision.**
   - See Step 4, above, and recommendations, below, for improvement of DTNT and DTBT.
5. **Decision to treat until mechanical opening of the infarct-related artery (IRA) using PCI (balloon time).**

Steps 3 to 5 comprise DTBT. Optimal DTBT < 60 minutes and maximum DTBT is 90 minutes (413). Team planning is essential in order to keep this time period short.

IMPROVING DTNT AND DTBT

The following are important improvements that a health care facility can make for decreasing DTNT and DTBT (399,429, 436–440).

Prehospital

- Institute protocols and train personnel to minimize transport times.
- Train prehospital providers to identify patients with risk factors for CAD (those most likely to have AMI).
- Train prehospital providers to read ST elevation and ST depression on unipolar rhythm monitoring leads, including MCL leads (see Chapters 10 and 31).
- Train prehospital providers to alert ED personnel about patients with possible AMI.
- Treat all patients with suspicious CP with aspirin and sublingual NTG, unless there are contraindications.
- Consider use of prehospital 12-lead ECGs and prehospital thrombolysis (see Chapter 31).

Hospital

Door to Data (ECG)

- **By protocol, immediately place any patient with suspicion of myocardial ischemia, and record an ECG.**
- Patients suspected of ischemia should include, but are not limited to, the following:
  - **Age of 30 or more with a chief complaint of chest discomfort,** no matter how atypical (**429,430,**440).
  - **Age of 50 or more and a chief complaint of dyspnea, syncope, weakness, or rapid HR (430).**
  - **Unexplained discomfort** of the arms, neck, chin, jaw, epigastrium, or other region above the umbilicus.
    - Do not ignore the symptoms of the young, including **young women,** and do not dismiss a diagnostic ECG. Women and minorities are undertreated, and young women with AMI have a high mortality (441,442).
- AMI in the elderly, diabetics, and those with decreased mental functioning, foreign language, or communication difficulties may be **difficult to identify.** Be alert to their symptoms.
- Keep the ECG machine close at hand and know how to operate it. Do not depend on a technician.
- Have the ECG tracing brought immediately and directly to the physician in charge. **Do not** leave it at the patient's bedside or leave it for anyone else to interpret.
- If necessary for diagnosis, obtain previous ECGs quickly to look for diagnostic changes.
  - Keep your institutional ECGs on an electronic system so that previous ECGs can be retrieved immediately, without searching for a paper chart. Have a fax machine on hand so that you can obtain a previous ECG from another institution immediately.

Door to Data: Adjunctive Therapy

- **By protocol, nurses should perform the following** on patients with symptoms or signs suspicious for AMI:
  - Intravenous (IV), oxygen, cardiac monitor, aspirin, sublingual NTG.

Data to Decision

- **Learn how to read the difficult ECGs as well as the easy ones,** and learn how to use this book to recognize subtle AMIs, to recognize the look-alikes, and to evaluate the risk/benefit ratio of thrombolytic therapy.
- **Do not** delay thrombolytic therapy in order to consult the primary care physician (443) or a cardiologist, unless you cannot make the decision without help **(444).** The mission of this book is to help you make the reperfusion decision and act expediently.
- Institute and use protocols in order to make the choice of thrombolytic therapy versus PCI.
- Evaluate quickly for significant contraindications to thrombolysis (see Chapter 34).

Decision to Drug

For patients arriving from outside the hospital, administration of the drug was a mean of 35 minutes faster if done in the ED, not in the cardiac care unit (CCU) (445).

- Decide as an institution which thrombolytic drug you will use and then use only one to avoid confusion.
- Keep the thrombolytic drug on hand in the patient care area (not in the pharmacy) and know how to prepare it (443).
- Use a bolus thrombolytic drug that is easy and quick to administer, such as rPA or TNK-tPA.
- Do not delay the thrombolytic bolus for other medications or unnecessary procedures. Only the following procedures take precedence:
  - Assessment of airway, breathing, circulation (ABCs).
  - IV, oxygen, cardiac monitor, vital signs.
  - Correction of hemodynamically significant brady- or tachy-dysrhythmias.
  - Aspirin and sublingual NTG, ± morphine for severe discomfort.

Decreasing DTBT

- **For PCI to be preferred to thrombolytic therapy, there must be 24-hour cath lab availability with a response time < 30 minutes.**
- The availability of PCI adds another time-consuming complex decision **(431).** Use a simple protocol to avoid this delay.
- Call the interventional cardiologist first. Preliminary calls to a primary physician or a general cardiologist waste valuable time.
- **Insist** on a 5-minute call-back time for interventional cardiology.
- Transport patients directly to the cath lab from the ED. Transport to the CCU adds an unnecessary delay.
- Administer adjunctive medications in the ED while awaiting the cath lab team. In consultation with your interventional cardiologist, this may include half-dose thrombolytics, glycoprotein (GP) IIb–IIIa inhibitors, clopidogrel, and/or high-dose heparin.

CASE 32-1

The Miracle of Thrombolytic Therapy

History
This 57-year-old man presented with CP.

ECG 32-1A (Type 1a)
- Diagnostic of a **very large anterior AMI**, as demonstrated by the number of leads involved (11 of 12 leads, eight with ST elevation and three with ST depression) and the height of the ST segments (11 mm in V4).

Clinical Course
The patient did not respond to NTG. **He received tPA within 15 minutes of presentation.**

ECG 32-1B (Type 2)
Recorded 27 minutes after ECG 32-1A, V1–V6 only
- Complete resolution of ST segments.

- Terminal T-wave inversion: V2 (Wellens' syndrome) indicates at least some myocardial necrosis.

Clinical Course
The patient had a minimal CK-MB elevation of 15.9 IU/L (total CK 127 IU/L). A left ventriculogram showed normal LV function. Angiography showed severe LAD and circumflex stenosis but TIMI-3 flow.

Conclusion
ECG 32-1A is not a difficult ECG and the benefit-to-risk ratio was very high for this patient. Thus the thrombolytic decision was easy. A 15-minute DTNT is fast and is the result of a good system. Assuming that the reperfusion was due to thrombolytics rather than to aspirin and heparin administration or to a transient STEMI, the quick action of the emergency physician saved much myocardium and possibly a life.

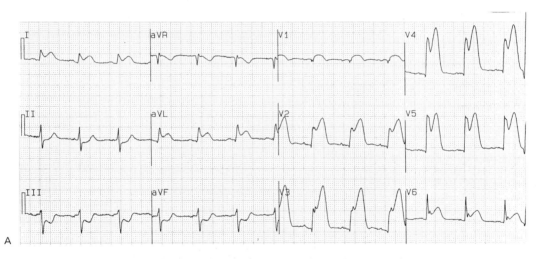

A

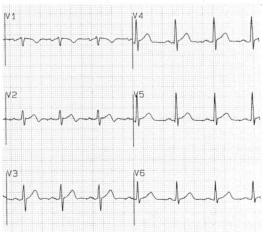

B

CASE 32-2

Symptom Onset to Balloon Time of 64 Minutes; DTBT of 30 Minutes

History
This 50-year-old man with a history of HTN had acute onset of CP at 08:50. He was found unconscious with respiratory effort at 09:00. After 5 to 10 minutes without cardiopulmonary resuscitation (CPR), resuscitation was begun and was successful after six defibrillations. He arrived at the ED unconscious but hemodynamically stable at 10:24.

Clinical Course
The ECG (not shown) revealed an obvious anterolateral AMI, similar to ECG 32-1a, above, and the patient was transported immediately to the cath lab after initiation of

aspirin, heparin, and lidocaine. Angiography was initiated at 09:45 and PCI opened a proximal LAD occlusion at 09:54, for a time of 64 minutes from **symptom onset** to intervention, and a DTBT of 30 minutes. Echocardiography on the day of admission showed severe anterior, lateral, septal, and apical WMA with severely decreased LV function. However, convalescent WMAs were mild with only mildly decreased LV function. The patient had full neurologic recovery.

Comment
Coordinated teams can act quickly to minimize DTBT.

ANNOTATED BIBLIOGRAPHY

National Heart Attack Alert Program Coordinating Committee 60 Minutes to Treatment Working Group. Rapid identification and treatment of patients with acute myocardial infarction, 1994.
  Findings: This is an excellent review (429), with detailed discussion and analyses, of the importance of early treatment, the reasons for delay, and areas for systematic improvement.

Time to Treatment and Outcomes
See annotation of Newby et al. (58) in Chapter 3.

Al-Mubarak N, et al. Consultation before thrombolytic therapy in acute myocardial infarction, 1999.
  Methods: Al-Mubarak et al. (444) analyzed data from the National Registry of Myocardial Infarction (NRMI)-II database from June 1994 to April 1996 (see Appendix C).
  Findings: Of 57,398 AMI patients with prehospital symptom onset who received thrombolytics, 36,368 patients (64%) were treated only after, and 20,730 (36%) were treated without, consultation with another physician. Baseline characteristics of the two groups showed statistically significant but clinically small difference. DTNT was 49 minutes versus 35 minutes and data-to-decision interval was 21 minutes versus 11 minutes in the consult versus no-consult groups ($p < 0.0001$). Multivariate analysis indicated that consultation was associated with greater in-hospital mortality even after adjustment for the minimally greater prevalence of high-risk characteristics in the consult group (OR 1.15, 1.04 to 1.26). Consultations were obtained more frequently in patients who were in health maintenance organizations, were of minority ethnic groups or advanced age, or had greater prehospital delay, pulmonary edema, a prior history of coronary revascularization, or an ECG with BBB or "normal" findings.

Cannon CP, et al. Relationship of symptom onset-to-balloon time and door-to-balloon time with mortality in patients undergoing angioplasty for acute myocardial infarction, 2000.
  Methods: Cannon et al. (428) analyzed NRMI-2 data (see Appendix C) on 27,080 AMI patients who underwent primary angioplasty.
  Findings: Median DTBT was 116 minutes. Symptom-onset-to-balloon-time did not correlate with in-hospital mortality, but DTBT did correlate. However, compared with patients with a DTBT < 60 minutes, multivariate relative mortality odds for those with DTBT = 60 to 120 minutes were as follows: 1.15 (0.88 to 1.49); for those with DTBT = 121 to 150 minutes: 1.41 (OR: 1.08 to 1.84); and for those

with DTBT = 151 to 180 minutes: 1.62 (OR: 1.23 to 2.14). For patients with a DTBT > 180 minutes, mortality odds did not increase more (1.61, OR: 1.25 to 2.08). Therefore **DTBT was strongly and independently associated with mortality.**
  Comment: Another study using NRMI data found that **mean** DTBT was 120 minutes for high-volume, 131 for medium-volume, and 145 for low-volume hospitals (33).

Berger PB, et al. Relationship between delay in performing direct coronary angioplasty and early clinical outcome in patients with acute myocardial infarction: results from the GUSTO-IIb trial, 1999.
  Methods: Berger et al. (427) analyzed data from the GUSTO-IIb trial (446) (see Chapter 36), in which 1,138 patients with STEMI were randomized to thrombolytics or angioplasty.
  Findings: Among 565 patients who underwent angioplasty, mean DTBT was 76 minutes. Thirty-day mortality was 1% for patients with DTBT < 60 minutes, 3.7% for DTBT of 61 to 75 minutes, 4.0% for DTBT of 76 to 90 minutes, and 6.4% for DTBT > 90 minutes. **Time to treatment with primary angioplasty, as with thrombolytic therapy, is a critical determinant of mortality.**

Shortening the Time from AMI Symptom Onset Until Care-Seeking by the Patient
Luepker RV, et al. Effect of a community intervention on patient delay and emergency medical service use in acute coronary heart disease, 2000.
  Methods: Luepker et al. (422) randomly assigned 10 matched pairs of communities to a broad-based community educational intervention designed to reduce patient delay from AMI symptom onset until EMS activation.
  Findings: At 18 months, there was no significant difference in delay time (time from symptom onset to ED arrival or to EMS use). The mean time was 140 minutes. However, there was a 20% increase in appropriate use of EMS services by patients with CP in the intervention communities.

Blohm M, et al. Consequences of a media campaign focusing on delay in acute myocardial infarction, 1992; Gazpoz J-M, et al. Impact of a public campaign on pre-hospital time delays in suspected acute myocardial infarction, 1993.
  Methods: Blohm et al. (420) and Gazpoz et al. (421), in Switzerland and Sweden, respectively, studied the effects of media campaigns that encourage people with symptoms of myocardial ischemia to seek medical attention. There were, respectively, 921 and 1,140 AMI patients who presented before the campaign, and 632 and 1,337 who presented during it.

Findings: Gazpoz et al. documented a **median** time decrease in delay from 195 minutes before the campaign to 155 minutes after, and a **mean** decrease from 9 hours, 10 minutes to 5 hours, 10 minutes. Blohm et al. documented a **median** decrease from 3 hours (before the media campaign) to 2 hours, 40 minutes during the campaign, and for AMI patients, a time of arrival of less than 3 hours was achieved in 50% before and 57% during the campaign. Infarct size as measured by CK-MB was significantly decreased. Both studies document a modest increase in presentations for noncardiac CP.

Shortening Time to Treatment (DTNT and DTBT)

Pell ACH, et al. Effect of "fast track" admission for acute myocardial infarction on delay to thrombolysis, 1992.

Methods: Pell et al. (434) developed a "fast track" ED evaluation and treatment plan at their hospital in England. Patients with AMI symptoms were immediately triaged to and evaluated by a physician who then administered thrombolytics to appropriate patients as quickly as possible.

Findings: DTNT was reduced by approximately 40 minutes when compared with the 2 years before implementation of the "fast-track" evaluation.

Cummings P. Improving the time to thrombolytic therapy for myocardial infarction by using a quality assurance audit, 1992.

Findings: Cummings (433) describes a quality assurance audit of time to treatment, with subsequent provision of findings to emergency physicians. DTNT at baseline was 63 minutes. After 2 years of the audit and feedback process, DTNT had been reduced to 38 minutes. Percentage of patients treated within 1 hour of presentation increased during this time from 45% to 96%.

Graff M, et al. Triage of patients for a rapid (5-minute) electrocardiogram: a rule based on presenting chief complaints, 2000.

Methods: Graff et al. (430) used a model set of patients to develop a rule for ordering "stat" protocol ECGs on patients according to presenting complaint and then tested the rule on a validation set.

Findings: AMI was diagnosed in 193 patients. Five chief complaints were most useful in identifying them: age > 30 years with CP and age > 50 years with syncope, weakness, tachycardia, and dyspnea. In the validation set, 142 patients had a final diagnosis of AMI. The rule performed better than CP in identifying patients in whom a "stat" ECG is necessary (93.7% versus 67.4% sensitivity for AMI) while only mod-

estly increasing the number of patients who undergo a "stat" ECG (6.3% to 7.3% of all ED patients). In thrombolytic patients, implementation of the rule was associated with a decrease in door-to-ECG time from 10.0 to 6.3 minutes, and a decrease in DTNT from 36.9 to 26.1 minutes.

Comment The time improvement was 11 minutes in a system that was already very fast.

Gilutz H, et al. The "door-to-needle blitz" in acute myocardial infarction: the impact of a CQI project, 1998.

Methods: Gilutz et al. (432) instituted a Continuous Quality Improvement (CQI) project. They grouped patients whose DTNT was > 45 minutes versus DTNT < 45 minutes.

Findings: The **most discrepant time interval** between the groups was "door-to-decision" time (36 versus 13 minutes), followed by "decision to treatment" time (26 versus 11 minutes). Subsequent efforts at shortening these intervals improved mean DTNT and are described in the paper.

Fesmire FM, et al. Diagnostic and prognostic importance of comparing the initial to the previous electrocardiogram in patients admitted for suspected acute myocardial infarction, 1991.

Methods: Fesmire et al. (73) studied 258 suspected AMI patients admitted to the hospital.

Findings: Patients with suspected AMI and a positive ECG (previous infarction, acute injury, ischemia, strain, LVH, LBBB, paced rhythm) were six times more likely to have AMI if the current ECG demonstrated changes from a previous ECG than if it showed no changes. **Prompt comparison with a previous ECG** to detect diagnostic changes may be critical for decreasing time to treatment.

Doorey A, et al. Dangers of delay of initiation of either thrombolysis or primary angioplasty in acute myocardial infarction with increasing use of primary angioplasty, 1998.

Methods: Doorey et al. (431) compared DTNTs and interviewed physicians about 37 AMI patients treated at their institution over 12 months when angioplasty first became available.

Findings: As angioplasty use increased, DTNT for thrombolytic patients increased from a mean time of 29 minutes (53% treated in less than 30 minutes) to 48 minutes (14% treated in less than 30 minutes). Mean DTBT was 134 minutes. Emergency physicians documented confusion about the best therapy (thrombolytic versus angioplasty) in 42% of all cases.

33

TIME WINDOW FOR REPERFUSION THERAPY

KEY POINTS

- The greatest benefit of reperfusion occurs in the first hour after coronary occlusion (the "golden hour").
- Thrombolytics are clearly and markedly beneficial when given within 6 hours of symptom onset and are still beneficial UP TO 12 hours.
- Time from symptom onset means time from onset of CONSTANT (as opposed to stuttering) symptoms.
- The ECG may be as important as the history in establishing the time of onset of coronary occlusion and in determining whether or not it is too late for reperfusion.
- High ST elevation, tall upright T waves, and ABSENCE of deep, well-formed Q waves may be diagnostic of RECENT onset of coronary occlusion even when not consistent with the history.
- Angioplasty may be indicated well beyond 12 hours.

GENERAL BACKGROUND

In AMI, time is myocardium. Animal studies indicate that myocardial infarction is nearly complete at 6 hours after coronary artery occlusion. Clinical trials have established the efficacy of thrombolytics up to 12 hours after symptom onset, and the earlier the better (30,31). Human and animal data indicate that salvage is nonlinear, with greater proportional salvage at earlier reperfusion. Thus the concept of the "golden hour," similar to trauma care but defined here as the first hour after coronary occlusion, has been promulgated (31). (See Chapters 31 and 32 for discussion of systems that reduce time to treatment.) Table 33-1 demonstrates mortality reduction as a function of time from symptom onset to thrombolytic administration (31). Further, as Bourke et al. (447) and Rapaport (448) have argued, the benefit of treatment from 6 to 24 hours has probably been underestimated in randomized clinical trials because of 30-day mortality endpoints. Most of the theoretical benefit of late thrombolysis, especially prevention of ventricular dilatation, would manifest **after** 30 days and thus would not be evident in the major trials.

Unfortunately, studies of the efficacy of thrombolysis do not specify whether "onset of symptoms" means onset of **constant** symptoms or onset of **any** symptoms. In evaluating STEMI, **time since onset of coronary occlusion** is not always easy to establish. Time since onset of occlusion is termed **"acuteness"** (90,458); "high" acuteness = short time interval since onset and "low" acuteness = long time interval since onset. We know that (a) preinfarction angina may continue for days before total coronary occlusion; (b) coronary occlusion is dynamic and occurs with spontaneous occlusion

TABLE 33.1. TIME TO THROMBOLYSIS AND MORTALITY REDUCTION

Time window	Lives saved per 1,000 patients treated (Number ± SD, CI)
0–1 hour	65 ± 14 (38–93)
1–2 hours	37 ± 9 (20–55)
2–3 hours	26 ± 6 (14–37)
3–6 hours	29 ± 5 (19–40)
6–12 hours	18 ± 6 (7–29)
12–24 hours	9 ± 7 (–5–22)

Reproduced with permission of The Lancet Ltd. From Boersma E, Maas AC, Deckers JW, et al. Early thromblytic treatment in acute myocardial infarction: reappraisal of the golden hour. *Lancet* 1996;348:771–775.

and reperfusion and with corresponding ST segment changes; and (c) myocardial risk area and infarction may be affected by collateral blood flow (91,159,341). Since intermittent anginal symptoms may be present long before the onset of infarction, **it is important to ascertain time since onset of CONSTANT symptoms.** Otherwise, patients with high acuteness but intermittent symptoms of longer duration may be inappropriately denied reperfusion therapy.

Assessment of acuteness based on historical data is not always clear. Patient histories are often vague and unreliable. Long duration of constant symptoms may occur with reversible ischemia; conversely, ischemia may be asymptomatic ("silent"). Additionally, pain onset does not always correlate well with angiographically proven occlusion. Women and diabetics, particularly, present with atypical histories. Historical data may be difficult to obtain if the patient speaks a foreign language or there are other communication difficulties. **Fortunately, the ECG may aid in determination of acuteness.** In fact, the ECG may be as important as the history in determining whether there remains viable myocardium that may be salvaged with reperfusion (180,340,**449**). The ECG, when it manifests **high ST elevation, high upright T waves, and absence of QS waves, may be diagnostic of recent occlusion** unless it contradicts a very clear history. On the other hand, **low ST elevation and T-wave inversion suggest spontaneous reperfusion or prolonged duration of occlusion,** the latter especially in the presence of QS waves.

TIME AND BENEFIT

Thrombolytics are definitely highly beneficial when symptoms have been present from **0 to 6 hours.** Thrombolytics are also **beneficial** when symptoms have been present for **6 to 12 hours,** although the relative benefit is less (Tables 33-1 and 33-

2). If **major** relative contraindications are present, consider limiting thrombolysis in the 6- to 12-hour group to those patients with moderate to large AMI (450).

Role of the ECG in Determining Acuteness

The following ECG characteristics aid in the determination of acuteness (time since coronary occlusion) especially when the history of symptom onset is vague or symptoms are atypical (180,**340**).

- **High ST elevation** (> 4 mm) **with tall, upright T waves** (higher than the ST elevation) indicates high acuteness **regardless** of historical time of symptom onset.
- **Tall upright T waves** correlate with **high** acuteness (180,**449**).
- **Flat or inverted T waves** correlate with **low** acuteness (more distant onset).
- **QS waves** correlate with **low** acuteness.
- **QR** waves, especially in anterior AMI, may be present very early (53% appear in the first hour) (92). **Q waves, especially QR waves, should NOT dissuade you from thrombolytic therapy** (see Case 11-1).

See Cases 33-1 through 33-8. (See also Case 8-13, in which prolonged occlusion as indicated by history is supported by QS waves and T-wave inversions.)

Role of Troponin

A minimally elevated troponin may be seen within 4 hours of onset of occlusion, but a very high troponin level is unlikely to represent early AMI. Few data exist, but a very high initial troponin level probably indicates prolonged occlusion or spontaneous reperfusion and, in equivocal situations, may sway the decision away from thrombolytic therapy (Case 33-8).

TABLE 33.2. DIFFERENCE IN NUMBERS OF LIVES SAVED PER 1,000 TREATED AS A FUNCTION OF TIME TO TREATMENT (45,000 PATIENTS PRESENTING WITH ST ELEVATION OR BBB ON THE ECG)

Time to thrombolytic administration	Mean number of lives saved per 1,000 treated
Up to 1 hour (mean, 0.98 hours)	39 (range, 28–62)
1–3 hours (mean, 2.5 hours)	30 (range, 25–36)
3–6 hours (mean, 4.79 hours)	27 (range, 21–33)
6–12 hours (mean, 9.11 hours)	21 (range, 14–28)
12–24 hours (mean, 17.48 hours)	12 (range, 1–14)

Reproduced with permission of The Lancet Ltd. From FTT Collaborative Group. Indications for fibrinolytic therapy in suspected acute myocardial infarction: collaborative overview of early mortality and major morbidity results from all randomised trials of more than 1000 patients. *Lancet* 1994;343:311–322.

CASE 33-1

Diabetic with 12 Hours of CP and ECG Diagnostic of AMI of Moderately High Acuteness

History

This 51-year-old man with long history of diabetes mellitus (DM) presented with 12 hours of typical CP. No previous ECG was available.

ECG 33-1 (Type 1a)

■ High voltage in aVL (> 12 mm): possible LVH.

■ Inferior Q waves: II, III, and aVF, are consistent with old inferior MI.

■ ST elevation: up to 3 mm at the J point, V1–V6; > 4 mm at 80 ms after the J point, V2.

Tall, acute T waves without inversion: up to 8 mm, V2.

■ QS waves: V3–V6, suggest that the AMI has been ongoing for at least several hours.

■ Persistent R wave: V2.

Clinical Course

This ECG is **consistent** with a history of 12 hours of AMI. The AMI is large, with persistent ST elevation and ongoing CP. There are no significant contraindications. Thrombolytics or

angiography ± PCI is indicated. A consulting cardiologist was reluctant to perform angioplasty, believing that the duration of occlusion was not apparent and that this could be a ventricular aneurysm. However, the **T waves are too tall and peaked** for either aneurysm (see Chapter 23) or completed AMI. The patient underwent successful immediate direct stent placement of an acutely occluded mid-LAD lesion. AMI was confirmed and the rise and fall of CK levels was typical for a 12-hour AMI. Echocardiography later that day revealed no aneurysm, but did show a severe anterior WMA with EF of 30% to 35%. The next day there was "significant recovery of anterior WMA," with 40% to 45% EF.

Conclusion

High ST elevation and tall T waves without inversion are findings of high acuteness (not older than 12 hours); they are **not consistent** with completed or old MI, or with aneurysm, even in the presence of Q waves. Reperfusion therapy probably helped to salvage significant myocardium.

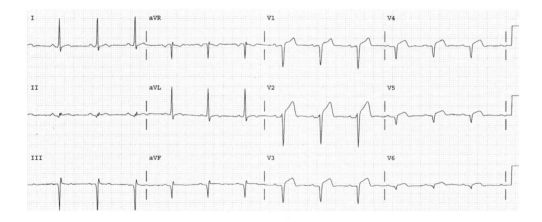

CASE 33-2

Seven Hours of CP, but the ECG Manifests High Acuteness, with Posterior AMI and Later Development of Inferior ST Elevation

History

This 68-year-old man with a history of right coronary artery (RCA) and LAD angioplasty 3 years prior presented at 14:37, 7 hours after the onset of stuttering CP.

ECG 33-2A (Type 1b)

At 14:37

- Junctional tachycardia.
- Pathologic Q waves: II, III, aVF are indicative of **old** inferior MI.

- ST depression: V2–V5, maximum in V2–V3, is **highly suspicious** of acute posterior MI, although this **ST depression may be due to supraventricular tachycardia.**
- ST elevation: minimal, aVL, V6, is **suspicious** for lateral AMI.

Clinical Course

Clinicians observed the patient and recorded a right-sided ECG 48 minutes later.

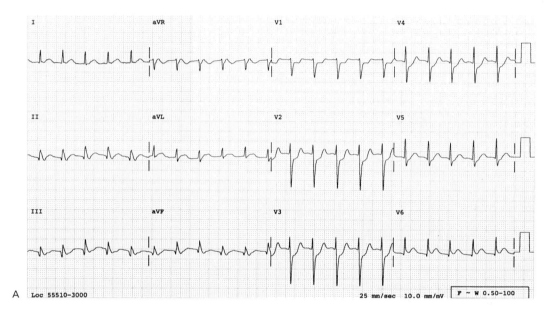

(continued on next page)

CASE 33-2

Seven Hours of CP, but the ECG Manifests High Acuteness, with Posterior AMI and Later Development of Inferior ST Elevation *(continued)*

ECG 33-2B (Type 1a)

At 15:25, is a right-sided ECG. (Limb leads are not altered when recording a right-sided ECG.)

- Sinus rhythm, HR = 92.
- ST elevation: II, III, aVF, is diagnostic of **inferior AMI.** The acuteness of this AMI is now very evident. There is **no ST depression in aVL because it is obscured** by the reciprocal electrical effect of **inferolateral AMI.** (This is **not** pericarditis.)
- ST depression: V1R–V6R, is **highly suspicious** for **posterior AMI.**

Clinical Course

Successful thrombolysis facilitated immediate resolution of ST abnormalities. Because of postinfarction angina, the patient was taken 2 days later for angiography. A 99% proximal circumflex lesion was successfully stented.

Conclusion

Measure time since onset of **constant pain,** not intermittent or stuttering pain, and recognize that some ECG findings can **only** be very acute, regardless of when symptoms began.

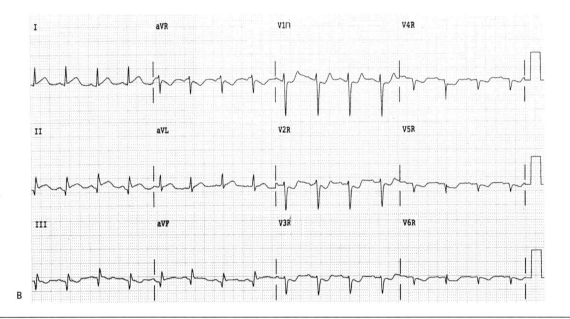

CASE 33-3

Fourteen Hours of CP and ECG Findings Are Consistent with Low Acuteness

History
This 51-year-old schizophrenic man at a nursing home complained of epigastric pain. He was given antacids but was "too shy to complain any more" until he had suffered symptoms for 14 hours. He was asymptomatic at presentation.

ECG 33-3 (Type 1d)
- ST elevation: low, 1 mm, V1–V4 and T-wave inversions: V2–V5, shallow, indicate long duration of occlusion (low acuteness).
- QS pattern: V1–V3, indicates long duration of occlusion (low acuteness).

Clinical Course
Biomarkers when the patient was admitted to the cardiac care unit (CCU) returned at CK = 490 IU/L and cardiac troponin I (cTnI) = 5.3 ng/mL. CK and cTnI peaked 19 hours after pain onset at 817 IU/L and 31 ng/mL, respectively. Angiography performed subsequent to recurrent ST elevation revealed a 100% proximal LAD occlusion and distal LAD filling via collaterals. A stent was successfully placed and ST segments normalized.

Conclusion
When the history and ECG are both consistent with a time course > 12 hours, thrombolytics are not indicated.

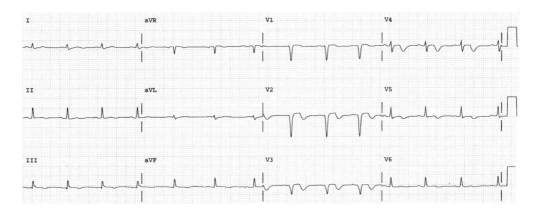

CASE 33-4

Two Days of Constant CP; the ECG Reveals High Acuteness

History
This 68-year-old man presented with 48 hours of CP that waxed and waned but never completely resolved.

ECG 33-4 (Type 1a)
- High ST elevation: V1–V5, > 6 mm in V2; and absence of T-wave inversion indicate **high acuteness.**
- QR pattern: V1–V4 (persistence of R waves also supports high acuteness).
- Q waves: III, aVF (old inferior MI).

Clinical Course
Reperfusion therapy is indicated. Angiography revealed a 100% acutely occluded proximal LAD lesion and a chronic 100% RCA occlusion. PCI successfully opened the LAD. Initial cTnI and CK returned at 4.3 ng/mL and 682 IU/L, respectively. CK peaked at 3,200 IU/L at 8 hours after successful reperfusion, confirming that the AMI was not 48 hours old. Echocardiography revealed anterior and lateral hypokinesis, with akinesis of the distal septum and apex, and moderately decreased LV function.

Conclusion
If the ECG shows high acuteness, 48 hours of even constant symptoms should not necessarily dissuade from reperfusion therapy, including thrombolytics.

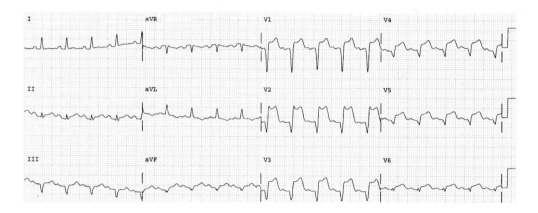

CASE 33-5

Eight Hours of CP; the ECG Revealed Moderately High Acuteness

History
This 81-year-old woman with history of DM and HTN presented with 8 hours of CP.

ECG 33-5 (Type 1a)
- ST elevation: II, III, aVF; and reciprocal depression: aVL, are diagnostic of **inferior AMI.**
- QR wave: II, III, aVF suggest infarction of at least several hours duration.
- No T-wave inversions.
- ST depression: V2–V3 is diagnostic of **posterior AMI;** R waves are not yet enlarged.

Clinical Course
With such a large inferoposterior AMI and ongoing pain and ST deviation, **reperfusion therapy is indicated.** Angiography ± PCI is preferable but thrombolytics are indicated if a cath lab is unavailable. Despite successful angioplasty and stenting of an occluded dominant RCA, the patient developed cardiogenic shock and died by 48 hours.

Conclusion
Neither Q waves nor 8 hours of symptoms should dissuade from reperfusion therapy.

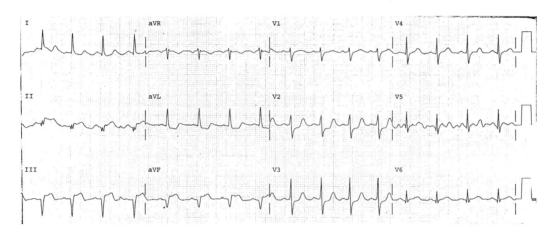

CASE 33-6

Two Days of CP and ECG Findings Are Indicative of Low Acuteness

History
This 53-year-old man presented with 2 days of constant chest tightness, with only brief relief 24 hours prior.

ECG 33-6 (Type 1d)
- Low ST elevation and QS waves with T-wave inversions: II, III, aVF indicate an **inferior AMI** of long duration (**low acuteness**).
- Minimal ST depression: V2–V4, and large T waves: V2–V3 are **suspicious** for evolving posterior AMI.

Clinical Course
Despite both symptoms and ECG findings of low acuteness, physicians gave thrombolytics. Fortunately, the patient experienced neither bleeding complications nor significant complications of AMI.

Conclusion
If it is too late by both symptoms and ECG findings, thrombolytics confer risk with little benefit. Angiography ± PCI is the preferred alternative for ongoing symptoms.

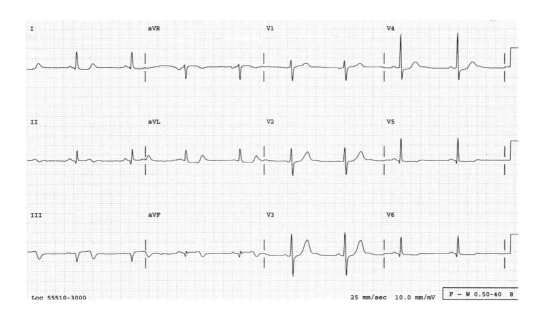

Loc 55510-3000   25 mm/sec   10.0 mm/mV   F ~ W 0.50-40 8

CASE 33-7

Anterior AMI with 12 Hours of CP and ECG Findings Consistent with Low Acuteness

History

This 68-year-old woman presented with 12 hours of CP, its constancy uncertain.

ECG 33-7 (Type 1d)

■ ST elevation, 3.5 mm; QS waves; and terminal T-wave inversions: V2–V4, are diagnostic of a well-developed **anterior AMI,** consistent with the history of 12 hours of continuous CP.

Clinical Course

Immediate echocardiography confirmed a WMA but could not aid in the remaining critical question: Is it too late for thrombolytics? Thrombolytics were administered. The first CK, drawn at the moment of presentation, was the peak (2,000 IU/L), which confirmed at least 12 hours of occlusion. Angiography performed due to postinfarction angina confirmed 100% mid-LAD occlusion and a 90% first diagonal stenosis. Convalescent echocardiography revealed a dyskinetic anterior wall and the ST segments remained 4 mm elevated for at least a week. Thus there is a high likelihood of ventricular aneurysm formation (see Chapter 23).

Conclusion

Once T waves are inverted and R waves gone, it may be too late for thrombolysis. Echocardiography cannot help determine the duration or acuity of AMI, as a WMA will be present whether the MI is 2 or 24 hours old. Immediate echocardiography may delay therapy if used for such a purpose.

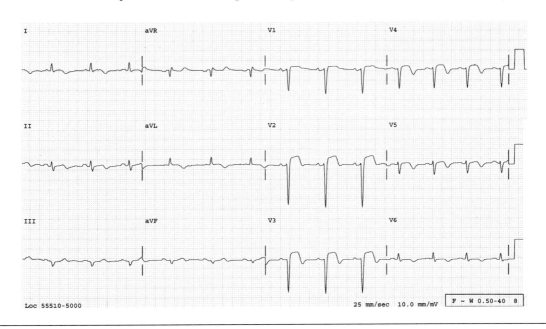

CASE 33-8

History and T-Wave Inversions Support Either Long Duration of Occlusion or Spontaneous Reperfusion; Confirmed by High Initial Troponin

History
This 31-year-old male smoker presented with 36 hours of constant sharp and reproducible CP. Clinicians recorded an ECG as a precautionary afterthought.

ECG 33-8 (Type 1d)
- ST elevation, QS waves, and deep T-wave inversion: V2–V6, are diagnostic of **acute or subacute anterolateral MI.** The T-wave inversions indicate long duration or spontaneous reperfusion. The depth of T wave inversion supports spontaneous reperfusion. ST segments remain elevated 3 to 4 mm, but the **presence of QS waves** supports **late** spontaneous reperfusion.

Clinical Course
By both clinical and ECG criteria, it is too late for thrombolytics. The admission cTnI returned at 78 ng/mL, CK was 3,437 IU/L, and all subsequent levels were lower, thus confirming subacute MI (prolonged occlusion). No reperfusion therapy was undertaken. A later echocardiogram revealed severe anterior, lateral, septal, and apical WMAs. The patient insisted on leaving without further work-up.

Conclusion
QS waves with deep terminal T-wave inversions are most consistent with late spontaneous reperfusion. This, in addition to the symptom duration, suggests that the AMI is too far progressed to benefit from thrombolytics.

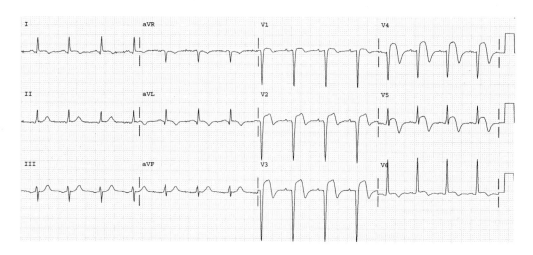

ANNOTATED BIBLIOGRAPHY

Background
Possible Mechanisms of Benefit of Late Reperfusion: Animal studies have indicated that myocardium is nearly 100% necrotic after 6 hours with no blood flow. Despite this, there is benefit to late reperfusion (more than 6 hours from symptom onset). Possible mechanisms include (a) the myocardium at risk may have collateral flow keeping it viable for more than 6 hours; (b) reperfusion of an IRA that provides collateral flow to other myocardial areas may preserve those zones if there is subsequent occlusion of another coronary artery; (c) collateral circulation to remote ischemic zones may be restored (447,448,450, **451,**452,**453**); (d) reduced mural thrombus formation (454); (e) better healing, scarring, and ventricular remodeling of the infarct zone thus limiting long-term LV dilatation and aneurysm formation (**101**) (the most important long-term prognostic factor after MI is **end-systolic volume**) (452,455); and (f) greater long-term electrical stability of the infarct zone (**456**).

There are also ways in which late reperfusion may be harmful. These include myocardial stunning, microvascular damage, and intramyocardial hemorrhage, which may lead to increased risk of myocardial rupture (448).

Time from Symptom Onset to Thrombolysis
Boersma E, et al. Early thrombolytic treatment in acute myocardial infarction: reappraisal of the golden hour, 1996.

Methods: Boersma et al. (31) analyzed all 22 placebo-controlled thrombolytic trials from 1983 to 1993 with at least 100 patients. They analyzed data with regard to time intervals of 0 to 1, 1 to 2, 2 to 3, 3 to 6, 6 to 12, and 12 to 24 hours after onset of symptoms. Some of the large trials included were GISSI-1, ISIS-2, LATE (see Appendix C), and EMERAS (see later). ISIS-3 (103) and USIM (457), having uncertain indications for thrombolysis, were analyzed separately. The 22 trials included 50,246 patients, 5,762 of whom were randomized within 2 hours of symptom onset, and 10,435 from 2 to 3 hours. Nonlinear regression was used to analyze for proportional mortality reduction.

Findings: See Table 33-1 for mortality benefit. The reduction in mortality was nonlinear, with added proportional benefit at earlier thrombolytic administration, which supports the notion of the "golden hour."

FTT Collaborative Group. Indications for fibrinolytic therapy in suspected acute myocardial infarction: collaborative overview of early mortality and major morbidity results from all randomised trials of more than 1,000 patients, 1994.

Methods: The FTT collaborative group study (30), which includes data from GISSI (29) and ISIS-2 (102) (see Appendix C), included patients who presented **without ST elevation or BBB on the ECG.** In contrast to Boersma et al. (31) above, they did not divide the data into hourly intervals up to 3 hours and they did not perform nonlinear regression.

Findings: There was a linear relation between time since onset and mortality reduction, with 1.6 lives saved per 1,000 patients per hour of delay. Data from the 45,000 patients who were eligible by standard ECG criteria is shown in Table 33-2.

Late Thrombolysis

LATE Study Group. Late assessment of thrombolytic efficacy (LATE) study with alteplase 6 to 24 hours after onset of acute myocardial infarction, 1993.

Methods: The LATE Study (169) (see Appendix C) collected data from 5,711 patients with suspected AMI and ECG changes including ST elevation of 1 mm inferior or 2 mm precordial or ST depression or T-wave inversion or new Q waves or new BBB or equivocal ECG changes with elevated cardiac enzymes. Patients were randomized to tissue plasminogen activator (tPA) or placebo at 6 to 24 hours after symptom onset. All patients received aspirin, 46% received IV heparin, and 18% received subcutaneous heparin.

Findings: ST elevation manifested in 55%. Patients treated **6 to 12 hours** from symptom onset had a 35-day mortality of 8.9% for tPA therapy and 12.0% for placebo, with a relative reduction of 25.6% (*p* = 0.0229, 95% CI of 6.3% to 45%) and an **absolute reduction of 3.1%, or 31 per 1,000 treated.** Among patients with an unequivocal diagnosis of AMI and who were **treated within 3 hours of arrival, the benefit was still greater and extended into the 12- to 24-hour group.** Among all patients treated from 12 to 24 hours from symptom onset, there was no statistically significant difference in mortality. In a subgroup analysis, treatment of undifferentiated inferior AMI from 6 to 12 hours after symptom onset showed no benefit (450). Inferior AMI subgroup analysis is not available for the other studies above. The 6-month rate of excess nonfatal disabling stroke was equal for tPA and placebo.

EMERAS. Randomised trial of late thrombolysis in patients with suspected acute myocardial infarction, 1993.

Methods: The EMERAS trial (451) randomized 4,534 patients presenting from 6 to 24 hours after AMI symptom onset to streptokinase (SK) or placebo. ECG changes were not necessary for entry.

Findings: Of 4,534 patients, 67% had ST elevation, 82% received aspirin, 23% received IV heparin, and 14% received subcutaneous heparin. Antiplatelet and anticoagulant use was comparable between the two groups. Among the 2,080 patients presenting 7 to 12 hours from symptom onset there was a nonsignificant reduction (14%) of in-hospital mortality for the SK group (11.7% versus 13.2%, CI: −33% to +12%). There was a nonsignificant increase of in-hospital mortality for the SK group in patients presenting 13 to 24 hours after symptom onset. The lack of efficacy extends to the subgroup of patients with ST elevation.

Mechanisms of Late Thrombolysis

Steinberg JS, et al. Effects of thrombolytic therapy administered 6 to 24 hours after myocardial infarction on the signal-averaged ECG. Results of a multicenter randomized trial, 1994.

Methods: Steinberg et al. (456) analyzed data on signal-averaged ECGs of 310 patients in the LATE trial (see above [169] and Appendix C), 160 of whom received placebo and 150 of whom received tPA, and also from the prespecified subgroup of 185 patients with ST elevation.

Findings: Of patients with ST elevation, those who received tPA had a 52% (CI: 4% to 77%) reduction in signal-averaged ECG abnormality compared with those who received placebo. **This suggests that late thrombolysis produces a more electrically stable myocardium.**

Topol EJ, et al. A randomized trial of late reperfusion therapy for acute myocardial infarction, 1992.

Methods: The TAMI-6 study (101) randomized 197 AMI patients with symptom duration of 6 to 24 hours to tPA or placebo. Patients underwent angiography within 24 hours and were followed for 6 months, at which time ejection fraction (EF) was assessed by gated blood pool scintigraphy.

Findings: By 24 hours, the IRA was patent in 65% in the tPA group and 25% in the placebo group. At 6 months, the IRA was patent in 59% of both groups and there was no difference in EF or WMAs. However, in the placebo group, **end diastolic volume had increased from an acute phase mean of 127 mL to 159 mL;** cavity size did not increase among the tPA patients.

ECG Analysis in Late Thrombolysis

Anderson ST, et al. Electrocardiographic phasing of acute myocardial infarction, 1992; Wilkins ML, et al. An electrocardiographic acuteness score for quantifying the timing of a myocardial infarction to guide decisions regarding reperfusion therapy, 1995.

Methods: Wilkins et al. (458) and Anderson et al. (459) used a phasing system for the ECG in STEMI as follows:

1A: Tall T, > 1 mV (10 mm), without abnormal Q wave
1B: Positive T without abnormal Q wave
2A: Tall T, > 1 mV (10 mm), with abnormal Q wave
2B: Positive T without abnormal Q wave
3: Abnormal Q wave with flat T **or** terminal T-wave inversion ≥ 0.05 mV
4: Abnormal Q wave with middle T-wave inversion ≥ 0.05 mV
U: ST elevation without abnormal Q wave with any T-wave inversion ≥ 0.05 mV

From these, they developed an acuteness score:
Formula:

$$\frac{4\ (\#\ leads\ 1A) + 3\ (\#\ leads\ 1B) + 2\ (\#\ leads\ 2A) + (\#\ leads\ 2B)}{\#\ leads\ with\ 1A,\ 1B,\ 2A,\ or\ 2B}$$

Patients with AMI from the MITI trial (399) had a prehospital- and a hospital-recorded ECG. Entry criteria were: no confounding ECG factors, the two ECGs were recorded within 2 hours, and had no thrombolytic therapy between the two ECGs.

Findings: One hundred fifty-four patients met the entry criteria. Two thirds of ECGs were recorded in a 30 to 60 minute time period. The mean acuteness score was higher for the first ECG, though with wide standard deviations (3.56 ± 0.55 versus 3.19 ± 0.54).

Comment: The data does serve to illustrate that even over a 30 to 60 minute time period, the ECG evolves in a predictable manner, and that **tall upright T waves correlate with acuteness and flat or inverted T waves and Q waves correlate with lack of acuteness.**

Corey KE, et al. Combined historical and electrocardiographic timing of acute anterior and inferior myocardial infarcts for prediction of reperfusion achievable size limitation, 1999.

Methods: Corey et al. (340) applied the acuteness score developed by Wilkins et al. (458) (see above) to the ECGs of 395 patients from four thrombolytic trials. Patients fulfilled several criteria, the most important of which were: (a) a report of the historical time of symptom onset; and (b) tomographic thallium-201 imaging 7 weeks after admission to measure final AMI size. Scores ranged from 1 (least acute) to 4 (most acute).

Findings: Patients with the highest acuteness scores had the greatest limitation of infarct size. For anterior AMI, a high acuteness score (≥ 3) correlated with a 50% smaller **final** anterior infarct size compared with the patients with low acuteness scores, despite a greater time interval from symptom onset to treatment. A low acuteness score (< 3) correlated with 50% **larger** final inferior infarct size in spite of shorter delay since time of symptom onset. This correlation may occur because: (a) patients may not have given an accurate history; (b) pain prior to presentation may have been stuttering, thus reflecting UA and not AMI; or (c) patients with a high acuteness score may have had good collateral circulation, which slows infarction. **Thus the ECG acuteness score added the most value in situations of data disagreement,** such as when: (a) the history in an anterior AMI indicated a time since symptom onset of more than 2 hours but the acuteness score was high; or (b) the history in an inferior AMI indicated a time since symptom onset of less than 2 hours but the acuteness score was low.

Comment: **Determining AMI duration from ECG morphology and from symptom duration are equally important.**

Hochrein J, et al. Higher T-wave amplitude associated with better prognosis in patients receiving thrombolytic therapy for acute myocardial infarction (a GUSTO-1 substudy), 1998.

Methods: Hochrein et al. (180) hypothesized that higher T waves would be a marker for earlier AMI and thus a marker for better outcome after reperfusion with thrombolytic therapy. They analyzed data from GUSTO-I (see Appendix C).

Findings: Patients with tall T waves, as defined by more than the 98th percentile of the upper limit of normal, had lower 30-day mortality (5.2% versus 8.6%, $p = 0.001$), less CHF (15% versus 24%, $p < 0.001$), and less cardiogenic shock (6.1% versus 8.6%, $p = 0.023$) than patients without tall T waves. Differences remained significant after controlling for multiple baseline variables. Patients with tall T waves had significantly shorter symptom duration, but tall T waves were prognostic even after controlling for symptom duration. Thus **tall T waves are an independent marker of benefit from thrombolytics.**

Herz I, et al. The prognostic implications of negative T waves in the leads with ST segment elevation on admission in acute myocardial infarction, 1999.

Methods: Herz et al. (449) assessed the prognostic significance of T waves in 2,853 patients with STEMI treated with thrombolysis. Only patients with ongoing symptoms and ST elevation were included. They divided patients into four groups: those who were "admitted" 2 hours or less from symptom onset with negative (T−) ($n = 252$) or positive (T+) ($n = 2,601$) T waves, and those who were admitted more than 2 hours from onset with (T−) or (T+).

Findings: (T−) was associated with 0 mortality (0/52) if admission occurred within 2 hours of symptom onset but 10.2% mortality (20/196) if admission was more than 2 hours from symptom onset. (T+) was associated with 5.0% mortality (36/726) if within 2 hours, and 5.4% (100/1836) if after 2 hours. **The authors believe that those who have early (T−) have spontaneous reperfusion and low mortality and those with late (T−) have more advanced AMI.**

Future Study

The ACTOR study (453) ("Aggressive versus conservative treatment of the infarct-related artery after acute MI") will randomize patients with persistently occluded arteries and no persistent symptoms or other reason for revascularization to late mechanical revascularization versus conservative therapy. Three-year follow-up is planned to determine if the benefits of very late reperfusion (including limitation of dilatation, better scar formation, better collateral flow, and more electrical stability) will lead to better outcomes.

34

THROMBOLYTIC STROKE RISK AND CONTRAINDICATIONS

KEY POINTS

■ Thrombolytics are underused, despite proven efficacy, in part due to the risk of ICH.

■ More patients would survive neurologically intact if physicians were more aggressive with therapy.

■ Although angioplasty may be preferable, if available, thrombolytics are NOT contraindicated in the elderly (more than 75 years of age) and are of GREAT BENEFIT.

■ Overall, in patients who present within 6 hours of symptom onset with ST elevation or BBB, tPA saves approximately 40 lives per 1,000 treated and will lead to two excess disabling strokes per 1,000.

GENERAL BACKGROUND

Intracranial hemorrhage (ICH), or hemorrhagic stroke, is the most feared complication of thrombolytic therapy (see Case 35-1). However, this risk must be accepted in order to save lives with thrombolytics. As difficult as it is when our therapy may lead to such an unfortunate outcome, we must always bear in mind that **if we take this risk more frequently than we do at present, we will save more lives.**

Analysis of Thrombolytic Stroke Risk

The vast majority of data comparing thrombolytics to placebo involves SK. Much data regarding efficacy and effects of tPA must therefore be derived indirectly. Although thrombolytic therapy increases the risk of hemorrhagic stroke, it also **decreases the risk of ischemic stroke,** which results from cardiogenic cerebral embolism from mural thrombus that may form after untreated, completed AMI. Although the overall excess stroke rate for thrombolytics (primarily SK) over placebo is four per 1,000, two of these four strokes were fatal and are included in mortality data (**30**). Furthermore, although the overall excess **nonfatal** stroke rate is only about **two per 1,000** patients treated, the **overall excess nonfatal but DISABLING stroke rate** is only about **one per 1,000** (**30**). Depending on the time since onset, **SK therapy resulted in 20 to 40 lives**

saved per 1,000 AMI patients treated (**30**). The LATE study (**169**) (see Chapter 33) found no excess disabling stroke for tPA over placebo at 6 months. GUSTO-1 (**86**) found 0.1% more nonfatal disabling stroke in the tPA group (0.6%) than in the SK group (0.5%), despite having 0.23% more intracranial bleeds in the tPA group. Combining these results, we estimate **the overall excess nonfatal but disabling stroke rate for tPA versus placebo to be two per 1,000.** Sleight made the same estimate (**308**) without the benefit of final results from LATE and GUSTO. When one considers that approximately **nine more lives** are saved per 1,000 treated with tPA than with SK (**86**) such that approximately 30 to 48 lives are saved per 1,000 treated with tPA versus placebo, **a very high benefit-to-risk ratio of tPA** is apparent. For patients with a large AMI, the number of lives saved with thrombolytic therapy is even greater than 30 to 48 per 1,000 treated; for patients with smaller AMI, the number is less.

Advanced Age

Despite consensus that thrombolytics are indicated for elderly patients (**308,460,461,462,463**) and evidence of benefit from thrombolytics equal to that of younger patients (**27,29,102, 291,308,365,463,464,465**) **elderly patients are consistently inappropriately denied thrombolytic therapy** (**25,27,28,464,466,467**). Elderly patients do have a high risk of hemorrhagic stroke (**86,469**). However, because AMI in the elderly is associated with very high mortality, the **absolute** number of lives saved per 1,000 elderly treated with thrombolytics equals that seen in younger patients even though the **relative** reduction is less (**29,102,463**). Although benefit was disputed in a single flawed but highly publicized nonrandomized retrospective study of 30-day mortality (**32**), a later study of the same data concluded that 1-year mortality was lower with thrombolytics. This was true especially for "ideal" thrombolytic candidates, defined as patients without contraindications who present less than 6 hours from symptom onset (**291**). More importantly, prospectively, randomized data proves the benefit of thrombolytics in the elderly: a recent reanalysis of data from the Fibrinolytic Therapy Trialists (FTT) collaborative group shows a **mortality reduction for those more than 75 years of age from 29.4% to 26.0%, or 34 lives saved per 1,000 treated** (**463**). Additionally, most data are from trials of SK versus placebo, not tPA. Thus the benefit-to-risk ratio from thrombolytic therapy is greater than most physicians appreciate, and **most elderly patients could benefit from being treated more aggressively** (470). A patient with a 5% risk of ICH due to thrombolytics but with a high-risk (large) AMI has a much better chance of surviving neurologically intact with early administration of thrombolytics than without it.

Heparin

Use of IV heparin is essential to obtain the maximal benefit from tPA, although it does add some risk of bleeding (**86**). Subcutaneous heparin adds little or no risk of ICH, but is rarely used today because it is less effective than IV heparin (98,103, **471**). To reduce the risk of serious hemorrhage with tPA, rPA, or TNK-tPA, **low-dose weight-based heparin is recommended.** The dosage is 60 U/kg bolus (maximum of 4,000 U), followed by 12 U/kg/hr (maximum 1,000 U/hr), targeting a prothrombin time (PTT) of 1.5 to 2 times control (105).

It appears now that enoxaparin, in an initial dose of 30 mg IV, followed by 1 mg/kg subcutaneously every 12 hours for 7 days, is superior to unfractionated heparin (471.5).

HEMORRHAGIC STROKE RISK

Table 34-1 summarizes the most recent data on the absolute risk for combinations of risk factors, but only in patients more than 65 years of age. The following were independently associated with ICH: **age 75 years or more, female sex, African-American ethnicity, prior stroke, systolic BP ≥ 160, use of tPA compared with other thrombolytics, International Normalized Ratio (INR) 4.0 or more or PTT of more than 24 seconds, and low weight (< 65 kg for females, < 80 kg for males)** (472).

Table 34-2 shows absolute risks as found in an earlier, smaller study (**473**).

Table 34-3 shows only adjusted OR (**469**), which must be multiplied by an index risk to obtain an absolute risk for any given patient. However, it allows calculation for patients with a history of stroke. The risk of ICH for a male under 65 years of age with no history of stroke who receives tPA (**index risk**) is well under 0.52%, perhaps **0.4% (86)**. The **OR × index risk = approximate risk of stroke.**

■ According to this table, a male 70 years of age, of weight > 80 kg, with no history of stroke, who receives tPA, has an estimated risk of ICH of **0.4% × 3.66 (from Table 34-3) = 1.46%.**

Tables 34-1, 34-2, and 34-3 provide very different estimates of risk of ICH after thrombolytic therapy for AMI in a community setting, as calculated and shown in Table 34-4.

As described earlier, it is important to remember that a significant number of these patients who received thrombolytics **avoided having a cardiogenic cerebral embolism** due to

TABLE 34.1. RISK STRATIFICATION SCALE OF INDEPENDENT PREDICTORS OF ICH IN PATIENTS OVER AGE 65[a]

Number of risk factors	Number in each group	Rate of intracranial hemorrhage
0 or 1	6,651	0.69%
2	10,509	1.02%
3	9,074	1.63%
4	4,298	2.49%
≥5	1,071	4.11%

Adapted from Brass LM, Lichtman JH, Wang Y, et al. Intracranial hemorrhage associated with thrombolytic therapy for elderly patients with acute myocardial infarction. *Stroke* 2000;31:1802–1811, with permission.
[a]Risk factors included: age ≥75 years, female sex, African-American ethnicity, prior stroke, systolic BP ≥160, use of tPA compared with other thrombolytics, international normalized ratio (INR) ≥4.0 or PTT time >24 seconds, and low weight (<65 kg for females, <80 kg for males).

TABLE 34.2. ABSOLUTE RISK (PERCENTAGE) OF ICH AFTER THROMBOLYTIC THERAPY[a]

Risk factor	Age <65	Age 66–75	Age 76–85	Age >85
0 other risk factors	0.3%	1.0%	1.5%	2.3%
1	1.0%	1.3%	2.0%	2.9%
2	1.3%	2.2%	3.3%	5.0%

Adapted from Simoons ML, Maggioni AP, Knatterud G, et al. Individual risk assessment for intracranial haemorrhage during thrombolytic therapy. *Lancet* 1993;342:1523–1528, with permission. Copyright The Lancet Ltd., 1993.
[a]Independent risk factors in this study include: HTN on admission, low body weight, and use of tPA.

TABLE 34.3. ADJUSTED ORs FOR ICH AFTER THROMBOLYTIC THERAPY[a]

	Male, no history of stroke	Female, no history of stroke	Male, history of stroke	Female, history of stroke
<65 years	1.00 (index)	2.46	5.09	12.5
65–74 years	3.66	4.91	6.99	9.38
≥75 years	6.42	8.31	6.98	9.04

Reproduced with permission of the American College of Physicians. From Gurwitz JH, Gore JM, Goldberg RJ, et al. Risk for intracranial hemorrhage after tissue plasminogen activator treatment for acute myocardial infarction. *Ann Intern Med* 1998;129:597–604.
[a]Absolute risks are unavailable in this study.

TABLE 34.4. RISK OF ICH: CONTRASTING RISK ESTIMATES FOR EXAMPLE PATIENTS (USING TABLES 34-1, 34-2, AND 34-3)

	Table 34-1	Table 34-2	Table 34-3
Male of age 70 years, >80 kg, with no other risk factors, who receives tPA	0.69%	1.3%	1.46%
Female of age 70 years, >65 kg, with no other risk factors, who receives tPA	1.02%	1.3%	1.96%

mural thrombus formation after completed AMI. This is not reflected in the data because all patients received thrombolytics. In patients with high risk of stroke, angiography ± PCI is the preferred method of reperfusion, if available.

CONTRAINDICATIONS TO THROMBOLYTICS

Table 34-5 lists absolute, relative, and minor contraindications to thrombolytic therapy (429,**472,474,**475–478,**479**). **Note:** The risk of thrombolytic therapy during pregnancy is unknown.

MANAGEMENT
Advanced Age

Do not deny patients more than 75 years of age thrombolytic therapy based on age alone. Although the benefits of angioplasty are believed to be greater in the elderly than in younger patients, research has not supported this (480). Nevertheless,

TABLE 34.5. CONTRAINDICATIONS TO THROMBOLYTICS

ABSOLUTE CONTRAINDICATIONS
History of **hemorrhagic stroke or known cerebral aneurysm**
Active, serious, noncompressible **bleeding**
Cerebral infarct within 2 months
Known **intracranial neoplasm**
Cranial or spinal surgery within 14 days

MAJOR RELATIVE CONTRAINDICATIONS
Persistent HTN > 180/110
Cerebral infarct within 2–6 months
Symptomatic **gastrointestinal bleed** within 14 days
Significant **head trauma** within 10–14 days
■ Do a head CT scan prior to treatment
Major surgery or trauma within 10–14 days

SIGNIFICANT RELATIVE CONTRAINDICATIONS
HTN > 180/110 at presentation but able to lower to <180/110
Warfarin use in the presence of minor bleeding
(e.g., occult blood in stool)
Significant bleeding diathesis (INR > 4.0 or PTT > 24 seconds);
RR = 2.15, CI: 1.1–4.2 **(472)**
CPR chest compressions **with evidence of injury**
Noncompressible vessel puncture
■ Use femoral access in a patient who needs a central line and who
may need thrombolytics
Nasotracheal intubation
■ Use orotracheal access in any patient who may need
thrombolytics **(474)**
Remote thrombotic stroke

MINOR CONTRAINDICATIONS
CPR chest compressions, with no physical evidence of injury (475)
Warfarin use with INR < 4.0
Minor bleeding (e.g., occult blood in stool)
■ Routine occult blood testing of stool is not required (429)

INCONSEQUENTIAL
Active menstruation (476–478)
Diabetic retinopathy (**479**)
History of previous MI
History of stent or angioplasty
History of CABG

as with younger patients, if angioplasty is available, the procedure is performed at a high-volume institution, and the DTBT is less than 60 minutes, angioplasty is preferable (see Chapter 36) (33,**291,**481). **If angioplasty is not available on a timely basis, do NOT withhold thrombolytics because of advanced age** if there are no significant contraindications and co-morbidity **(291)**. For a large AMI, even elderly patients with relative contraindications should receive thrombolytics (see Chapter 35).

Altered Mental Status After Cardiac Arrest

It is very unusual for a cardiac arrest due to ventricular fibrillation or ventricular tachycardia to result from ICH and even more rare for a patient with primary ICH to have a Type 1a or 1b ECG. In the rare event that these two factors coincide, however, the prognosis is grim, regardless of management. Such a cardiac arrest should be assumed to be of cardiac etiology, and altered mental status should be assumed to be the result of hypoxia while in arrest.

■ **Do not delay therapy unnecessarily by doing computed tomography (CT) of the head** before thrombolysis unless the history or physical exam provides **clear evidence of significant head trauma** from a fall after arrest. If there is significant suspicion of head trauma or primary ICH, **angiography ± PCI** is indicated, if available.

Challenging Management Issues

The following are challenging management issues presented by thrombolytic complications. See also Table 34-6 for management of severe bleeding and reversal of thrombolytic state (482).

ICH

Seventy-three percent of episodes of ICH occur **within 24 hours of treatment (469)** and 82% of patients manifest a

TABLE 34.6. TREATMENT OF SEVERE BLEEDING

1. Apply compression when possible.
2. Discontinue heparin and antiplatelet drugs. Administer protamine to reverse heparin.
3. Draw a thrombin time and a PTT.
4. Administer fluids and packed red cells for hypovolemia.
5. Give at least 10 units cryoprecipitate and 2–4 units of fresh frozen plasma.
6. Check fibrinogen; if the patient is still bleeding and fibrinogen is <1.0 g/L, transfuse 10 more units of cryoprecipitate.
7. Give epsilon aminocaproic acid (fibrinolytic inhibiter) for:
   a. Any intracranial bleeding
   b. Continued **life-threatening** bleeding, even with persistent coronary occlusion
   Dose: 5 g IV, then 0.5–1.0 g per hour
   Caution: this may cause refractory thrombosis or recurrent coronary thrombosis
8. Consider administering 10 units of platelets for continued bleeding, especially if GP IIb–IIIa inhibitors have been used.

TABLE 34.7. INCIDENCE OF STROKE IN GUSTO-1

	SK and IV heparin	SK and subcutaneous heparin	Accelerated tPA
All ages combined			
ICH	0.54%	0.49%	0.72%
Any stroke	1.40%	1.22%	1.55%
30-day mortality	7.4%	7.2%	6.3%
Death or disabling stroke	**7.9%**	**7.7%**	**6.9%**
Age <75 years	Both SK groups together		Accelerated tPA
Any ICH	0.42%		0.52%
Any stroke	1.08%		1.20%
Mortality	5.5%		4.4%
Death or disabling stroke	**6.0%**		**5.0%**
Age >75 years			
ICH	1.23%		2.08%
Any stroke	3.05%		3.93%
Mortality	20.6%		19.3%
Death or disabling stroke	**21.5%**		**20.2%**

Adapted with permission from GUSTO investigators. An international trial comparing four thrombolytic strategies for acute myocardial infarction. *N Engl J Med* 1993;329:673–682.

decreased level of consciousness (LOC) as the initial physical finding (483). The onset of symptoms and signs is gradual and leads to a maximum deficit within 6 hours (483). Neurosurgical evacuation is beneficial (484).

- **Observe all patients who receive thrombolytics for any signs of neurologic deterioration.** A brief, hourly neurologic screen by a nurse is probably adequate. If there is deterioration, **send immediately for brain imaging studies.**

Nasopharyngeal Bleeding

- **Avoid nasotracheal intubation, if possible,** in anyone who may be a thrombolytic candidate. If bleeding occurs, patients may require emergent airway management or nasal packing (474). The Combitube airway has been effective at securing the airway and for tamponade of bleeding. Cricothyrotomy is not contraindicated (485).

Bleeding from IV Access Sites

- **Avoid obtaining access at noncompressible sites.** Use the femoral approach to obtain central venous access. **If bleeding occurs, apply compression;** this should be adequate. Severe bleeding from central access sites may require reversal of the thrombolytic state.

Hemopericardium

Patients with pericarditis or aortic dissection that is misdiagnosed as AMI are at particular risk for hemopericardium. Any patient with AMI may develop or present with myocardial rupture.

- Consider the diagnosis and use bedside echocardiography for fast and simple confirmation (369). Once diagnosed, hemopericardium is readily treatable (370).

Gastrointestinal Bleeding

- Treat with standard medical therapy (proton-pump inhibitor, somatostatin) and endoscopic banding or coagulation. If this fails or bleeding is severe and life-threatening, treat by reversing the thrombolytic state.

Severe Bleeding

See Table 34-6 (482).

For incidence of stroke in GUSTO-1, see Table 34-7.

ANNOTATED BIBLIOGRAPHY

Stroke Risk and Thrombolytics

Brass LM, et al. Intracranial hemorrhage associated with thrombolytic therapy for elderly patients with acute myocardial infarction: results from the Cooperative Cardiovascular Project, 2000.
    Methods: Brass et al. (472) used Medicare data, with all patients more than 65 years of age, to identify all patients from nearly all acute-care hospitals in the United States who received thrombolytics for AMI during a 9-month period in 1994–1995. Charts of all 31,732 patients were reviewed.
    Findings: The overall rate of ICH in these patients was 1.43% (455 of 31,732). Table 34-1 shows independent predictors of ICH, with a risk stratification scale.

Simoons ML, et al. Individual risk assessment for intracranial hemorrhage during thrombolytic therapy, 1993.
    Methods: Simoons et al. (473) used data from 16 small studies to compare 150 patients with documented ICH to 294 matched controls.
    Findings: Multivariate analysis identified four factors as independent predictors of ICH: (a) age more than 65 years (OR = 2.2; range, 1.4 to 3.5); (b) weight < 70 kg (OR = 2.1; range, 1.2 to 3.2); (c) elevated BP at admission (≥ 165 systolic or ≥ 95 diastolic, or both) (OR = 2.0; range, 1.2 to 3.2); and (d) administration of tPA (OR = 1.6; range, 1.0 to 2.5). Table 34-2 lists the absolute risks.

Gurwitz JH, et al. Risk for intracranial hemorrhage after tissue plasminogen activator treatment for acute myocardial infarction, 1998.
    Methods: Gurwitz et al. (469) analyzed NRMI-2 data (see Appendix C) from 71,073 AMI patients treated with tPA.

Findings: ICH occurred in 673 patients (0.95%). Of 625 patients confirmed by CT or magnetic resonance imaging (MRI), 331 (53%) died while hospitalized for the ICH and 158 of the remaining 294 patients (25.3% of all ICH patients, 54% of survivors) had some neurologic deficit on discharge. Independent variables associated with higher risk of ICH were **age** (65 to 74 years, OR = 2.71; ≥ 75 years, OR = 4.34), **sex** (female, OR = 1.59), history of **stroke** (OR = 1.9), African-American **ethnicity** (OR = 1.70 versus European-American), **systolic BP** (140 to 159 mm Hg, OR = 1.33; ≥ 160 mm Hg, OR = 1.48), **diastolic BP** (≥ 100 mm Hg, OR = 1.40), and **tPA dose** (≥ 1.5 mg/kg, OR = 1.49). Age, sex, and history of stroke had a complex relationship that is best illustrated by the combined adjusted ORs in Table 34-3. Unfortunately, the absolute risk for a male less than 65 years of age with no history of stroke was neither published and nor obtainable. Thus the absolute risks for any of the multivariable categories cannot be calculated.

GUSTO Investigators. An international randomized trial comparing four thrombolytic strategies for acute myocardial infarction, 1993.
    Methods: The GUSTO-1 trial (86) (see Appendix C) compared four thrombolytic regimens in 41,021 AMI patients.
    Findings: Table 34-7 shows the risk of stroke. The risk of ICH after thrombolysis was much greater in patients more than 75 years of age. Nonetheless, note in Table 34-7 that the elderly had lower mortality when given tPA, which had a higher incidence of ICH.

Gore JM, et al. Stroke after thrombolysis: mortality and functional outcomes in the GUSTO-1 trial, 1995.
    Methods: Gore et al. (486) analyzed data from the GUSTO-1 trial as described earlier (86).
    Findings: Of all cases of stroke, 41% were fatal, 31% were disabling, 24% were nondisabling; the remaining percentage is unknown. There were no significant differences between thrombolytic regimens. The type of stroke affected outcomes. ICH was 60% fatal and 25% disabling, whereas nonhemorrhagic infarctions were 17% fatal and 40% disabling.

Berkowitz SD, et al. Incidence and predictors of bleeding after contemporary thrombolytic therapy for myocardial infarction, 1997.
    Methods: Berkowitz et al. (487) analyzed data from the GUSTO-1 trial as described earlier (86).
    Findings: Age more than 75 years, lighter body weight, female sex, and African-American ethnicity were independent predictors of bleeding complications. Overall, 1.2% suffered "severe bleeding" and 11.4% experienced moderate bleeding at various sites.

FTT Collaborative Group. Indications for fibrinolytic therapy in suspected acute myocardial infarction: collaborative overview of early mortality and major morbidity results from all randomised trials of more than 1,000 patients, 1994.
    Methods: The FTT Collaborative Group (30) (see Appendix C) compiled data from nine studies. Of 58,600 suspected AMI patients, 10,783 patients were randomized to trials of tPA versus placebo and the remainder were randomized to an SK-related thrombolytic or placebo.
    Findings: Four extra strokes occurred per 1,000 patients treated with a thrombolytic. Of these four strokes per 1,000 treated, two were fatal and **are already included in mortality data,** one was disabling, and one was not disabling. Thus the risk of excess stroke is four in 1,000, or 0.4%, but the risk of excess disabling stroke in the survivors is only 0.1%, or one in 1,000.

LATE Study Group. Late assessment of thrombolytic efficacy (LATE) study with alteplase 6 to 24 hours after onset of acute myocardial infarction, 1993.
    Methods: The LATE trial (169) (see Chapter 33) randomized AMI patients with 6 to 24 hours of symptoms to tPA or placebo; 46% received IV heparin.
    Findings: Treatment with tPA resulted in 0.5% excess nonfatal strokes by Day 35. Among patients with obvious diagnoses and thrombolytic treatment within 3 hours, the rate of excess nonfatal stroke was only 0.25%. **The 6-month rate of excess nonfatal disabling stroke was equal for tPA and placebo.**

ISIS-2 Collaborative Group. Randomised trial of intravenous streptokinase, oral aspirin, both, or neither among 17,187 cases of suspected acute myocardial infarction: ISIS-2, 1988.
    Methods: ISIS-2 (102) randomized 17,187 patients with up to 24 hours of AMI symptoms (mean, 5 hours) to SK or placebo; 3,411 patients were more than 70 years of age. Aspirin use was dependent on a second randomization (see Appendix C).
    Findings: The SK group had a higher incidence of ICH but a lower risk of overall stroke than in the placebo group (0.71% versus 0.78%) (*p* = NS). This was due to decreased incidence of myocardial necrosis-related cerebral embolism. The number of disabled patients at discharge was higher in the placebo group. Findings were not broken down by age. These numbers are included in the FTT data above (30).

Maggioni AP, et al. The risk of stroke in patients with acute myocardial infarction after thrombolytic and antithrombotic treatment, 1992.
    Methods: Maggioni et al. (471) analyzed stroke data from 20,768 patients randomized to tPA or SK in the GISSI-2 and International Study Group trials. The trials also compared subcutaneous heparin to placebo.
    Findings: SK was associated with an overall stroke incidence of 0.94% versus 1.14% (0.36% hemorrhagic stroke) for tPA. **Subcutaneous heparin was not associated with an increased risk of ICH.**

Age of More Than 75 Years Is NOT a Contraindication for Thrombolysis

GISSI-1 (29) and ISIS-2 (102) (see Appendix C) were the only placebo-controlled thrombolytic trials that randomized significant numbers of elderly patients (age more than 70 to 75 years) who presented during the 0- to 6-hour time window for reperfusion. An unknown number, however, were also in the 6- to 12-hour (GISSI-1) and 6- to 24-hour (ISIS-2) groups.

GISSI. Effectiveness of intravenous thrombolytic treatment in acute myocardial infarction, 1986.
    Methods: GISSI-1 (29) randomized 1,215 patients more than 75 years of age who presented within 12 hours (unknown number within 6 hours) to SK or placebo; only 14% of all patients received aspirin.
    Findings: Mortality was 33.1% for placebo and 28.9% for SK, with 42 lives saved for every 1,000 treated (*p* = NS).

ISIS-2 Collaborative Group. Randomised trial of intravenous streptokinase, oral aspirin, both, or neither among 17,187 cases of suspected acute myocardial infarction: ISIS-2, 1988.
    Methods: See the ISIS-2 (102) annotation, above.
    Findings: Mortality for age beyond 70 years was 21.6% for SK and 18.2% for placebo, with 34 lives saved per 1,000 treated (*p* < 0.05).

FTT Collaborative Group. Indications for fibrinolytic therapy in suspected acute myocardial infarction: collaborative overview of early mortality and major morbidity results from all randomised trials of more than 1,000 patients, 1994.
    Comment: As pointed out by Reikvam et al. (488), **data from the initial report of the FTT collaborative group** (30) **should NOT be used for evaluation of thrombolytic efficacy in the elderly.** This study was a meta-analysis of nine trials of thrombolytic versus placebo, many of which excluded patients more than 75 years of age. Five studies included elderly patients. GISSI-1 (29) and ISIS-2 (102), as described earlier, showed benefit for the elderly despite inclusion of many patients who presented more than 6 hours after the onset of symptoms. ISIS-3 (103), EMERAS (451), and LATE (169) trials inappropriately dilute these positive data. ISIS-3 only compared thrombolytics to placebo in patients whose indication for thrombolytics was unclear, whether due to presentation more than 6 hours after symptom onset or due to lack of ST elevation. EMERAS and LATE included only patients with more than 6 hours of symptoms, and ST elevation was not required for entry. **The FTT data were recently reanalyzed.** Approximately 3,300 patients more than 75 years of age who presented less than 12 hours after symptom onset and with either ST elevation or BBB were randomized to thrombolytic or placebo. Thirty-five day-mortality was reduced from 29.4% to 26.0% (*p* = 0.03) or **34 lives saved per 1,000 treated** (463).

Maggioni AP, et al. Age-related increase in mortality among patients with first myocardial infarctions treated with thrombolysis, 1993.

> *Methods:* Maggioni et al. (365) analyzed data on 9,720 patients with first AMI enrolled in the GISSI-2 trial (98), which compared SK and tPA.

> *Findings:* Mortality for patients more than 80 years of age was 31.9%. All these patients received a thrombolytic drug.

Thiemann DR, et al. Lack of benefit for intravenous thrombolysis in patients with myocardial infarction who are older than 75 years, 2000.

> *Methods:* Thiemann et al. (32) analyzed data from the Cooperative Cardiovascular Project (CCP), in which all patients were more than 65 years of age.

> *Findings:* Of 2,673 patients 76 to 86 years of age who presented with STEMI within **12 hours** of symptom onset, **only 60% received thrombolytics.** Multivariate analysis indicated that patients who received thrombolytics had worse outcomes overall compared with those who received no reperfusion therapy (hazard ratio = 1.29 to 1.38).

> *Comment:* **Although the authors conclude that thrombolytics are unwarranted for the elderly, this is not convincing.** They did not analyze for an ideal cohort, nor did they analyze for 1-year mortality, as does the following study of the same data (291).

Berger AK et al. Thrombolytic therapy in older patients, 2000.

> *Methods:* Berger et al. (291) analyzed CCP data and compared outcomes of patients treated with thrombolytics or angioplasty with those of patients who received no reperfusion therapy. They defined an **"ideal cohort"** as patients with neither relative nor absolute contraindications to thrombolytics, minimal comorbidity, and time to thrombolysis of less than 6 hours.

> *Findings:* Of 37,983 patients more than 65 years of age who presented **less than 12 hours** after symptom onset with ST elevation or LBBB, **only 37.8% received thrombolytics and 4.2% underwent angioplasty.** Overall unadjusted 30-day and 1-year mortality, respectively was 20.6% and 36.9% in the nonreperfusion group, 13.5% and 19.5% in the thrombolytics group, and 13.0% and 19.3% in the angioplasty group. **Adjusted 1-year mortality (but not 30-day mortality) for all patients in all age groups was significantly lower in the thrombolytic group.**

> Of the 16,305 patients in the "ideal cohort," **only 52% received thrombolytics**, 4.3% underwent angioplasty, and 43.7% received no therapy. Unadjusted 1-year mortality was 15.8% for the thrombolytic group and 29.4% for the nonreperfusion group. Adjusted 1-year mortality OR was 0.85 for those who received thrombolytics, which **showed benefit in all age groups.**

Krumholz HM, et al. Thrombolytic therapy for eligible elderly patients with acute myocardial infarction, 1997.

> *Methods:* Krumholz et al. (28) analyzed earlier CCP data. "Eligibility" was conservatively defined as presentation within 6 hours with a diagnostic ECG and no contraindications.

> *Findings:* Elderly patients were grossly undertreated (see Chapter 3 and Table 3-1). Only 109 of 289 (38%) eligible patients of age 75 to 84 years and only 18 of 110 (16%) eligible patients more than 85 years of age received any kind of reperfusion therapy.

Sleight P. Is there an age limit for thrombolytic therapy? 1993.

> *Methods and Findings:* Sleight (308) reviewed data from thrombolytic trials and calculated (in 1993) that the elderly (those more than 75 years of age) would suffer one or two excess nonfatal strokes per 1,000 elderly treated, but with approximately 20 to 30 fewer deaths per 1,000 treated. He estimated a 0.1% rate of excess disabling stroke for tPA over SK, or about two per 1,000 versus placebo.

Krumholz HM, et al. Cost effectiveness of thrombolytic therapy with streptokinase in elderly patients with suspected myocardial infarction, 1992.

> *Methods:* Krumholz et al. (462) applied an economic model to data from GISSI and ISIS-2.

> *Findings:* Cost of SK treatment of an AMI patient per year of life saved was $21,200 for an 80-year-old, $22,400 for a 75-year-old, and $21,600 for a 70-year-old patient. This compares favorably with such therapies as treatment of HTN and hypercholesterolemia in patients with established coronary disease.

Tresch DD, et al. Comparison of elderly and younger patients with out-of-hospital chest pain: clinical characteristics, acute myocardial infarction, therapy, and outcomes, 1996.

> *Methods:* Tresch et al. (464) stratified their database of 2,482 CP patients with prehospital ECGs into groups less than 70 years (younger), 70 to 80 years (elderly), and more than 80 years of age (very elderly).

> *Findings:* Hospital mortality among elderly patients who ruled in for AMI was double that of the younger. Use of thrombolytics was associated with a 50% decrease in mortality for all age groups, but was used in only 17% of elderly, compared with 50% of younger patients.

Despite Evidence of Thrombolytic Efficacy, the Elderly Continue to be Undertreated

Gurwitz JH, et al. Recent age-related trends in the use of thrombolytic therapy on patients who have had acute myocardial infarction, 1996.

> *Methods:* Gurwitz et al. (466) analyzed NRMI-1 data (see Appendix C) on 350,755 AMI patients.

> *Findings:* After adjusting for initial ECG diagnosis, ECG factors, time from symptom onset to hospital presentation, sex, and year of presentation (years 1 to 4 of the study), the OR for patients 75 to 84 years of age to receive thrombolytics as compared with patients less than 55 years of age was 0.27 (CI, 0.26 to 0.28), and for those 85 years of age or more, 0.09 (CI, 0.08 to 0.10). This improved slightly over the 4 years of the study. In year 1, 16.0% of patients 75 to 84 years of age received thrombolytics, as compared with 21.4% in year 4 (a 33.8% relative increase in use). Among patients 85 years of age or more, the proportion treated increased very minimally, from 5.3% to 9.1% over this same period (a 71.7% relative increase in use). **The increase in use of thrombolytics in the elderly was minimal despite a consensus even at that time that age is not a contraindication to thrombolytic therapy** (308,460–462).

Berger AK, et al. Primary coronary angioplasty versus thrombolysis for the management of acute myocardial infarction in elderly patients, 1999.

> *Methods:* Berger et al. (27) provide **further evidence that the elderly are being denied reperfusion therapy.** They analyzed Medicare data (patients more than 65 years of age) from 80,356 consecutive patients eligible for reperfusion therapy.

> *Findings:* Only 12,941 (44.7%) of 28,955 **ideal** candidates, with symptoms < 6 hours, ST elevation or LBBB, and no contraindications received reperfusion therapy. Only 7,742 (15%) of 51,401 patients who presented from 6 to 12 hours, who were otherwise ideal candidates, received reperfusion therapy. Mortality for patients who received reperfusion therapy versus those who did not was 11.8% versus 17.6% at 30 days and 17.2% versus 33.1% at 1 year, respectively.

Krumholz HM, et al. Relationship of age with eligibility for thrombolytic therapy and mortality among patients with suspected acute myocardial infarction, 1994.

> *Methods:* Krumholz et al. (55) analyzed data from the Multicenter Chest Pain Study, undertaken in the "prethrombolytic era."

> *Findings:* Of 1,584 AMI patients whose data on ECG findings and time to presentation were available, 746 were more than 65 years of age. The proportion of patients who arrived within 6 hours and had diagnostic (Type 1a) ECGs was 34% in patients less than 65 years of age and only 18% for those more than 75 years of age. Of patients more than 65 years of age, 12% had contraindications to thrombolytics.

General Contraindications for Thrombolytic Therapy

Doorey AJ, et al. Review: thrombolytic therapy of acute myocardial infarction. Keeping the unfulfilled promises, 1992.

> *Methods:* Doorey et al. (460) reviewed literature on thrombolytic therapy of AMI.

> *Findings:* The authors concluded that contraindications for thrombolytic therapy were much too strict and calculated that if thrombolytics were given (appropriately) more liberally, there would be a 61% increase in use and a tripling of lives saved per year. **Age was singled out as a clinical factor that should not be a contraindication.**

Mahaffey KW, et al. Diabetic retinopathy should not be a contraindication to thrombolytic therapy for acute myocardial infarction: review of ocular hemorrhage incidence and location in the GUSTO-I trial, 1997.

Methods: Mahaffey et al. (479) analyzed GUSTO-1 data (see Appendix C).

Findings: Of 6,011 patients with DM, none had intraocular hemorrhage due to thrombolysis. The authors concluded that diabetic retinopathy should not be considered a contraindication.

Mohammad S, et al. Hemopericardium with cardiac tamponade after intravenous thrombolysis for acute myocardial infarction, 1996.

Methods: Mohammad et al. (370) reported **two patients with hemopericardium and tamponade** from a group of 26 AMI patients treated with thrombolytics over an 8-month period.

Findings: There was apparently no investigation to determine if the underlying cause was pericarditis or myocardial rupture. Both patients responded promptly to pericardiocentesis and pericardial catheter drainage. The authors suggest that this rarely reported complication may occur more frequently with increasing use of thrombolytics and aggressive anticoagulant regimens.

Roppolo LP, et al. Nasotracheal intubation in the emergency department, revisited, 1999.

Methods: Roppolo et al. (474) reviewed complications of 105 nasotracheal intubation attempts in the ED.

Findings: Two patients had severe epistaxis, both of whom had received thrombolytics for AMI. Both occurred 24 hours after administration and were controlled with nasal packing.

Mahaffey KW, et al. Neurosurgical evacuation of intracranial hemorrhage after thrombolytic therapy for acute myocardial infarction: experience from the GUSTO-I trial, 1999.

Methods: Mahaffey et al. (484) analyzed GUSTO-1 data (see Appendix C).

Findings: Of the 268 patients with ICH due to thrombolysis, 222 patients did not undergo neurosurgical evacuation, 65% of whom died. Of 46 patients who did undergo surgery, 35% died. This nonrandomized study could have very obvious biases.

35

SUMMARY OF BENEFIT/RISK ANALYSIS

KEY POINTS

- Assess the risk of AMI based on clinical and ECG factors.
- Assess the risk of thrombolytic therapy.
- The benefit/risk ratio is usually underestimated, and patients are most commonly UNDERTREATED.

There are patients who have ECGs diagnostic of AMI but for whom the risks of thrombolytic therapy exceed the benefits. However, remember that the greatest risk to most patients is UNDERTREATMENT, which is an error of omission, not overtreatment, which is an error of commission (470).

BENEFITS

When weighing the risks of thrombolytic therapy, know the benefits. A high-risk AMI is worth a higher risk of adverse events from thrombolysis than a low-risk AMI. For example, an 85-year-old patient with risk factors for ICH may have a 5% risk of ICH from thrombolytics, but the risk of death from an anterior AMI is 30% to 40%. Thrombolytic administration may be worth the risk of bleeding, unless angioplasty is immediately available.

Factors for which there is increased benefit of reperfusion in AMI include (a) **shorter time** since onset; (b) **greater ST elevation** and presence in **more leads;** (c) **anterior** location; (d) inferior AMI with **RV, posterior, or lateral involvement;** (e) **reciprocal ST depression;** and (f) **history of previous MI** in a different location (111).

SUMMARY OF CONSIDERATIONS

- Is there **history of previous Q-wave MI** in the **same** location? Infarction of the myocardium in **that** coronary distribution may indicate less mortality benefit from thrombolytics (29,102).
- Is **lateral AMI** being overlooked?
- Is **posterior AMI** being overlooked? Did you record posterior leads?
- Is **RV AMI** being overlooked?

- Is **anterior ST elevation due to AMI** being **misinterpreted** as early repolarization?
- Is ST segment elevation due to ventricular aneurysm, pericarditis, early repolarization, BBB, LVH, or hyperkalemia?
- Did you compare the ECG with **previous ECGs?**
- Is there an **inferior AMI?** Although thrombolytics are indicated for uncomplicated inferior AMI, mortality benefit has not been demonstrated in small inferior AMIs (29,30). Thus for a patient with late presentation or major contraindications, risks may be too great.
- If the ECG is **nondiagnostic** (Types 1c, 2, 3, or 4), are you recording **serial ECGs?**
- Is there **severe heart failure** (Killip Class III or IV) or **cardiogenic shock?** If so, angioplasty is preferable if available.

ARE YOU BEING TOO CONSERVATIVE?

Are you denying reperfusion therapy to the patient:

- Who is **elderly?**
- With typical symptoms and **LBBB?**
- With **ST elevation in only two leads** or even unequivocally diagnostic in just one lead?
- With **already formed Q waves** (**not** deep QS waves and low ST elevation due to ventricular aneurysm)?
- With **no CP,** even with an unequivocally diagnostic ECG?
- With history of **CABG?**
- With **high risk of stroke** despite a very large AMI?
- Who presented **6 to 12 hours** after CP onset, even though the AMI is **large** and the **ST segments remain very elevated and T waves upright?**
- Because symptoms have been present for **more than 12 hours?** Have you considered that the onset of **infarction** (as opposed to angina) **may be more recent?**
- Because he or she had a **previous MI?** Mortality benefit of thrombolytics is equivalent or greater in patients with previous MI (30,102).

See Cases 35-1 to 35-3 for examples of risk/benefit considerations. See Chapter 34 for discussion of thrombolytic contraindications and risk. (See also Case 16-5, of a patient who was inappropriately denied cardiac catheterization because he was taking coumadin and Cases 17-10 and 17-11, in which the benefit of reperfusion therapy for an extensive AMI clearly outweighs nearly any risk.)

CASE 35-1

Elderly Woman with Anterior Ventricular Aneurysm Had CP, Increased Anterior ST Elevation, and Acute High Lateral MI: The Woman in This Case Received Thrombolytics and Died of ICH

History

This 75-year-old woman presented with 1 hour of CP. She had no relative or absolute contraindications to thrombolytics, specifically no history of stroke of any kind and no HTN.

ECG 35-1A (Type 1c)

■ QS waves with 2 mm ST elevation: V2–V3, and shallow T-wave inversion: V1–V6, consistent with anterior ventricular aneurysm.

ECG 35-1B (Type 1a)

Twenty minutes later

■ **Increased ST elevation:** V2–V3 and "pseudonormalization" of T-waves: V1–V5. A new infarction in the area of the old QS-wave MI would receive moderate benefit from reperfusion.

■ **New ST elevation:** V4 and aVL; and **reciprocal depression:** II, III, aVF, are diagnostic of a new lateral AMI, which would benefit significantly from reperfusion.

Clinical Course

Angiography ± PCI is preferable, if available, but thrombolytics are definitely indicated if a cath lab is unavailable. The patient received thrombolytics with successful reperfusion but died of ICH.

Conclusion

Taking necessary risks may sometimes result in a bad outcome. It is important to remember that this patient had a **high risk of both death and stroke without thrombolysis.**

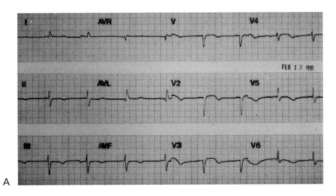

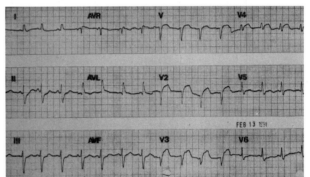

CASE 35-2

Shock, Hemetemesis, and Inferoposterior AMI (No ECG Shown)

History

This 49-year-old man was vomiting blood. His pH was 6.70. He was intubated, paralyzed, and volume- and blood-resuscitated. Preresuscitation hemoglobin/hematocrit were 4.0/12.0. BP = 50/palp and P = 120.

Clinical Course

His ECG (not shown) revealed a large inferoposterior AMI. Thrombolytics are absolutely contraindicated. Even angioplasty, with the need for heparin, is contraindicated until the bleeding can be controlled. The patient rapidly underwent endoscopic banding of esophageal varices, with

continued volume and blood-product administration, and then underwent successful angioplasty of a 100% occluded circumflex. CK peaked at 2,296 IU/L and cTnI peaked at 185 ng/mL, 8 hours after arrival. Echocardiography revealed a moderately severe inferoposterior WMA. The patient walked out of the hospital several days later.

Conclusion

Thrombolytic therapy is absolutely contraindicated. However, after banding, taking the risk of anticoagulation during PCI was potentially lifesaving.

CASE 35-3

Inferior QS Morphology and New ST Elevation: Patient Received Thrombolytics and Had Noncerebral Bleeding Complications

History
This 74-year-old, non-English-speaking woman with end-stage renal disease (ESRD), HTN, and anterolateral "subendocardial MI" presented with weakness and left arm pain.

ECG 35-3 (Type 1c)
- ST elevation: 1 mm, II, III, aVF; with reciprocal depression: aVL.
- QS waves: II, III, aVF, with small Q waves V4–V6. The QS waves and low ST elevation could be **inferior ventricular aneurysm, subacute AMI (of more than 12 hours duration), or AMI in the location of an old MI.**

Clinical Course
The patient was admitted to the CCU and received SK. Q waves were later noted to be preexisting, but the ST ele-

vation was new. She developed **bleeding complications that required reversal of the SK.** Biomarkers were negative. There was neither angiography nor echocardiography.

Conclusion
This ECG is classic for inferior ventricular aneurysm. **The indication for thrombolytics is borderline at best.** From a prospective viewpoint, even if the ST elevation is new, the benefit of thrombolytics is minimal for acute MI (new ST elevation) in the same location as a previous QS wave inferior MI. The negative biomarkers are interesting: Was this a "transient ST elevation AMI" without necrosis, or was the ST elevation not a result of coronary occlusion? **Fortunately, the bleeding complications were minor.**

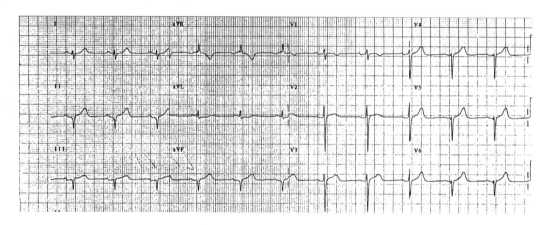

ANNOTATED BIBLIOGRAPHY

See also Chapter 34 annotations on stroke risk.

Selker HP, et al. Patient-specific predictions of outcomes in myocardial infarction for real-time emergency use: a thrombolytic predictive instrument, 1997.
Methods: Selker et al. (419) utilized original data from 13 clinical trials and registries on 4,911 AMI patients at 107 U.S. hospitals to develop a thrombolytic predictive instrument (TPI).
Findings: The TPI predicts, for an individual patient, the effect of thrombolysis on the probability of key clinical outcomes, acute mortality, long-term mortality, cardiac arrest, and serious complications of thrombolytic therapy such as hemorrhagic stroke and major bleeding. It is designed for incorporation into an ECG machine, such that, upon detection of significant ST-elevation, predictions are computed and printed on the ECG header.

36

REPERFUSION THERAPY FOR STEMI

RAO HARIS NASEEM, TIMOTHY D. HENRY, AND STEPHEN W. SMITH

Disruption of an atherosclerotic plaque and resultant intraluminal thrombosis plays a fundamental role in the pathogenesis of AMI (345). Early and complete reperfusion of the occluded artery, with either thrombolytic therapy or angioplasty or both, limits the extent of myocardial necrosis, preserves global and regional myocardial function, and reduces morbidity and mortality (489–492). Summaries of the comparative merits of various reperfusion therapies follow.

THROMBOLYTIC THERAPY

Thrombolytic Agents: SK and tPA

Both SK (29,98,102,103) and tPA (98,103) have been shown to significantly reduce mortality in AMI. IV and intracoronary administration are equally efficacious (493). Although 90-minute patency rates are higher with tPA (100,494), patency rates at 24 hours are equal. Front-loaded tPA given with IV heparin has a lower 30-day mortality than SK (6.4% versus 7.3%) (86).

- Front-loaded tPA is administered as a 15-mg bolus, then 0.75 mg/kg (not to exceed 50 mg) over 30 minutes, followed by 0.5 mg/kg (not to exceed 35 mg) over the next 60 minutes.

Third-Generation Thrombolytic Agents: Reteplase and Tenecteplase

Both TNK-tPA and rPA are important third-generation thrombolytics that can be administered in bolus form and are therefore convenient to use with less chance of error. TNK-tPA has a longer half-life (20 versus 4 minutes), better fibrin specificity, and higher resistance to inhibition by plasminogen-activator inhibitor-I than rPA. TNK-tPA and rPA have equivalent 30-day survival compared with front-loaded tPA in STEMI (362,412). Compared with tPA: (a) TNK-tPA had a slightly but significantly lower incidence of noncerebral bleeds and need for transfusion (412); and (b) rPA was associated with small increase in ICH in patients more than 75 years of age (362). TNK-tPA and rPA have never been directly compared.

- Administer TNK-tPA at (approximately) 0.5 mg/kg (minimum 30 mg, maximum 50 mg) in a single 5-second injection (see package insert for exact dosing).
- Administer rPA in two 10-U boluses 30 minutes apart, regardless of weight.

PERCUTANEOUS CORONARY INTERVENTION

Prompt direct reperfusion of an occluded artery using PCI is an excellent method of myocardial reperfusion; DTBT should be less than 60 minutes. PCI involves the use of guidewires to mechanically open an occluded coronary artery and includes angioplasty and stenting. Clinical trials comparing angioplasty with thrombolytic therapy have produced conflicting results. Some indicate that angioplasty is superior (495,496,497); others show no difference (446,498). In the largest randomized, placebo-controlled trial to compare angioplasty with thrombolytic therapy, angioplasty demonstrated a mild short-term benefit over thrombolysis. However, 6-month follow-up data showed no significant difference (446). Although no conclusive data demonstrates greater efficacy of angioplasty, in all comparative studies published before July 2000, time to angioplasty was approximately 1.5 to 2 hours and lacked adjunctive stenting and abciximab. When DTBT time is less than 60 minutes, angioplasty is likely to result in better outcomes (427) (see Chapter 32), but such timeliness is rare (33,428).

A small comparative trial showed significantly greater myocardial salvage with angioplasty used in conjunction with abciximab and stenting than with thrombolysis (499). Similarly, most studies show stenting to be slightly superior to angioplasty for primary treatment of STEMI (500–502). The addition of abciximab to PCI for STEMI improved combined endpoints at 30 days (500,503) but not at 6 months (500). Additionally, NRMI data (see Appendix C) suggest that, at low-volume hospitals (16 procedures or less per year), thrombolytic mortality is equivalent to that of angioplasty (5.9% versus 6.2%), whereas at moderate-volume hospitals (17 to 48 procedures/year), and especially at high-volume hospitals (49 procedures per year or more), angioplasty results in significantly lower mortality (5.9% versus 4.5%, and 5.4% versus 3.4%, respectively) (33,481).

Angiography ± PCI, if promptly available, is superior to thrombolytics when:

- The diagnosis is in question.
- The patient is hemodynamically unstable, as in cardiogenic shock (504,505).
- There are conditions that increase risks of thrombolysis, including an age of more than 75 years (27,291,506).
- There is inadequate response to thrombolytics (see Chapter 27, on rescue angioplasty).

Very-high-dose heparin (300 U/kg) administered before angioplasty results in higher patency rates than placebo (507, 508). However, antiplatelet agents such as GPIIb-IIIa inhibitors and clopidogrel are usually favored over very-high-dose heparin as adjunctive therapy with angioplasty (499).

COMBINATION THERAPIES

Thrombolytics and PCI

Initial trials of routine angioplasty performed after full dose thrombolytic therapy showed no additional benefit and indicated increased adverse effects (**509**,510,511,512). However, data from a randomized study of 600 patients indicates that **half-dose tPA** (50-mg bolus) **followed by immediate angiography ± angioplasty** is safe and effective; strongly consider this combination for any patient who cannot be guaranteed to have balloon inflation within 60 minutes of presentation (**513**).

Thrombolytics and GP IIb/IIIa Platelet Receptor Blockers

Abciximab is a GP IIb/IIIa platelet receptor blocker. **Half-dose tPA given in conjunction with abciximab,** with heparin and aspirin, resulted in a high rate of TIMI-3 flow at 90 minutes (77% versus 62% for front-loaded tPA) (**514**) and a high rate of complete (defined as > 70%) ST resolution (59%, versus 37% for tPA alone) (515). However, abciximab also resulted in a slightly higher rate of hemorrhage when given with low-dose heparin (7% major hemorrhage versus 6% for tPA alone), but **not** with **very-low-dose** heparin (1% major hemorrhage) (**514**). Patients in the very-low-dose group were too few to draw firm conclusions, however; thus this therapy cannot be recommended as of April 2001. Doses were as follows:

- Dose of abciximab with tPA: (bolus 0.25 mg/kg and 12-hour infusion of 0.125 µg/kg/min).
- Dose of tPA with abciximab: 15 mg bolus, then 35 mg over 60 minutes.
- Very-low-dose heparin: 30 U/kg bolus, then 4 U/kg/hr.
- Aspirin, of course, should be included.

Thrombolytics with Enoxaparin and/or Abciximab—Recent Studies

Two major randomized studies released shortly before publication are relevant. In GUSTO V (515.5), half-dose reteplase plus abciximab (in the above dose) was approximately equivalent to reteplase alone.

In ASSENT-3 (471.5), patients were randomized to 3 different treatments: full-dose TNK-tPA in combination with enoxaparin (30 mg IV plus 1 mg/kg subcutaneously every 12 hours for 7 days), ½-dose TNK-tPA in combination with abciximab (in the above dose), and standard full-dose TNK-tPA with unfractionated heparin. The former two regimens had similar outcomes, in both cases significantly better than standard unfractionated heparin. Given its ease of use, enoxaparin with full-dose thrombolytics may be the preferred choice.

RESCUE ANGIOPLASTY

Rescue angioplasty, also called "salvage angioplasty," may be useful in a subset of AMI patients for whom thrombolytic therapy fails. Rescue angioplasty results in improved LV function and 30-day mortality compared with conservative therapy, with no significant difference in adverse events (**323**,324,360). We recommend rescue angioplasty for large infarctions with no reliable ECG evidence of reperfusion at 1 hour following thrombolytic therapy (see Chapter 27).

ANGIOPLASTY AFTER SUCCESSFUL THROMBOLYSIS

After successful thrombolysis, unless there is spontaneous or provokable ischemia, neither immediate nor delayed angioplasty confers mortality benefit (**509,511,512**).

ANNOTATED BIBLIOGRAPHY

De Wood MA, et al. Prevalence of total coronary occlusion during the early hours of transmural myocardial infarction, 1980.
  Methods: In a landmark study, De Wood et al. (345) performed angiography on 322 AMI patients at each of four time intervals following symptom onset.
  Findings: Occlusion of coronary arteries was 87.3% at 4 hours, 85.3% at 4 to 6 hours, 68.4% at 6 to 8 hours, and 64.9% at 12 to 24 hours. De Wood et al. conclude that total coronary occlusion is high after AMI and decreases over time.

ISIS-2 and GISSI-1
See Appendix C.

Other Clinical Trials
Chesebro JH, et al. Thrombolysis in Myocardial Infarction (TIMI) Trial, Phase I: a comparison between intravenous tissue plasminogen activator and intravenous streptokinase: clinical findings through hospital discharge, 1987.
  Methods: TIMI investigators (100) conducted a double-blind, placebo-controlled trial of 290 patients with AMI and symptom duration of less than 7 hours. They performed initial angiography and then randomized patients to SK, 1.5 million units over 1 hour or tPA, 80 mg over 3 hours. They then performed angiography at 10, 20, 30, 45, 60, 75, and 90 minutes after drug administration to assess IRA patency.
  Findings: Total IRA occlusion at baseline was found in 232 of 290 AMI patients, of whom 113 received tPA and 119 had received SK. Ninety-minute IRA patency was found in 62% in the tPA group versus only 31% of the SK group.

GISSI-2. A factorial randomised trial of alteplase versus streptokinase and heparin versus no heparin among 12,490 patients with acute myocardial infarction, 1990; ISIS-3. A randomised comparison of streptokinase versus tissue plasminogen activator versus anistreplase and of aspirin plus heparin versus aspirin alone among 41,299 cases of suspected acute myocardial infarction, 1992.
  Methods: GISSI-2 (98) and ISIS-3 (103) were the first two large multicenter, randomized, placebo-controlled mortality studies that compared tPA with SK in the treatment of STEMI.
  Findings: Neither study showed a significant difference between thrombolytic drugs.
  Comment: Adjunctive heparin was administered subcutaneously. There are theoretical reasons why IV heparin is necessary for full efficacy of tPA. The GUSTO trial was undertaken to better assess this effect.

GUSTO. An international randomized trial comparing four thrombolytic strategies for acute myocardial infarction, 1993.

See Appendix C.

TNK-tPA and rPA

Data below clearly show that both rPA and TNK-tPA are comparable to tPA in safety and efficacy profile and are much easier to administer.

GUSTO III trial. A comparison of reteplase with alteplase for acute myocardial infarction, 1997.
> *Methods:* GUSTO-III (362) randomized 15,000 patients with STEMI to either rPA or tPA. The primary endpoint was 30-day mortality.
> *Findings:* Thirty-day mortality rates were 7.47% in the rPA group and 7.24% in the tPA group, with no significant difference in bleeding complications.

ASSENT-2. Single-bolus tenecteplase compared with front-loaded alteplase in acute myocardial infarction, 1999.
> *Methods:* ASSENT-2 (412) randomized 16,949 patients to either front-loaded alteplase (tPA) or a single bolus injection of weight-adjusted TNK-tPA (approximately 0.5 mg/kg).
> *Findings:* Thirty-day mortality was similar in the two treatment groups (6.15% versus 6.18%). There were significantly fewer minor bleeds and need for transfusion in the TNK-tPA group.

Thrombolytic Therapy Versus Primary Angioplasty

Stone GW, et al. Predictors of in-hospital and 6-month outcome after acute myocardial infarction in the reperfusion era: the Primary Angioplasty in Myocardial Infarction (PAMI) trial, 1995; Stone GW, et al. Outcome of different reperfusion strategies in patients with former contraindications to thrombolytic therapy: a comparison of primary angioplasty and tissue plasminogen activator, 1996.
> *Methods:* PAMI investigators (495) randomized 395 patients who presented within 12 hours of the onset of STEMI to either primary angioplasty (195 patients) or IV tPA (200 patients). The tPA was dosed at 100 mg over 3 hours (not front-loaded).
> *Findings:* The primary endpoint of the study, combined death or nonfatal reinfarction at 6 months, was 16.8% in the tPA group and 8.5% in the angioplasty group. The only variables independently associated with freedom from complication were young age and treatment with angioplasty. Patients more than 70 years of age and those with more than 4 hours of symptoms had the greatest benefit of angioplasty over thrombolytics (506).

Zijlstra F, et al. A comparison of immediate coronary angioplasty with intravenous streptokinase in acute myocardial infarction, 1993.
> *Methods:* Zijlstra et al. (497) randomized 142 AMI patients to either immediate angioplasty or thrombolytic therapy with SK.
> *Findings:* Patients who underwent angioplasty had better outcomes with regard to IRA patency, residual stenotic lesions, LV function, and recurrent myocardial ischemia and infarction.

Gibbons RJ, et al. Immediate angioplasty compared with the administration of a thrombolytic agent followed by conservative treatment for myocardial infarction, 1993.
> *Methods:* Gibbons et al. (498) randomized 108 AMI patients to receive tPA (**not** front-loaded) or primary PCI.
> *Findings:* There was no significant difference in myocardial salvage between the two groups.

GUSTO IIb. A clinical trial comparing primary coronary angioplasty with tissue plasminogen activator for acute myocardial infarction, 1997.
> *Methods:* GUSTO-IIb (446) randomized 1,138 patients with STEMI to primary angioplasty or front-loaded tPA, as in the GUSTO trial described earlier (86); 1,012 of these patients were also randomized to heparin or hirudin treatment in a factorial design.
> *Findings:* The composite endpoint was death, nonfatal reinfarction, and nonfatal disabling stroke. At 30 days, 9.6% of the angioplasty group versus 13.7% of the tPA group had reached the composite endpoint, but at 6 months there was no significant difference.

Magid DJ, et al. Relation between hospital primary angioplasty volume and mortality for patients with acute MI treated with primary angioplasty versus thrombolytic therapy, 2000.
> *Methods:* Magid et al. (33) studied NRMI data from 1994 to 1999 (see Appendix C). They stratified hospitals by volume of angioplasty procedures (16 per year or less, 17 to 48 per year, or 49 or more per year) and analyzed outcomes for nontransferred AMI patients treated with angioplasty or thrombolytic therapy. A total of 62,299 patients received either treatment.
> *Findings:* Mortality was lower for patients who underwent angioplasty versus those receiving thrombolytics at high (3.4% versus 5.4%) and intermediate (4.5% versus 5.9%) volume hospitals, but not at low volume hospitals (6.2% versus 5.9%). Mean DTBT at the high-, intermediate-, and low-volume hospitals was 120, 131, and 145 minutes, respectively. Angioplasty patients had much less need for subsequent revascularization (12% to 20% versus 54% to 61%) and a lower incidence of stroke (0.4% to 0.5% versus 0.9% to 1.1%) than patients who received thrombolytics.

Hochman JS, et al. Early revascularization in acute myocardial infarction complicated by cardiogenic shock, 1999; Hochman JS, et al. One-year survival following early revascularization for cardiogenic shock, 2001.
> *Methods:* Hochman et al. (504) randomized 302 AMI patients with cardiogenic shock to either emergency revascularization (CABG or angioplasty) or initial medical stabilization.
> *Findings:* There was no 30-day mortality difference, but 6-month and 12-month mortality (505) was lower in the revascularization group. The median time from onset of cardiogenic shock to randomization was **6 hours,** which could seriously compromise the efficacy of revascularization. **Immediate** PCI for cardiogenic shock is doubtless much more effective.

Immediate Angioplasty After Successful Thrombolysis: No Additional Benefit

Topol EJ, et al. A randomized trial of immediate versus delayed elective angioplasty after intravenous tissue plasminogen activator in acute myocardial infarction (TAMI trial), 1987.
> *Methods:* Topol et al. (509) randomized 188 patients with a patent but severely stenotic vessel after successful thrombolytic therapy to either immediate or delayed angioplasty.
> *Findings:* Immediate angioplasty conferred no benefit, and was, in fact, associated with more adverse events.

TIMI Study Group. Comparison of invasive and conservative strategies after treatment with intravenous tissue plasminogen activator in acute myocardial infarction: results of the Thrombolysis in Myocardial Infarction (TIMI) phase II trial, 1989.
> *Methods:* In TIMI-II (511), 3,262 STEMI patients who received thrombolytics were randomized to undergo, within 18 to 48 hours, an invasive strategy (angiography with angioplasty, if indicated), or a conservative strategy (procedures undertaken only for spontaneous or inducible ischemia). Reinfarction or death within 42 days was the primary endpoint of the study.
> *Findings:* The primary endpoint occurred in 10.9% of the patients randomized to the invasive strategy and in 9.7% of the patients randomized to the conservative strategy.

de Bono DP. The European Cooperative Study Group trial of intravenous recombinant tissue-type plasminogen activator (rt-PA) and conservative therapy versus rt-PA and immediate coronary angioplasty, 1988.
> *Methods:* de Bono et al. (512) randomized 367 STEMI patients who received thrombolytics to either ischemia-guided therapy or an early invasive strategy.
> *Findings:* Lower mortality was reported in the conservative group (3%) than in the invasive group (7%), and the incidence of recurrent ischemia, bleeding complications, hypotension, and ventricular fibrillation was higher in the invasive group.

Combined Use of Thrombolytics and PCI

Ross AM, et al. A randomized trial comparing primary angioplasty with a strategy of short-acting thrombolysis and immediate planned rescue angioplasty in acute myocardial infarction: the PACT trial. PACT Investigators. Plasminogen-activator Angioplasty Compatibility Trial, 1999.

Methods: Ross et al. (513) randomized 606 patients to half-dose tPA (50 mg as a bolus) or placebo, along with aspirin and heparin. This was followed by immediate planned angiography and angioplasty if necessary.

Findings: Both mean door-to-drug time and mean drug-to-contrast-injection were 49 minutes. Patency (TIMI-3 flow) at contrast injection was 61% in the tPA group versus 34% in the placebo group. Convalescent EF was highest (62.4%) with a patent IRA at contrast injection or when produced by angioplasty within 1 hour of medication delivery (62.5%), but was only 57.3% if balloon inflation was performed more than 1 hour after drug injection, which occurred in 88%.

Abciximab

Antman EM, et al. Abciximab facilitates the rate and extent of thrombolysis: results of the thrombolysis in myocardial infarction (TIMI) 14 trial, 1999.

Methods: The TIMI-14 trial (514) randomized STEMI patients to full-dose tPA or to reduced-dose tPA with abciximab (a GP IIb/IIIa inhibitor). All patients received aspirin. Heparin was given in varying doses.

Findings: Percentage of patients with TIMI-3 flow rates was higher in the group that received 50 mg of tPA plus abciximab with low-dose heparin, both at 60 minutes (72% versus 43%) and 90 minutes (77% versus 62%). Major hemorrhage occurred in 6% with tPA alone and 7% in the combined group. The very-low-dose heparin group ($n = 70$) had only 1% incidence of major hemorrhage. The rate of TIMI-3 flow at 90 minutes was 69% in this group.

37

REPERFUSION THERAPY FOR ACUTE CORONARY SYNDROMES WITHOUT ST ELEVATION (UA/NSTEMI)

M. BILAL MURAD, TIMOTHY D. HENRY, AND STEPHEN W. SMITH

UA/NSTEMI is never an indication for thrombolytic therapy (29,30,**99**,102,**163**). However, it may be an indication for **emergency angiography ± PCI** if symptoms of ischemia are **refractory to medical management (163,166)**, especially if any of the following are present:

- Hypotension, shock, pulmonary edema, new or worsening mitral regurgitation murmur.
- Presence of objective measures of ischemia, including ST depression, T-wave inversion, elevated troponin, or new echocardiographic WMA.

MEDICAL THERAPY FOR UA/NSTEMI

- Antiplatelet therapy: aspirin or clopidogrel in rare cases of aspirin allergy.
- Sublingual NTG, followed by IV NTG for HTN, CHF, or refractory ischemia.
- Antithrombotic therapy: unfractionated heparin (UF) or low molecular weight heparin (LMWH). Enoxaparin is superior **(163,166,516–518)**. However, interventional experience with enoxaparin is limited, as is its use in conjunction with GP IIb-IIIa inhibitors. Hirudin (lepirudin) is modestly more effective than UFH **(519,520)**.

- Beta-blockers: esmolol or metoprolol. Metoprolol dose is 15 mg IV in three divided doses 5 minutes apart, then 50 mg orally.
- Potent antiplatelet therapy: Although there are conflicting results in major noninterventional studies **(521–525)**, a trial of GP IIb-IIIa inhibitors is indicated for refractory ischemia. If PCI is planned, a GP IIb-IIIa inhibitor is indicated and highly effective **(526)**.
- Correction of secondary (nonthrombotic) causes of ischemia such as hypovolemia, anemia, hypoxemia, catecholamine overload, and toxic exposure such as carbon monoxide.

Persistent ischemia despite optimal medical therapy is an indication for PCI (11,163,527–529). If medical therapy is initially effective, it appears from two trials **(148,528)** that an early invasive management strategy (PCI within 48 hours) is preferred to an early conservative strategy, particularly if there is ST depression or a positive troponin **(148)**. Further discussion of management of UA/NSTEMI is beyond the scope of this book.

See Case 37-1. See also Cases 8-5 and 8-6, of UA/NSTEMI presenting with ST depression. See Cases 5-3, 6-4, 8-13, and 12-3, of transient ST elevation followed by Wellens' syndrome; Case 21-1 for cocaine-associated CP presenting with reversible T-wave inversion; and Cases 31-1 and 31-3 for Wellens' syndrome preceded by suggestive prehospital rhythm strips. See also Figure 8-6 of Wellens' syndrome.

CASE 37-1

NSTEMI Presenting As Pulmonary Edema with Dynamic ST Depression

History
This 77-year-old man with no previous cardiopulmonary disease had a sudden onset of dyspnea. On exam, he had bilateral rales and no other evidence of fluid overload. A chest film confirmed pulmonary edema. BP = 130/70.

ECG 37-1A (Type 2)
- No ST elevation.
- ST depression: 1 to 2 mm in V3–V6, with upright T waves, consistent with either anterior (LAD) UA/NSTEMI or posterior (circumflex/obtuse marginal first diagonal) STEMI. It is not necessarily posterior STEMI because it is not maximal in V2–V3.

Clinical Course
The patient was treated with aspirin, heparin, metoprolol, NTG, and tirofiban, and symptoms improved.

ECG 37-1B (Type 3)
Recorded 38 minutes after treatment, V1–V6 only
- ST depression: almost completely resolved.

Clinical Course
Echocardiography revealed an inferoposterior WMA and normal LV function, cTnI peaked at 6.7 ng/mL, and angiography revealed diffuse CAD with no obvious culprit lesion. Stenoses were: first, second, and third obtuse marginals, 70% each; LAD, 40%; left main, 40%; RCA, 30%; posterior descending, 80%; and small proximal first diagonal, 70%.

Conclusion
Lateral precordial ST depression may represent either nonocclusive ischemia or a reciprocal view of posterior injury. In either case, it may resolve with antiplatelet, antithrombotic, and anti-ischemic therapy without reperfusion therapy.

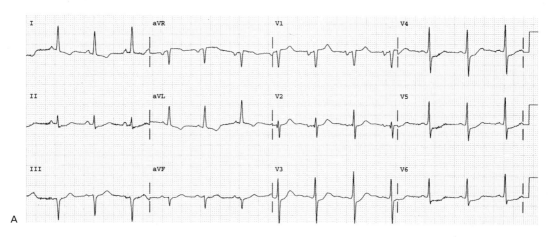

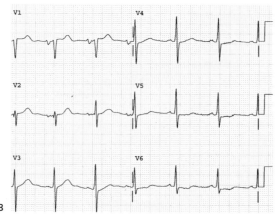

ANNOTATED BIBLIOGRAPHY

Management: General Information

Braunwald E, et al. ACC/AHA guidelines for the management of patients with unstable angina and non–ST-segment elevation myocardial infarction, 2000.

Findings: This 92-page article by Braunwald et al. provides detailed discussion of the standard of care for UA/NSTEMI (11).

Emergent Coronary Angiography

Background: We are unaware of any trial of invasive versus conservative management of UA/NSTEMI in patients with **ischemia refractory to medical management**. Trials have excluded such refractory patients because they should undergo angiography with or without revascularization. Whether **patients who respond to medical management** should undergo PCI is more controversial, as the following studies illustrate.

The TIMI-IIIb (163), DANAMI (529), VANQWISH (527), and FRISC II (528) trials compared early invasive versus conservative strategies in ACS. In TIMI-IIIb, the clinical endpoints of death or nonfatal infarction after 6 weeks and 1 year were similar in both groups with UA/NSTEMI. By 1 year, 58% of patients in the conservative arm and 64% in the invasive arm had undergone revascularization. There were no differences in the rates of MI or death at 1 year, but recurrent ischemia and rehospitalization rates were lower with the invasive strategy (163). These trials were conducted before the use of stenting and GP IIb/IIIa inhibitors, which reduces postprocedural complication rates and improves long-term outcomes in UA/NSTEMI. Similarly, the FRISC II trial showed benefit of an early invasive approach. A direct comparison between early conservative and early invasive strategies using GP IIb/IIIa inhibitors (TIMI 18-TACTICS trial) was recently completed and shows significant benefit from the invasive arm (148).

The TIMI investigators. A randomised comparison of tissue-type plasminogen activator versus placebo and early invasive versus early conservative strategies in unstable angina and non–Q-wave myocardial infarction, 1995.
See Chapter 8 for annotations of TIMI-IIIA (99) and TIMI-IIIB (163, 166).

VANQWISH investigators. Outcomes in patients with acute non–Q-wave myocardial infarction randomly assigned to an invasive as compared with a conservative management strategy, 1998.

Methods: The VANQUISH study (527) randomized 920 patients with UA/NSTEMI to early invasive management (*n* = 462) or conservative management (*n* = 458). Invasive management involved diagnostic catheterization and intervention, if indicated, soon after randomization. Conservative treatment involved medical management with cardiac catheterization guided by spontaneous or inducible ischemia on noninvasive stress testing.

Findings: The early invasive strategy was associated with increased early mortality and of the combined end-point of death or MI at 30 days and at 1 year, but there were no long-term differences in outcome between groups. The greater mortality in the invasive arm was due to a high 11.6% surgical mortality rate at 30 days. There were no deaths related to angioplasty. Of interest, only 44% of patients in the invasive arm (lower than the conservative arm of TIMI-IIIb) and 33% in the conservative arm underwent revascularization, which highlights the differences between strategies in clinical trials.

FRISC II Investigators. Invasive compared with noninvasive treatment in unstable coronary-artery disease: FRISC II prospective randomized multi-center study, 1999.

Methods: FRISC II (528) was a prospective, randomized trial in which 2,457 patients with UA/NSTEMI were assigned to an early invasive or noninvasive strategy and to either in-hospital UFH or dalteparin for 3 months. Coronary angiography and revascularization, if needed, were performed within the first 7 and 10 days, respectively.

Findings: In-hospital treatment with dalteparin lowered the 30-day event rate compared with UFH in patients randomized to the conservative strategy. However, there was no additional benefit to continuation of dalteparin for 6 weeks after discharge. Randomization to the early invasive strategy achieved a 21% reduction in mortality compared with the early conservative strategy group (9.5% versus 12.5%). For the invasive and noninvasive groups, respectively, 1-year mortality was 2% versus 4% (*p* = 0.016), incidence of AMI was 9% and 12%, and hospital readmission was 37% versus 57%.

(TACTICS)-TIMI 18 investigators. Comparison of early invasive versus conservative strategies in patients with unstable angina and non-ST elevation myocardial infarction treated with the glycoprotein IIb/IIIa inhibitor tirofiban, 2001.

Methods: Cannon et al. (148) treated 2,220 patients with UA/NSTEMI and either ECG changes (ST deviation, or T-wave inversion > 3 mm), elevated biomarkers, or documented history of CAD with aspirin, heparin, and tirofiban. Patients were randomized to an early invasive (4 to 48 hours) or selectively invasive (for those with spontaneous or provokable ischemia only) management. The primary composite endpoint was **death, MI, or recurrent hospitalization for ACS** within 6 months.

Findings: Of 2,220 patients, 27% met entry criteria only by history of CAD. Of those in the conservative group, 51% underwent catheterization during the initial hospitalization. Early invasive strategy reduced the primary endpoint and the rate of **MI or death** (15.9% versus 19.4% and 7.3% versus 9.5%, respectively). The best independent predictors of benefit from an early invasive strategy were ST changes, elevated troponin, and no prior use of aspirin.

Aspirin in UA/NSTEMI

Antiplatelet Trialists' Collaboration. Collaborative review of randomized trials of antiplatelet therapy I. Prevention of death, MI, and stroke by prolonged antiplatelet therapy in various categories of patients, 1994.

Methods: This study was a meta-analysis of trials evaluating aspirin use in ACS (530).

Findings: After an episode of UA or MI, aspirin was found to lower the risk of MI by 60% at 3 months and by 52% at 2 years.

Unfractionated Heparin in UA/NSTEMI

Oler A, et al. Adding heparin to aspirin reduces the incidence of myocardial infarction and death in patients with unstable angina: a meta-analysis, 1996.

Methods: This study was a meta-analysis of trials comparing the efficacy of heparin added to aspirin versus aspirin alone for UA/NSTEMI (531).

Findings: Adding heparin to aspirin lowers the risk of **MI or death** by 33% compared with aspirin alone.

Enoxaparin in UA/NSTEMI

Cohen M, et al. A comparison of low-molecular-weight heparin with unfractionated heparin for unstable coronary artery disease, 1997.

Methods: The ESSENCE study (516) randomized 3,171 UA/NSTEMI patients in a double-blind, placebo-controlled design to enoxaparin (1 mg/kg twice daily subcutaneously) or UFH for 2 to 8 days. All patients received aspirin. The study enrolled a largely low-risk group, 56% of whom had a normal ECG on admission.

Findings: Enoxaparin achieved a modest 15% relative risk reduction (RRR) in death, MI, or refractory angina at 30 days (19.8% versus 23.3%; *p* = 0.016) and at 1 year (22.8% versus 26.6%; RRR 14%) compared with UFH. Enoxaparin was significantly more effective than UFH in higher-risk patients with ST depression and lowered the need for revascularization at 30 days (27% versus 32.2%; *p* = 0.001). Patients who underwent unplanned angioplasty did not experience an increase in major bleeding risk compared with UFH.

Antman EM, et al. Enoxaparin prevents death and cardiac ischemic events in unstable angina/non–Q-wave MI: results of the TIMI-11B trial, 1999b.

Methods: The TIMI-11B trial (517) randomized 3,910 UA/NSTEMI patients, 83% with ECG changes (75% with ST depression) and 40% with elevated cTnI, to UFH (70 U/kg, then 15 U/kg/hour) or enoxaparin (30 mg IV bolus, then 1 mg/kg subcutaneous twice daily) for 3 to 8 days of treatment or until hospital discharge. Enoxaparin-treated patients received it as outpatients for 43 days. The composite endpoint was defined as **death, MI, or recurrent angina.**

Findings: Study entry to first dose was 11 hours. For the UFH group and the enoxaparin group, respectively, 14.5% versus 12.4% (p = 0.048) (8 days) and 19.7% versus 17.3% (p = 0.048) (43 days) reached the composite endpoint.

Antman EM, et al. Assessment of the treatment effect of enoxaparin for unstable angina/NQMI:TIMI 11B-ESSENCE meta-analysis, 1999a.
  Methods: Antman et al. (518) did a meta-analysis of TIMI-11B (517) and ESSENCE (516) described earlier. The combined endpoint was death, MI, and urgent revascularization.
  Findings: There was no difference at 2 days between UFH and enoxaparin in the combined endpoint. However, at Days 8, 14, and 43 there was a statistically significant 20% reduction in the combined endpoint, mostly in **MI and urgent revascularization.**

Lindahl B, et al. Troponin T identifies patients with unstable coronary artery disease who benefit from long-term antithrombotic protection. Fragmin in Unstable Coronary Artery Disease (FRISC) Study Group, 1997.
  Methods: Lindahl et al. (385) compared the benefit of low-molecular-weight heparin (dalteparin) in 644 patients with ACS with cTnT ≥ versus ≤ 0.1 μg/mL.
  Findings: The benefit of LMWH is particularly marked in, and possibly limited to, those patients with cTnT ≥ 0.1. At 6 days, death or MI was reduced from 6.0% to 2.5% in the 317 patients with positive cTnT (versus a reduction from 2.4% to 0% in 327 patients with cTnT of less than 0.1 μg/L). At 40 days, the reduction was 14.2% to 7.4% versus a nonsignificant increase from 4.7% to 5.7% in the group with cTnT of less than 0.1 μg/l.

Hirudin

GUSTO IIa Investigators. A comparison of recombinant hirudin with heparin for the treatment of acute coronary syndromes, 1996.
  Methods: The GUSTO IIa trial (520) compared the clinical efficacy of hirudin versus UFH for ACS in 12,142 patients. Patients with STEMI (n = 4,131) also received thrombolytics.
  Findings: The risk of **death or MI,** regardless of ST-segment status, was significantly lower in the hirudin group (1.3% versus 2.1%; p = 0.001) at 24 hours, but not at 30 days (8.9% versus 9.8%; p = 0.06). Hirudin was associated with a higher risk of ICH (0.2% versus 0.02%) and moderate bleeding complications compared with UFH.

OASIS-2 Investigators. Effects of recombinant hirudin (lepirudin) compared with heparin on death, MI, refractory angina, and revascularization procedures in patients with acute myocardial ischemia without ST elevation: a randomized trial, 1999.
  Methods: OASIS-2 (519) randomized 10,141 patients with UA/NSTEMI to UFH or lepirudin for 72 hours in a double-blind trial.
  Findings: At 7 days, lepirudin lowered the risk of death, MI, or refractory angina by 10% to 15% compared with UFH (5.6% versus 6.7%; p = 0.012), suggesting the modest superiority of lepirudin. However, this benefit is incurred at the cost of increase in major but not life-threatening bleeding (0.8% versus 0.3% for UFH, p = 0.001).

GP IIb–IIIa Inhibitors: Tirofiban, Eptifibatide, Abciximab

Kong DF, et al. Clinical outcomes of therapeutic agents that block the platelet glycoprotein IIb/IIIa integrin in ischemic heart disease, 1998.
  Methods: Kong et al. (522) identified randomized, blinded, controlled trials of parenteral GP IIb/IIIa antagonists through MEDLINE and **categorized them separately, based on whether the primary intent at study entry was (a) percutaneous revascularization; or (b) medical treatment of UA/NSTEMI, with revascularization reserved for refractory angina.** ORs were calculated for 16 trials, and the outcome of 32,135 patients in four trials was evaluated. The four trials were PRISM (523), PRISM-PLUS (524), PURSUIT (525), and PARAGON (532). PCI was discouraged until after drug administration for at least 48 hours, and early outcome data allowed evaluation without the early confounding influence of PCI.
  Findings: For the combined endpoint of **death, MI or revascularization,** there was a highly significant benefit favoring GP IIb/IIIa inhibitors, with every trial showing statistically significant RRRs. This was primarily due to reductions in rates of non–Q-wave MI. For every 1,000 patients in PCI and medical therapy trials combined, GP IIb/IIIa inhibitors caused 27 fewer events at 48 to 96 hours, 30 fewer events at

30 days, and 23 fewer events at 6 months. **There was no significant reduction in mortality.** In the subset of patients undergoing PCI in the EPIC trial (Evaluation of c7E3 for Prevention of Ischemic Complications), abciximab reduced the risk of death compared with placebo by 72% at 6 months (1.8% versus 6.6%; p = 0.018), and by 60% at 3 years (5.1% versus 12.7%; p = 0.01).

PRISM Study Investigators. A comparison of aspirin plus tirofiban with aspirin plus heparin for unstable angina, 1998.
  Methods: The PRISM study (523) randomized 3,232 patients with UA/NSTEMI and ECG changes, in double-blind fashion, to UFH or tirofiban.
  Findings: The composite end-point of death, MI or refractory ischemia at 48 hours was 32% lower in the tirofiban group (3.8% versus 5.6% with UFH; p = 0.01). There was no difference in the incidence of ischemia or MI between groups at 30 days, but tirofiban reduced the absolute mortality rate by 1.3% (2.3% versus 3.6% with UFH; p = 0.02).

PRISM-PLUS Study Investigators: Inhibition of the platelet GP IIb/IIIa receptor with tirofiban in unstable angina and non–Q wave MI, 1998.
  Methods: The PRISM-PLUS trial (524) randomized 1,915 patients with UA/NSTEMI and ECG changes in a placebo-controlled, double-blind study of tirofiban, UFH, or both.
  Findings: The arm with tirofiban alone was stopped prematurely. The primary composite endpoint of **death, MI, or refractory ischemia** within 7 days of enrollment was lower among patients who received combination therapy than among those who received UFH alone (13% versus 18%; relative risk 0.68; p = 0.004). This benefit was maintained at 30 days and at 6 months.

PURSUIT Trial Investigators, Inhibition of platelet GP IIb/IIIa with eptifibatide in patients with acute coronary syndromes, 1998.
  Methods: The PURSUIT trial (525) randomized 10,948 UA/NSTEMI patients with ECG changes to eptifibatide or placebo in double-blind fashion for up to 72 hours, or up to 96 hours if coronary intervention was performed.
  Findings: Patients who received eptifibatide had an absolute reduction of 1.5% in the primary endpoint of **death or MI** at 30 days compared with placebo (14.2% versus 15.7%; p = 0.04).

CAPTURE Investigators. Randomized placebo-controlled trial of abciximab before and during coronary intervention in refractory unstable angina: the CAPTURE study, 1997.
  Methods: The CAPTURE study (526) randomized 1,265 patients with refractory angina (pain at rest with ECG changes while on IV NTG and UFH) in a placebo-controlled, open-label trial, to abciximab or placebo for 18 to 24 hours before angiography and continued for 1 hour after angioplasty.
  Findings: The primary composite end-point, which was **death, MI, or urgent revascularization at 30 days,** occurred in 11.3% of the abciximab group compared with 15.9% of the placebo group (p = 0.012). The RR of **death or MI** among patients with **elevated cTnT** was 0.32 among patients treated with abciximab compared with patients on placebo (p = 0.002). **Abciximab reduced the risk of preprocedural MI by 70%, postangioplasty MI by 52%, and death or MI at 30 days by 47%, respectively.** In patients without elevated cTnT, there was no benefit of treatment with respect to the RR of death or MI at 6 months.

Simooons, ML. GUSTO IV ACS: Effect of glucoprotein IIb/IIIa receptor blocker abeiximab on outcome in patients with acute coronary syndromes without early revascularization, 2001.
  Methods: GUSTO-IV-ACS (521) included 7,800 patients with ACS **and** either a positive cTnI or cTnT **or** ST depression of at least 0.5 mm, **and** no plans for coronary intervention. Patients were blindly randomized to placebo or to abciximab for either 24 or 48 hours, along with aspirin and heparin.
  Findings: Of 7,800 patients, 97% received aspirin and either heparin or low-molecular-weight heparin. Surprisingly, given the previous findings of greater efficacy for abciximab than tirofiban or eptifibatide in other situations, and the proven efficacy for these agents for UA/NSTEMI, there was no difference between abciximab and placebo in primary endpoint of death or MI at 30 days.

38

ADJUNCTIVE MEDICATIONS IN REPERFUSION THERAPY FOR AMI

FARHANA KAZZI AND STEPHEN W. SMITH

There are numerous pharmacologic agents that are important for the convalescent period and/or for secondary prevention of STEMI. Many of these agents are important very **early in the course of STEMI,** in addition to thrombolytics or PCI. They include (a) **nitrates** such as sublingual NTG and IV NTG; (b) **antiplatelet agents,** particularly **aspirin,** but also including clopidogrel and GP IIb/IIIa inhibitors; (c) **anticoagulants,** particularly **heparin** and **enoxaparin;** (d) **beta-adrenergic blockers,** particularly **metoprolol;** (e) **magnesium;** (f) **angiotensin converting enzyme (ACE) inhibitors;** and (g) **angiotensin receptor antagonists.**

Certain subsets of patients with STEMI have a high, intermediate, or low risk of death, related in part to convalescent LV function. Prolongation of life in this heterogeneous group of patients is a major goal of secondary prevention strategies. In addition to the pharmacologic agents mentioned earlier, **antiarrhythmic drugs, calcium channel blockers,** and especially **lipid-lowering drugs** may be important in the convalescent period and for secondary prevention of MI. These treatments may reduce mortality by 5% to 30% (533).

NITRATES: SUBLINGUAL NTG AND IV NTG

Some patients with AMI have a component of coronary spasm, and NTG may safely open the IRA. A number of small studies in the prethrombolytic era demonstrated an improvement in mortality and major cardiovascular morbidity following early administration of IV NTG. A meta-analysis of these early trials showed reduction in odds of death after AMI by 35% (534). However, in the context of routine thrombolytic therapy and use of aspirin, recent trials of prolonged administration of transdermal or oral NTG within 24 hours of onset have shown no reduction in mortality (62,535). When these data are pooled, there is a small relative reduction in mortality, representing four lives saved per 1,000 patients treated (62).

Data from animal studies, small nonrandomized trials, and randomized trials have indicated **detrimental impact of IV NTG on tPA efficacy** (59–61). These studies indicated that IV NTG lowered reperfusion rates by increasing hepatic blood flow and, subsequently, tPA metabolism. The American College of Cardiology/American Heart Association (AHA) does not recommend routine use of intravenous nitrates but does recommend IV NTG for AMI with recurrent ischemia, CHF, or HTN (105). In summary:

- **Administer sublingual NTG** (up to three tablets or spray every 5 minutes) **immediately** to all patients with suspected AMI with a systolic BP > 90, except in patients who have taken sildenafil (Viagra®) within 24 hours (536).
- **Routine use of IV NTG** with thrombolytics is **not** recommended. Routine use of IV NTG in conjunction with PCI **may** be beneficial. Initial dose is 10 units/minute, with subsequent titration to BP and pain.

Administer IV NTG in AMI with recurrent ischemia, elevated BP or CHF.

ANTIPLATELET AGENTS: ASPIRIN, CLOPIDIGREL, AND GP IIb/IIIa INHIBITORS

Aspirin reduces the mortality of AMI. It has been proven to be much safer than thrombolytic therapy and of equal importance (102). A dose of **160 mg to 325 mg** should be given to **all patients with possible AMI,** with a daily dose of 81 mg to 325 mg indefinitely thereafter (105).

Clopidigrel inhibits adenosine diphospate (ADP)-mediated platelet aggregation and is safer than ticlodipine for long-term use. Clopidigrel should be used with reperfusion therapy **when aspirin is contraindicated,** primarily in cases of aspirin allergy that manifests as asthma. Clopidogrel is often added to aspirin when PCI is planned; a 300 mg loading dose may be given with the approval of the interventional cardiologist. Clopidigrel has an overall safety profile similar to that of medium-dose aspirin (537).

GP IIb/IIIa inhibitors, including **abciximab,** are platelet receptor blockers or antagonists. As discussed in Chapter 36, they may be useful in conjunction with **half-dose thrombolytics** (514,515,515.5). They are indicated **prior to PCI,** including PCI for STEMI. Long-term use of oral agents has not yet shown similar benefit for secondary prevention of MI.

ANTICOAGULANTS: HEPARIN AND HIRUDIN

GISSI-2 (98) and ISIS-3 (103) showed no mortality difference between SK and tPA using subcutaneous heparin; however, the GUSTO-1 trial showed **tPA with IV heparin** to be the most effective regimen (86). IV Heparin is therefore routinely recommended with fibrin-specific thrombolytic agents such as tPA and rPA in order to maintain coronary patency and to minimize the risk of reocclusion due to rethrombosis.

ISIS-3 (103) and GISSI-2 (98) showed that adjunctive subcutaneous heparin in combination with SK does not improve outcome, and GUSTO-1 showed that, in conjunction with SK, IV over subcutaneous heparin conferred no benefit. However, **in patients who receive SK and are at high risk of systemic emboli (such as those with large anterior AMI, LV thrombus, atrial fibrillation, or history of embolic stroke), subcutaneous heparin is recommended** (105).

Doses are as follows:

- With **tPA, rPA,** or **TNK-tPA,** administer **IV heparin** in a dose of 60 U/kg bolus (maximum of 4,000 U), followed by 12 U/kg/hr (maximum 1,000 U/hr), to be continued for at least 48 hours.
  The low molecular weight heparin **enoxparin** (30 mg IV plus 1 mg/kg subcutaneously every 12 hours for 7 days) in conjunction with full-dose TNK-tpA, was shown to be superior to unfractionated heparin (471.5).
- With **SK, anistreplase, urokinase** or nonspecific fibrinolytic agents, in patients at high risk of systemic emboli, administer **subcutaneous heparin** in a dose of **12,500 U twice daily** during hospitalization.
- With **primary angioplasty, high-dose heparin** (10,000 U, or 100 U/kg IV bolus, followed by a maintenance infusion of 1,000 U/kg) is recommended to produce an activated clotting time (ACT) of 300 to 350 seconds during the procedure. When abciximab is used with heparin during percutaneous revascularization, a lower dose of heparin is used, with target ACT between 150 and 300 seconds.

Although newer direct antithrombin inhibitors such as **hirudin** and its synthetic analog lepirudin initially showed promising results in early trials in AMI and UA/NSTEMI, large-scale trials had to be halted secondary to excess risk of ICH in patients treated with thrombolytic agents (520,538). Therefore **their use is not recommended** for STEMI in conjunction with thrombolytics.

Routine use of **warfarin** is **not recommended.** The ACC/AHA suggests 3-month use of warfarin for patients with high embolic risk such as those with anterior wall MI, severe LV dysfunction, CHF, history of prior systemic or pulmonary emboli, and echocardiographic evidence of a mural thrombus (105).

BETA-ADRENERGIC BLOCKERS: METROPOLOL, ESMOLOL

Beta-adrenergic blockers, or beta-blockers, can decrease myocardial oxygen demand by reducing HR, systemic arterial pressure, and myocardial contractility. In the prethrombolytic era, use of beta-blockers was shown to have a favorable influence on infarct size and diminish short-term mortality (539). In subjects receiving concomitant thrombolytic therapy, IV beta-blockers decrease the incidence of nonfatal reinfarction and recurrent angina. They may also reduce mortality if given within 2 hours of symptom onset (511). Chronic administration of beta-blockers decreases mortality by reducing the incidence of sudden and

nonsudden cardiac death. Although overall trial data do not establish a basis of therapy beyond 2 years, patients in some studies were followed with sustained benefit for up to 6 years.

- **Beta-blockers should be routinely administered in STEMI** and continued indefinitely.
- Administer **metoprolol** 5 mg every 5 minutes for three doses, followed by 50 mg orally.
  - **Alternatively,** administer **esmolol** in a 500 μg/kg bolus, followed by 50 μg/kg/min. Esmolol can be turned off if adverse events are likely. You may rebolus and increase drip if the patient's HR is not controlled.
- **Contraindications** include significant **asthma,** clinically significant **bradycardia** (HR < 60), **second- or third-degree heart block, PR interval > 0.24 second, hypotension** (systolic BP < 100 mmHg), and severe peripheral vascular disease (105).
- Beta-blockers should be used cautiously in patients with insulin-dependent diabetes and moderately or severely depressed LV function.

MAGNESIUM

Cardioprotective effects of magnesium include vasodilatation, reduction of platelet aggregation, stabilization of cell membranes, and protection of myocardial cells from catecholamine-induced myocardial necrosis (533). A meta-analysis of several small, randomized trials published from 1984 to 1991 indicated that magnesium conferred a significant mortality benefit, and the LIMIT-2 trial subsequently reported a 24% reduction in mortality and 25% lower incidence of CHF with magnesium treatment (540). These trials were contradicted by results of ISIS-4, however, which indicated no mortality benefit and even the possibility of harm (62). These differences could be due to the relatively late administration of magnesium and a low control group mortality of 7.2% in ISIS-4 (541). The MAGIC trial will be a large, randomized study to test for benefit of magnesium administration in early stages of reperfusion in high-risk patients, defined as an age of 65 years or more, or patients with contraindications to reperfusion.

- **Check serum magnesium in all AMI patients and administer early magnesium** to AMI patients who are not eligible for thrombolytic therapy and to those with a magnesium level of less than 2.0 mEq/L (105).
- **Dose:** 2 grams over 5 to 15 minutes, followed by 18 grams over 24 hours.

ANGIOTENSIN-CONVERTING ENZYME INHIBITORS

ACE inhibitors reduce LV dysfunction and dilatation, decrease incidence and slow progression of CHF, and significantly reduce mortality after AMI, especially in patients with anterior AMI or prior history of CHF (62,63,535). Initiation of ACE inhibitor therapy during the first few days to weeks after myocardial infarction in selected patients and the continuation of that therapy over the long term has been shown to significantly decrease mortality in several large randomized trials (542). Use of **IV** ACE inhibitors within 24 hours of AMI may be **harmful,** however, especially in high-risk elderly patients, as they may cause early hypotensive reactions (543).

- **Administer ACE inhibitors within the first 24 hours** of suspected or established AMI. This is especially important in patients with anterior AMI **or** clinical CHF **or** EF < 40%. Give **lisinopril:** 5 mg po, 5 mg after 24 hours, and 10 mg daily thereafter if well tolerated.
- **Continue oral ACE inhibitors for 4 to 6 weeks** in all patients with AMI and no contraindications. Continue longer in patients with a history of LV dysfunction, with or without symptoms (105).
- **Contraindications:** systolic BP < 100, after use of beta-blockers.
- **Avoid** intravenous enalapril.

ANGIOTENSIN RECEPTOR ANTAGONISTS

Angiotensin receptor antagonists have not been studied in large, post-MI clinical trials. Data from HTN and CHF trials suggest therapeutic equivalence with ACE inhibitors with fewer side effects. Although routine use is not recommended in post-MI patients, these agents should be considered a suitable alternative for ACE inhibitor-intolerant patients.

PHARMACOLOGIC AGENTS FOR CONVALESCENCE AND SECONDARY PREVENTION OF AMI

In addition to the pharmacologic agents mentioned earlier, **antiarrhythmic drugs, calcium channel blockers,** and especially **lipid-lowering drugs** may be important in the convalescent period and for secondary prevention of AMI.

Antiarrhythmic Agents

From 4% to 18% of AMI patients have potentially fatal ventricular fibrillation within the first 24 to 48 hours (544). This led to the prophylactic administration of class I antiarrhythmic drugs, predominantly IV lidocaine. A meta-analysis of randomized trials of prophylactic lidocaine in the prethrombolytic era revealed a significant reduction in peri-infarct ventricular fibrillation, benefits of which were offset by deaths associated with asystole and electromechanical dissociation (544). However, a more recent review of lidocaine use in the thrombolytic era (GUSTO-I and GUSTO-IIb trials) showed no increased incidence of adverse events (545).

- **Administer lidocaine** only in cases of malignant ventricular dysrhythmias or to prevent their recurrence.
- **Initial dose:** 1.0 to 1.5 mg/kg bolus, additional boluses of 0.5 to 0.75 mg/kg every 5 to 10 minutes up to a total of 3 mg/kg, followed by infusion of 1 to 4 mg/min.

Calcium Channel Blockers

Calcium channel blockers have antianginal, vasodilatory, and antihypertensive properties. Individual trials and meta-analyses of therapy with these agents, however, have not indicated mortality benefits when administered during or after AMI (533). Clinical trials with short-acting nifedipine (a dihydropyridine) have not shown benefit in reduction of mortality or reinfarction, and indeed, have shown an adverse trend (546). Data on long-acting nifedipine and other dihydropyridines, such as felodipine and amlodipine, are scant. Clinical trials with verapamil have shown only a trend toward reduction in reinfarction and marginal effects on mortality (547). Large clinical trials indicate that diltiazem has no mortality benefit and is actually harmful in patients with CHF and pulmonary edema (548).

- **Calcium channel blockers are not recommended for routine use in AMI patients,** except in patients for whom beta-blockers are ineffective or contraindicated, such as bronchospastic patients; in this case they are used for relief of ongoing ischemia or control of rapid ventricular response with atrial fibrillation. Short-acting nifedipine is generally contraindicated (105).

Lipid-Lowering Therapy

Secondary prevention of myocardial infarction has focused on effects of lipid-lowering drugs and diet to lower cholesterol. Recently, the Scandinavian Simvastatin Survival Study (4S) showed significant reduction of total and cardiovascular mortality in patients with CAD and moderate hypercholestrolemia (mean baseline low density lipid, LDL = 188 mg/dL) who used simvistatin (549). These results were replicated in the Cholesterol and Recurrent Events (CARE) trial, which studied the effects of pravastatin on coronary events after MI in patients with average cholesterol levels (mean baseline LDL = 139 mg/dL) (550). Similar results were observed in the Long-Term Intervention with Pravastatin in Ischemic Disease (LIPID) trial (551). A complete blood lipid profile is recommended in all infarct patients, either at the time of admission or within the first 24 hours. Otherwise, there is a minimum 4-week waiting period after infarction to allow stabilization of lipid fractions. During this interim all patients should be treated with the AHA Step II diet, which is a low-cholesterol, low-saturated-fat diet. If plasma LDL cholesterol remains > 130 mg/dL, drug therapy should be initiated with the goal of achieving LDL levels < 100 mg/dL (105).

Appendix A

ABBREVIATIONS

ABCs, airway, breathing, circulation
ACC, American College of Cardiology
ACEP, American College of Emergency Physicians
ACI-TIPI, Acute Cardiac Ischemia Time Insensitive Predictive Instruments
ACS, acute coronary syndrome
AHA, American Heart Association
AIVR, accelerated idioventricular rhythm
ALS, advanced life support
AMI, acute myocardial infarction
ATP, adenosine triphosphate
AV, atrioventricular
BBB, bundle branch block
BP, blood pressure
b.p.m., beats per minute
CABG, coronary artery bypass graft
CACP, cocaine-associated chest pain
CAD, coronary artery disease
cath, catheterization
CCP, Cooperative Cardiovascular Project
CCU, cardiac care unit
CHF, congestive heart failure
CI, confidence interval
CK-MB, creatine kinase-MB
COPD, chronic obstructive pulmonary disease
CP, chest pain
CPR, cardiopulmonary resuscitation
CQI, Continuous Quality Improvement
CT, computed tomography
CTFC, corrected TIMI frame count
cTnI, cardiac troponin I
cTnT, cardiac troponin T
DM, diabetes mellitus
DTBT, door-to-balloon-time
DTNT, door-to-needle-time
ECG, electrocardiogram
ECSG, European Cooperative Study Group
ED, emergency department
EF, ejection fraction
EMS, emergency medical service
ESRD, end-stage renal disease
ETT, exercise tolerance testing
FTT, Fibrinolytic Therapy Trialists
FWR, free wall rupture

GP, glycoprotein
HR, heart rate
HTN, hypertension
ICH, intracranial hemorrhage
INR, international normalized ratio
IRA, infarct related artery
IVCD, intraventricular conduction delay
LAD, left anterior descending artery
LAFB, left anterior fascicular block
LBBB, left bundle branch block
LD, lactate dehydrogenase
LMWH, low molecular weight heparin
LOC, level of consciousness
LPFB, left posterior fascicular block
LV, left ventricle (ventricular)
LVH, left ventricular hypertrophy
MAR, myocardium at risk
MCL, modified chest leads
MI, myocardial infarction
MRI, magnetic resonance imaging
MS, myocardial salvage
NPV, negative predictive value
NRMI, National Registry of Myocardial Infarction
NSTEMI, non-ST—elevation MI
NTG, nitroglycerine
OR, odds ratio
PCI, percutaneous coronary intervention
PDA, posterior descending artery
PIRP, post-infarction regional pericarditis
PMR, papillary muscle rupture
PPV, positive predictive value
PSVT, paroxysmal supraventricular tachycardia
PTT, prothrombin time
PVC, premature ventricular contraction
RBBB, right bundle branch block
RCA, right coronary artery
rPA, reteplase
RR, risk ratio or relative risk
RRR, relative risk reduction
RV, right ventricle (ventricular)
RVH, right ventricular hypertrophy
SA, sinoatrial
SECG, serial ECGs
SK, streptokinase

SOB, shortness of breath
SR, septal rupture
STEMI, ST elevation MI
TNK-tPA, tenecteplase tissue plasminogen activator
tPA, tissue plasminogen activator

UA/NSTEMI, unstable angina/non-ST elevation myocardial infarction
UFH, unfractionated heparin
WMA, wall motion abnormality
WPW, Wolff-Parkinson-White

Appendix B

GLOSSARY

Acute coronary syndrome (ACS) Any symptomatic atherosclerotic plaque rupture or coronary thrombotic event, whether resulting in ischemia or infarction. ACS consists of a constellation of signs, symptoms, ECG findings, and/or biochemical markers indicating acute thrombotic event, or acute increase in the size and occlusiveness of an atherosclerotic plaque, in a coronary artery. It includes most acute myocardial infarction (AMI) and unstable angina (UA). ACS usually leads to at least brief cardiac ischemia, but cardiac ischemia may be due to many conditions other than ACS.

Akinesia Lack of myocardial wall motion.

Asymmetrically inverted T waves The magnitude of the slope of the downward limb of the T wave is less than the magnitude of the slope of the upward limb.

Condordant Description applied when the QRS complex and the ST-T complex are in the same direction. In the setting of left bundle branch block (LBBB) and, to a lesser extent, left ventricular hypertrophy (LVH) with ST-T abnormalities, this is a sign of AMI.

Delta waves Slurring of the QRS upstroke seen in Wolff-Parkinson-White (WPW) syndrome.

Discordant Description applied when the QRS complex and the ST-T complex are in opposite directions. This is the normal condition in LBBB and, to a lesser extent, in LVH with ST-T abnormalities.

Dyskinesia Myocardial wall motion that is in the wrong direction, usually bulging out in systole. This is different from aneurysm, which implies bulging out even in diastole. Contrast also with hypokinesia and akinesia.

Early transition R waves appearing in more rightward precordial leads than normal: R/S ratio greater than 1 in V2 or V3, whereas normal is V3 or V4.

Epicardial coronary artery The large coronary arteries that are commonly referred to only as coronary artery. These are called epicardial because they run on the outside surface of the heart, and they are in distinction to smaller branches and arterioles that penetrate the myocardium.

First diagonal coronary artery Branch of the left anterior descending artery (LAD) that supplies the lateral wall of the heart.

Hypokinesia Decreased myocardial wall motion, but in the right direction.

"Inadvertent" thrombolytic therapy Thrombolysis given appropriately (as determined by appropriate use of criteria and benefit/risk analysis) to patients who, in retrospect, are proven not to have ST elevation AMI (STEMI).

J point Junction of the QRS and ST segments.

J wave Notch or slur at the J point, suggestive of early repolarization.

Left dominant coronary system Coronary system in which the circumflex artery supplies the posterior descending artery, which supplies the inferior wall.

Millivolts (mV) On the standard ECG, 1.0 mV of amplitude = 10 mm of amplitude.

Minor myocardial damage New term for minimal elevation of troponin after an episode of acute coronary syndrome that does not meet creatine kinase (CK) criteria for AMI. This may also be the result of other disease processes that lead to minimal myocyte necrosis.

Myocardial blush Appearance on an angiogram of diffuse and faint highlighting of the myocardium by contrast.

Myocardial stunning Transient, reversible **postischemic** myocardial dysfunction with relatively normal blood flow. This may be due to coronary disease and/or acute coronary syndrome but also may occur in circumstances of very high circulating catecholamines due to a variety of critical illnesses. In this situation it is probably due to vasospasm of small vessels, due to sympathetic activation, but it is unlikely to be due to epicardial coronary vasospasm (150). Although it is not necessarily due to an unstable coronary atherosclerotic plaque or to coronary occlusion, it may manifest with typically ischemic ECG findings and reversible ultrasonic regional wall motion abnormality (WMA).

Non–ST-elevation acute coronary syndrome (NSTE-ACS) This is the same as unstable angina/non–ST-elevation MI (UA/NSTEMI). It contrasts with ST-elevation MI (STEMI).

Obtuse marginal coronary artery Branch of the circumflex artery supplying the posterolateral wall of the heart.

Percutaneous coronary intervention (PCI) A procedure that uses guide wires, angiographic visualization, balloons, and stents to open coronary artery occlusions and dilate stenoses.

Posterior descending artery Coronary artery that supplies the inferior wall. In a right dominant system, it is the distal right coronary artery (RCA). In a left dominant system, it is the distal circumflex artery.

Primary intracranial hemorrhage (ICH) ICH that is the initial or primary problem. This contrasts with hemorrhage resulting from trauma after a fall due to cardiac arrest, or hemorrhage due to thrombolytic therapy.

Primary ST-T abnormalities ECG abnormalities that are not due to abnormal depolarization.

QRS distortion In conjunction with ST elevation, this indicates J-point at a height of 50% or more of the height of R wave OR disappearance of the S wave in leads with Rs configuration.

Relative index CK-MB level, in mass units of ng/mL, divided by total CK level, which is measured in international units per liter (IU/L). See Case 14-5.

Right ventricular hypertrophy (RVH) Is present if one or more of the following criteria are met and the QRS duration is < 120 ms: right axis deviation of +110°, R/S ratio in V1 > 1, R wave in V1 ≥ 7 mm, S wave in V1 < 2 mm, qR pattern in V1, rSR′ in V1 with R′ > 10 mm. See Chou (2).

Secondary ST-T abnormalities Due to abnormalities of depolarization, which have an abnormal QRS (e.g. LVH, LBBB, WPW, RVH).

Subacute MI Completed AMI. ST segments have generally stabilized, often with some T-wave inversion.

Symmetrically inverted T waves The magnitude of the slopes of the downward limb and the upward limb of the T wave are nearly equal.

Terminal T-wave inversion Inversion of the latter part of the T wave, as opposed to inversion of the entire T wave. This has biphasic morphology and happens when the T wave inverts with the ST segment still somewhat elevated.

TIMI flow grade Classification used by the Thrombolysis in Myocardial Infarction (TIMI) trial group to indicate perfusion of an infarct-related artery (IRA) that improved from visual grade 0 or 1 (total occlusion or penetration without perfusion) to grade 2 or 3 (partial or full reperfusion).

TIMI myocardial perfusion (TMP) grade An angiographic method to assess filling and clearance of contrast in the myocardium that is graded from 0 to 3. TMP grade 0 = no myocardial perfusion, grade 1 refers to no clearance of injected contrast, grade 2 refers to slow clearance, and grade 3 refers to normal clearance.

Troponin (cardiac troponin I and T, cTnI and cTnT) Protein released from damaged myocardium, and is now used as definition of AMI. "Positive" troponin refers to a level above the laboratory's reference range for a particular assay, and depending on the assay, ranges from 0.1 ng/mL to 0.8 ng/mL. The upper level of the reference range at the time these cases were collected was 0.8 ng/mL.

Unstable angina (UA) Acute coronary syndrome that does not result in troponin elevation. It may present without ECG changes, with transient ST elevation, or with ST depression or T-wave inversion.

Wellens' syndrome Ischemic symptoms and anterior T-wave inversion indicating high risk of anterior AMI due to tight proximal LAD stenosis. Described by Wellens in 1982. Morphology is identical to early reperfusion of anterior AMI resulting in T-wave inversion. Thus the probable pathophysiology is spontaneous reperfusion of occluded tight LAD stenosis. The same process has also been described for the inferior leads and inferior AMI.

Wolff-Parkinson-White syndrome (WPW) Highly complex, but to state in brief: it is the presence of a bypass tract that conducts the impulse from the atrium faster than the AV node, thus leading to premature excitation of the ventricle ("preexcitation"), which often manifests on the ECG as a shortened P-R interval and a "delta" wave (slurring of the upstroke of the R wave). It often leads to repolarization abnormalities such as ST depression and T-wave inversion.

Wraparound LAD LAD that wraps around the apex of the heart to reach and supply the inferior wall.

Appendix C

ACRONYMS AND DESCRIPTIONS OF FREQUENTLY CITED CLINICAL TRIALS

Acronym	Full Name
ASSENT	Assessment of the Safety and Efficacy of a New Thrombolytic (412)
CAPTURE	C7E3 Fab Anti-Platelet Therapy in Unstable Refractory Angina (526)
DANAMI	DANish Trial in Acute Myocardial Infarction (529)
ECSG	European Cooperative Study Group (515,552)
EMIP	European Myocardial Infarction Project (403)
FRISC	Fast Revascularization during InStability in Coronary artery disease (528,553)
FTT	Fibrinolytic Therapy Trialists' Collaborative Group (30)
GISSI	Gruppo Italiano per lo Studio della Sopravvivenza nell'Infarto Miocardico (29,63,98,535)
GREAT	Grampian Region Early Anistreplase Trial (423)
GUSTO	Global Use of Streptokinase and Tissue Plasminogen Activator for Occluded Coronary Arteries (86,362,446,515.5,520,521)
ISIS	International Study of Infarct Survival (62,102,103,539)
LATE	Late Assessment of Thrombolytic Efficacy (169)
MITI	Myocardial Infarction Triage and Intervention Trial (405,554)
OASIS	Organization to Assess Strategies for Ischemic Syndromes (519)
PAMI	Primary Angioplasty in Myocardial Infarction (502,555)
PRISM	Platelet Receptor Inhibition in ischemic SyndroMe (523)
PRISM-PLUS	Platelet Receptor Inhibition in ischemic SyndroMe in Patients Limited by Unstable Signs and symptoms (524)
PURSUIT	Platelet Glycoprotein IIb-IIIa in Unstable Angina: Receptor Suppression Using Integrilin Therapy (525)
TACTICS	Treat Angina with Aggrastat and determine Cost of Therapy with an Invasive or Conservative Strategy (148)
TAMI	Thrombolysis and Angioplasty in Myocardial Infarction (101,558–560)
TIMI	Thrombolysis in Myocardial Infarction (99,100,163,166,325,360,494,511)
USIM	Urochinasi per la Sistemica nell' Infarto Miocardico (457)
VANQWISH	Veterans Affairs Non-Q Wave Infarction Strategies in Hospital (527)

GISSI-1 (29,56)(109)(110)(462)

- **Time period:** February 1984 to June 1985; publication February 1986.
- **Setting:** 176 CCUs in Italy.
- **Design:** Randomized, unblinded trial of IV SK versus control for treatment of AMI.
- **Patients:** 11,806 patients.
- **Inclusion criteria:** Admission within 12 hours of AMI symptom onset; CP and ST elevation or depression ≥ 1 mm in ≥ **one** limb leads **or** ≥ 2 mm in **one** or more precordial leads.
- **Exclusion criteria:** No contraindications to thrombolytics (no excess bleeding risk).
- **Intervention:** Patients received 1.5 million units of SK in 100 mL saline over 1 hour. Aspirin and IV heparin were administered, respectively, in only **13%** and 20% of patients.
- **Primary endpoint:** **Overall** 21-day in-hospital mortality, as calculated by **intention-to-treat analysis** (an analysis of all patients randomized to the treatment, whether or not they actually received it); long-term follow-up indicated overall one-year mortality.
- **Findings:** SK treatment produced an 18% reduction of overall hospital mortality at 21 days (10.7% versus 13% in controls). The greatest benefit from thrombolytics was conferred if treatment was within 3 hours of symptom onset, with an overall mortality reduction of 23%. Statistically significant in-hospital mortality benefit occurred up to 6 hours, and a nonsignificant benefit was found for patients with 6 to 9 hours (14.1% versus 12.6%) and 9 to 12 hours (15.8% versus 13.6%) of symptoms. Long-term follow-up of 98.3% of the patients recruited showed persistence of beneficial effects on mortality at 12 months (17.2% in the SK group versus 19% in controls), especially among patients treated within 3 hours (15.1% versus 17.3%) and in those treated in 3 to 6 hours (18.3% versus 21.2%).

- **Conclusions:** IV infusion of 1.5 million U SK is safe for patients with no positive contraindications who present within 6 hours of pain onset. Pooled analyses (retrospective) suggest that the period of benefit may exceed 6 hours.
- **Comment:** ST elevation was required in only one lead. Post-hoc subgroup analyses did not show **mortality** benefit for those with ST elevation in three leads or less (109).

ISIS-2 (102)

- **Time period:** March 5, 1985 to December 31, 1987; published August 1988.
- **Setting:** 417 hospitals in 16 Europe and North America.
- **Design:** Randomized, placebo controlled, 2 × 2 factorial trial of IV SK, oral aspirin, both, or neither for treatment of AMI.
- **Inclusion criteria:** Fundamental criterion: **the responsible physician was uncertain whether treatment with SK or aspirin was indicated;** there were no contraindications to SK; patient presentation within **24 hours** of suspected AMI symptom onset; **no ECG changes were required for inclusion.** See **Comment**, below.
- **Intervention:** Patients were randomized to Group 1: SK alone, 1.5 million U infused over 1 hour, starting immediately; Group 2: oral aspirin alone, 162.5 mg in enteric-coated tablets, with one given immediately and one daily for 1 month; Group 3: both SK and aspirin, as above; and Group 4: neither treatment. Heparin was not required and received no comment.
- **Primary endpoint:** 35-day **vascular** mortality.
- **Findings:** 17,187 **patients** were entered. Overall 5-week vascular mortality was 8% for patients who received aspirin and SK, 9.2% for SK alone, 9.4% for aspirin alone, and 13% for double placebo, with 28 lives saved per 1,000 patients treated with SK. For those with ST elevation or BBB, mortality was 8.9% for aspirin plus SK and 16.1% for double placebo. Five-week vascular mortality for patients treated between 4.5 and 12 hours of symptom onset was 10.4% for SK versus 12.1% for placebo, with 17 lives saved per 1,000 treated (CI: 1 to 29). For earlier treatment, 30-day mortality reduction was 40% when treatment was within 1.5 hours of symptom onset, 35% at 1.5 to 2.5 hours, 30% at 2.5 to 3.5 hours, 32% at 3.5 to 4.5 hours, and 14% at 4.5 to 12 hours.
- **Comment:** Physicians were required to only include patients for whom they did **not** recognize a definite indication for SK. Thus the exact mix of patients is uncertain and many patients with very subtle STEMI and **without** STEMI were included. Therefore the beneficial effects of SK are **underestimated.**

ECSG (84)(110)(552)

- **Time period:** Study launched May 1986; publication November 1988.
- **Setting:** 26 European referral centers.
- **Design:** Randomized, double-blind, placebo-controlled trial of tPA for treatment of AMI.

- **Patients:** Treatment group: 355 patients; control group: 366 patients.
- **Inclusion criteria:** CP typical of myocardial ischemia; presentation within 5 hours of symptom onset; **ST elevation** (measured 60 msec after the J point) ≥ 2 mm in two or more limb leads or leads V5 and V6 **or** ST elevation ≥ 3 mm in two or more precordial leads **or** ST depression ≥ 2 mm in two precordial leads together with ST elevation ≥ 1 mm in two limb leads or V5–V6.
- **Endpoints:** LV function at 10 to 22 days, enzymatic infarct size, clinical course, and survival to 3-month follow-up.
- **Intervention:** All patients received aspirin 250 mg and bolus heparin 5,000 IU immediately (and continued for 10 to 22 days, until angiography), then either 100 mg tPA over 3 hours or placebo administered in the same fashion. Beta-blockers were given at discharge.
- **Findings:** Mortality was reduced by 51% at 14 days and by 36% at 3 months in patients treated with tPA. Among those treated within 3 hours of MI, overall mortality was reduced by 82% at 14 days and 59% at 3 months. In-hospital cardiovascular complications at 14 days were less for patients who received tPA than in controls. Enzymatic size of infarct was 20% less, EF was 2.2% higher, and end-diastolic and end-systolic volumes were smaller in treated patients by 6.0 mLs and 5.8 mLs, respectively.
- **Conclusions:** Recombinant tPA with heparin and aspirin reduced infarct size, preserved LV function, and reduced complications and mortality from cardiac causes but increased the risk of bleeding complications.

GUSTO-1 (86)

- **Time period:** December 27, 1990 to February 22, 1993.
- **Setting:** 1,081 hospitals in 15 countries in North America and Europe and in Israel, Australia, and New Zealand.
- **Design:** Randomized trial of four thrombolytic regimens for treatment of AMI: SK plus subcutaneous heparin; SK plus IV heparin; tPA plus IV heparin; and tPA plus SK plus IV heparin (all patients received aspirin).
- **Patients:** 41,021 patients total.
- **Inclusion criteria:** Presentation < 6 hours of symptom onset; CP of ≥ 20 minutes; and ECG changes including ≥ 0.1 mV ST elevation in two or more limb leads or ≥ 0.2 mV ST elevation in two or more contiguous precordial leads.
- **Intervention:** Group 1: SK 1.5 million U over 60 minutes with subcutaneous (SQ) heparin 12,500 U twice daily, starting 4 hours after administration of SK; Group 2: SK 1.5 million U over 60 minutes, with IV heparin bolus 5,000 U and 1,000 U per hour, with dose adjusted to raise the PTT to 60 to 85 seconds; Group 3: accelerated tPA, given in a bolus of 15 mg, 0.75 mg/kg over 30 minutes (up to 50 mg), and 0.5 mg/kg (up to 35 mg) over the next 60 minutes, with the same IV heparin regimen; and Group 4: IV tPA 1.0 mg/kg (up to 90 mg) over 60 minutes, with 10% given as bolus dose, plus SK 1.0 million U over 60 minutes, given simultaneously through different catheters, plus IV heparin as above. SQ heparin was given for 7 days or until discharge and IV heparin

was given for at least 48 hours or more at investigators' discretion. All patients received chewable aspirin ≥ 160 mg as soon as possible, followed by a daily dose of 160 to 325 mg. Patients with no contraindications received IV atenolol 5 mg in 2 divided doses followed by oral therapy of 50 to 100 mg once daily.

■ *Primary endpoint:* **Overall** 30-day mortality; also, combined endpoints of death and nonfatal stroke, death and nonfatal hemorrhagic stroke, and death and nonfatal disabling stroke.

■ *Findings:* (There were multiple substudies and subgroup analyses which are mentioned in various chapters of this book.) Thirty-day mortality was 7.2% for SK and SQ heparin; 7.4% for SK with IV heparin, 6.3% for accelerated tPA with IV heparin, and 7.0% for tPA and SK with IV heparin. This indicates a mortality reduction of 14% for accelerated tPA versus the two SK only strategies. Incidence of intracranial hemorrhage was higher with accelerated tPA and tPA plus SK (0.72% and 0.94%, respectively) than for SK with SQ or IV heparin (0.49% versus 0.54%). Death or nonfatal disabling stroke was significantly lower in the accelerated tPA group than in the SK-only groups (6.9% versus 7.7% in SK plus SQ heparin, and 7.9% in the SK plus IV heparin).

■ *Conclusions:* Accelerated tPA plus IV heparin offers improved survival benefit over previous standard thrombolytic regimens.

LATE (167)(169)

(See Chapter 33.)

■ *Time period:* April 1989 to February 1992.
■ Setting: 230 centers in Australia, Canada, Europe, and the United States.
■ *Design:* Randomized, double-blind placebo controlled study of IV tPA for those patients for whom the **decision to initiate** thrombolysis was between **6 and 24 hours** of symptom onset.
■ *Patients:* 5,711 patients; 31% **arrived** < 6 hours after CP onset, 39% arrived at 6 to 12 hours, and 30% arrived > 12 hours later.
■ *Inclusion criteria:* CP of suspected myocardial origin for 30 minutes or more; treatment initiated 6 to 24 hours after CP onset; and one or more of the following ECG changes: (a) ST elevation ≥ 1 mm in two or more limb leads or ≥ 2 mm in two or more precordial leads (note: 55% of all patients had ST elevation so defined), (b) ST depression of ≥ 2 mm in at least two leads, (c) pathologic Q waves, or (d) abnormal T-wave inversion in at least two leads and thought to represent a non–Q-wave MI. Patients with old or equivocal ECG changes or BBB were included if cardiac enzymes were elevated. The original protocol required **admission** more than 6 hours after CP onset, but this was removed in June 1990 (**treatment** still required to be from 6 to 24 hours). At this time, the upper age limit of 75 years was also removed and IV heparin for 48 hours was advised for all patients.

■ *Primary endpoint:* **Overall** mortality up to 6 months as calculated by **intention-to-treat analysis.** Follow-up was from 6 months to 1 year.
■ *Intervention:* Patients were randomized to receive: IV tPA 10-mg bolus, 50-mg infusion in 1 hour, and 20 mg in each of the next 2 hours; or matching placebo. All patients received immediate and daily aspirin (75 to 360 mg, according to local practice). After June 1990, IV heparin was strongly advised for the first 48 hours.
■ *Findings:* Prespecified 35-day mortality for those receiving treatment within 12 hours of symptom onset was 8.9% for tPA versus 11.8% for placebo. Relative reduction in 35-day mortality was not significant for those treated 12 to 24 hours after symptom onset, but subgroup analysis indicates that some patients may benefit after 12 hours. Treatment with alteplase resulted in an excess of hemorrhagic strokes, but by 6 months, **incidence of disability was equal.**
■ *Conclusions:* The time window for thrombolytic therapy with alteplase should extend at least 12 hours post-symptom onset. Study authors suggest that LATE findings and ISIS-2 data suggest that, for some patients, benefit may extend to 24 hours.

FTT Collaborative Group (30)(463)

■ Time: 1994 publication of collaborative overview of nine clinical trials of different lengths from March 1982 to February 1992.
■ *Setting:* Multinational, nine trials: GISSI, ISAM (Intravenous Streptokinase in Acute Myocardial Infarction), AMES (APSAC Intervention Mortality Study), ISIS-2, ASSET (Anglo-Scandinavian Study of Early Thrombolysis), USIM (Urochinasi per via Sistemica nell'Infarto Miocardico), ISIS-3, EMERAS (Estudio Multicentrico Estreptoquinasa Republicas de America del Sur), and LATE.
■ *Design:* Collaborative overview of nine randomized clinical trials of thrombolysis versus control. Six trials were randomized, placebo controlled and three randomized patients to thrombolytic therapy or "open" control (both physician and patient knew whether a thrombolytic had been given).
■ *Patients:* 58,600 patients.
■ Inclusion criteria: Clinical trials of more than 1,000 patients randomized to thrombolysis or control.
■ *Intervention:* SK (four trials), anistreplase (one trial), tPA (two trials), urokinase (one trial), and a random choice of SK, tPA, or anistreplase in one. Aspirin was given to all patients in four trials and to 50% of patients in one trial.
■ *Findings:* At 35 days, among patients presenting with ST elevation or BBB up to at least 6 hours from onset of symptoms, thrombolytic therapy prevented 30 deaths per 1,000 treated, and treatment between 6 and 12 hours prevented 20 deaths per 1,000 treated. Thrombolysis was associated with approximately four more strokes per 1,000 treated on days 0 to 1; of these, two were associated with early death and were included in the overall mortality reduction, one was disabling, and one was not.
■ *Conclusions:* This collaborative overview indicated that thrombolysis was beneficial to a much wider range of patients than routinely perceived at time of publication.

- **Comment:** FTT collaborative group should not be used to assess the efficacy of thrombolytics in patients more than 75 years of age; see the second annotation of FTT data (229) in Chapter 34, under the annotated bibliography heading of "Age of More Than 75 Years Is NOT a Contraindication for Thrombolysis."

NRMI-2 (33,245,414,469,481)

- **Time period:** NRMI-2 began with patients admitted in June 1994 and is ongoing.
- **Setting:** More than 1,480 U.S. hospitals as of September 1996 (469).
- **Design:** Voluntary registry of cross-sectional data on patients hospitalized with **confirmed AMI**. Data accuracy is nearly identical to that of the more rigorous **CCP** database from Medicare (561). Registry hospitals are larger than nonparticipating hospitals (27% have more than 350 beds versus 8%), are more likely to be affiliated with a medical school (36% versus 17%), and more often have a cardiac care unit (CCU) (73% versus 31%), a cath lab (72% versus 23%), and a cardiac surgery program (39% versus 11%).
- **Patients:** As of March 1998, 772,586 patients had been included in the registry (481).
- **Inclusion criteria:** Confirmed diagnosis of AMI based on at least one of: CK; ECG evidence of AMI; enzymatic, scintigraphic, or autopsy evidence of MI; or a diagnosis of MI according to the International Classification of Diseases, Ninth Revision, Clinical Modification (code 410.X1).
- **Methods:** Participating hospitals are encouraged to enter consecutive AMI patients regardless of treatment or outcome. Detailed data is entered on individual data forms by a study coordinator at each hospital and forms are processed at an independent central data collection center.
- **Findings:** Various. Findings are listed under individual papers throughout the book.

REFERENCES

1. Goldberger AL. *Myocardial infarction: electrocardiographic differential diagnosis.* St. Louis: Mosby, 1991:386 pp.
2. Chou TC, Knilans TK. *Electrocardiography in clinical practice.* Philadelphia: WB Saunders, 1996.
3. Bayes de Luna A. *Clinical electrocardiography: a textbook.* New York: Futura, 1993.
4. Josephson ME. *Clinical cardiac electrophysiology: techniques and interpretations.* Philadelphia: Lea & Febiger, 1993.
5. Coumel P, Garfein OB. *Electrocardiography: past and future.* New York: The New York Academy of Sciences, 1990.
6. Dunn MI, Lipman BS. Lipman-Massie: *Clinical electrocardiography.* Chicago: Year Book, 1989.
7. Chung EK. *Fundamentals of electrocardiography.* Baltimore: University Park Press, 1984.
8. Goldman MJ. *Principles of clinical electrocardiography.* Los Altos, CA: Lange Medical Publishing, 1982.
9. Beckwith JR, McGuire LB. *Basic electrocardiography and vectorcardiography.* New York: Raven Press, 1982.
10. Burch GE, DePasquale NP. *A history of electrocardiography.* Chicago: Year Book, 1964.
11. Braunwald E, for the Committee on the Management of Patients with Unstable Angina. ACC/AHA guidelines for the management of patients with unstable angina and non-ST-segment elevation myocardial infarction. *J Am Coll Cardiol* 2000;36:970–1062.
12. Joint European Society of Cardiology/American College of Cardiology Committee. Myocardial infarction redefined: a consensus document of the Joint European Society of Cardiology/American College of Cardiology committee for the redefinition of myocardial infarction. *J Am Coll Cardiol* 2000;36:959–969.
13. Ohman EM, Armstrong PW, Christenson RH, et al. Cardiac troponin T levels for risk stratification in acute myocardial ischemia. *N Engl J Med* 1996;335:332–337.
14. Antman EM, Tanasijevic MJ, Thompson B, et al. Cardiac-specific troponin I levels to predict the risk of mortality in patients with acute coronary syndromes. *N Engl J Med* 1996;335:1342–1349.
15. Smith SW. ST elevation acute myocardial infarction: a critical but difficult electrocardiographic diagnosis. *Acad Emerg Med* 2001;8:382–385.
16. Fesmire FM. Which chest pain patients benefit from continuous ST-segment monitoring with automated serial ECG? *Ann Emerg Med* 1999;34:S4–S5.
17. Menown IB, Mackenzie G, Adgey AA. Optimizing the initial 12-lead electrocardiographic diagnosis of acute myocardial infarction. *Eur Heart J* 2000;21:275–283.
18. Rouan GW, Lee TH, Cook EF, et al. Clinical characteristics and outcome of acute myocardial infarction in patients with initially normal or nonspecific electrocardiograms (a report from the Multicenter Chest Pain Study). *Am J Cardiol* 1989;64:1087–1092.
19. Fesmire FM, Percy RF, Wears RL, et al. Initial ECG in Q wave and non–Q wave myocardial infarction. *Ann Emerg Med* 1989;18:741–746.
20. Rude RE, Poole WK, Muller J, et al. Electrocardiographic and clinical criteria for recognition of acute myocardial infarction based on analysis of 3,697 patients. *Am J Cardiol* 1983;52:936–942.
21. Karlson BW, Herlitz J, Wiklund O, et al. Early prediction of acute myocardial infarction from clinical history, examination and electrocardiogram in the emergency room. *Am J Cardiol* 1991;68:171–175.
22. Slater DK, Hlatky MA, Mark DB, et al. Outcome in suspected acute myocardial infarction with normal or minimally abnormal admission electrocardiographic findings. *Am J Cardiol* 1987;60:766–770.
23. Krone RJ, Greenberg H, Dwyer EMJ, et al. Long-term prognostic significance of ST segment depression during acute myocardial infarction. The Multicenter Diltiazem Postinfarction Trial Research Group. *J Am Coll Cardiol* 1993;22:361–367.
24. Fesmire FM, Percy RF, Wears RL, et al. Risk stratification according to the initial electrocardiogram in patients with suspected acute myocardial infarction. *Arch Int Med* 1989;149:1294–1297.
25. Barron HV, Bowlby LJ, Breen T, et al. Use of reperfusion therapy for acute myocardial infarction in the United States: data from the National Registry of Myocardial Infarction 2. *Circulation* 1997;97:1150–1156.
26. Lincoff A, Topol EJ, Califf RM, et al. Significance of a coronary artery with thrombolysis in myocardial infarction grade 2 flow "patency" (outcome in the Thrombolysis and Angioplasty in Myocardial Infarction Trials). *Am J Cardiol* 1995;75:871–876.
27. Berger AK, Schulman KA, Gersh BJ, et al. Primary coronary angioplasty vs. thrombolysis for the management of acute myocardial infarction in elderly patients. *JAMA* 1999;282:341–348.
28. Krumholz HM, Murillo JE, Chen J, et al. Thrombolytic therapy for eligible elderly patients with acute myocardial infarction. *JAMA* 1997;277:1683–1688.
29. GISSI (Gruppo Italiano per lo Studio Della Sopravvvivenza nell'Infarto Miocardico). Effectiveness of intravenous thrombolytic treatment in acute myocardial infarction. *Lancet* 1986;1:397–401.
30. Fibrinolytic Therapy Trialists' (FTT) Collaborative Group. Indications for fibrinolytic therapy in suspected acute myocardial infarction: collaborative overview of early mortality and major morbidity results from all randomised trials of more than 1000 patients. *Lancet* 1994;343:311–322.
31. Boersma E, Maas ACP, Deckers JW, et al. Early thrombolytic treatment in acute myocardial infarction: reappraisal of the golden hour. *Lancet* 1996;348:771–775.
32. Thiemann DR, Coresh J, Schulman SP, et al. Lack of benefit for intravenous thrombolysis in patients with myocardial infarction who are older than 75 years. *Circulation* 2000;101:2239–2246.
33. Magid DJ, Calonge BN, Rumsfeld JS, et al. Relation between hospital primary angioplasty volume and mortality for patients with acute MI treated with primary angioplasty vs. thrombolytic therapy. *JAMA* 2000;284:3131–3138.
34. Boisjolie CR, Sharkey SW, Cannon CP, et al. Brief reports: impact of a thrombolysis research trial on time to treatment for acute myocardial infarction in the emergency department. *Am J Cardiol* 1995;76:396–398.
35. Jayes RL, Larsen GC, Beshansky J, et al. Physician electrocardiogram reading in the emergency department: accuracy and effect on triage decisions. *J Gen Intern Med* 1992;7:392.
36. Brady WJ, Perron A, Ullman E. Errors in emergency physician interpretation of ST-segment elevation in emergency department chest pain patients. *Acad Emerg Med* 2000;7:1256–1260.
37. Brady WJ, Perron AD, Chan T. Electrocardiographic ST segment ele-

vation: correct identification of AMI and non-AMI syndromes by emergency physicians. *Acad Emerg Med* 2001;8:349–360.

38. Hirvonen TP, Halinen MO, Kala RA, et al. Delays in thrombolytic therapy for acute myocardial infarction in Finland. Results of a national thrombolytic therapy delay study. Finnish Hospitals' Thrombolysis Survey Group. *Eur Heart J* 1998;19:885–992.

39. Sharkey SW, Berger CR, Brunette DD, et al. Impact of the electrocardiogram on the delivery of thrombolytic therapy for acute myocardial infarction. *Am J Cardiol* 1994;73:550–553.

40. Berger AK, Radford MJ, Krumholz HM. Factors associated with delay in reperfusion therapy in elderly patients with acute myocardial infarction: analysis of the cooperative cardiovascular project. *Am Heart J* 2000;139:985–992.

41. Massel D, Dawdy JA, Melendez LJ. Strict reliance on a computer algorithm or measurable ST segment criteria may lead to errors in thrombolytic therapy eligibility. *Am Heart J* 2000;140:221–216.

42. Tighe M, Kellett J, Corry E, et al. The early diagnosis of acute myocardial infarction: comparison of a simple algorithm with a computer program for electrocardiogram interpretation. *Ir J Med Sci* 1996;165:159–163.

43. Elko P, Warner RA. Using directly acquired digital ECG data to optimize the diagnostic criteria for anterior myocardial infarction. *J Electrocardiol* 1994;27(Suppl):10–13.

44. Elko P, Rowlandson I. A statistical analysis of the ECG measurements used in computerized interpretation of acute anterior myocardial infarction with applications to interpretive criteria development. *J Electrocardiol* 1993;25(Suppl):113–119.

45. Elko P, Weaver WD, Kudenchuk PJ, et al. The dilemma of sensitivity versus specificity in computer-interpreted acute myocardial infarction. *J Electrocardiol* 1992;24(Suppl):2–7.

46. Kudenchuk PJ, Ho MT, Weaver WD, et al. Accuracy of computer-interpreted electrocardiography in selecting patients for thrombolytic therapy. *J Am Coll Cardiol* 1991;17:1486–1491.

47. Rowlandson I, Kudenchuk PJ, Elko P. Computerized recognition of acute infarction: criteria advances and test results. *J Electrocardiol* 1990;23(Suppl):1–5.

48. Ryan TJ, Anderson JL, Antman EM, et al. ACC/AHA Guidelines for the management of patients with acute myocardial infarction: a report of the American College of Cardiology/American Heart Association Task Force on Practice Guidelines (Committee on Management of Acute Myocardial Infarction). *J Am Coll Cardiol* 1996;28: 1328–1428.

49. Midgette AS, Wong JB, Beshansky JR, et al. Cost-effectiveness of streptokinase for acute myocardial infarction. *Med Decis Making* 1994;14:108–117.

50. Bayer AJ, Chadha JS, Farag RR, et al. Changing presentation of myocardial infarction with increasing old age. *J Am Geriatr Soc* 1986; 34:263–266.

51. Muller RT, Gould LA, Betzu R, et al. Painless myocardial infarction in the elderly. *Am Heart J* 1990;119:202–204.

52. Canto JG, Shlipak MG, Roger WJ, et al. Prevalence, clinical characteristics, and mortality among patients with myocardial infarction presenting without chest pain. *JAMA* 2000;283:3223–3229.

53. Miller PF, Sheps DS, Bragdon EE, et al. Aging and pain perception in ischemic heart disease. *Am Heart J* 1990;120:22–30.

54. Sigurdsson E, Thorgeirsson G, Sigfusson N. Unrecognized myocardial infarction: epidemiology, clinical characteristics, and the prognostic role of angina pectoris. The Reykjavik Study. *Ann Intern Med* 1995;122:96–102.

55. Krumholz HM, Friesinger GC, Cook EF, et al. Relationship of age with eligibility for thrombolytic therapy and mortality among patients with suspected acute myocardial infarction. *J Am Geriatr Soc* 1994;42:127–131.

56. GISSI. Long-term effects of intravenous thrombolysis in acute myocardial infarction: final report of the GISSI study. *Lancet* 1987; 2:871–874.

57. Lee TH, Weisberg MC, Brand DA, et al. Candidates for thrombolysis among emergency room patients with acute chest pain: potential true- and false-positive rates. *Ann Int Med* 1989;110:957–962.

58. Newby LK, Rutsch WR, Califf RM, et al. Time from symptom onset to treatment and outcomes after thrombolytic therapy. GUSTO-1 Investigators. *J Am Coll Cardiol* 1996;27:1646–1655.

59. Mehta JL, Nicolini FA, Nichols WW, et al. Concurrent nitroglycerine administration decreases thrombolytic potential of tissue-type plasminogen activator. *J Am Coll Cardiol* 1991;17:805–811.

60. Nicolini FA, Ferrini D, Ottani F, et al. Concurrent nitroglycerin therapy impairs tissue-type plasminogen activator-induced thrombolysis in patients with acute myocardial infarction. *Am J Cardiol* 1994; 74:662–666.

61. Romeo F, Rosano GM, Martuscelli E, et al. Concurrent nitroglycerin administration reduces the efficacy of recombinant tissue-type plasminogen activator in patients with acute anterior wall myocardial infarction. *Am Heart J* 1995;130:692–697.

62. ISIS-4 (Fourth International Study of Infarct Survival) Collaborative Group. ISIS-4: a randomised factorial trial assessing early oral captopril, oral mononitrate, and intravenous sulphate in 58,050 patients with suspected acute myocardial infarction. *Lancet* 1995;345:669–685.

63. GISSI-3 (Gruppo Italiano per lo Studio della Sopravvivenza nell'Infarto Miocardico). Effects of lisinopril and transdermal glyceryl trinitrate singly and together on 6-week mortality and ventricular function after acute myocardial infarction. *Lancet* 1994;343:1115–1122.

64. Tandberg D, Kastendieck KD, Meskin S. Observer variation in measured ST-segment elevation. *Ann Emerg Med* 1999;34:448–452.

65. Brady WJ. ST segment elevation in ED adult chest pain patients: etiology and diagnostic accuracy for AMI. *J Emerg Med* 1998;16: 797–798.

66. Chapman GD, Ohman EM, Topol EJ, et al. Minimizing the risk of inappropriately administering thrombolytic therapy (Thrombolysis and Angioplasty in Myocardial Infarction [TAMI] study group). *Am J Cardiol* 1993;71:783–787.

67. Singer AJ, Brogan GX, Valentine SM, et al. Effect of duration from symptom onset on the negative predictive value of a normal ECG for exclusion of acute myocardial infarction. *Ann Emerg Med* 1997;29: 575–579.

68. Huey BL, Beller GA, Kaiser D, et al. A comprehensive analysis of myocardial infarction due to left circumflex artery occlusion: comparison with infarction due to right coronary artery and left anterior descending artery occlusion. *J Am Coll Cardiol* 1988;12:1156–1166.

69. Berry C, Zalewsky A, Kovach R, et al. Surface electrocardiogram in the detection of transmural myocardial ischemia during coronary artery occlusion. *Am J Cardiol* 1989;63:21–26.

70. Christian TF, Clements IP, Gibbons RJ. Noninvasive identification of myocardium at risk in patients with acute myocardial infarction and nondiagnostic electrocardiograms with technetium-99m-sestamibi. *Circulation* 1991;83:1615–1620.

71. Matetzky S, Friemark D, Feinberg MS, et al. Acute myocardial infarction with isolated ST-segment elevation in posterior chest leads V7–V9: "hidden" ST-segment elevations revealing acute posterior infarction. *J Am Coll Cardiol* 1999;34:748–753.

72. Agarwal JB, Khaw K, Aurignac F, et al. Importance of posterior chest leads in patients with suspected myocardial infarction, but nondiagnostic, routine 12-lead electrogram. *Am J Cardiol* 1999;83:323–326.

73. Fesmire FM, Percy RF, Wears RL. Diagnostic and prognostic importance of comparing the initial to the previous electrocardiogram in patients admitted for suspected acute myocardial infarction. *South Med J* 1991;84:841–846.

74. Cragg DR, Friedman HZ, Bonema JD, et al. Outcome of patients with acute myocardial infarction who are ineligible for thrombolytic therapy. *Ann Int Med* 1991;115:173–177.

75. Brush JE, Brand DA, Acampora D, et al. Use of the initial electrocardiogram to predict in-hospital complications of acute myocardial infarction. *N Engl J Med* 1985;312:1137–1141.

76. Christian TF, Miller TD, Bailey KR, et al. Exercise tomographic thallium-201 imaging in patients with severe coronary artery disease and normal electrocardiograms. *Ann Intern Med* 1994;121:825–832.

77. Pope JH, Aufderheide TP, Ruthazer R, et al. Missed diagnosis of acute cardiac ischemia in the emergency department. *N Engl J Med* 2000; 342:1163–1170.

78. Lee TH, Rouan GW, Weisberg MC, et al. Clinical characteristics and natural history of patients with acute myocardial infarction sent home from the emergency room. *Am J Cardiol* 1987;60:219–224.

79. McCarthy BD, Beshansky JR, D'Agostino RB, et al. Missed diagnosis of acute myocardial infarction in the emergency department: results from a multicenter study. *Ann Emerg Med* 1993;22:579–582.

80. Smith SW. ECG abnormality in acute myocardial infarction. *Ann Emerg Med* 1998;31:136–137.

81. Charles MA, Bensinger TA, Glasser SP. Atrial injury current in pericarditis. *Arch Int Med* 1973;131:657–662.

82. Shipley R, Hallaran W. The four lead electrocardiogram in 200 normal men and women. *Am Heart J* 1936;11:325.

83. Bush HS, Ferguson JJ, Angelini P, et al. Twelve-lead electrocardiographic evaluation of ischemia during percutaneous transluminal coronary angioplasty and its correlation with acute reocclusion. *Am Heart J* 1991;121:1591–1599.

84. Willems JL, Willems RJ, Willems GM, et al. Significance of initial ST segment elevation and depression for the management of thrombolytic therapy in acute myocardial infarction. *Circulation* 1990;82: 1147–1158.

85. Tamura A, Mikuriya Y, Kataoka H, et al. Emergent coronary angiographic findings of patients with ST depression in the inferior or lateral leads, or both, during anterior wall acute myocardial infarction. *Am J Cardiol* 1995a;76:516–517.

86. GUSTO Investigators. An international randomized trial comparing four thrombolytic strategies for acute myocardial infarction. *N Engl J Med* 1993;329:673–682.

87. Kosuge M, Kimura K, Ishikawa T, et al. Value of ST-segment elevation pattern in predicting infarct size and left ventricular function at discharge in patients with reperfused acute anterior myocardial infarction. *Am Heart J* 1999;137:522–527.

87.5 Brady WJ, Syverud SA, Beagle C, et al. Electrocardiographic ST segment elevation: the diagnosis of acute myocardial infarction by morphologic analysis of the ST segment. *Acad Emerg Med* 2001;8: 961–967.

88. Soo CS. Tall precordial T waves with depressed ST take-off: an early sign of acute myocardial infarction? *Singapore Med J* 1995;36: 236–237.

89. Ohman EM, Califf RM, Topol EJ, et al. Consequences of reocclusion after successful reperfusion therapy in acute myocardial infarction. *Circulation* 1991;84:1454–1455.

90. Wilkins ML, Anderson ST, Pryor AD, et al. Variability of acute ST-segment predicted myocardial infarct size in the absence of thrombolytic therapy. *Am J Cardiol* 1994;74:174–177.

91. Hackett D, Davies G, Chierchia S, et al. Intermittent coronary occlusion in acute myocardial infarction: value of combined thrombolytic and vasodilator therapy. *N Engl J Med* 1987;317:1055–1059.

92. Raitt MH, Maynard C, Wagner GS, et al. Appearance of abnormal Q waves early in the course of acute myocardial infarction: implications for efficacy of thrombolytic therapy. *J Am Coll Cardiol* 1995;25: 1084–1088.

93. Bar FW, Volders PG, Hoppener B, et al. Development of ST-segment elevation and Q- and R-wave changes in acute myocardial infarction and the influence of thrombolytic therapy. *Am J Cardiol* 1996;77: 337–343.

94. Oliva PB, Hammill SC, Edwards WD. Electrocardiographic diagnosis of postinfarction regional pericarditis: ancillary observations regarding the effect of reperfusion on the rapidity and amplitude of T wave inversion after acute myocardial infarction. *Circulation* 1993;88: 896–904.

95. Mills RM, Young E, Gorlin R, et al. Natural history of S-T segment elevation after acute myocardial infarction. *Am J Cardiol* 1975;35: 609–614.

96. Sequeira RF, Lemberg L. The electrocardiogram read as nonspecific ST-T waves. *ACC Curr J Rev* 1995;5:36–40.

97. Hollander JE, Lozano M, Goldstein E, et al. Variations in the electrocardiograms of young adults: are revised criteria for thrombolysis needed? *Acad Emerg Med* 1994;1:94–102.

98. GISSI-2 (Gruppo Italiano per lo Studio Della Sopravvivenza nell'Infarto Miocardico). GISSI-2: A factorial randomised trial of alteplase versus streptokinase and heparin versus no heparin among 12,490 patients with acute myocardial infarction. *Lancet* 1990;336:65–71.

99. TIMI IIIA. Early effects of tissue-type plasminogen activator added to conventional therapy on the culprit coronary lesion in patients presenting with ischemic cardiac pain at rest: results of the Thrombolysis in Myocardial Ischemia (TIMI IIIA) trial. *Circulation* 1993;87: 38–52.

100. Chesebro JH, Knatterud G, Roberts R, et al. Thrombolysis in Myocardial Infarction (TIMI) Trial, Phase I: a comparison between intravenous tissue plasminogen activator and intravenous streptokinase: clinical findings through hospital discharge. *Circulation* 1987; 76:142–154.

101. Topol EJ, Califf RM, Vandormael M, et al. A randomized trial of late reperfusion therapy for acute myocardial infarction. Thrombolysis and Angioplasty in Myocardial Infarction-6 (TAMI-6) Study Group. *Circulation* 1992;85:2090–2099.

102. ISIS-2 (Second International Study of Infarct Survival) Collaborative Group. Randomised trial of intravenous streptokinase, oral aspirin, both, or neither among 17,187 cases of suspected acute myocardial infarction: ISIS-2. *Lancet* 1988;2:349–360.

103. ISIS-3 (Third International Study of Infarct Survival) Collaborative Study Group. ISIS-3: a randomised comparison of streptokinase vs. tissue plasminogen activator vs anistreplase and of aspirin plus heparin vs aspirin alone among 41,299 cases of suspected acute myocardial infarction. *Lancet* 1992;339:753–770.

104. Prineas RJ, Crow RS, Blackburn H. The Minnesota Code manual of electrocardiographic findings: standards and procedures for measurement and classification. Littleton, MA: PSG, Inc., 1982, 228.

105. Ryan TJ, Antman EM, Brooks NH, et al. 1999 update: ACC/AHA guidelines for the management of patients with acute myocardial infarction. *J Am Coll Cardiol* 1999;34:890–911.

106. Otto LA, Aufderheide TP. Evaluation of ST segment elevation criteria for the prehospital electrocardiographic diagnosis of acute myocardial infarction. *Ann Emerg Med* 1994;23:17–24.

107. Hands ME, Lloyd BL, Robinson JS, et al. Prognostic significance of electrocardiographic site of infarction after correction for enzymatic size of infarction. *Circulation* 1986;73:885–891.

108. Stone PH, Raabe DS, Jaffe AS, et al. Prognostic significance of location and type of MI: independent adverse outcome associated with anterior location. *J Am Coll Cardiol* 1988;11:453–463.

109. Mauri F, Gasparini M, Barbonaglia L, et al. Prognostic significance of the extent of myocardial injury in acute myocardial infarction treated by streptokinase. (The GISSI trial). *Am J Cardiol* 1989;63:1291–1295.

110. Selvester RH. The 12-lead ECG and the initiation of thrombolytic therapy for acute myocardial infarction. *J Electrocardiol* 1993;26 (Suppl):114–121.

111. Bar FW, Vermeer F, de Zwaan C, et al. Value of admission electrocardiogram in predicting outcome of thrombolytic therapy in acute myocardial infarction. *Am J Cardiol* 1987;59:6–13.

112. Peterson ED, Hathaway WR, Zabel KM, et al. Prognostic significance of precordial ST segment depression during inferior myocardial infarction in the thrombolytic era: results in 16,521 patients. *J Am Coll Cardiol* 1996;28:305–312.

113. Christian TF, Gibbons RJ, Clements IP, et al. Estimates of myocardium at risk and collateral flow in acute myocardial infarction using electrocardiographic indexes with comparison to radionuclide and angiographic measures. *J Am Coll Cardiol* 1995;26:388–393.

114. Hick JL, Clements IP, Gibbons RJ. Clinical utility of the electrocardiogram for prediction of myocardium at risk in acute myocardial infarction. Unpublished data.

115. Birnbaum Y, Kloner RA, Sclarovsky S, et al. Distortion of the terminal portion of the QRS on the admission electrocardiogram in acute myocardial infarction and correlation with infarct size and long-term prognosis (Thrombolysis in Myocardial Infarction 4 Trial). *Am J Cardiol* 1996;78:396–403.

116. Hathaway WR, Peterson ED, Wagner GS, et al. Prognostic significance of the initial electrocardiogram in patients with acute myocardial infarction. GUSTO-I Investigators. Global Utilization of Streptokinase and t-PA for Occluded Coronary Arteries. *JAMA* 1998;279: 387–381.

117. Vermeer F, Simoons ML, Bar FW, et al. Which patients benefit most from early thrombolytic therapy with intracoronary streptokinase? *Circulation* 1999;74:1379–1389.

118. Birnbaum Y, Herz I, Sclarovsky S, et al. Prognostic significance of the admission electrocardiogram in acute myocardial infarction. *J Am Coll Cardiol* 1996;27:1128–1132.

119. Hasdai D, Porter A, Birnbaum Y, et al. Predicting postinfarction left ventricular dysfunction based on the configuration of the QRS complex and ST segment in the initial ECG of patients with a first anterior wall myocardial infarction. *Cardiology* 1996;87:125–128.

120. Garcia-Rubira JC, Perez-Leal I, Garcia-Martinez JT, et al. The initial electrocardiogram pattern is a strong predictor of outcome in acute myocardial infarction. *Int J Cardiol* 1995;51:301–305.

121. Madias JE. The "giant R waves" ECG pattern of hyperacute phase of myocardial infarction. *J Electrocardiol* 1993;26:77–82.

122. Lee KL, Woodlief LH, Topol EJ, et al. Predictors of 30-day mortality in the era of reperfusion for acute myocardial infarction: results from an international trial of 41,021 patients. *Circulation* 1995;91:1659–1668.

123. Gwechenberger M, Schreiber W, Kittler H, et al. Prediction of early complications in patients with acute myocardial infarction by calculation of the ST score. *Ann Emerg Med* 1911;30:563–570.

124. Nixdorff J, Erbel R, Rupprecht HJ, et al. Sum of ST-segment elevations on admission electrocardiograms in acute myocardial infarction predicts left ventricular dilation. *Am J Cardiol* 1996;77:1237–1241.

125. Sugiura T, Nagahama Y, Takehana K, et al. Prognostic significance of precordial ST-segment changes in acute inferior wall myocardial infarction. *Chest* 1904;111:1039–1044.

126. Aldrich HR, Wagner NB, Boswick, et al. Use of initial ST-segment deviation for prediction of final electrocardiographic size of acute myocardial infarcts. *Am J Cardiol* 1988;61:749–753.

127. Kornreich F, Montague TJ, Pentti MR. Location and magnitude of ST changes in acute myocardial infarction by analysis of body surface maps. *J Electrocardiol* 1992;25(Suppl):15–19.

128. Hasdai D, Sclarovsky S, Solodky A, et al. Prognostic significance of maximal precordial ST segment depression in right (V1 to V3) versus left (V4 to V6) leads in patients with inferior wall acute myocardial infarction. *Am J Cardiol* 1994;74:1081–1084.

129. Birnbaum Y, Herz I, Sclarovsky S, et al. Prognostic significance of precordial ST segment depression on admission electrocardiogram in patients with inferior wall myocardial infarction. *J Am Coll Cardiol* 1996;28:313–318.

130. Kontos MC, Desai PV, Jesse RL, et al. Usefulness of the admission electrocardiogram for identifying the infarct-related artery in inferior wall acute myocardial infarction. *Am J Cardiol* 1997;79:182–184.

131. Chia BL, Yip JW, Tan HC, et al. Usefulness of ST elevation II/III ratio and ST deviation in lead I for identifying the culprit artery in inferior wall acute myocardial infarction. *Am J Cardiol* 2000;86:341–343.

132. Birnbaum Y, Sclarovsky S, Solodky A, et al. Prediction of the level of left anterior descending coronary artery obstruction during anterior wall acute myocardial infarction by the admission electrocardiogram. *Am J Cardiol* 1993;72:823–826.

133. Engelen DJ, Gorgens AP, Cheriex EC, et al. Value of the electrocardiogram in localizing the occlusion site in the left anterior descending coronary artery in acute myocardial infarction. *J Am Coll Cardiol* 1999;34:389–395.

134. Mittal SR, Tiwari D. Electrocardiographic diagnosis of infarction of the right ventricular anterior wall. *J Electrocardiol* 1996;29:119–122.

135. Haraphongse M, Tanomsup S, Kappagoda CT, et al. Significance of ST-segment depression in inferior leads in patients with acute anterior infarction. *Clin Invest Med* 1984;7:143–148.

136. Norell MS, Lyons JP, Gardener JE, et al. Significance of "reciprocal" ST segment depression: left ventriculographic observations during left anterior descending coronary angioplasty. *J Am Coll Cardiol* 1989;13:1270–1274.

137. Tamura A, Kataoka H, Mikuriya Y, et al. Inferior ST segment depression as a useful marker for identifying proximal left anterior descending artery occlusion during acute anterior myocardial infarction. *Eur Heart J* 1995b;16:1795–1799.

138. Shah PK. New insights into the electocardiogram of acute myocardial infarction. In: Gersh BJ, Rahimtoola SH, eds. *Acute myocardial infarction.* New York: Elsevier, 1991:128–143.

139. Ruddy TD, Yasuda T, Gold HK, et al. Anterior ST segment depression in acute myocardial infarction as a marker of greater inferior, apical, and posterolateral damage. *Am Heart J* 1986;112:1210–1216.

140. Edmunds JJ, Gibbons RJ, Bresnahan JF, et al. Significance of anterior ST depression in inferior wall acute myocardial infarction. *Am J Cardiol* 1994;73:143–148.

141. Wong CK, Freedman SB. Usefulness of continuous ST monitoring in inferior wall acute myocardial infarction for describing the relation between precordial ST depression and inferior ST elevation. *Am J Cardiol* 1993;72:532–537.

142. Savonitto S, Ardissino D, Granger CB, et al. Prognostic value of the admission electrocardiogram in acute coronary syndromes. *JAMA* 1999;281:707–713.

143. Shah A, Wagner GS, Califf RM, et al. Comparative prognostic significance of simultaneous versus independent resolution of ST segment depression relative to ST segment elevation during acute myocardial infarction. *J Am Coll Cardiol* 1997;30:1478–1483.

144. Shah A, Wagner GS, Green CL, et al. Electrocardiographic differentiation of the ST-segment depression of acute myocardial injury due to the left circumflex artery occlusion from that of myocardial ischemia of nonocclusive etiologies. *Am J Cardiol* 1997;80:512–513.

145. Roul G, Bareiss P, Germain P, et al. Isolated ST segment depression from V2 to V4 leads, an early electrocardiographic sign of posterior myocardial infarction. *Arch Mal Coeur Vaiss* 1991;84:1815–1819.

146. Lee HS, Cross SJ, Rawles JM, et al. Patients with suspected myocardial infarction who present with ST depression. *Lancet* 1993;342:1204–1207.

147. Schechtman KB, Capone RJ, Kleiger RE, et al. Risk stratification of patients with non–Q wave myocardial infarction: the critical role of ST segment depression. *Circulation* 1989;80:1148–1158.

148. Cannon CP, Weintraub WS, Demopoulos LA, et al. Comparison of early invasive and conservative strategies in patients with unstable coronary syndromes treated with the glycoprotein IIb/IIIa inhibitor tirofiban. (TACTICS-TIMI 18) *N Engl J Med* 2001;344:1879–1887.

149. Kono T, Morita H, Kuroiwa T, et al. Left ventricular wall motion abnormalities in patients with subarachnoid hemorrhage: neurogenic stunned myocardium. *J Am Coll Cardiol* 1994;24:636–640.

150. Sharkey SW. Reversible myocardial contraction abnormalities in patients with an acute noncardiac illness. *Chest* 1998;114:98–105.

151. Wasserburger RH, Alt WJ, Lloyd CJ. The normal RS-T segment elevation variant. *Am J Cardiol* 1961;8:184–192.

152. De Zwaan C, Bar FW, Janssen JHA, et al. Angiographic and clinical characteristics of patients with unstable angina showing an ECG pattern indicating critical narrowing of the proximal LAD coronary artery. *Am Heart J* 1989;117:657–665.

153. De Zwaan C, Bar FW, Wellens HJJ. Characteristic electrocardiographic pattern indicating a critical stenosis high in left anterior descending coronary artery in patients admitted because of impending myocardial infarction. *Am Heart J* 1982;103:730–736.

154. Tandy TK, Bottomy DP, Lewis J. Wellens' syndrome. *Ann Emerg Med* 1999;33:347–351.

155. Haines DE, Raabe DS, Gundel WD, et al. Anatomic and prognostic significance of new T-wave inversion in unstable angina. *Am J Cardiol* 1983;52:14–18.

156. Doevendans PA, Gorgels AP, van der Zee R, et al. Electrocardiographic diagnosis of reperfusion during thrombolytic therapy in acute myocardial infarction. *Am J Cardiol* 1995;75:1206–1210.

157. Wehrens XH, Doevendans PA, Ophuis TJ, et al. A comparison of electrocardiographic changes during reperfusion of acute myocardial infarction by thrombolysis or percutaneous transluminal coronary angioplasty. *Am Heart J* 2000;139:430–436.

158. Shah PK, Cercek B, Lew AS, et al. Angiographic validation of bedside markers of reperfusion. *J Am Coll Cardiol* 1993;21:55–61.

159. Krucoff MW, Croll MA, Pope JE, et al. Continuous 12-lead ST-segment recovery analysis in the TAMI 7 study. Performance of a noninvasive method for real-time detection of failed myocardial reperfusion. *Circulation* 1993;88:437–446.

160. Varat A. Non-transmural infarction: clinical distinction between patients with ST depression and those with T wave inversion. *J Electrocardiol* 1985;18:15–20.

161. Lee HS, Brooks N, Jennings K. Patients with suspected myocardial infarction presenting with ST segment depression (editorial). *Heart* 1997;77:493–494.

162. Raunio H, Rissanen V, Romppanen T, et al. Changes in the QRS complex and ST segment in transmural and subendocardial myocardial infarctions: a clinicopathologic study. *Am Heart J* 1979;98:176–184.

163. Anderson HV, Cannon CP, Stone PH, et al. One-year results of the Thrombolysis in Myocardial Infarction (TIMI) IIIB clinical trial: a randomised comparison of tissue-type plasminogen activator versus placebo and early invasive versus early conservative strategies in unstable angina and non–Q wave myocardial infarction. *J Am Coll Cardiol* 1995;26:1643–1650.

164. Roberts MJD, McNeill AJ, Dalzell GWN, et al. Double-blind randomized trial of alteplase versus placebo in patients with chest pain at rest. *Eur Heart J* 1993;14:1536–1542.

165. White HD, French JK, Norris RM, et al. Effects of streptokinase in patients presenting within 6 hours of prolonged chest pain with ST segment depression. *Br Heart J* 1995;73:500–505.

166. TIMI IIIB Investigators. Effects of tissue plasminogen activator and a comparison of early invasive and conservative strategies in unstable angina and non–Q-wave myocardial infarction. Results of the TIMI IIIB Trial. Thrombolysis in Myocardial Ischemia. *Circulation* 1994;89:1545–1556.

167. Langer A, Goodman SG, Topol EJ, et al. Late assessment of thrombolytic efficacy (LATE) study: prognosis in patients with non–Q wave myocardial infarction. *J Am Coll Cardiol* 1996;27:1327–1332.

168. Braunwald E, Cannon CP. Non–Q-wave and ST segment depression myocardial infarction: Is there a role for thrombolytic therapy? *J Am Coll Cardiol* 1996;27:1333–1334.

169. LATE Study Group. Late assessment of thrombolytic efficacy (LATE) study with alteplase 6–24 hours after onset of acute myocardial infarction. *Lancet* 1993;342:759–766.

170. Smith FM. The ligation of coronary arteries with electrocardiographic study. *Arch Intern Med* 1918;5:1–27.

171. Bayley RH, LaDue JS, York DJ. Electrocardiographic changes (local ventricular ischemia and injury) produced in the dog by temporary occlusion of a coronary artery, showing a new stage in the evolution of myocardial infarction. *Am Heart J* 1944;27:164–169.

172. Bohning A, Katz LN. Unusual changes in the electrocardiograms of patients with recent coronary occlusion. *Am J Med Sci* 1933;186:39–52.

173. Wood FC, Wolferth CC. Huge T-waves in precordial leads in cardiac infarction. *Am Heart J* 1934;9:706–721.

174. Graham GK, Laforet EG. An electrocardiographic and morphologic study of changes following ligation of the left coronary artery in human beings: a report of two cases. *Am Heart J* 1952;43:42–52.

175. Wachtel FW, Teich EM. Tall precordial T waves as the earliest sign in diaphragmatic wall infarction. *Am Heart J* 1956;51:917–920.

176. Pinto IJ, Nanda NC, Biswas AK, et al. Tall upright T waves in the precordial leads. *Circulation* 1967;36:708–716.

177. Dressler W, Roesler H. High T waves in the earliest stage of myocardial infarction. *Am Heart J* 1947;34:627–645.

178. Freundlich J. The diagnostic significance of tall upright T waves in the chest leads. *Am Heart J* 1956;52:749–767.

179. Collins MS, Carter JE, Dougherty JM, et al. Hyperacute T wave criteria using computer ECG analysis. *Ann Emerg Med* 1990;19:114–120.

180. Hochrein J, Sun F, Pieper KS, et al. Higher T-wave amplitude associated with better prognosis in patients receiving thrombolytic therapy for acute myocardial infarction (a GUSTO-1 substudy). Global Utilization of Streptokinase and Tissue plasminogen activator for Occluded Coronary Arteries. *Am J Cardiol* 1998;81:1078–1084.

181. Fesmire FM, Wharton DR, Calhoun FB. Instability of ST segments in the early stages of acute myocardial infarction in patients undergoing continuous 12-lead ECG monitoring. *Am J Emerg Med* 1995;13:158–163.

182. Fesmire FM. ECG diagnosis of acute myocardial infarction in the presence of left bundle-branch block in patients undergoing continuous ECG monitoring. *Ann Emerg Med* 1995;26:69–82.

183. Fesmire FM, Percy RF, Bardoner JB, et al. Usefulness of automated serial 12-lead ECG monitoring during the initial emergency department evaluation of patients with chest pain. *Ann Emerg Med* 1998;31:3–11.

184. Gibler WB, Runyon JP, Levy RC, et al. A rapid diagnostic and treatment center for patients with chest pain in the emergency department. *Ann Emerg Med* 1995;25:1–8.

185. Hedges JR, Young GP, Henkel GF, et al. Serial ECGs are less accurate than serial CK-MB results for emergency department diagnosis of myocardial infarction. *Ann Emerg Med* 1992;21:1445–1450.

186. Fesmire FM, Campbell M, Decker WW, et al. Clinical policy: critical issues in the evaluation and management of adult patients presenting with suspected acute myocardial infarction or unstable angina. *Ann Emerg Med* 2000;35:521–544.

187. Krucoff MW, Wagner NB, Pope JE, et al. The portable programmable microprocessor-driven real-time 12-lead electrocardiographic monitor: a preliminary report of a new device for the noninvasive detection of successful reperfusion or silent coronary reocclusion. *Am J Cardiol* 1990;65:143–148.

188. Mizutani M, Freedman SB, Barns E, et al. ST monitoring for myocardial ischemia during and after coronary angioplasty. *Am J Cardiol* 1990;66:389–393.

189. Krucoff MW, Jackson TR, Kehoe M, et al. Quantitative and qualitative ST segment monitoring during and after percutaneous and transluminal coronary angioplasty. *Circulation* 1990;81(Suppl):IV20–26.

190. Krucoff MW, Parente AR, Bottner RK, et al. Stability of multilead ST-segment "fingerprints" over time after percutaneous transluminal coronary angioplasty and its usefulness in detecting reocclusion. *Am J Cardiol* 1988;61:1232–1237.

191. Krucoff MW, Green CE, Satler LF, et al. Noninvasive detection of coronary artery patency using continuous ST-segment monitoring. *Am J Cardiol* 1986;57:916–922.

192. Fesmire FM, Bardoner JB. ST-segment instability preceding simultaneous cardiac arrest and AMI in a patient undergoing continuous 12-lead ECG monitoring. *Am J Emerg Med* 1994;12:69–76.

193. Silber SH, Leo PJ, Katapadi M. Serial electrocardiograms for chest pain patients with initial nondiagnostic electrocardiograms: implications for thrombolytic therapy. *Acad Emerg Med* 1996;3:147–152.

194. Zalenski RJ, Rydman RJ, Sloan EP, et al. The emergency department electrocardiogram and hospital complications in myocardial infarction patients. *Acad Emerg Med* 1996;3:318–325.

195. Jernberg T, Lindahl B, Wallentin L. ST-segment monitoring with continuous 12-lead ECG improves early risk stratification in patients with chest pain and ECG nondiagnostic of acute myocardial infarction. *J Am Coll Cardiol* 1999;34:1413–1419.

196. Holmvang L, Andersen K, Dellborg M, et al. Relative contributions of a single-admission 12-lead electrocardiogram and early 24-hour continuous electrocardiographic monitoring for early risk stratification in patients with unstable coronary artery disease. *Am J Cardiol* 1999;83:667–674.

197. Chou TC. Pseudoinfarction. *Cardiovasc Clin* 1973;5:199–218.

198. Barbagelata A, Califf RM, Sgarbossa EB, et al. Use of resources, quality of life, and clinical outcomes in patients with and without new Q waves after thrombolytic therapy for acute myocardial infarction (from the GUSTO-I trial). *Am J Cardiol* 2000;86:24–29.

199. Birnbaum Y, Chetrit A, Sclarovsky S, et al. Abnormal Q waves on the admission electrocardiogram of patients with first acute myocardial infarction: prognostic implications. *Clin Cardiol* 1997;20:477–481.

200. Khan ZU, Chou TC. Right ventricular infarction mimicking acute anteroseptal left ventricular infarction. *Am Heart J* 1996;132:1089–1093.

201. Geft IL, Shah PK, Rodriguez L, et al. ST elevations in leads V1 to V5 may be caused by right coronary artery occlusion and acute right ventricular infarction. *Am J Cardiol* 1984;53:991–996.

202. Kosuge M, Kimura K, Toshiyuki I, et al. Electrocardiographic criteria for predicting total occlusion of the proximal left anterior descending coronary artery in anterior wall acute myocardial infarction. *Clin Cardiol* 2001;24:33–38.

203. Lew AS, Hod H, Cercek B, et al. Inferior ST segment changes during acute anterior myocardial infarction: a marker of the presence or absence of concomitant inferior wall ischemia. *J Am Coll Cardiol* 1987;10:519–526.

204. Andersen HR, Falk E, Nielsen D. Right ventricular infarction: diagnostic accuracy of electrocardiographic right chest leads V3R to V7R investigated prospectively in 43 consecutive fatal cases from a coronary care unit. *Br Heart J* 1989;61:514–520.

205. Assali AR, Sclarovsky S, Herz I, et al. Comparison of patients with inferior wall acute myocardial infarction with versus without ST-segment elevation in leads V5 and V6. *Am J Cardiol* 1998;81:81–83.

206. O'Keefe JHJ, Sayed-Taha K, Gibson W, et al. Do patients with left circumflex coronary artery-related acute myocardial infarction without ST-segment elevation benefit from reperfusion therapy? (See comments.) *Am J Cardiol* 1995;75:718–720.

207. Zehender M, Kasper W, Schonthaler M, et al. Right ventricular infarction as an independent predictor of prognosis after acute inferior myocardial infarction. *N Engl J Med* 1993;328:981–988.

208. Matetzky S, Freimark D, Chouraqui P, et al. Significance of ST segment elevations in posterior chest leads (V7–V9) in patients with acute inferior myocardial infarction: application for thrombolytic therapy. *J Am Coll Cardiol* 1998;31:506–511.

209. Shah PK, Pichler M, Berman DS, et al. Noninvasive identification of a high risk subset of patients with acute myocardial infarction. *Am J Cardiol* 1980;46:915–921.

210. Bates ER, Clemmensen PM, Califf RM, et al. Precordial ST segment depression predicts a worse prognosis in inferior infarction despite reperfusion therapy. The Thrombolysis and Angioplasty in Myocardial Infarction (TAMI) Study Group. *J Am Coll Cardiol* 1990;16:1538–1544.

211. Kulkarni AU, Brown R, Ayoubi M, et al. Clinical use of posterior electrocardiographic leads: a prospective electrocardiographic analysis during coronary occlusion. *Am Heart J* 1996;131:736–741.

212. Veldkamp RF, Sawchak S, Pope JE, et al. Performance of an automated real-time ST segment analysis program to detect coronary occlusion and reperfusion. *J Electrocardiol* 1996;29:257–263.

213. Figueras J, Curos A, Cortadellas J, et al. Relevance of electrocardiographic findings, heart failure, and infarct size in assessing risk and timing of left ventricular free wall rupture during acute myocardial infarction. *Am J Cardiol* 1995;76:543–547.

214. Zalenski RJ, Rydman RJ, Sloan EP, et al. Value of posterior and right ventricular leads in comparison to the standard 12-lead electrocardiogram in evaluation of ST-segment elevation in suspected acute myocardial infarction. *Am J Cardiol* 1997;79:1579–1585.

215. Andersen HR, Nielsen D, Hanse LG. The normal right chest electrocardiogram. *J Electrocardiol* 1987;20:27–32.

216. Simon R, Angehrn W. Right ventricular involvement in infero-posterior myocardial infarct: clinical significance of ECG diagnosis. *Schweiz Med Wochenschr* 1993;123:1499–1507.

217. Erhardt LR, Sjogren A, Wahlberg I. Single right-sided precordial lead in the diagnosis of right ventricular involvement in inferior myocardial infarction. *Am Heart J* 1976;91:571–576.

218. Zehender M, Kasper W, Kauder E, et al. Eligibility for and benefit of thrombolytic therapy in inferior myocardial infarction: focus on the prognostic importance of right ventricular infarction. *J Am Coll Cardiol* 1994;24:362–369.

219. Mak KH, Chia BL, Tan AT, et al. Simultaneous ST segment elevation in lead V1 and depression in lead V2: a discordant ECG pattern indicating right ventricular infarction. *J Electrocardiol* 1994;27:203–207.

220. Andersen HR, Neilson D, Lund O, et al. Prognostic significance of right ventricular infarction diagnosed by ST elevation in right chest leads V3R to V7R. *Int J Cardiol* 1989;23:349–356.

221. Bowers TR, O'Neill WW, Grines CL, et al. Effect of reperfusion on biventricular function and survival after right ventricular infarction. *N Engl J Med* 1998;338:933–940.

222. Shiraki H, Yoshikawa T, Anzai T, et al. Association between preinfarction angina and a lower risk of right ventricular infarction. *N Engl J Med* 1998;338:941–948.

223. Dell'Italia LJ. Reperfusion for right ventricular infarction. *N Engl J Med* 1998;338:978–980.

224. Chou TC, van der Bel-Kahn J, Allen J, et al. Electrocardiographic diagnosis of right ventricular infarction. *Am J Med* 1981;70:1175–1180.

225. Oraii S, Maleki I, Tavakolian AA, et al. Prevalence and outcome of ST-segment elevation in posterior electrocardiographic leads during acute myocardial infarction. *J Electrocardiol* 1999;32:275–278.

226. Melendez LJ, Jones DT, Salcedo JR. Usefulness of three additional electrocardiographic chest leads (V7, V8, V9) in the diagnosis of acute myocardial infarction. *Can Med Assoc J* 1978;119:745–748.

227. Taha B, Reddy S, Agarwal J, et al. Normal limits of ST segment measurements in posterior ECG leads. *J Electrocardiol* 1998;31(Suppl):178–179.

228. Brady WJ, Hwang V, Sullivan R. A comparison of 12- and 15-lead ECGs in ED chest pain patients: impact on diagnosis, therapy, and disposition. *Am J Emerg Med* 2000:18:239–243.

229. Boden WE, Kleiger RE, Gibson RS, et al. Electrocardiographic evolution of posterior acute myocardial infarction: importance of early precordial ST-segment depression. *Am J Cardiol* 1987;59:782–787.

230. Rich MW, Imburgia M, King TR, et al. Electrocardiographic diagnosis of remote posterior wall myocardial infarction using unipolar posterior lead V9. *Chest* 1989;96:489–493.

231. Lim R, Wilson DT. Abolition of electrocardiographic pattern of left ventricular aneurysm by posterior myocardial infarction. *Br J Clin Pract* 1990;44:328–329.

232. Go AS, Barron HV, Rundle AC, et al. Bundle-branch block and in-hospital mortality in acute myocardial infarction. National Registry of Myocardial Infarction. *Ann Int Med* 1998;129:690–697.

233. Scheidt S, Killip T. Bundle-branch block complicating acute myocardial infarction. *JAMA* 1972;222:919–924.

234. Newby KH, Pisano O, Krucoff MW, et al. Incidence and clinical relevance of the occurrence of bundle-branch block in patients treated with thrombolytic therapy. *Circulation* 1996;94:2424–2428.

235. Hiss RG, Lamb LE. Electrocardiographic findings in 122,043 individuals. *Circulation* 1962;25:947–961.

236. Sgarbossa EB, Pinski SL, Topol EJ, et al. Acute myocardial infarction and complete bundle branch block at hospital admission: clinical characteristics and outcome in the thrombolytic era. *J Am Coll Cardiol* 1998;31:105–110.

237. Roth A, Miller HI, Glick A, et al. Rapid resolution of new right bundle branch block in acute anterior myocardial infarction patients after thrombolytic therapy. *Pacing Clin Electrophysiol* 1993;16:13–18.

238. Hod H, Goldbourt U, Behar S. Bundle branch block in acute Q-wave inferior wall myocardial infarction: a high risk subgroup of interior myocardial infarction patients. The SPRINT Study Group. Secondary Prevention Reinfarction Israeli Nifedipine Trial. *Eur Heart J* 1995;16:471–477.

239. Freedman RA, Alderman EL, Sheffield L, et al. Bundle branch block in patients with chronic coronary artery disease: angiographic correlates and prognostic significance. *J Am Coll Cardiol* 1987;10:73–80.

240. Schneider JF, Thomas HE, Kreger BE, et al. Newly acquired right bundle-branch block: the Framingham Study. *Ann Int Med* 1901;92:37–44.

241. Edhouse JA, Sakr M, Angus J, et al. Suspected myocardial infarction and left bundle branch block: electrocardiographic indicators of acute ischaemia. *J Accid Emerg Med* 1999;16:331–335.

242. Hands ME, Cook EF, Stone PH, et al. Electrocardiographic diagnosis of myocardial infarction in the presence of complete left bundle branch block. *Am Heart J* 1988;116:23–31.

242.5. Cannon CP, McCabe CH, Stone PW, et al. The electrocardiogram predicts one-year outcome of patients with unstable angina and non-Q-wave myocardial infarction: results of the TIMI III Registry ECG Ancillary Study. *J Am Coll Cardiol* 1997;30:133–140.

243. Kontos MC, McQueen RH, Jesse RL, et al. Can myocardial infarction be rapidly identified in emergency department patients who have left bundle branch block? *Ann Emerg Med* 2001;37:431–438.

244. Li SF, Walden PL, Marcilla O, et al. Electrocardiographic diagnosis of myocardial infarction in patients with left bundle branch block. *Ann Emerg Med* 1999;36:561–566.

245. Shlipak MG, Go AS, Frederick PD. Treatment and outcomes of left bundle-branch block patients with myocardial infarction who present without chest pain. *J Am Coll Cardiol* 2000;36:706–712.

246. Sgarbossa EB, Pinski SL, Barbagelata A, et al. Electrocardiographic diagnosis of evolving acute myocardial infarction in the presence of left bundle-branch block. *N Engl J Med* 1996;334:481–487.

247. Wackers FJT. The diagnosis of myocardial infarction in the presence of left bundle branch block. *Cardiol Clinics* 1987;5:393–401.

248. Cannon A, Freedman SB, Bailey BP, et al. ST-Segment changes during transmural myocardial ischemia in chronic left bundle branch block. *Am J Cardiol* 1989;64:1216–1217.

249. Stark KS, Krucoff MW, Schryver B, et al. Quantification of ST-segment changes during coronary angioplasty in patients with left bundle branch block. *Am J Cardiol* 1991;67:1219–1222.

250. Brady WJ, Aufderheide TP. Left bundle branch block pattern complicating the electrocardiographic evaluation of acute myocardial infarction. *Acad Emerg Med* 1997;4:56–62.

251. Ackermann RJ, Vogel RL. Electrocardiographic diagnosis of acute myocardial infarction in the presence of left bundle-branch block (letter; comment). *N Engl J Med* 1996;335:131–133.

252. Shlipak MG, Lyons WL, Go AS, et al. Should the electrocardiogram be used to guide therapy for patients with left bundle-branch block and suspected myocardial infarction? *JAMA* 1999;281:714–719.

253. Ozment A, Garvey L, Littmann L, et al. An analysis of ECG criteria for acute myocardial infarction in the presence of left bundle branch block (abstract). *Acad Emerg Med* 1999;6:423–424.

254. Sokolove PE, Sgarbossa EB, Amsterdam EA, et al. Interobserver agreement in the electrocardiographic diagnosis of acute myocardial infarction in patients with left bundle branch block. *Ann Emerg Med* 2000;36:566–572.

255. Wellens HJ. Acute myocardial infarction and left bundle-branch block—can we lift the veil? (editorial; comment). *N Engl J Med* 1996; 334:528–529.

256. Melgarejo MA, Galcera TJ, Garcia A, et al. The incidence, clinical characteristics, and prognostic significance of a left bundle-branch block associated with an acute myocardial infarct. *Rev Esp Cardiol* 1999;52:245–252.

257. Byrne J. Electrocardiographic diagnosis of acute myocardial infarction in the presence of left bundle-branch block (letter; comment). *N Engl J Med* 1996;335:132–133.

258. Levenson J. Electrocardiographic diagnosis of acute myocardial infarction in the presence of left bundle-branch block (letter; comment). *N Engl J Med* 1996;335:132–133.

259. Sgarbossa EB, Pinski SL, Gates KB, et al. Early electrocardiographic diagnosis of acute myocardial infarction in the presence of ventricular paced rhythm. GUSTO-I investigators. *Am J Cardiol* 1996;77:423–424.

260. Sgarbossa EB. Recent advances in the electrocardiographic diagnosis of myocardial infarction: left bundle branch block and pacing. *Pace* 1996;19:1370–1379.

261. Kozlowski FH, Brady WJ, Aufderheide TP, et al. The electrocardiographic diagnosis of acute myocardial infarction in patients with ventricular paced rhythms. *Acad Emerg Med* 1998;5:52–57.

262. Mehta MC, Jain AC. Early repolarization on scalar electrocardiogram. *Am J Med Sci* 1995;309:305–311.

263. Kambara H, Phillips J. Long-term evaluation of early repolarization syndrome (normal variant RS-T segment elevation). *Am J Cardiol* 1976;38:157–161.

264. Ginzton LE, Laks MM. The differential diagnosis of acute pericarditis from the normal variant: new electrocardiographic criteria. *Circulation* 1982;65:1004–1009.

265. Marriott HJL. *ECG Challenge Pack: 78 ECG's for Advanced Review.* Windermere, FL: Trinity Press, 1999.

266. Amin M, Gabelman G, Karpel J, et al. Acute myocardial infarction and chest pain syndromes after cocaine use. *Am J Cardiol* 1990;66: 1434–1437.

267. Kontos MC, Schmidt KL, Nicholson CS, et al. Myocardial perfusion imaging with technetium-99m sestamibi in patients with cocaine-associated chest pain. *Ann Emerg Med* 1999;33:639–645.

268. Zimmerman JL, Dellinger RP, Majid PA. Cocaine-associated chest pain. *Ann Emerg Med* 1991;20:611–615.

269. Hollander JE, Hoffman RS, Gennis P, et al. Prospective multicenter evaluation of cocaine-associated chest pain. *Acad Emerg Med* 1994;1:330–339.

270. Weber JE, Chudnofsky CR, Boczar M, et al. Cocaine-associated chest pain: How common is myocardial infarction? *Acad Emerg Med* 2000; 7:873–877.

271. Gitter MJ, Goldsmith SR, Dunbar DN, et al. Cocaine and chest pain: clinical features and outcome of patients hospitalized to rule out myocardial infarction. *Ann Int Med* 1992;115:277–282.

272. Hollander JE, Lozano M, Fairwether P, et al. "Abnormal" electrocardiograms in patients with cocaine-associated chest pain are due to "normal" variants. *J Emerg Med* 1994;12:199–205.

273. Hollander JE. Current concepts: the management of cocaine-associated myocardial ischemia. *N Engl J Med* 1995;333:1267–1272.

274. Feldman JA, Fish SS, Beshansky JR, et al. Acute cardiac ischemia in patients with cocaine-associated complaints: results of a multicenter trial. *Ann Emerg Med* 2000;36:469–476.

275. Mittleman MA, Mintzer MD, Maclure M, et al. Triggering of myocardial infarction by cocaine. *Circulation* 2000;99:2737–2741.

276. Hollander JE, Hoffman RS, Gennis P, et al. Cocaine-associated chest pain: one year follow-up. *Acad Emerg Med* 1995;2:179–184.

277. Tokarski GF, Paganussi P, Urbanski R, et al. An evaluation of cocaine-induced chest pain. *Ann Emerg Med* 1990;19:1088–1092.

278. Feldman BA, Bui LD, Mitchell PM, et al. The evaluation of cocaine-induced chest pain with acute myocardial perfusion imaging. *Acad Emerg Med* 1999;6:103–109.

279. McLaurin M, Apple FS, Henry TD, et al. Cardiac troponin I and T concentrations in patients with cocaine-associated chest pain. *Ann Clin Biochem* 1996;33:183–186.

280. Lange RA, Cigarroa RG, Flores ED, et al. Potentiation of cocaine-induced coronary vasoconstriction by beta-adrenergic blockade. *Ann Int Med* 1990;112:897–903.

281. Hollander JE, Wilson LD, Leo PJ, et al. Complications from the use of thrombolytic agents in patients with cocaine-associated chest pain. *J Emerg Med* 1996;14:731–736.

282. Hollander JE, Hoffman RS. Cocaine-induced myocardial infarction: an analysis and review of the literature. *J Emerg Med* 1992;10: 169–177.

283. Selker HP, Beshansky J, Griffith JL, et al. Use of the Acute Cardiac Time-Insensitive Predictor Instrument (ACI-TIPI) to assist with triage of patients with chest pain or other symptoms suggestive of acute cardiac ischemia: a multicenter, controlled clinical trial. *Ann Int Med* 1998;129:845–855.

284. Hollander JE, Hoffman RS, Burstein JL, et al. Cocaine-associated myocardial infarction. Mortality and complications. Cocaine-Associated Myocardial Infarction Study Group. *Arch Int Med* 1995;155: 1081–1086.

285. Khoury NE, Borzak S, Gokli A, et al. "Inadvertent" thrombolytic administration in patients without myocardial infarction: clinical features and outcome. *Ann Emerg Med* 1996;28:289–293.

286. Larsen GC, Griffith JL, Beshansky JR, et al. Electrocardiographic left ventricular hypertrophy in patients with suspected acute cardiac ischemia: its influence on diagnosis, triage, and short-term prognosis. *J Gen Intern Med* 1994;9:666–676.

287. Myers G. QRS-T patterns in multiple precordial leads that may be mistaken for myocardial infarction. *Circulation* 1950;1:844–859.

288. Khan IA, Ajatta FO, Ansari AW. Persistent ST segment elevation: a new ECG finding in hypertrophic cardiomyopathy. *Am J Emerg Med* 1999;17:296–299.

289. Selzer A, Ebnother CL, Packard P, et al. Reliability of electrocardiographic diagnosis of left ventricular hypertrophy. *Circulation* 1958;17: 255–265.

290. Miller DH, Kligfield P, Schreiber TL, et al. Relationship of prior myocardial infarction to false-positive electrocardiographic diagnosis of acute injury in patients with chest pain. *Arch Intern Med* 1987;147: 257–261.

291. Berger AK, Radford MJ, Wang Y, et al. Thrombolytic therapy in older patients. *J Am Coll Cardiol* 2000;36:366–374.

292. Moyer JB, Hiller GI. Cardiac aneurysm: clinical and electrocardiographic analysis. *Am Heart J* 1951;41:340–358.

293. Ford RV, Levine HD. The electrocardiographic clue to ventricular aneurysm. *Ann Int Med* 1951;34:998–1016.

294. Schlichter J, Hellerstein HK, Katz LN. Aneurysm of the heart: a com-

parative study of one hundred and two proved cases. *Medicine* 1954; 33:43–86.

295. Pipilis GA, Wosika PH. Unipolar precordial electrocardiogram in ventricular aneurysm. *JAMA* 1951;145:147–152.

296. Dubnow MH, Burchell HB, Titus JL. Postinfarction ventricular aneurysm. *Am Heart J* 1965;70:753–760.

297. Visser CA, Kan G, David GK, et al. Echocardiographic-cineangiographic correlation in detecting left ventricular aneurysm: a prospective study of 422 patients. *Am J Cardiol* 1982;50:337–341.

298. Visser CA, Kan G, Meltzer RS, et al. Incidence, timing and prognostic value of left ventricular aneurysm formation after myocardial infarction: a prospective, serial echocardiographic study of 158 patients. *Am J Cardiol* 1986;57:729–732.

299. Arvan S, Varat MA. Persistent ST-segment elevation and left ventricular wall abnormalities: a two-dimensional echocardiographic study. *Am J Cardiol* 1984;53:1542–1546.

300. Cokkinos DV, Hallman GL, Cooley DA, et al. Left ventricular aneurysm: analysis of electrocardiographic features and postresection changes. *Am Heart J* 1971;82:149–157.

301. Kontny F, Hegrenaes L, Lem P, et al. Left ventricular thrombosis and arterial embolism after thrombolysis in acute anterior myocardial infarction: predictors and effects of adjunctive antithrombolytic therapy. *Eur Heart J* 1993;14:1489–1492.

302. Abraham JS, Wilson M, Scripcariu V, et al. Microembolism from aortic aneurysm and ventricular thrombus: a complication of intravenous streptokinase. *Postgrad Med J* 1994;70:756–758.

303. Miller RR, Amsterdam EA, Bogren HG, et al. Electrocardiographic and cineangiographic correlations in assessment of the location, nature, and extent of abnormal left ventricular segmental contraction in coronary artery disease. *Circulation* 1974;49:447–454.

304. Bhatnagar SK. Observations of the relationship between left ventricular aneurysm and ST segment elevation in patients with a first acute anterior Q wave myocardial infarction. *Eur Heart J* 1994;15: 1500–1504.

305. Millaire A, de Groote P, Decoulx E, et al. Outcome after thrombolytic therapy of nine cases of myopericarditis misdiagnosed as myocardial infarction. *Eur Heart J* 1995;16:333–338.

306. Sarda L, Colin P, Boccara F, et al. Myocarditis in patients with clinical presentation of myocardial infarction and normal coronary arteries. *J Am Coll Cardiol* 2001;37:786–792.

307. Spodick DH. The electrocardiogram in acute pericarditis: distributions of morphologic and axial changes in stages. *Prog Cardiovasc Dis* 1974;33:470–474.

308. Sleight P. Is there an age limit for thrombolytic therapy? *Am J Cardiol* 1993;72:30G–33G.

309. Juneja R, Kothari SS, Saxena A, et al. Intrapericardial streptokinase in purulent pericarditis. *Arch Dis Child* 1999;80:275–277.

310. Kahn JK. Inadvertent thrombolytic therapy for cardiovascular diseases masquerading as acute coronary thrombosis. *Clin Cardiol* 1993;16:67–71.

311. Huang CH, Wu CC, Lee YT. Thrombolytic therapy complicated hyperacute cardiac tamponade in a patient with purulent pericarditis. *Int J Cardiol* 1996;55:209–210.

312. Tilley WS, Harston WE. Inadvertent administration of streptokinase to patients with pericarditis. *Am J Med* 1986;81:541–544.

313. Ferguson DW, Dewey RC, Plante DA. Clinical pitfalls in the noninvasive thrombolytic approach to presumed acute myocardial infarction. *Can J Cardiol* 1986;2:146–151.

314. Blankenship JC, Almquist AK. Cardiovascular complications of thrombolytic therapy in patients with a mistaken diagnosis of acute myocardial infarction. *J Am Coll Cardiol* 1989;14:1579–1582.

315. Eriksen UH, Molgaard H, Ingerslev J, et al. Fatal haemostatic complications due to thrombolytic therapy in patients falsely diagnosed as acute myocardial infarction. *Eur Heart J* 1992;13:840–843.

316. Barrington WW, Smith JE, Himmelstein SI. Cardiac tamponade following treatment with tissue plasminogen activator: an atypical hemodynamic response to pericardiocentesis. *Am Heart J* 1991;121: 1227–1229.

317. Heymann TD, Culling W. Cardiac tamponade after thrombolysis. *Postgrad Med J* 1994;70:455–456.

318. Shah A, Wagner GS, O'Connor CM, et al. Prognostic implications of TIMI flow grade in the infarct related artery compared with continuous 12-lead ST-segment resolution analysis. Reexamining the "gold standard" for myocardial reperfusion treatment. *J Am Coll Cardiol* 2000;35:666–672.

319. Claeys MJ, Bosmans J, Veenstra L, et al. Determinants and prognostic implications of persistent ST-segment elevation after primary angioplasty for acute myocardial infarction: importance of microvascular reperfusion injury on clinical outcome. *Circulation* 1999;99: 1972–1977.

320. Van't Hof AW, Liem A, de Boer MJ, et al. Clinical value of 12-lead electrocardiogram after successful reperfusion therapy for acute myocardial infarction. Zwolle Myocardial Infarction Study Group. *Lancet* 1997;350:615–619.

321. Dissman R, Schroder R, Busse U, et al. Early assessment of outcome by ST segment analysis after thrombolytic therapy in acute myocardial infarction. *Am Heart J* 1994;128:851–857.

322. Schroder R, Wegscheider K, Schroder K, et al. Extent of early ST segment elevation resolution: a strong predictor of outcome in patients with acute myocardial infarction and a sensitive measure to compare thrombolytic regimens. A substudy of the International Joint Efficacy Comparison of Thrombolytics (INJECT) trial. *J Am Coll Cardiol* 1995;26:1657–1664.

323. Ross AM, Lundergan CF, Rohrbeck SC, et al. Rescue angioplasty after failed thrombolysis: technical and clinical outcomes in a large thrombolysis trial. *J Am Coll Cardiol* 1998;31:1511–1517.

324. Ellis SG, da Silva ER, Spaulding CM, et al. Review of immediate angioplasty after fibrinolytic therapy for acute myocardial infarction. *Am Heart J* 2000;139:1046–1053.

325. The TIMI Study Group. The thrombolysis in myocardial infarction (TIMI) trial. *N Engl J Med* 1985;312:932–936.

326. Gibson CM, Cannon CP, Murphy SA, et al. Relationship of TIMI myocardial perfusion grade to mortality after administration of thrombolytic drugs. *Circulation* 2000;101:125–130.

327. Cannon CP, Braunwald E. GUSTO, TIMI and the Case for Rapid Reperfusion (editorial). *Acta Cardiologica* 1994;49:1–8.

328. Lenderink T, Maarten L, Van Es GA, et al. Benefit of thrombolytic therapy is sustained throughout five years and is related to TIMI perfusion grade 3 but not grade 2 flow at discharge. Clinical investigation and reports. *Circulation* 1995;92:1110–1116.

329. Van't Hof AW, Liem A, Suryapranata H, et al. Angiographic assessment of myocardial reperfusion in patients treated with primary angioplasty for acute myocardial infarction: myocardial blush grade. Zwolle Myocardial Infarction Study Group. *Circulation* 1998;97:2 303–2306.

330. Von Essen R, Merx W, Effert S. Spontaneous course of ST-segment elevation in acute anterior myocardial infarction. *Circulation* 1979;59:105–112.

331. Klootwijk P, Langer A, Meij S, et al. Non-invasive prediction of reperfusion and coronary artery patency by continuous ST segment monitoring in the GUSTO-I trial. *Eur Heart J* 1996;17:689–698.

332. Dissman R, Linderer T, Goerke M, et al. Sudden increase of the ST segment elevation at a time of reperfusion predicts extensive infarcts in patients with intravenous thrombolysis. *Am Heart J* 1993;126:832–839.

333. Figueras J, Bermejo B. Additional elevation of the ST segment: a possible early electrocardiographic marker of experimental myocardial reperfusion. *Cardiovasc Res* 1996;32:1141–1147.

334. Figueras J, Cortadellas J. Further elevation of the ST segment during the first hour of thrombolysis: a possible early marker of reperfusion. *Eur Heart J* 1995;16:1807–1813.

335. Clements IP. *The electrocardiogram in acute myocardial infarction.* Armonk, NY: Futura, 1998.

336. Matetzky S, Barabash GI, Shahar A, et al. Early T wave inversion after thrombolytic therapy predicts better coronary perfusion: clinical and angiographic study. *J Am Coll Cardiol* 1994;24:378–383.

337. Mikell FL, Petrovich J, Snyder M, et al. Reliability of Q-wave formation and QRS score in predicting regional and global left ventricular performance in acute myocardial infarction with successful reperfusion. *Am J Cardiol* 1986;57:923–926.

338. Hohnloser SH, Zabel M, Kasper W, et al. Assessment of coronary

artery patency after thrombolytic therapy: accurate prediction using the combined analysis of three noninvasive markers. *J Am Coll Cardiol* 1991;18:44–49.

339. Califf RM, O'Neill WW, Stack RS, et al. Failure of simple clinical measurements to predict perfusion status after intravenous thrombolysis. *Ann Int Med* 1988;108:658–662.

340. Corey KE, Maynard C, Pahlm O, et al. Combined historical and electrocardiographic timing of acute anterior and inferior myocardial infarcts for prediction of reperfusion achievable size limitation. *Am J Cardiol* 1999;83:826–831.

340.5. Barbash GI, Birnbaum Y, Boggerts K, et al. Treatment of reinfarction after thrombolytic therapy for acute myocardial infarction: an analysis of outcome and treatment choices in GUSTO-I and ASSENT-2. *Circulation* 2001;103:954–960.

341. Krucoff MW, Croll MA, Pope JE, et al. Continuously updated 12-lead ST-segment recovery analysis for myocardial infarct artery patency assessment and its correlation with multiple simultaneous early angiographic observations. *Am J Cardiol* 1993;71:145–151.

342. Gibson CM, Cannon CP, Daley WL, et al. The TIMI frame count: a quantitative method of assessing coronary artery flow. *Circulation* 1996;93:879–888.

343. Gibson CM, Murphy SA, Rizzo MJ, et al. Relationship between TIMI frame count and clinical outcomes after thrombolytic administration. *Circulation* 1999;99:1945–1950.

344. Saran RK, Been M, Furniss SS. Reduction in ST segment elevation after thrombolysis predicts either coronary reperfusion or preservation of left ventricular function. *Br Heart J* 1990;64:113–117.

345. De Wood MA, Spores J, Notske R, et al. Prevalence of total coronary occlusion during the early hours of transmural myocardial infarction. *N Engl J Med* 1980;303:897–902.

346. Veldkamp RF, Green CL, Wilkins ML, et al. Comparison of continuous ST-segment recovery analysis with methods using static electrocardiograms for noninvasive patency assessment during acute myocardial infarction. Thrombolysis and Angioplasty in Myocardial Infarction (TAMI) 7 Study Group. *Am J Cardiol* 1994;73:1069–1074.

347. Hackworthy RA, Vogel MB, Harris PJ. Relationship between changes in ST segment elevation and patency of the infarct-related coronary artery in acute myocardial infarction. *Am Heart J* 1986;112:279–284.

348. Clemmensen P, Ohman EM, Sevilla DC, et al. Changes in standard electrocardiographic ST-segment elevation predictive of successful reperfusion in acute myocardial infarction. *Am J Cardiol* 1990;66:1407–1411.

349. Gorgels AP, Vos MA, Letsh IS, et al. Usefulness of the accelerated idioventricular rhythm as a marker for myocardial necrosis and reperfusion during thrombolytic therapy in acute myocardial infarction. *Am J Cardiol* 1988;61:231–235.

350. Goldberg S, Urban P, Greenspon A, et al. Limitation of infarct size with thrombolytic agents: electrocardiographic indexes. *Circulation* 1983;68:I77–I82.

351. Miller FC, Krucoff MW, Satler LF, et al. Ventricular arrhythmias during reperfusion. *Am Heart J* 1986;112:928–932.

352. Gore JM, Ball SP, Corrao JM, et al. Arrhythmias in the assessment of coronary artery reperfusion following thrombolytic therapy. *Chest* 1988;94:727–730.

353. Gressin V, Louvard Y, Pezzano M, et al. Holter recording of ventricular arrhythmias during intravenous thrombolysis for acute myocardial infarction. *Am J Cardiol* 1992;69:152–159.

354. Dellborg M, Topol EJ, Swedberg K. Dynamic QRS complex and ST segment vectorcardiographic monitoring can identify vessel patency in patients with acute myocardial infarction treated with reperfusion therapy. *Am Heart J* 1991;122:94–948.

355. Von Essen R, Schmidt W, Uebis R, et al. Myocardial infarction and thrombolysis: electrocardiographic short term and long term results using precordial mapping. *Br Heart J* 1985;54:6–10.

356. Badir BF, Nasmith JB, Dutoy JL, et al. Continuous ST segment recording during thrombolysis in acute myocardial infarction: a report on orthogonal ECG monitoring. *Can J Cardiol* 1995;11:545–552.

357. Ellis SG, da Silva ER, Heyndricks G, et al. Randomized comparison of rescue angioplasty with conservative management of patients with early failure of thrombolysis for acute anterior myocardial infarction. *Circulation* 1994;90:2280–2284.

358. McKendall GR, Forman S, Sopko G, et al. Value of rescue percutaneous transluminal coronary angioplasty following unsuccessful thrombolytic therapy in patients with acute myocardial infarction. Thrombolysis in Myocardial Infarction Investigators. *Am J Cardiol* 1995;76:1108–1111.

359. Anonymous. Outcome of attempted rescue coronary angioplasty after failed thrombolysis for acute myocardial infarction. The CORAMI Study Group. Cohort of Rescue Angioplasty in Myocardial Infarction. *Am J Cardiol* 1994;74:172–174.

360. Gibson CM, Cannon CP, Greene RM, et al. Rescue angioplasty in the Thrombolysis in Myocardial Infarction (TIMI) 4 trial. *Am J Cardiol* 1997;80:21–26.

361. Miller JM, Smalling R, Ohman EM, et al. Effectiveness of early coronary angioplasty and abciximab for failed thrombolysis (reteplase or alteplase) during acute myocardial infarction (results from the GUSTO-III trial). Global Use of Strategies to Open occluded coronary arteries. *Am J Cardiol* 1999;84:779–784.

362. GUSTO III. A comparison of reteplase with alteplase for acute myocardial infarction. *N Engl J Med* 1997;337:1118–1123.

363. Langer A, Krucoff MW, Klootwijk P, et al. Prognostic significance of ST segment shift early after resolution of ST elevation in patients with myocardial infarction treated with thrombolytic therapy: the GUSTO-I ST Segment Monitoring Substudy. *J Am Coll Cardiol* 1998;31:783–789.

364. Dissman R, Schroder R, Bruggemann T, et al. Early recurrence of ST-segment elevation in patients with initial reperfusion during thrombolytic therapy: impact on in-hospital reinfarction and long-term vessel patency. *Coron Artery Dis* 1994;5:745–753.

365. Maggioni AP, Maseri A, Fresco C, et al. Age-related increase in mortality among patients with first myocardial infarctions treated with thrombolysis. *N Engl J Med* 1993;329:1442–1448.

366. Oliva PB, Hammill SC, Edwards WD. Cardiac rupture, a clinically predictable complication of acute myocardial infarction: report of 70 cases with clinicopathologic correlations. *J Am Coll Cardiol* 1993;22:720–726.

367. Honan MB, Harrell FE, Reimer K, et al. Cardiac rupture, mortality and the timing of thrombolytic therapy: a meta-analysis. *J Am Coll Cardiol* 1990;16:359–367.

368. Figueras J, Cortadellas J, Calvo F, et al. Relevance of delayed hospital admission on development of cardiac rupture during acute myocardial infarction: study in 225 patients with free wall, septal or papillary muscle rupture. *J Am Coll Cardiol* 1998;32:135–139.

369. Plummer D, Dick C, Ruiz E, et al. Emergency department two-dimensional echocardiography in the diagnosis of nontraumatic cardiac rupture. *Ann Emerg Med* 1994;23:1333–1342.

370. Mohammad S, Austin SM. Hemopericardium with cardiac tamponade after intravenous thrombolysis for acute myocardial infarction. *Clin Cardiol* 1996;19:432–434.

371. Figueras J, Cortadellas J, Evangelista A, et al. Medical management of selected patients with left ventricular free wall rupture during acute myocardial infarction. *J Am Coll Cardiol* 1997;29:512–518.

372. Purcaro A, Constantini C, Ciampani N, et al. Diagnostic criteria and management of subacute ventricular free wall rupture complicating acute myocardial infarction. *Am J Cardiol* 1997;80:397–405.

373. Guron CW, Hagman M, Hartford M, et al. Echocardiography allows early detection and long-term survival after infarct free wall rupture. *J Am Soc Echocardiogr* 1998;11:307–309.

374. Becker RC, Charlesworth A, Wilcox RG, et al. Cardiac rupture associated with thrombolytic therapy: impact of time to treatment in the Late Assessment of Thrombolytic Efficacy (LATE) Study. *J Am Coll Cardiol* 1995;25:1063–1068.

375. Kleiman NS, Terrin M, Mueller H, et al. Mechanisms of early death despite thrombolytic therapy: experience from the Thrombolysis in Myocardial Infarction Phase II (TIMI II). *J Am Coll Cardiol* 1992;19:1129–1135.

376. Aguirre FV, Younis LT, Chaitman BR, et al. Early and 1-year clinical outcome of patients evolving non–Q-wave versus Q-wave myocardial

infarction after thrombolysis. Results from the TIMI II trial. *Circulation* 1995;91:2541–2548.

377. Kleiman NS, White HD, Ohman EM, et al. Mortality within 24 hours of thrombolysis for myocardial infarction. The importance of early reperfusion. *Circulation* 1912;90:2658–2665.

378. Becker RC, Gore JM, Lambrew C, et al. A composite view of cardiac rupture in the United States National Registry of Myocardial Infarction. *J Am Coll Cardiol* 1996;27:1321–1326.

379. Becker RC, Hochman JS, Cannon CP, et al. Fatal cardiac rupture among patients treated with thrombolytic agents and adjunctive thrombin antagonists: observation from the Thrombolysis and Thrombin Inhibition in Myocardial Infarction 9 Study. *J Am Coll Cardiol* 1999;33:479–487.

380. Wu AHB, Apple FS, Gibler WB, et al. National Academy of Clinical Biochemistry Standards of Laboratory Practice: Recommendations for use of cardiac markers in coronary artery disease. *Clin Chem* 1999; 45:1121.

381. Apple FS. Tissue specificity of cardiac troponin I, cardiac troponin T and creatine kinase MB. *Clin Chim Acta* 1999;284:151–159.

382. Apple FS. Clinical and analytical standardization issues confronting cardiac troponin I. *Clin Chem* 1999;45:18–20.

383. Hamm CW, Goldmann BU, Heeschen C, et al. Emergency room triage of patients with acute chest pain by means of rapid testing for cardiac troponin T or troponin I. *N Engl J Med* 1997;337: 1648–1653.

384. Hamm CW, Heeschen C, Goldmann BU, et al. Value of troponins in predicting therapeutic efficacy of abciximab in patients with unstable angina. *J Am Coll Cardiol* 1998;31:185A.

385. Lindahl B, Venge P, Wallentin L. Troponin T identifies patients with unstable coronary artery disease who benefit from long-term antithrombotic protection. Fragmin in Unstable Coronary Artery Disease (FRISC) Study Group. *J Am Coll Cardiol* 1997;29:43–48.

386. Stubbs P, Collinson P, Moseley D, et al. Prognostic significance of admission troponin T concentrations in patients with myocardial infarction. *Circulation* 1996;94:1291–1297.

387. Zimmerman J, Fromm R, Meyer D, et al. Diagnostic marker cooperative study for the diagnosis of myocardial infarction. *Circulation* 1999;99:1671–1677.

388. Falahati A, Sharkey SW, Christenson RH, et al. Implementation of serum cardiac troponin I as a marker for detection of acute myocardial infarction. *Am Heart J* 1999;137:332–337.

389. Apple FS, Falahati A, Paulsen PR, et al. Improved detection of minor ischemic myocardial injury with measurement of serum cardiac troponin I. *Clin Chem* 1997;43:2047–2051.

390. Apple FS. Biochemical markers of thrombolytic success. *Scand J Clin Lab Invest* 1999;59:60–66.

391. Apple FS, Sharkey SW, Henry TD. Early serum cardiac troponin I and T concentrations following successful thrombolysis for acute myocardial infarction. *Clin Chem* 1995;41:1197–1198.

392. Apple FS. Value of soluble markers for the diagnosis of reperfusion after thrombolysis. In: Kaski JC, Holt DW, eds. *Myocardial damage: early detection by novel biochemical markers.* London: Kluwer Academic Publishers, 1998:149–158.

393. Mohler ER, Ryan T, Segar DS, et al. Clinical utility of troponin T levels and echocardiography in the emergency department. *Am Heart J* 1998;135:253–260.

394. Colon PJ, Guarisco JS, Murgo J, et al. Utility of stress echocardiography in the triage of patients with atypical chest pain from the emergency department. *Am J Cardiol* 1998;82:1282–1284, A 10.

395. Slater J, Brown RJ, Antonelli TA, et al. Cardiogenic Shock due to cardiac free-wall rupture or tamponade after acute myocardial infarction: a report from the SHOCK trial registry. *Circulation* 2000;36: 1117–1122.

396. Sabia P, Afrookteh A, Touchstone D, et al. Value of regional wall motion abnormality in the emergency room diagnosis of acute myocardial infarction: a prospective study using two-dimensional echocardiography. *Circulation* 1991;84:185–192.

397. Kontos MC, Arrowood JA, Paulsen WH, et al. Early echocardiography can predict cardiac events in emergency department patients with chest pain. *Ann Emerg Med* 1905;31:550–557.

398. Kontos MC, Arrowood JA, Jesse RL, et al. Comparison between 2-dimensional echocardiography and myocardial perfusion imaging in the emergency department in patients with possible myocardial ischemia. *Am Heart J* 1998;136:724–733.

399. Weaver WD, Cerqueira MD, Hallstrom AP, et al. Prehospital-initiated vs. hospital-initiated thrombolytic therapy. *JAMA* 1993;270: 1211–1216.

400. Rawles JM. Quantification of the benefit of earlier thrombolytic therapy: five-year results of the Grampian Region Early Anistreplase Trial (GREAT). *J Am Coll Cardiol* 1997;30:1181–1186.

401. Schuster CJ, Tebbe U. (Prehospital thrombolytic therapy in acute myocardial infarction) German. *Anaesthesist* 1997;46:829–839.

402. Linderer T, Schroder R, Arntz R, et al. Prehospital thrombolysis: beneficial effects of very early treatment on infarct size and left ventricular function. *J Am Coll Cardiol* 1993;22:1304–1310.

403. European Myocardial Infarction Project Group. Prehospital thrombolytic therapy in patients with suspected acute myocardial infarction. *N Engl J Med* 1993;329:383–389.

404. Benson NH, Maningas PA, Krohmer JR, et al. Guidelines for the prehospital use of thrombolytic agents. *Ann Emerg Med* 1994;23: 1047–1048.

405. Brouwer MA, Martin JS, Maynard C, et al. Influence of early prehospital thrombolysis on mortality and event-free survival (the Myocardial Infarction Triage and Intervention [MITI] Randomized Trial). MITI Project Investigators. *Am J Cardiol* 1996;78:497–502.

406. Morrison LJ, Verbeek PR, McDonald AC, et al. Mortality and prehospital thrombolysis for acute myocardial infarction. *JAMA* 2000; 283:2686–2692.

407. Rawles JM. Myocardial salvage with early anistreplase treatment. *Clin Cardiol* 1997;20:III6–III10.

408. Kereiakes DJ, Gibler WB, Martin LH, et al. Relative importance of emergency medical system transport and the prehospital electrocardiogram on reducing hospital time delay to therapy for acute myocardial infarction; a preliminary report from the Cincinnati Heart Project. *Am Heart J* 1992;123:835–840.

409. Castaigne AD, Herve C, Duval-Moulin AM, et al. Prehospital use of APSAC: results of a placebo-controlled study. *Am J Cardiol* 1989;64: 30A–33A.

410. Schofer J, Buttner J, Geng G, et al. Prehospital thrombolysis in acute myocardial infarction. *Am J Cardiol* 1990;66:1429–1433.

411. Roth A, Barbash GI, Hod H, et al. Should thrombolytic therapy be administered in the Mobile Intensive Care Unit in patients with evolving myocardial infarction? *J Am Coll Cardiol* 1990;15:932–936.

412. Assessment of the Safety and Efficacy of a New Thrombolytic (ASSENT-2) investigators. Single-bolus tenecteplase compared with front-loaded alteplase in acute myocardial infarction: the ASSENT-2 double-blind randomised trial. *Lancet* 1999;354:722.

413. Aufderheide TP, Bossaert LL, Field J, et al. Acute Coronary Syndromes. Proceedings of the international guidelines 2000 conference for cardiopulmonary resuscitation and emergency cardiovascular care. *Ann Emerg Med* 2001;37:163S–181S.

414. Canto JG, Rogers WJ, Bowlby LJ, et al. The pre-hospital electrocardiogram in acute myocardial infarction: Is its full potential being realized? National Registry of Myocardial Infarction 2 Investigators. *J Am Coll Cardiol* 1997;29:498–505.

415. Foster DB, Dufendach JH, Barkdoll CM, et al. Prehospital recognition of AMI using independent nurse/paramedic 12-lead ECG evaluation: impact on in-hospital times to thrombolysis in a rural community hospital. *Am J Emerg Med* 1994;12:25–31.

416. Kudenchuk PJ, Maynard C, Cobb LA, et al. Utility of the prehospital electrocardiogram in diagnosing acute coronary syndromes. *J Am Coll Cardiol* 1998;32:17–27.

417. Pozen MW, D'Agostino RB, Selker HP, et al. A predictive instrument to improve Coronary-Care-Unit admission practices in acute ischemic heart disease. *N Engl J Med* 1984;310:1273–1278.

418. Aufderheide TP, Rowlandson I, Lawrence SW, et al. Test of the Acute Coronary Ischemia Time-Insensitive Predictive Instrument (ACI-TIPI) for prehospital use. *Ann Emerg Med* 1996;27:193–198.

419. Selker HP, Griffith JL, Beshansk JR, et al. Patient-specific predictions of outcomes in myocardial infarction for real-time emergency use: a

thrombolytic predictive instrument. *Ann Int Med* 1997;127:538–556.

420. Blohm M, Herlitz J, Hartford M, et al. Consequences of a media campaign focusing on delay in acute myocardial infarction. *Am J Cardiol* 1992;69:411–413.

421. Gazpoz J-M, Unger P-F, Urban P, et al. Impact of a public campaign on pre-hospital time delays in suspected acute myocardial infarction. *Circulation* 1993;88:1–13. Abstract.

422. Luepker RV, Raczynski JM, Osganian S, et al. Effect of a community intervention on patient delay and emergency medical service use in acute coronary heart disease. *JAMA* 2000;284:60–67.

423. GREAT Group. Feasibility, safety, efficacy of domiciliary thrombolysis by general practitioners: Grampian Region Early Anistreplase Trial. *BMJ* 1992;305:548–553.

424. Rawles J. Magnitude of benefit from earlier thrombolytic treatment in acute myocardial infarction: new evidence from Grampian Region Early Anistreplase Trial (GREAT). *BMJ* 1996;312:212–215.

425. Rawles J. Halving of mortality at 1 year by domiciliary thrombolysis in the Grampian Region Early Anistreplase Trial (GREAT). *J Am Coll Cardiol* 1994;23:1–5.

426. Maynard C, Weaver WD, Lambrew C, et al. Factors influencing the time to administration of thrombolytic therapy with recombinant tissue plasminogen activator (data from the National Registry of Myocardial Infarction). *Am J Cardiol* 1995;76:548–552.

427. Berger PB, Ellis SG, Holmes DR, et al. Relationship between delay in performing direct coronary angioplasty and early clinical outcome in patients with acute myocardial infarction: results from the global use of strategies to open occluded arteries in Acute Coronary Syndromes (GUSTO-IIb) trial. *Circulation* 1999;100:14–20.

428. Cannon CP, Gibson CM, Lambrew CT, et al. Relationship of symptom onset-to-balloon-time and door-to-balloon time with mortality in patients undergoing angioplasty for acute myocardial infarction. *JAMA* 2000;283:2941–2947.

429. National Heart Attack Alert Program Coordinating Committee 60 Minutes to Treatment Working Group. Rapid identification and treatment of patients with acute myocardial infarction. *Ann Emerg Med* 1994;23:311–329.

430. Graff L, Palmer AC, LaMonica P, et al. Triage of patients for a rapid (5-minute) electrocardiogram: a rule based on presenting chief complaints. *Ann Emerg Med* 2000;36:554–560.

431. Doorey A, Patel S, Reese C, et al. Dangers of delay of initiation of either thrombolysis or primary angioplasty in acute myocardial infarction with increasing use of primary angioplasty. *Am J Cardiol* 1998;81:1173–1177.

432. Gilutz H, Battler A, Rabinowitz I, et al. The "door-to-needle blitz" in acute myocardial infarction: the impact of a CQI project. *Jt Comm J Qual Improv* 1998;24:323–333.

433. Cummings P. Improving the time to thrombolytic therapy for myocardial infarction by using a quality assurance audit. *Ann Emerg Med* 1992;21:1107–1110.

434. Pell ACH, Miller HC, Robertson CE, et al. Effect of "fast track" admission for acute myocardial infarction on delay to thrombolysis. *BMJ* 1992;304:83–87.

435. Cannon CP, Goldhaber SZ. The importance of rapidly treating patients with acute myocardial infarction. Editorial. *Chest* 1995;107:598–600.

436. Califf RM, Newby LK. How much do we gain by reducing time to reperfusion therapy? *Am J Cardiol* 1996;78:8–15.

437. Brophy JM, Diodati JG, Bogaty P, et al. The delay to thrombolysis: an analysis of hospital and patient characteristics. *CMAJ* 1998;158:475–480.

438. Senior J, Patel N. Reducing thrombolytic therapy time delays in the emergency department. *J Qual Clin Pract* 1999;18:99–107.

439. Lambrew CT, Bowlby LJ, Rogers WJ, et al. Factors influencing the time to thrombolysis in acute myocardial infarction. Time to Thrombolysis Substudy of the National Registry of Myocardial Infarction-1. *Arch Int Med* 1997;157:2577–2582.

440. Palmer DJ, Cox KL, Dear K, et al. Factors associated with delay in giving thrombolytic therapy after arrival at hospital. *Med J Aust* 1998;168:111–114.

441. Vaccarino V, Parsons L, Every NR, et al. Sex-based differences in early mortality after myocardial infarction. *N Engl J Med* 1999;341:217–225.

442. Wexler LF. Studies of acute coronary syndromes in women — lessons for everyone. *N Engl J Med* 1999;341:275–276.

443. Gonzalez ER, Jones LA, Ornato JP, et al. Hospital delays and problems with thrombolytic administration in patients receiving thrombolytic therapy: a multicenter prospective assessment. *Ann Emerg Med* 1992;21:1215–1221.

444. Al-Mubarak N, Rogers WJ, Lambrew CT, et al. Consultation before thrombolytic therapy in acute myocardial infarction. *Am J Cardiol* 1999;83:89–93.

445. Sharkey SW, Brunette DD, Ruiz E, et al. An analysis of time delays preceding thrombolysis for acute myocardial infarction. *JAMA* 1989;262:3171–3174.

446. GUSTO IIb (Global Use of Strategies to Open Occluded Arteries in Acute Coronary Syndromes Angioplasty Substudy Investigators). A clinical trial comparing primary coronary angioplasty with tissue plasminogen activator for acute myocardial infarction. *N Engl J Med* 1997;336:1621–1628.

447. Bourke JP, Young AA, Richards DAB, et al. Reduction in incidence of inducible ventricular tachycardia after myocardial infarction by treatment with streptokinase during infarct evolution. *J Am Coll Cardiol* 1990;16:1703–1710.

448. Rapaport E. Early versus late opening of coronary arteries: the effect of timing. *Clin Cardiol* 1990;13:VIII18–VIII22.

449. Herz I, Birnbaum Y, Zlotikamien B, et al. The prognostic implications of negative T-waves in the leads with ST segment elevation on admission in acute myocardial infarction. *Cardiology* 1999;92:121–127.

450. Bates ER. Late thrombolysis in acute myocardial infarction. Abstract and commentary for: LATE Study Group. Late assessment of thrombolytic efficacy (LATE) with alteplase 6–24 hours after onset of acute myocardial infarction. *ACP J Club* 1994;120:72–74.

451. EMERAS (Estudio Multicentro Estreptoquinasa Republicas de America del Sur). Randomised trial of late thrombolysis in patients with suspected acute myocardial infarction. *Lancet* 1993;342:767–772.

452. White H. Mechanism of late benefit in ISIS-2. *Lancet* 1988;2:914.

453. Anonymous. The late open artery hypothesis at the crossroad. The ACTOR study: aggressive versus conservative treatment of the infarct-related artery after acute MI. ACTOR Study Group. *Giornale Italiano di Cardiologia* 1999;29:1–10.

454. Eigler N, Maurer G, Shah PK. Effect of early systemic thrombolytic therapy on left ventricular mural thrombus formation in acute anterior myocardial infarction. *Am J Cardiol* 1984;54:261–263.

455. White HD, Norris RM, Brown MA, et al. Left ventricular end systolic volume as the major determinant of survival after recovery from myocardial infarction. *Circulation* 1987;76:44–51.

456. Steinberg JS, Hochman JS, Morgan CD, et al. Effects of thrombolytic therapy administered 6 to 24 hours after myocardial infarction on the signal-averaged ECG. Results of a multicenter randomized trial. LATE Ancillary Study Investigators. Late Assessment of Thrombolytic Efficacy. *Circulation* 1994;90:746–752.

457. Rossi P, Bolognese L. Comparison of intravenous urokinase plus heparin versus heparin alone in acute myocardial infarction. *Am J Cardiol* 1991;68:585–592.

458. Wilkins ML, Pryor AD, Maynard C, et al. An electrocardiographic acuteness score for quantifying the timing of a myocardial infarction to guide decisions regarding reperfusion therapy. *Am J Cardiol* 1995;75:617–620.

459. Anderson ST, Wilkins ML, Weaver WD, et al. Electrocardiographic phasing of acute myocardial infarction. *J Electrocardiology* 1992;25(Suppl):3–5.

460. Doorey AJ, Michelson EL, Topol EJ. Review: thrombolytic therapy of acute myocardial infarction. Keeping the unfulfilled promises. *JAMA* 1992;268:3108–3114.

461. Topol EJ, Califf RM. Thrombolytic therapy for elderly patients. *N Engl J Med* 1999;327:45–47.

462. Krumholz HM, Pasternak RC, Weinstein MC, et al. Cost effectiveness of thrombolytic therapy with streptokinase in elderly patients with suspected myocardial infarction. *N Engl J Med* 1992;327:7–13.

463. White HD. Thrombolytic therapy in the elderly. *Lancet* 2000;356: 2028–2030.

464. Tresch DD, Brady WJ, Aufderheide TP. Comparison of elderly and younger patients with out-of-hospital chest pain. Clinical characteristics, acute myocardial infarction, therapy, and outcomes. *Arch Int Med* 1996;156:1089–1093.

465. Morgan B, Emerman CL. Effect of age on myocardial infarction and thrombolysis. *Am J Emerg Med* 1903;13:196–198.

466. Gurwitz JH, Gore JM, Goldberg RJ, et al. Recent age-related trends in the use of thrombolytic therapy on patients who have had acute myocardial infarction. *Ann Int Med* 1996;124:283–291.

467. Rosenthal GE, Fortinsky RH. Differences in the treatment of patients with acute myocardial infarction according to patient age. *J Am Geriatr Soc* 1994;42:826–832.

468. Wasserburger RH, Corliss RJ. Prominent precordial T waves as an expression of coronary insufficiency. *Am J Cardiol* 1965;16:195–205.

469. Gurwitz JH, Gore JH, Goldberg RJ, et al. Risk for intracranial hemorrhage after tissue plasminogen activator treatment for acute myocardial infarction. *Ann Int Med* 1998;129:597–604.

470. Hillegass WB, Jollis JG, Granger CB, et al. Intracranial hemorrhage risk and new thrombolytic therapies in acute myocardial infarction. *Am J Cardiol* 1994;73:444–449.

471. Maggioni AP, Franzosi MG, Santoro E, et al. The risk of stroke in patients with acute myocardial infarction after thrombolytic and antithrombotic treatment. *N Engl J Med* 1992;327:1–6.

471.5. ASSENT-3 Investigators. Efficacy and safety of tenecteplase in combination with enoxaparin, abciximab, or unfractionated heparin: the ASSENT-3 randomised trial in acute myocardial infarction. *Lancet* 2001;358:605–613.

472. Brass LM, Lichtman JH, Wang Y, et al. Intracranial hemorrhage associated with thrombolytic therapy for elderly patients with acute myocardial infarction: results from the Cooperative Cardiovascular Project. *Stroke* 2000;31:1802–1811.

473. Simoons ML, Maggioni AP, Knatterud G, et al. Individual risk assessment for intracranial hemorrhage during thrombolytic therapy. *Lancet* 1993;342:1523–1528.

474. Roppolo LP, Vilke GM, Chan TC, et al. Nasotracheal intubation in the emergency department, revisited. *J Emerg Med* 1999;17:791–799.

475. Scholz KH, Tebbe U, Herrmann C, et al. Frequency of complications of cardiopulmonary resuscitation after thrombolysis during acute myocardial infarction. *Am J Cardiol* 1992;69:724–728.

476. Sekyema YF, Baltazar RF. Is thrombolytic therapy safe during active menstruation? *J Emerg Med* 1995;13:345–348.

477. Karnash SL, Granger CB, White HD, et al. Treating menstruating women with thrombolytic therapy: insights from the global utilization of streptokinase and tissue plasminogen activator for occluded coronary arteries (GUSTO-I) trial. *J Am Coll Cardiol* 1995;26:1651–1656.

478. Lee DW, Garza JL. Front-loaded infusion therapy of rT-PA during active menstruation. A case report. *Angiology* 1994;45:311–314.

479. Mahaffey KW, Granger CB, Toth CA, et al. Diabetic retinopathy should not be a contraindication to thrombolytic therapy for acute myocardial infarction: review of ocular hemorrhage incidence and location in the GUSTO-I trial. Global Utilization of Streptokinase and t-PA for Occluded Coronary Arteries. *J Am Coll Cardiol* 1997; 30:1606–1610.

480. Holmes DR, White HD, Pieper KS, et al. Effect of age on outcome with primary angioplasty versus thrombolysis. *J Am Coll Cardiol* 1999;33:412–419.

481. Canto JG, Every NR, Magid DJ, et al. The volume of primary angioplasty procedures and survival after acute myocardial infarction. *N Engl J Med* 2000;342:1573–1580.

482. Califf RM, Fortin DF, Tenaglia AN, et al. Clinical risks of thrombolytic therapy. *Am J Cardiol* 1992;69:12A–20A.

483. Sloan MA, Price TR, Petito CK, et al. Clinical features and pathogenesis of intracerebral hemorrhage after rt-PA and heparin therapy for acute myocardial infarction: the Thrombolysis in Myocardial Infarction (TIMI) II Pilot and Randomized Clinical Trial combined experience. *Neurology* 1995;45:649–658.

484. Mahaffey KW, Granger CB, Sloan MA, et al. Neurosurgical evacuation of intracranial hemorrhage after thrombolytic therapy for acute myocardial infarction: experience from the GUSTO-I trial. *Am Heart J* 1999;138:493–499.

485. Walls RM, Pollack CV, et al. Successful cricothyrotomy after thrombolytic therapy for acute myocardial infarction: a report of two cases. *Ann Emerg Med* 2000;35:188–191.

486. Gore JM, Granger CB, Simoons ML, et al. Stroke after thrombolysis: mortality and functional outcomes in the GUSTO-1 trial. *Circulation* 1995;92:2811–2818.

487. Berkowitz SD, Granger CB, Pieper KS, et al. Incidence and predictors of bleeding after contemporary thrombolytic therapy for myocardial infarction. *Circulation* 1997;95:2508–2516.

488. Reikvam A, Abdelnoor M. Thrombolytic therapy for acute myocardial infarction in older patients. *Lancet* 1996;347:840.

489. Smalling WR, Fuentes F, Mathews MW, et al. Sustained improvements in left ventricular function and mortality by intracoronary streptokinase administration during evolving myocardial infarction. *J Am Coll Cardiol* 1986;7:729–742.

490. Serrays PW, Simoons ML, Suryapranata H, et al. Preservation of global and regional left ventricular function after early thrombolysis in acute myocardial infarction. *J Am Coll Cardiol* 1986;7:729–742.

491. GUSTO-I Angiographic Investigators. The effects of tissue plasminogen activator, streptokinase or both on coronary artery patency, ventricular function, and survival after acute myocardial infarction. *N Engl J Med* 1993;329:673–682.

492. Simes RJ, Topol EJ, Holmes DR, et al. Link between the angiographic substudy and mortality outcomes in a large randomized trial of myocardial reperfusion: Importance of early and complete infarct artery reperfusion. *Circulation* 1995;91:1923–1928.

493. Yusuf S, Collins R, Peto R, et al. Intravenous and intracoronary fibrinolytic therapy in acute myocardial infarction: overview of results on mortality, reinfarction and side-effects from 33 randomized controlled trials. *Eur Heart J* 1985;6:556–85.

494. TIMI. The thrombolysis in myocardial infarction (TIMI) trial: Phase 1 findings. *N Engl J Med* 1984;312:936.

495. Stone GW, Grines CL, Browne KF, et al. Predictors of in-hospital and 6-month outcome after acute myocardial infarction in the reperfusion era: the Primary Angioplasty in Myocardial Infarction (PAMI) trial. *J Am Coll Cardiol* 1995;25:370–377.

496. Grines CL, Browne KF, Marco J, et al. A comparison of immediate angioplasty with thrombolytic therapy for acute myocardial infarction. *N Engl J Med* 1993;328:673–679.

497. Zijlstra F, de Boer MJ, Hoorntje JC, et al. A comparison of immediate coronary angioplasty with intravenous streptokinase in acute myocardial infarction. *N Engl J Med* 1993;328:680–684.

498. Gibbons RJ, Holmes DR, Reeder GS, et al. Immediate angioplasty compared with the administration of a thrombolytic agent followed by conservative treatment for myocardial infarction. *N Engl J Med* 1993;328:685–691.

499. Schomig A, Kastrati A, Dirschinger J, et al. Coronary stenting plus platelet glycoprotein IIb/IIIa blockade compared with tissue plasminogen activator in acute myocardial infarction. Stent versus thrombolysis for occluded coronary arteries in patients with acute myocardial infarction. *N Engl J Med* 2000;343:385–391.

500. Stone GW. Results of the CADILLAC trial, Transvascular Cardiovascular Therapeutics XI: Frontiers in Interventional Cardiology, Washington, DC., 2000.

501. Grines CL, Cox DA, Stone GW, et al. Coronary angioplasty with or without stent implantation for acute myocardial infarction. *N Engl J Med* 1999;341:1949–1956.

502. Stone GW, Brodie BR, Griffin JJ, et al. Clinical and angiographic follow-up after primary stenting in acute myocardial infarction: the Primary Angioplasty in Myocardial Infarction (PAMI) stent pilot trial. *Circulation* 1999;99:1548–1554.

503. Neumann FJ, Kastrati A, Schmitt C, et al. Effect of glycoprotein IIb/IIIa receptor blockade with abciximab on clinical and antiographic restenosis rate after the placement of coronary stents following acute myocardial infarction. *J Am Coll Cardiol* 2000;35:915–921.

504. Hochman JS, Sleeper LA, Webb JG, et al. Early revascularization in acute myocardial infarction complicated by cardiogenic shock. *N Engl J Med* 1999;341:625–634.

505. Hochman JS, Sleeper LA, White HD, et. al. One-year survival following early revascularization for cardiogenic shock. *JAMA* 2001; 285:190–192.

506. Stone GW, Grines CL, Browne KF, et al. Outcome of different reperfusion strategies in patients with former contraindications to thrombolytic therapy: a comparison of primary angioplasty and tissue plasminogen activator. *Cath Cardiovasc Diagn* 1996;39:333–339.

507. Barga JC, Esteves FP, Esteves JP, et al. Confirmation that heparin is an alternative means of promoting early reperfusion. *Coron Artery Dis* 1998;9:335–338.

508. Verheugt FW, Liem A, Zijlstra F, et al. High dose bolus heparin as initial therapy before primary angioplasty for acute myocardial infarction: results of the Heparin in Early Patency (HEAP) pilot study. *J Am Coll Cardiol* 1998;31:289–293.

509. Topol EJ, Califf RM, George BS, et al. A randomized trial of immediate versus delayed elective angioplasty after intravenous tissue plasminogen activator in acute myocardial infarction. *N Engl J Med* 1987; 317:581–588.

510. Simoons JL, Arnold AER, Betriu A. Thrombolysis with tissue plasminogen activator in acute myocardial infarction. *Lancet* 1988;1: 197–203.

511. TIMI Study Group. Comparison of invasive and conservative strategies after treatment with intravenous tissue plasminogen activator in acute myocardial infarction: results of the Thrombolysis in Myocardial Infarction (TIMI) phase II trial. *N Engl J Med* 1989;320: 618–627.

512. De Bono DP. The European Cooperative Study Group trial of intravenous recombinant tissue-type plasminogen activator (rt-PA) and conservative therapy versus rt-PA and immediate coronary angioplasty. *J Am Coll Cardiol* 1988;12:20A–23A.

513. Ross AM, Coyne KS, Reiner JS, et al. A randomized trial comparing primary angioplasty with a strategy of short-acting thrombolysis and immediate planned rescue angioplasty in acute myocardial infarction: the PACT trial. PACT investigators. Plasminogen-Activator Angioplasty Compatibility Trial. *J Am Coll Cardiol* 1999;34:1954–1962.

514. Antman EM, Giugliano RP, Gibson CM, et al. Abciximab facilitates the rate and extent of thrombolysis: results of the thrombolysis in myocardial infarction (TIMI) 14 trial. *Circulation* 1999;99: 2720–2732.

515. De Lemos JA, Antman EM, Gibson CM, et al. Abciximab improves both epicardial flow and myocardial reperfusion in ST-elevation myocardial infarction. Observations from the TIMI 14 trial. *Circulation* 2000;101:239–243.

515.5. GUSTO-V Investigators. Reperfusion therapy for acute myocardial infarction with fibrinolytic therapy or combination reduced fibrinolytic therapy and platelet glycoprotein IIb/IIIa inhibition: the GUSTO-V randomised trial. *Lancet* 2001;357:1905–1914.

516. Cohen M, Demers C, Gurfinkel E, et al. A comparison of low-molecular weight heparin with unfractionated heparin for unstable coronary artery disease. *N Engl J Med* 1997;337:447–452.

517. Antman EM, McCabe CH, Gurfinkel EP, et al. Enoxaparin prevents death and cardiac ischemia events in unstable angina/non-Q-wave MI: Results of the TIMI-11B trial. *Circulation* 1999b;12:1593–1601.

518. Antman EM, Cohen M, Radley D, et al. Assessment of the treatment effect of enoxaparin for unstable angina/NQMI: TIMI 11B-ESSENCE meta-analysis. *Circulation* 1999a;100:1602–1608.

519. OASIS-2 Investigators. Effects of recombinant hirudin (lepirudin) compared with heparin on death, MI, refractory angina, and revascularization procedures in patients with acute myocardial ischemia without ST elevation: a randomized trial. *Lancet* 1999;353:429–438.

520. GUSTO-IIa Investigators. Randomized trial of intravenous heparin versus recombinant hirudin for acute coronary syndromes. *Circulation* 1994;90:1631–1637.

521. Simoons ML. GUSTO IV-ACS Investigators. Effect of glycoprotein IIb/IIIa receptor blocker abciximab on outcome in patients with acute coronary syndromes without early revascularization: the GUSTO IV-ACS randomised trial. *Lancet* 2001;357(9272):1915–1924.

522. Kong DF, Califf RM, Miller DP, et al. Clinical outcomes of therapeutic agents that block the platelet glycoprotein IIb/IIIa integrin in ischemic heart disease. *Circulation* 1998;98:2829–2835.

523. PRISM Study Investigators. A comparison of aspirin plus tirofiban with aspirin plus heparin for unstable angina. *N Engl J Med* 1998; 338:1498–1505.

524. PRISM-PLUS Study Investigators. Inhibition of the platelet GP IIb/IIIa receptor with tirofiban in unstable angina and non–Q wave MI. *N Engl J Med* 1998;338:1488–1497.

525. PURSUIT Trial Investigators. Inhibition of platelet GP IIb/IIIa with eptifibatide in patients with acute coronary syndromes. *N Engl J Med* 1998;339:436–443.

526. CAPTURE Investigators. Randomized placebo-controlled trial of abciximab before and during coronary intervention in refractory unstable angina: the CAPTURE study. *Lancet* 1997;349:1429–1435.

527. Boden WE, O'Rourke RA, Crawford MH, et al. for the VAN-QWISH Investigators. Outcomes in patients with acute non–Q wave myocardial infarction randomly assigned to an invasive as compared with a conservative management strategy. *N Engl J Med* 1998;338: 1785–1792.

528. FRISC II Investigators. Invasive compared with non-invasive treatment in unstable coronary artery disease: FRISC II prospective randomized multi-center study. *Lancet* 1999;354:708–715.

529. Madsen JK, Grande P, Saunamaki K, et al. Danish multicenter randomized study of invasive versus conservative treatment in patients with inducible ischemia after thrombolysis in acute myocardial infarction (DANAMI). *Circulation* 1997;96:748–755.

530. Antiplatelet Trialists Collaboration. Collaborative review of randomized trials of anti-platelet therapy I. Prevention of death, MI, and stroke by prolonged anti-platelet therapy in various categories of patients. *BMJ* 1994;308:81–106.

531. Oler A, Whooley MA, Oler J, et al. Adding heparin to aspirin reduces the incidence of myocardial infarction and death in patients with unstable angina: a meta-analysis. *JAMA* 1996;276:811–815.

532. The PARAGON Investigators. International, randomized, controlled trial of lamifiban (a platelet glycoprotein IIb/IIIa inhibitor), heparin, or both in unstable angina. *Circulation* 1998;97:2386–2395.

533. Hennekens CH, Albert CM, Godfried SL, et al. Adjunctive drug therapy of acute myocardial infarction: evidence from clinical trials. *N Engl J Med* 1996;335:1660–1667.

534. Jugdutt BI, Warnica JW. Intravenous nitroglycerine therapy to limit myocardial infarction size, expansion and complications: effect of timing, dosage and infarct location. *Circulation* 1998;78:906–919.

535. GISSI-3 (Gruppo Italiano per lo Studio della Sopravvivenza nell'Infarto Miocardico). Six-month effects of early treatment with lisinopril and transdermal glyceryltrinitrate singly and together withdrawn six weeks after acute myocardial infarction: the GISSI-3 trial. *J Am Coll Cardiol* 1996;27:337–344.

536. Cheitlin MD, Hutter AMJ, Brindis RG, et al. Use of sildenafil (Viagra) in patients with cardiovascular disease. *Circulation* 1999;100:2389.

537. CAPRIE Steering Committee. A randomized blinded trial of clopidogrel versus aspirin in patients at risk of ischemic events (CAPRIE). *Lancet* 1996;348:1329–1339.

538. Antman EM. Hirudin in acute myocardial infarction. Safety report from the thrombolysis and thrombin inhibitors in myocardial infarction (TIMI) 9A trial. *Circulation* 1994;90:1624–1630.

539. ISIS-1 (First International Study of Infarct Survival) Collaborative Group. Randomised trial of intravenous atenolol among 16,027 cases of suspected acute myocardial infarction. *Lancet* 1986;2:57–66.

540. Woods KL, Fletcher S. Long-term outcome after intravenous magnesium sulphate in suspected acute myocardial infarction: the second Leicester Intravenous Magnesium Intervention Trial (LIMIT-2). *Lancet* 1994;343:816–819.

541. Antman EM. Magnesium in acute myocardial infarction: timing is critical. *Circulation* 1995;92:2367–2372.

542. Pfeffer MA, Braunwald E, Moye LA, et al. Effects of captopril on mortality and morbidity in patients with left ventricular dysfunction after myocardial infarction: results of the Survival and Ventricular Enlargement Trial—the SAVE investigators. *N Engl J Med* 1992;327:669–677.

543. Swedberg K, Held P, Kjeshus J, et al. Effects of the early administration of enalapril on mortality in patients with acute myocardial infarction: results of the Cooperative New Scandinavian Enalapril Survival Study II (Consensus II). *N Engl J Med* 1992;327:669–677.

phylactic lidocaine
ction. *Am Heart J*

phylactic lidocaine
outcomes from two
D-IIb Investigators.

y administration of
ion: the Secondary
study. *Arch Int Med*

l Infarction. Effects
er acute myocardial
9–785.

search Group. The
n after myocardial

. Randomized trial
onary heart disease:
). *Lancet* 1994;344:

or Cholesterol and
pravastatin in coro-
s with average cho-
9.

Ischemic Disease
lar events and death
road range of initial
1357.

asminogen activator

and size of infarct, left ventricular function, and survival in acute myocardial infarction. *BMJ* 1988;297:1374–1379.

553. Wallentin L, Lagerqvist B, Husted S, et al., for the FRISC II Investigators. Outcome at 1 year after an invasive compared with a noninvasive strategy in unstable coronary-artery disease: the FRISC II invasive randomised trial. *Lancet* 2000;356:9–16.

554. Weaver WD, Eisenberg MS, Martin JS, et al. Myocardial infarction triage and intervention project, Phase I: patient characteristics and feasibility of prehospital initiation of thrombolytic therapy. *J Am Coll Cardiol* 1990;15:925–931.

555. Stone GW, Brodie BR, Griffin JJ, et al. Prospective, multicenter study of the safety and feasibility of primary stenting in acute myocardial infarction: in-hospital and 30-day results of the PAMI stent pilot trial. *J Am Coll Cardiol* 1998;31:23–30.

556. Califf RM, Topol EJ, Stack RS, et al. Evaluation of combination thrombolytic therapy and timing of cardiac catheterization in acute myocardial infarction—phase 5 randomized trial. TAMI Study Group. *Circulation* 1991;83:1543–1556.

557. Califf RM, Topol EJ, George BS, et al. Characteristics and outcome of patients in whom reperfusion with intravenous tissue-type plasminogen activator fails: results of the Thrombolysis and Angioplasty in Myocardial Infarction (TAMI) 1 Trial. *Circulation* 1988;77:1090–1099.

558. Ellis SG, Lincoff AM, George BS, et al. Randomized evaluation of coronary angioplasty for early TIMI 2 flow after thrombolytic therapy for the treatment of acute myocardial infarction: a new look at an old study. The Thrombolysis and Angioplasty in Myocardial Infarction (TAMI) Study Group. *Coron Artery Dis* 1994;5:611–615.

559. Every NR, Frederick PD, Robinson M, et al. A comparison of the national registry of myocardial infarction 2 with the cooperative cardiovascular project. *J Am Coll Cardiol* 1999;33:1886–1894.

INDEX

Note:Page numbers followed by "f" indicate figures; those followed by "t" indicate tables.